Nursing Care Plans
& Documentation
Nursing Diagnoses and Collaborative Problems

Nursing Care Plans & Documentation

Nursing Diagnoses and Collaborative Problems

Lynda Juall Carpenito-Moyet, R.N., M.S.N., C.R.N.P.

Family Nurse Practitioner
ChesPenn Health Services
Chester, Pennsylvania

Nursing Consultant
Mullica Hill, New Jersey

EDITION 5

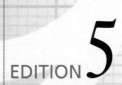
Wolters Kluwer | Lippincott Williams & Wilkins
Health

Philadelphia • Baltimore • New York • London
Buenos Aires • Hong Kong • Sydney • Tokyo

Senior Acquisitions Editor: Jean Rodenberger
Managing Editor: Michelle Clarke
Production Editor: Mary Kinsella
Director of Nursing Production: Helen Ewan
Senior Managing Editor / Production: Erika Kors
Design Coordinator: Joan Wendt
Manufacturing Coordinator: Karin Duffield
Indexer: Coughlin Indexing Services, Inc.
Production Services / Compositor: Circle Graphics

5th Edition

Library of Congress Cataloging-in-Publication Data

Carpenito-Moyet, Lynda Juall.
    Nursing care plans & documentation : nursing diagnoses and collaborative problems /
Lynda Juall Carpenito-Moyet.—5th ed.
        p. ; cm.
    Includes bibliographical references and index.
    ISBN 978-0-7817-7064-4 (alk. paper)
    1. Nursing care plans. 2. Nursing assessment. 3. Nursing diagnosis. I. Title. II. Title: Nursing care plans and documentation.
  [DNLM: 1. Patient Care Planning. 2. Nursing Process. 3. Nursing Records. WY 100
C294n 2008]
    RT49.C38 2008
    610.73—dc22

                                                                                                2008016029

Care has been taken to confirm the accuracy of the information presented and to describe generally accepted practices. However, the author, editors, and publisher are not responsible for errors or omissions or for any consequences from application of the information in this book and make no warranty, expressed or implied, with respect to the currency, completeness, or accuracy of the contents of the publication. Application of this information in a particular situation remains the professional responsibility of the practitioner; the clinical treatments described and recommended may not be considered absolute and universal recommendations.

The author, editors, and publisher have exerted every effort to ensure that drug selection and dosage set forth in this text are in accordance with the current recommendations and practice at the time of publication. However, in view of ongoing research, changes in government regulations, and the constant flow of information relating to drug therapy and drug reactions, the reader is urged to check the package insert for each drug for any change in indications and dosage and for added warnings and precautions. This is particularly important when the recommended agent is a new or infrequently employed drug.

Some drugs and medical devices presented in this publication have Food and Drug Administration (FDA) clearance for limited use in restricted research settings. It is the responsibility of the health care provider to ascertain the FDA status of each drug or device planned for use in his or her clinical practice.

To My Mother: Elizabeth Julia Juall

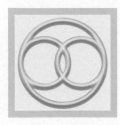

Every year brings me a new appreciation and admiration for this woman

In her 80s (close to 90) there is not much she does not do

She has role-modeled unconditional love, respect for all, forgiveness, and independence

She is determined she can, and she does!

She is one generation of my family's Hungarian Woman Warriors, and I proudly walk in their footprints, carry their swords to battle injustice, and cherish deeply our loved ones.

Love your daughter
Lynda

Current Contributors

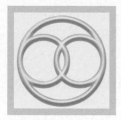

John Dugan, R.N., B.S.N.
Manager, Intensive Care Unit
Carondelet Health Network
St. Joseph's Hospital
Tucson, Arizona

(Cardiovascular and Peripheral Vascular Disorders)

Gloria J. Gdovin, R.N., M.S.N., C.C.R.N.
Clinical Nurse Educator, Critical Care
Carondelet Health Network
St. Joseph's Hospital
Tucson, Arizona

[Stroke, Multiple Sclerosis, Neurogenic Bladder, Fractures, Osteomyelitis, Neoplastic Disorders, Pressure Ulcers, Immobility, HIV-Aids, Systemic Lupus, Glaucoma, (Surgical Procedures: Abdominal Aortic Aneurysm Repair, Amputation, Arterial Bypass, Breast Surgery, Carotid Endarectomy, Coronary Bypass Graft, Radical Prostatectomy, Thoracic Surgery, Total Joint Replacement, Urostomy)]

Susan Laureen Jones, R.N., B.S.N., C.C.R.N.
Clinical Specialist, Inpatient Neuroscience
Carondelet Health Network
St. Joseph's Hospital
Tucson, Arizona

[Cancer End-Stage, Alcohol Withdrawal, Thermal Injuries, Spinal Cord Injury, Seizures, Parkinson Disease, Myasthenia Gravis, Guillain-Barré, Inflammatory Joint Disease, Renal and Urinary Disorders, Peritoneal Dialysis, Hemodialysis, Sexual Assault, (Surgical Procedures: Generic Surgery, Nephrectomy, Enucleation, Cranial Surgery, Cataract Extraction, Laryngectomy, Ileostomy, Fractured Hip and Femur, Neck Dissection, Laminectomy, Hysterectomy, Colostomy)]

Tracy Schreiner, R.N., M.S.N., M.B.A.
President, Schreiner Consulting
Adjunct Faculty
Grand Canyon University
Phoenix, Arizona
Chamberlain College of Nursing
Chamberlin, Ohio

[Respiratory Disorders, Osteoporosis, Osteomyelitis, (Diagnostic and Therapeutic Procedures: Anticoagulant Therapy, Casts, Chemotherapy, Corticosteroid Therapy, Enteral Nutrition, Long-Term Venous Access, Pacemaker Insertion, Radiation Therapy, Total Parenteral Nutrition)]

Previous Contributors

Caroline M. Alterman, M.S.N., C.N.S.
Director, Spinal Cord Injury Program, Lakeshore Rehabilitation Hospital, Birmingham, Alabama

(Spinal Cord Injury, 2nd ed.)

Elizabeth Brady-Avis, R.N., M.S.N., C.C.R.N.
Clinical Nurse Specialist, Thomas Jefferson University Hospital, Philadelphia, Pennsylvania

(Mechanical Ventilation, Asthma)

Sharon Buckingham, B.S.N.
Staff Nurse, ICU, Huron Valley Hospital, Milford, Michigan

(Hypertension, Cirrhosis, 2nd ed.)

Gerald A. Burns, M.S.N.
Clinical Nurse Specialist/Case Manager, Harper Hospital, Detroit, Michigan

(Human Immunodeficiency Virus/Acquired Immunodeficiency Syndrome)

Ann Delengowski, R.N., M.S.N.
Oncology Clinical Nurse Specialist, Thomas
    Jefferson University Hospital, Philadelphia,
    Pennsylvania

(Leukemia, Sickle Cell Anemia, 2nd ed.)

Mary Ann Ducharme, R.N., M.S.N.,
    C.C.R.N.
Case Manager/Clinical Nurse Specialist, Harper
    Hospital, Detroit, Michigan

(Hemodynamic Monitoring, Peritoneal Dialysis)

Rita Dundon, R.N., M.S.N., C.S., O.C.N.
Clinical Nurse Specialist, Henry Ford Hospital,
    Detroit, Michigan

*[Cancer (Initial Diagnosis), Chemotherapy, End-Stage
Cancer, Long-Term Venous Access Devices]*

Doris R. Fleming, M.S.N., R.N.,
    C.S., C.D.E.
Clinical Nurse Specialist, Harper Hospital,
    Detroit, Michigan

(Diabetes Mellitus)

Andrea Sampson Haggood,
    M.S.N., R.N.
Clinical Nurse Specialist/Case Manager,
    Oncology and Otorhinolaryngology, Harper
    Hospital, Detroit, Michigan

(Tracheostomy, Neck Dissection, Laryngectomy, 2nd ed.)

Evelyn Howard, R.N., C.N.N.
Director, Renal Dialysis, St. Vincent Infirmary
    Medical Center, Little Rock, Arkansas

(Acute Renal Failure, Chronic Renal Failure, 2nd ed.)

Debra J. Lynn-McHale, R.N., M.S.N.,
    C.S., C.C.R.N.
Clinical Nurse Specialist, Surgical Cardiac Care
    Unit, Thomas Jefferson University Hospital,
    Philadelphia, Pennsylvania

*(Coronary Artery Bypass Graft, Percutaneous
Transluminal Coronary Angioplasty)*

JoAnn Maklebust, M.S.N., R.N., C.S.
Clinical Nurse Specialist/Wound Care, Case
    Manager/General and Reconstructive Surgery,
    Harper Hospital, Detroit, Michigan

*(Colostomy, Ileostomy, Urostomy, Pressure Ulcers,
Inflammatory Bowel Disease, Neurogenic Bladder)*

Amy Ottariano, R.N., M.S.N.
Clinical Nurse Specialist, Intermediate Cardiac
    Care Unit, Thomas Jefferson University
    Hospital, Philadelphia, Pennsylvania

(Thoracic Surgery, 2nd ed.)

Rhonda R. Panfilli, R.N., M.S.N.
Coordinator, Case Management, Grace Hospital,
    Detroit Medical Center, Detroit, Michigan

(Obesity)

Gayle Vandendool Parker, R.N., B.S.N.
Nursing Practice Coordinator, London
    Psychiatric Hospital, London, Ontario, Canada

(Alcohol Withdrawal)

Joy Ross, R.N.
London Psychiatric Hospital, London,
    Ontario, Canada

(Sexual Assault)

Rose B. Shaffer, R.N., M.S.N., C.C.R.N.
Clinical Nurse Specialist, Intermediate Cardiac
    Care Unit, Thomas Jefferson University
    Hospital, Philadelphia, Pennsylvania

(Cardiac Catheterization, Pacemaker Insertion)

Ellen Stefanosky, R.N., M.S.N.
Transplant Coordinator, Thomas Jefferson
    University Hospital, Philadelphia,
    Pennsylvania

(Renal Transplant, 2nd ed.)

Patricia A. Vaccaro, R.N., M.S.N.
Clinical Nurse Facilitator, Burn Center, Lehigh
    Valley Hospital, Allentown, Pennsylvania

(Thermal Injuries, 2nd ed.)

Donna J. Zazworsky, R.N., M.S.
Professional Nurse Case Manager, Carondelet St.
    Mary's Hospital, Tucson, Arizona

(Multiple Sclerosis)

Preface

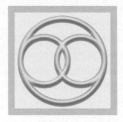

Nursing is primarily assisting individuals, sick or well, in activities that contribute to health or its recovery, or to a peaceful death, and that they perform unaided when they have the necessary strength, will, or knowledge. Nursing also helps individuals carry out prescribed therapy and to be independent of assistance as soon as possible (Henderson, 1960).

Historically, nurses have represented the core of the health care delivery system (including acute, long-term, and community agencies), but their image continues to be one of individuals whose actions are dependent on physician supervision. Unfortunately, what Donna Diers wrote over 15 years ago is still relevant today: "Nursing is exceedingly complicated work since it involves technical skill, a great deal of formal knowledge, communication ability, use of self, timing, emotional investment, and any number of other qualities. What it also involves—and what is hidden from the public—is the complex process of thinking that leads from the knowledge to the skill, from the perception to the action, from the decision to the touch, from the observation to the diagnosis. *Yet it is this process of nursing care, which is at the center of nursing's work, that is so little described . . .*" (Diers, 1981, p. 1, emphasis supplied).

Physicians regularly and openly explain the measures they plan to the public, especially to clients and their families. Nurses, however, often fail to consistently explain their plan of care to clients and family. This book provides both a framework for nurses to provide responsible nursing care and guidelines for them to document and communicate that care. These care plans should not be hand-written. They must be reference documents for practicing nurses. Write or free text the different care the client needs in addition to the standard.

The focus of *Nursing Care Plans and Documentation* is independent nursing care—the management of client situations that the nurse can treat legally and independently. It will assist students in transferring their theoretical knowledge to clinical practice; it can help experienced nurses provide care in a variety of unfamiliar clinical situations. This book also incorporates the findings of a validation study, a description of which (method, subjects, instrument findings) is presented in the section titled *Validation Project*, following the Preface. These findings should be very useful for practicing nurses, students of nursing, and departments of nursing.

The Bifocal Clinical Practice Model underpins this book and serves to organize the nursing care plans in Unit II. Chapter 1 describes and discusses the Bifocal Clinical Practice Model, which differentiates nursing diagnoses from other problems that nurses treat. In this chapter, nursing diagnoses and collaborative problems are explained and differentiated. The relationship of the type of diagnosis to outcome criteria and nursing interventions is also emphasized.

Efficient and appropriate documentation of nursing care is outlined in Chapter 2. Legal issues, standards, and regulatory agencies and their effect on nursing documentation are discussed. The chapter explains a documentation system from admission to discharge. Sample forms are used to emphasize efficient, professional charting. This chapter also includes a discussion of priority diagnoses and case management. The elements of critical pathways are explained with examples. Directions on how to create critical pathways using the care plans in Unit II are discussed and illustrated.

Chapter 3 gives an overview of the 11 steps in care planning and takes the reader through each phase of this process.

Chapter 4 explores the issues and human responses associated with illness and hospitalization, and describes the coping strategies of the client and family. A discussion of Bandura's self-efficacy theory and its application to management of therapeutic regimens is also presented.

Chapter 5 focuses on the surgical experience and related nursing care to discuss the human response to the experience. Preoperative assessment and preparation are described for preadmitted and same-day-admission surgical clients. The nursing responsibilities in the postanesthesia recovery room are described, and the related documentation forms are included. This chapter also outlines the integration of the nursing process in caring for same-day surgery clients; again, the corresponding forms that will help the nurse to do this are included.

New to this edition is Chapter 6. This chapter focuses on Moral Distress in nurses. This new NANDA nursing diagnosis has the nurse as the focus, not the client. The clinical reality of Moral

Distress in nursing will be explored, and strategies for preventing and reducing Moral Distress will be presented. Self-Assessment of Health Behaviors will help the nurse with a self-evaluation of his or her life style. End-of-Life Decisions will be explored and strategies for promoting these decisions in one's personal life and with clients will be discussed. A reproducible Living Will document is available for distribution with instructions on how to use it.

Unit II presents care plans that represent a compilation of the complex work of nursing in caring for individuals (and their families) experiencing medical disorders or surgical interventions or undergoing diagnostic or therapeutic procedures. It uses the nursing process to present the type of nursing care that is expected to be necessary for clients experiencing similar situations. The plans provide the nurse with a framework for providing initial, or essential, care. This is the nursing care known to be provided when a certain clinical situation is present—for example, preoperative teaching for clients awaiting surgery or the management of fatigue in individuals with arthritis. As the nurse intervenes and continues to assess, additional diagnoses, goals, and interventions can be added to the initial plan. Even though the type of care that is warranted for clients in certain clinical situations is predictable, the nurse must still assess the individual for additional responses. The fifth edition features extensive revisions or additions to the goals/outcome criteria in each care plan and, when possible, research findings or the work of expert clinicians were incorporated.

The intent of this book is to assist the nurse to identify the responsible care that nurses are accountable to provide. The incorporation of recent research findings further enhances the applicability of the care plans. By using the Bifocal Clinical Practice Model, the book clearly defines the scope of independent practice. The author invites comments and suggestions from readers. Correspondence can be directed to the publisher or to the author's address.

REFERENCES

Diers, D. (1981). Why write? Why publish? *Image*, 13, 991–997

Henderson, V. & Nite, G. (1960). *Principles and practice of nursing* (5th ed.). New York: Macmillan, p. 14.

Validation Project

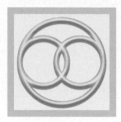

Background

In 1984, this author published diagnostic clusters under medical and surgical conditions (Carpenito, 1984). These diagnostic clusters represented nursing diagnoses and collaborative problems described in the literature for a medical or surgical population. After the initial diagnostic clusters were created, they were reviewed by clinicians who practiced with specific corresponding populations.

Since 1984, numerous other authors (Holloway, 1988; Doenges, 1991; Sparks, 1993; Ulrich, 1994) have generated similar groupings. To date none of the clusters have been studied to determine their frequency of occurrence. In other words, are some diagnoses in the diagnostic cluster treated more frequently than others?

Reasons for Study

In the last 10 years, the health care delivery system has experienced numerous changes. Specifically, clients are in the acute care setting for shorter periods. These client populations all share a high acuity. This acuity is represented with multiple nursing diagnoses and collaborative problems. However, do all these diagnoses have the same priority? Which diagnoses necessitate nursing interventions during the length of stay?

Care planning books report a varied number of diagnoses to treat under a specific condition. For example, in reviewing a care plan for a client with a myocardial infarction, this author found the following number of diagnoses reported: Ulrich, 16; Carpenito, 11; Doenges, 7; Holloway, 4. When students review these references, how helpful are lists ranging from 4 to 16 diagnoses? How many diagnoses can nurses be accountable for during a client's length of stay?

The identification of nursing diagnoses and collaborative problems that nurses treat more frequently than others in certain populations can be very useful data to:

• Assist nurses with decision making
• Determine the cost of nursing services for population sets
• Plan for resources needed
• Describe the specific responsibilities of nursing

Novice nurses and students can use these data to anticipate the initial care needed. They can benefit from data reported by nurses experienced in caring for clients in specific populations.

These data should not eliminate an assessment of an individual client to evaluate if additional nursing diagnoses or collaborative problems are present and establish priority for treatment during the hospital stay. This individual assessment will also provide information to delete or supplement the care plan found in this book. The researched data will provide a beginning focus for care.

By identifying frequently treated nursing diagnoses and collaborative problems in client populations, institutions can determine nursing costs based on nursing care provided. Nurse administrators and managers can plan for effective use of staff and resources. Knowledge of types of nursing diagnoses needing nursing interventions will also assist with matching the level of preparation of nurses with appropriate diagnoses.

To date, the nursing care of clients with medical conditions or postsurgical procedures has centered on the physician-prescribed orders. The data from this study would assist departments of nursing to emphasize the primary reason why clients stay in the acute care setting—*for treatment of nursing diagnoses and collaborative problems.* The purpose of this study is to identify which nursing diagnoses and collaborative problems are most frequently treated when a person is hospitalized with a specific condition.

Method

Settings and Subjects

The findings presented are based on data collected from August 1993 to March 1994. The research population consisted of registered nurses with over 2 years' experience in health care agencies in the United States and Canada. A convenience sample of 18 institutions represented five U.S. geographical regions (Northeast, Southeast, North-Midwest, Northwest, Southwest) and Ontario province in Canada. The display lists the participating institutions. The target number of R.N. responses was 10 per condition from each institution. The accompanying table illustrates the demographics of the subjects.

Instrument

A graphic rating scale was developed and pilot-tested to measure self-reported frequencies of interventions provided to clients with a specific condition. Each collaborative problem listed under the condition was accompanied by the question:

When you care for clients with this condition, how often do you monitor for this problem?
Each nursing diagnosis listed under the condition was accompanied by the question:

When you care for clients with this condition, how often do you provide interventions for this nursing diagnosis?

The respondent was asked to make an X on a frequency scale of 0% to 100%. Scoring was tabulated by summing the scores for each question and calculating the median.

PARTICIPATING INSTITUTIONS

Allen Memorial Hospital
1825 Logan Avenue
Waterloo, Iowa 50703

Carondelet St. Joseph's Hospital
350 N. Wilmont Road
Tucson, AZ 85711-2678

The Evanston Hospital
Burch Building
2650 Ridge Avenue
Evanston, IL 60201

Huron Valley Hospital
1601 East Commerce Road
Milford, MI 48382-9900

Lehigh Valley Hospital
Cedar Crest & I-78
Allentown, PA 18105-1556

Memorial Medical Center of Jacksonville
3625 University Blvd., South
Jacksonville, FL 32216

Presbyterian Hospital
200 Hawthorne Lane
Charlotte, NC 28233-3549

St. Francis Medical Center
211 St. Francis Drive
Cape Girardeau, MO 63701

St. Joseph Hospital
601 N. 30th Street
Omaha, NE 68131

St. Peter Community Hospital
2475 Broadway
Helena, MT 39601

San Bernardino County Medical Center
780 E. Gilbert Street
San Bernardino, CA 92415-0935

Sioux Valley Hospital
1100 South Euclid Avenue
Sioux Falls, SD 57117-5039

University of Minnesota Hospital
420 Delaware Street, S.E.
Minneapolis, MN 55455

University of New Mexico Hospital
2211 Lomas Blvd., N.E.
Albuquerque, NM 87131

Victoria Hospital
800 Commissioners Road, East
London, Canada N6A 4G5

Wills Eye Hospital
900 Walnut Street
Philadelphia, PA 19107

Wilmer Ophthalmological Institute
Johns Hopkins Hospital
Baltimore, MD 21287-9054

Winthrop-University Hospital
259 First Street
Mineola, NY 11501

Data Collection

Prior to data collection, the researcher addressed the requirements for research in the institution. These requirements varied from a review by the nursing department's research committee to a review by the institutional review board (IRB).

After the approval process was completed, each department of nursing was sent a list of the 72 conditions to be studied and asked to select only those conditions that were regularly treated in their institution. Only those questionnaires were sent to the respective institutions. Study institutions received a packet for those selected conditions containing 10 questionnaires for each condition. Completed questionnaires were returned by the nurse respondent to the envelope and the envelope sealed by the designated distributor. Nurse respondents were given the option of putting their questionnaire in a sealed envelope prior to placing it in the larger envelope.

Since two of the study institutions did not treat ophthalmic conditions, questionnaires related to these conditions were sent to two institutions specializing in these conditions.

Findings

Of the 19 institutions that agreed to participate, 18 (including the two ophthalmic institutions) returned the questionnaires. The target return was 160 questionnaires for each condition. The range of return was 29% to 70%, with the average rate of return 52.5%.

Each condition has a set of nursing diagnoses and collaborative problems with its own frequency score. The diagnoses were grouped into three ranges of frequency: 75% to 100%—frequent; 50% to 74%—often; <50%—infrequent. Each of the 72 conditions included in the study and in this book has the nursing diagnoses and collaborative problems grouped according to the study findings.

Future Work

This study represents the initial step in the validation of the nursing care predicted to be needed when a client is hospitalized for a medical or surgical condition. It is important to validate which nursing diagnoses and collaborative problems necessitate nursing interventions. Future work will include the identification of nursing interventions that have priority in treating a diagnosis, clarification of outcomes realistic for the length of stay, and evaluation and review by national groups of nurses.

DEMOGRAPHICS OF RESPONDENTS

Questionnaires	
Sent	9,920
Returned	5,299
% returned	53.4%
Average Age	39
Average Years in Nursing	15

Level of Nursing Preparation	
Diploma	22.7%
AD	25.7%
BSN	36.5%
MSN	12.4%
PhD	1.5%
No indication	1.2%

REFERENCES

Carpenito, L. J. (1984). *Handbook of nursing diagnosis.* Philadelphia: J. B. Lippincott.
Carpenito, L. J. (1991). *Nursing care plans and documentation.* Philadelphia: J. B. Lippincott.
Doenges, M., & Moorhouse, M. (1991). *Nurse's pocket guide: Nursing diagnoses with interventions.* Philadelphia: F. A. Davis.
Holloway, N. M. (1988). *Medical surgical care plans.* Springhouse, PA: Springhouse.
Sparks, S. M., & Taylor, C. M. (1993). *Nursing diagnoses reference manual.* Springhouse, PA: Springhouse.
Ulrich, S., Canale, S., & Wendell, S. (1994). *Medical-surgical nursing: Care planning guide.* Philadelphia: W. B. Saunders.

Acknowledgments

The Validation Project could not have been completed without the support of the following nurses who coordinated the data collection in their institutions:

Tammy Spier, R.N., M.S.N.
Department of Nursing Services
Department of Staff Development
Allen Memorial Hospital
Waterloo, Iowa

Donna Dickinson, R.N., M.S.
Carol Mangold, R.N., M.S.N.
Carondelet St. Joseph's Hospital
Tucson, Arizona

Kathy Killman, R.N., M.S.N.
Liz Nelson, R.N., M.S.N.
The Evanston Hospital
Evanston, Illinois

Margaret Price, R.N., M.S.N.
Lynn Bobel Turbin, R.N., M.S.N.
Nancy DiJanni, R.N., M.S.N.
Huron Valley Hospital
Milford, Michigan

Pat Vaccaro, R.N., B.S.N., C.C.R.N.
Deborah Stroh, R.N.
Mary Jean Potylycki, R.N.
Carolyn Peters, R.N.
Sue DeSanto, R.N.
Christine Niznik, R.N.
Carol Saxman, R.N.
Kelly Brown, R.N.
Judy Bailey, R.N.
Nancy Root, R.N.
Cheryl Bitting, R.N.
Carol Sorrentino, R.N.
Lehigh Valley Hospital
Allentown, Pennsylvania

Loretta Baldwin, R.N., B.S.N.
Karin Prussak, R.N., M.S.N., C.C.R.N.
Bess Cullen, R.N.
Debra Goetz, R.N., M.S.N.
Susan Goucher, R.N.
Sandra Brackett, R.N., B.S.N.
Barbara Johnston, R.N., C.C.R.N.
Lisa Lauderdale, R.N.
Randy Shoemaker, R.N., C.C.R.N.
Memorial Medical Center of Jacksonville
Jacksonville, Florida

Karen Stiefel, R.N., Ph.D.
Jerre Jones, R.N., M.S.N., C.S.
Lise Heidenreich, R.N., M.S.N., F.N.P., C.S.
Christiana Redwood-Sawyerr, R.N., M.S.N.
Presbyterian Hospital
Charlotte, North Carolina

Pauline Elliott, R.N., B.S.N.
St. Francis Medical Center
Cape Girardeau, Missouri

Dena Belfiore, R.N., Ph.D.
Dianne Hayko, M.S.R.N., C.N.S.
St. Joseph Hospital
Omaha, Nebraska

Jennie Nemec, R.N., M.S.N.
St. Peter Community Hospital
Helena, Montana

Eleanor Borkowski, R.N.
Tina Buchanan, R.N.
Jill Posadas, R.N.
Deanna Stover, R.N.
Margie Bracken, R.N.
Barbara Upton, R.N.
Kathleen Powers, R.N.
Jeanie Goodwin, R.N.
San Bernardino County Medical Center
San Bernardino, California

Kathy Karpiuk, R.N., M.N.E.
Monica Mauer, R.N.
Susan Fey, R.N.
Joan Reisdorfer, R.N.
Cheryl Wilson, Health Unit Coordinator
Gail Sundet, R.N.
Pat Halverson, R.N.
Ellie Baker, R.N.
Jackie Kisecker, R.N.
Cheri Dore-Paulson, R.N.
Kay Gartner, R.N.
Vicki Tigner, R.N.
Jan Burnette, R.N.
Maggie Scherff, R.N.
Sioux Valley Hospital
Sioux Falls, South Dakota

Keith Hampton, R.N., M.S.N.
University of Minnesota Hospital
Minneapolis, Minnesota

Eva Adler, R.N., M.S.N.
Jean Giddens, R.N., M.S.N., C.S.
Dawn Roseberry, R.N., B.S.N.
University of New Mexico Hospital
Albuquerque, New Mexico

Fran Tolley, R.N., B.S.N.
Vicky Navarro, R.N., M.A.S.
Wilmer Ophthalmological Institute
Johns Hopkins Hospital
Baltimore, Maryland

Heather Boyd-Monk, R.N., M.S.N.
Wills Eye Hospital
Philadelphia, Pennsylvania

Joan Crosley, R.N., Ph.D.
Winthrop-University Hospital
Mineola, New York

Carol Wong, R.N., M.Sc.N.
Cheryl Simpson, R.N.
Victoria Hospital
London, Canada

My gratitude also extends to each of the nurses who gave their time to complete the questionnaires.

A sincere thank you to Dr. Ginny Arcangelo, Director of the Family Nurse Practitioner Program at Thomas Jefferson University in Philadelphia, for her work as the methodology consultant to the project.

A study of this magnitude required over 9000 questionnaires to be produced, duplicated, and distributed. Over 100,000 data entries were made, yielding the findings found throughout this edition.

Contents

UNIT I

Introduction to Care Planning   1

UNIT II

Clinical Nursing Care Plans   55

Section 1 ▶ MEDICAL CONDITIONS   61

Section 2 ▶ SURGICAL PROCEDURES 463

Section 3 ▶ DIAGNOSTIC AND THERAPEUTIC PROCEDURES 667

Introduction to Care Planning

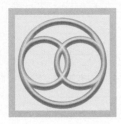

1

THE BIFOCAL CLINICAL PRACTICE MODEL

The classification activities of the North American Nursing Diagnosis Association International (NANDA-I) have been instrumental in defining nursing's unique body of knowledge. This unified system of terminology

• Provides consistent language for oral, written, and electronic communication
• Stimulates nurses to examine new knowledge
• Establishes a system for automation and reimbursement
• Provides an educational framework
• Allows efficient information retrieval for research and quality assurance
• Provides a consistent structure for literature presentation of nursing knowledge
• Clarifies nursing as an art and a science for its members and society
• Establishes standards to which nurses are held accountable

The inside cover of this text provides a list of nursing diagnoses grouped under conditions that necessitate nursing care.

Clearly, nursing diagnosis has influenced the nursing profession positively. Integration of nursing diagnosis into nursing practice, however, has proved problematic. Although references to nursing diagnosis in the literature have increased 100-fold since the first meeting in 1973 of the National Group for the Classification of Nursing Diagnoses (which later became NANDA-I), nurses have not seen efficient and representative applications. For example, nurses have been directed to use nursing diagnoses exclusively to describe their clinical focus. Nevertheless, nurses who strongly support nursing diagnosis often become frustrated when they try to attach a nursing diagnosis label to every facet of nursing practice. Some of the dilemmas that result from the attempt to label as nursing diagnoses all situations in which nurses intervene are as follows:

1. *Using nursing diagnoses without validation.* When the nursing diagnoses are the only labels or diagnostic statements the nurse can use, the nurse is encouraged to "change the data to fit the label." For example, using the Imbalanced Nutrition category for all clients who are given nothing-by-mouth status. Risk for Injury also frequently serves as a "wastebasket" diagnosis because all potentially injurious situations (e.g., bleeding) can be captured within a Risk for Injury diagnosis.
2. *Renaming medical diagnoses.* Clinical nurses know that an important component of their practice is monitoring for the onset and status of physiologic complications and initiating both nurse-prescribed and physician-prescribed interventions. Morbidity and mortality are reduced and prevented because of nursing's expert management.

   If nursing diagnoses are to describe all situations in which nurses intervene, then clearly a vast number must be developed to describe the situations identified in the International Code of Diseases (ICD-10). Table 1.1 represents examples of misuse of nursing diagnoses and the renaming of medical diagnoses. Examination of the substitution of nursing diagnosis terminology for medical diagnoses or pathophysiology in Table 1.1 gives rise to several questions:
   • Should nursing diagnoses describe all situations in which nurses intervene?
   • If a situation is not called a nursing diagnosis, is it then less important or scientific?
   • How will it serve the profession to rename medical diagnoses as nursing diagnoses?
   • Will using the examples in Table 1.1 improve communication and clarify nursing?
3. *Omitting problem situations in documentation.* If a documentation system requires the use of nursing diagnosis exclusively, and if the nurse does not choose to "change the data to fit a category" or "to rename medical diagnoses," then the nurse has no terminology to describe a critical component of nursing practice. Failure to describe these situations can seriously jeopardize nursing's effort to justify and affirm the need for professional nurses in all health care settings (Carpenito, 1983).

TABLE 1.1	Diagnostic Errors: Renaming Medical Diagnoses With Nursing Diagnosis Terminology	
Medical Diagnosis	**Nursing Diagnosis**
Myocardial Infarction	Decreased Cardiac Output
Shock	Decreased Cardiac Output
Adult Respiratory Distress	Impaired Gas Exchange
Chronic Obstructive Lung Disease	Impaired Gas Exchange
Asthma	Impaired Gas Exchange
Alzheimer's Disease	Impaired Cerebral Tissue Perfusion
Increased Intracranial Pressure	Impaired Cerebral Tissue Perfusion
Retinal Detachment	Disturbed Sensory Perception: Visual
Thermal Burns	Impaired Tissue Integrity
Incisions, Lacerations	Impaired Skin Integrity
Hemorrhage	Deficient Fluid Volume
Congestive Heart Failure	Excess Fluid Volume

Bifocal Clinical Practice Model

Nursing's theoretical knowledge derives from the natural, physical, and behavioral sciences, as well as the humanities and nursing research. Nurses can use various theories in practice, including family systems, loss, growth and development, crisis intervention, and general systems theories.

The difference between nursing and the other health care disciplines is nursing's depth and breadth of focus. Certainly the nutritionist has more expertise in the field of nutrition and the pharmacist in the field of therapeutic pharmacology than any nurse. Every nurse, however, brings a knowledge of nutrition and pharmacology to client interactions. The depth of this knowledge is sufficient for many client situations; when it is insufficient, consultation is required. No other discipline has this varied knowledge, explaining why attempts to substitute other disciplines for nursing have proved costly and ultimately unsuccessful. Figure 1.1 illustrates this varied expertise.

The Bifocal Clinical Practice Model (Carpenito, 1983) represents situations that influence persons, groups, and communities as well as the classification of these responses from a nursing perspective. The situations are organized into five broad categories: pathophysiologic, treatment-related, personal, environmental, and maturational (Figure 1.2). Without an understanding of such situations, the nurse will be unable to diagnose responses and intervene appropriately.

Clinically, these situations are important to nurses. Thus, as nursing diagnoses evolved, nurses sought to substitute nursing terminology for these situations; for example, Impaired Tissue Integrity for burns and High Risk for Injury for dialysis. Nurses do not prescribe for and treat these situations (e.g., burns and dialysis). Rather, they prescribe for and treat the *responses* to these situations.

The practice focus for clinical nursing is at the response level, not at the situation level. For example, a client who has sustained burns may exhibit a wide variety of responses to the burns and the treatments. Some responses may be predicted, such as High Risk for Infection; others, such as fear of losing a job, may not be predictable. In the past, nurses focused on the nursing interventions associated with treating burns rather than on those associated with the client's responses. *This resulted in nurses being described as "doers" rather than "knowers"; as technicians rather than scientists.*

Nursing Diagnoses and Collaborative Problems

The Bifocal Clinical Practice Model describes the two foci of clinical nursing: nursing diagnoses and collaborative problems.

> *A nursing diagnosis is a clinical judgment about individual, family, or community responses to actual or potential health problems/life processes. Nursing diagnosis provides the basis for selection of nursing interventions to achieve outcomes for which the nurse is accountable* (NANDA, 1990). *Collaborative problems are certain*

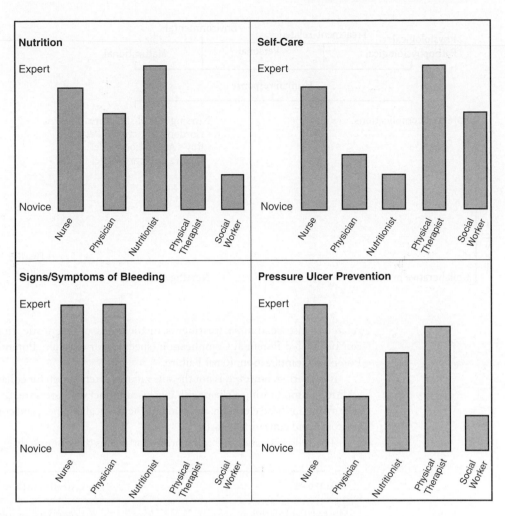

FIGURE 1.1
Knowledge of multidisciplines of selected topics.

physiologic complications that nurses monitor to detect onset or changes of status. Nurses manage collaborative problems using physician-prescribed and nursing-prescribed interventions to minimize the complications of the events (Carpenito, 1997). Figure 1.3 illustrates the Bifocal Clinical Practice Model.

The nurse makes independent decisions for both collaborative problems and nursing diagnoses. The difference is that in nursing diagnoses, nursing prescribes the definitive treatment to achieve the desired outcome, while in collaborative problems, prescription for definitive treatment comes from both nursing and medicine. Some physiologic complications (such as High Risk for Infection and Impaired Skin Integrity) are nursing diagnoses because nurses can order the definitive treatment. In a collaborative problem, the nurse uses surveillance to monitor for the onset and change in status of physiologic complications, and manages these changes to prevent morbidity and mortality. These physiologic complications are usually

Pathophysiological
Myocardial infarction
Borderline personality disorder
Burns

Treatment-related
Anticoagulants
Dialysis
Arteriogram

Personal
Dying
Divorce
Relocation

FIGURE 1.2
Examples of pathophysiologic, treatment-related, personal, environmental, and maturational situations.

Environmental
Overcrowded school
No handrails on stairs
Rodents

Maturational
Peer pressure
Parenthood
Aging

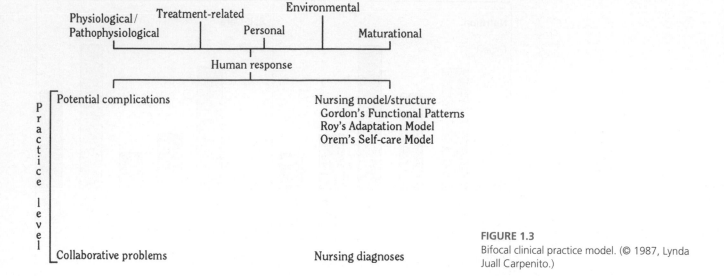

FIGURE 1.3
Bifocal clinical practice model. (© 1987, Lynda Juall Carpenito.)

related to disease, trauma, treatments, medications, or diagnostic studies. Thus, collaborative problems can be labeled Potential Complication (specify); for example, Potential Complication: Hemorrhage or Potential Complication: Renal Failure.

Monitoring, however, is not the sole nursing intervention for collaborative problems. For example, in addition to monitoring a client with increased intracranial pressure, the nurse also restricts certain activities, maintains head elevation, implements the medical regimen, and continually addresses the client's psychosocial and educational needs.

The following are some collaborative problems that commonly apply to certain situations:

Situation	Collaborative Problem
Myocardial Infarction	Potential Complication (PC): Dysrhythmias
Craniotomy	PC: Increased Intracranial Pressure
Hemodialysis	PC: Fluid/Electrolyte Imbalance
Surgery	PC: Hemorrhage
Cardiac Catheterization	PC: Allergic Reaction

If the situation calls for the nurse to monitor for a cluster or group of physiologic complications, the collaborative problems may be documented as

PC: Cardiac
or
PC: Post-op: Urinary retention
PC: Hemorrhage
PC: Hypovolemia
PC: Hypoxia
PC: Thrombophlebitis
PC: Renal insufficiency
PC: Paralytic ileus
PC: Evisceration

A list of common collaborative problems grouped under conditions that necessitate nursing care appears on the inside front and back covers. *Not all physiologic complications, however, are collaborative problems.* Nurses themselves can prevent some physiologic complications such as infections from external sources (e.g., wounds and catheters), contractures, incontinence, and pressure ulcers. Thus, such complications fall under the category of nursing diagnosis.

Nursing Interventions

Nursing interventions are treatments or actions that benefit a client by presenting a problem, reducing or eliminating a problem, or promoting a healthier response. Nursing interventions can be classified as either of two types: nurse-prescribed or physician-prescribed. Independent interventions are nurse-prescribed; delegated interventions are physician-prescribed. Both types of interventions, however, require independent nursing judgment. By law, the nurse must determine if it is appropriate to initiate an intervention regardless of whether it is independent or delegated (Carpenito, 1997).

Carpenito (1987) stated that the relationship of diagnosis to interventions is a critical element in defining nursing diagnoses. Many definitions of nursing diagnoses focus on the relationship of selected interventions to the diagnoses. A certain type of intervention appears to distinguish a nursing diagnosis from a medical diagnosis or other problems that nurses treat. The type of intervention distinguishes a nursing diagnosis from a collaborative problem and also differentiates between actual risk/high risk and possible nursing diagnoses. Table 1.2 outlines definitions of each type and the corresponding intervention focus. For example, for a nursing diagnosis of Impaired Tissue Integrity related to immobility as manifested by a 2-cm epidermal lesion on the client's left heel, the nurse would order interventions to monitor the lesion and to heal it. In another client with a surgical wound, the nurse would focus on prevention of infection and promotion of healing. High Risk for Infection would better describe the situation than Impaired Tissue Integrity. *Nursing diagnoses are not more important than collaborative problems, and collaborative problems are not more important than nursing diagnoses. Priorities are determined by the client's situation, not by whether it is a nursing diagnosis or a collaborative problem.*

A *diagnostic cluster* represents those nursing diagnoses and collaborative problems that have a high likelihood of occurring in a client population. The nurse validates their presence in the individual client. Figure 1.4 represents the diagnostic cluster for a client after abdominal surgery. Sections 1 and 2 contain diagnostic clusters for medical and surgical conditions or goals.

Goals/Outcome Criteria

In a nursing care plan, goals (outcome criteria) are "statements describing a measurable behavior of client/family that denote a favorable status (changed or maintained) after nursing care has been delivered" (Alfaro, 1989). Outcome criteria help to determine the success or appropriateness of the nursing care plan. If the nursing care plan does not achieve a favorable status even though the diagnosis is correct, the nurse must change the goal or change the plan. If neither option is indicated, the nurse confers with the physician for delegated orders. Nursing diagnoses should *not* represent situations that require physician orders

TABLE 1.2   Differentiation Among Types of Diagnoses

Diagnostic Statement	Corresponding Client Outcome or Nursing Goals	Focus of Intervention
Actual Diagnosis Three-part statement including nursing diagnostic label, etiology, and signs/symptoms	Change in client behavior moving toward resolution of the diagnosis or improved status	Reduce or eliminate problem
Risk/High-Risk Diagnosis Two-part statement including nursing diagnostic label and risk factors	Maintenance of present conditions	Reduce risk factors to prevent an actual problem
Possible Diagnosis Two-part statement including nursing diagnostic label and unconfirmed etiology or unconfirmed defining characteristics	Undetermined until problem is validated	Collect additional data to confirm or rule out signs/symptoms or risk factors
Collaborative Problems Potential or actual physiologic complication	Nursing goals	Determine onset or status of the problem Manage change in status

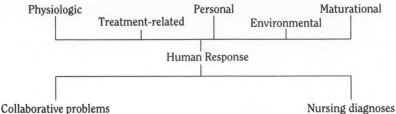

Abdominal surgery (postoperative)

Physiologic   Personal   Maturational
  Treatment-related   Environmental

Human Response

Collaborative problems   Nursing diagnoses

Potential complications

Hemorrhage
Hypovolemia/shock
Urinary retention
Peritonitis
Thrombophlebitis
Paralytic ileus
Evisceration
Dehiscence

Risk for Ineffective Respiratory Function related to immobility
  secondary to postanesthesia state and pain
Risk for Infection related to increased susceptibility
  to bacteria secondary to wound
Acute Pain related to surgical interruption of body structures,
  flatus, and immobility
Risk for Imbalanced Nutrition: Less than Body Requirements
  related to increased protein/vitamin requirements for
  wound healing and decreased intake secondary to pain,
  nausea, vomiting, and diet restrictions
Risk for Constipation related to decreased peristalsis
  secondary to immobility, effects of anesthesia,
  and narcotics
Activity Intolerance related to pain and weakness secondary
  to anesthesia, tissue hypoxia, and insufficient fluids/nutrients
Risk for Ineffective Therapeutic Regimen Management
  related to insufficient knowledge of care of operative site,
  restrictions (diet, activity), medications, signs and symptoms of
  complications, follow-up care

FIGURE 1.4
Diagnostic cluster for client recovering
from abdominal surgery.

for treatment. Otherwise how can nurses assume accountability for diagnosis and treatment? For example, consider a client with a nursing diagnosis:

High Risk for Impaired Cerebral Tissue Perfusion related to effects of recent head injury and these goals:

The client will demonstrate continued optimal cerebral pressure as evidenced by

• Pupils equally reactive to light and accommodation
• No change in orientation or consciousness

If this client were to exhibit evidence of increased intracranial pressure, would it be appropriate for the nurse to change the goals? What changes in the nursing care plan would the nurse make to stop the cranial pressure from increasing? Actually, neither action is warranted. Rather, the nurse should confer with the physician for delegated orders to treat increased intracranial pressure. When the nurse formulates client goals or outcomes that require delegated medical orders for goal achievement, the situation is not a nursing diagnosis but a collaborative problem. In this case, the client's problem would be described better as a collaborative problem:

Potential Complications: Increased Intracranial Pressure and the nursing goal:

The nurse will manage and minimize changes in increased intracranial pressure

Summary

The Bifocal Clinical Practice Model provides nurses with a framework to diagnose the unique responses of a client and significant others to various situations. Clear definition of the two dimensions of nursing enhances the use and minimizes the misuse of nursing diagnoses. The Bifocal Clinical Practice Model describes the unique knowledge and focus of professional nursing.

2 DOCUMENTATION OF NURSING CARE

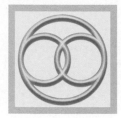

Legal Issues of Nursing Documentation

Historically, nurses have believed that the more information a nurse has charted, the better his or her legal defense will be in any litigation. Today nurses recognize that a comprehensive, streamlined documentation system actually can document more data in less time and space. Nursing documentation must be objective and comprehensive and must accurately reflect the status of the client and what has happened to him or her. If legally challenged, the nursing records represent what reasonably prudent nurses chart, and should demonstrate compliance with the institution's policy.

Unfortunately, most hospitals and other agencies have not seriously examined what documentation actually requires. Many nurses have been taught to write as much as possible; they operate under the philosophy "If it wasn't charted, it wasn't done." Does poor charting represent poor care? Inherent in this question are others: What is poor charting? By what standard is it poor? Does copious charting represent good care?

If a department of nursing does not establish specific policies for charting, then the charting in question can be held to standards from another department of nursing or from expert testimony. Case law does not determine the standards for nursing documentation, but instead passes a judgment regarding compliance with a standard.

Attributes of Nursing Documentation

The most important purpose of documentation is to communicate to other members of the health care team the client's progress and condition. In addition, nursing documentation is important:

- To define the nursing focus for the client or group
- To differentiate the accountability of the nurse from that of other members of the health care team
- To provide the criteria for reviewing and evaluating care (quality improvement)
- To provide the criteria for client classification
- To provide justification for reimbursement
- To provide data for administrative and legal review
- To comply with legal, accreditation, and professional standard requirements
- To provide data for research and educational purposes

Defining documentation as always hand-written or typed as free text (in a computer) is problematic. Documentation can take the form of a standard of care, a check marked on a form, or an initial on a flow record. The accompanying policy should direct that there is to be minimal or no writing unless an unusual or unsatisfactory situation has occurred.

Assessment

In assessment—the deliberate collection of data about a client, family, or group—the nurse obtains data by interviewing, observing, and examining. The two types of assessment are the initial screening interview and focus assessment.

Initial Screening Interview

The screening interview has two parts: functional patterns and physical assessment. It focuses on determining the client's present health status and ability to function. Figure 2.1 shows a nursing admission database. Examples of specific functional pattern assessment categories are as follows:

- Ability to bathe self
- Presence of confusion
- Spiritual practices
- Ability to control urination

**NURSING ADMISSION
DATA BASE**

Date _____ Arrival Time _____ Contact Person _____ Phone _____
ADMITTED FROM: ___ Home alone   ___Home with relative   ___Long-term care
                ___ Homeless   ___Home with_____   facility
                ___ ER   (Specify)   ___ Other _____
MODE OF ARRIVAL: ___ Wheelchair   ___ Ambulance   ___ Stretcher
REASON FOR HOSPITALIZATION: _____
_____

LAST HOSPITAL ADMISSION: Date _____ Reason _____
_____
PAST MEDICAL HISTORY: _____
_____

MEDICATION (Prescription/Over-the-Counter)	DOSAGE	LAST DOSE	FREQUENCY

HEALTH MAINTENANCE–PERCEPTION PATTERN
USE OF:
Tobacco: ___None ___Quit (date) ___Pipe ___Cigar ___<1 pk/day
            ___1–2 pks/day ___>2 pks/day Pks/year history _____
Alcohol: ___None ___Type/Amount ____/day ____/wk ___/month
Other Drugs ___No ___Yes Type _____ Use _____
Allergies (drugs, food, tape, dyes): _____ Reaction _____
_____

ACTIVITY/EXERCISE PATTERN
SELF-CARE ABILITY:
  0 = Independent   1 = Assistive device   2 = Assistance from others
  3 = Assistance from person and equipment   4 = Dependent/Unable

	0	1	2	3	4
Eating/Drinking					
Bathing					
Dressing/Grooming					
Toileting					
Bed Mobility					
Transferring					
Ambulating					
Stair Climbing					
Shopping					
Cooking					
Home Maintenance					

ASSISTIVE DEVICES: ___None ___Crutches ___Bedside commode ___Walker
                   ___Cane ___ Splint/Brace ___Wheelchair ___Other___

CODE: (1) Non-applicable (2) Unable to acquire
      (3) Not a priority at this time (4) Other (specify in notes)

FIGURE 2.1
Sample admission database. (Carpenito, L. J. [2004] *Nursing diagnosis: Application to clinical practice* [10th ed.]. Philadelphia: Lippincott Williams & Wilkins.)

The physical examination uses the skills of inspection, auscultation, and palpation to assess areas such as

- Pulse
- Skin condition
- Muscle strength
- Lung fields

After completing and recording the screening assessment, the nurse analyzes the data and asks questions such as:

- Does the client have a problem that requires nursing interventions (e.g., assistance with ambulation)?
- Is the client at risk for developing a problem (e.g., pressure ulcers)?
- Does the client's medical condition put him or her at high risk for complications (e.g., problems associated with increased blood glucose level in diabetes mellitus)?
- Do the prescribed treatments put the client at high risk for complications (e.g., phlebitis from IV therapy)?
- Is additional data collection needed?

Focus Assessment

Focus assessment involves the acquisition of selected or specific data as determined by the nurse and the client or family or as directed by the client's condition (Carpenito, 1983). The nurse can perform a focus assessment during the initial interview if the data suggest that he or she should ask additional questions. For example, on admission the nurse would question most clients about eating patterns. He or she also would ask a client

```
NUTRITION/METABOLIC PATTERN
Special Diet/Supplements _____
Previous Dietary Instruction: ___ Yes ___ No
Appetite:   ___ Normal ___ Increased ___ Decreased ___ Decreased taste sensation
            ___ Nausea ___ Vomiting ___ Stomatitis
Weight Fluctuations Last 6 Months: ___ None _____ lbs. Gained/Lost
Swallowing Difficulty (Dysphagia): ___ None ___ Solids ___ Liquids
Dentures: ___ Upper (_ Partial _ Full) ___ Lower (_ Partial _ Full)
          With Patient ___ Yes ___ No
Historty of Skin/Healing Problems ___ None ___ Abnormal Healing ___ Rash
                                  ___ Dryness ___ Excess Perspiration

ELIMINATION PATTERN
Bowel Habits ___ # BMs/day ___ Date of last BM ___ Within normal limits
             ___ Constipation ___ Diarrhea ___ Incontinence
             ___ Ostomy: Type ___ Appliance ___ Self care ___ Yes ___ No
Bladder Habits ___ WNL ___ Frequency ___ Dysuria ___ Nocturia ___ Urgency
               ___ Hematuria ___ Retention
  Incontinency: ___ No ___ Yes ___ Total ___ Daytime ___ Nighttime
                ___ Occasional ___ Difficulty delaying voiding
                ___ Difficulty reaching toilet
  Assistive Devices: ___ Intermittent catheterization
                     ___ Indwelling catheter ___ External catheter
                     ___ Incontinent briefs ___ Penile implant type _____

SLEEP/REST PATTERN
Habits: ___ hrs/night ___ AM nap ___ PM nap
        Feel rested after sleep ___ Yes ___ No
Problems ___ None ___ Early waking ___ Insomnia ___ Nightmares

COGNITIVE–PERCEPTUAL PATTERN
Mental Status: ___ Alert ___ Receptive aphasia ___ Poor historian
               ___ Oriented ___ Confused ___ Combative ___ Unresponsive
Speech: ___ Normal ___ Slurred ___ Garbled ___ Expressive aphasia
        Spoken Language _____ Interpreter _____
Language Spoken: ___ English ___ Spanish ___ Other _____
Ability to Read English: ___ Yes ___ No _____
Ability to Communicate: ___ Yes ___ No _____
Ability to Comprehend: ___ Yes ___ No _____
Level of Anxiety: ___ Mild ___ Moderate ___ Severe ___ Panic
Interactive Skills: ___ Appropriate ___ Other _____
Hearing: ___ WNL ___ Impaired ( _ Right _ Left) ___ Deaf ( _ Right _ Left)
         ___ Hearing Aid ___ Tinnitus
Vision: ___ WNL ___ Eyeglasses ___ Contact lens
        ___ Impaired ___ Right ___ Left
        ___ Blind ___ Right ___ Left
        ___ Cataract ___ Right ___ Left
        ___ Glaucoma
        ___ Prosthesis ___ Right _ Left
Vertigo: ___ Yes ___ No
Discomfort/Pain: ___ None ___ Acute ___ Chronic ___ Description _____
_____
Pain Management: _____

COPING STRESS TOLERANCE/SELF-PERCEPTION/SELF-CONCEPT PATTERN
Major concerns regarding hospitalization or illness (financial, self-care): _____
_____
Major loss/change in past year: ___ No ___ Yes _____
_____
Fear of violence_____ Yes_____No_____ Who_____
Outlook on future_____ (rate from 1 (poor) to 10 (very optimistic))

CODE: (1) Non-applicable (2) Unable to acquire
      (3) Not a priority at this time (4) Other (Specify in notes)
```

FIGURE 2.1 continued.

(continued on page 12)

with chronic obstructive pulmonary disease if dyspnea interferes with eating. This represents a focus assessment because the nurse would not ask every client if dyspnea affects food intake.

The nurse does certain focus assessments—such as vital signs, bowel and bladder function, and nutritional status—each shift for every client. (Section I presents a generic care plan for all hospitalized adults that includes these routine focus assessments.) The nurse determines the need for additional focus assessments based on the client's condition. For example, in a postoperative client, the nurse assesses and monitors the surgical wound and IV therapy.

Planning

The clinical purposes of documentation are to guide the caregiver and to record the client's status or response. Directions for nursing care originate in both nursing and medicine. Interventions prescribed by physicians are entered on various forms (e.g., Kardex or treatment and medication administration records). Nurses prescribe both routine interventions and those specific to the client. Routine or predictive nursing interventions can be found in nursing care standards. These client-specific interventions are listed in the addendum care plan.

Care plans (standards, addendum) serve the following purposes:

• They represent the priority set of diagnoses (collaborative problems or nursing diagnoses) for a client.
• They provide a "blueprint" to direct charting.
• They communicate to the nursing staff what to teach, observe, and implement.

SEXUALITY/REPRODUCTIVE PATTERN
LMP: _____ Gravida _____ Para_____
Menstrual Problems: ____ Yes ____ No _____
Last Pap Smear: ___Hx of abnormal PAP___
Monthly Self-Breast/Testicular Exam: ____ Yes ____ No
Sexual Concerns R/T Illness: _____
_____

ROLE-RELATIONSHIP PATTERN
Marital status_____
Occupation: _____
Employment Status: ____ Employed ____ Short-term disability
                    ____ Long-term disability ____ Unemployed
Support System: ____ Spouse ____ Neighbors/Friends ____ None
                ____ Family in same residence ____ Family in separate residence
                ____ Other _____
Family concerns regarding hospitalization: _____
_____

VALUE-BELIEF PATTERN
Religion: _____
Religious Restrictions: ____ No ____ Yes (Specify) _____
Request Chaplain Visitation at This Time: ____ Yes ____ No

PHYSICAL ASSESSMENT (Objective)
1. CLINICAL DATA
    Age _____ Height _____ Weight _____ (Actual/Approximate)
    Temperature _____
    Pulse: ____ Strong ____ Weak ____ Regular ____ Irregular
    Blood Pressure: Right Arm: ____ Left Arm ____ Sitting ____ Lying ____

2. RESPIRATORY/CIRCULATORY
    Rate _____
    Quality: ____ WNL ____ Shallow ____ Rapid ____ Labored ____ Other _____
    Cough: ____ No ____ Yes/Describe _____
    Auscultation:
      Upper rt lobes ___WNL ___Decreased ___Absent ___Abnormal sounds ___
      Upper lt lobes ___WNL ___Decreased ___Absent ___Abnormal sounds ___
      Lower rt lobes ___WNL ___Decreased ___Absent ___Abnormal sounds ___
      Lower lt lobes ___WNL ___Decreased ___Absent ___Abnormal sounds ___
    Right Pedal Pulse: ____ Strong ____ Weak ____ Absent
    Left Pedal Pulse ____ Strong ____ Weak ____ Absent

3. METABOLIC-INTEGUMENTARY
    SKIN:
      Color:____WNL ____Pale ____Cyanotic ____Ashen ____Jaundice ____Other ____
      Temperature: ____WNL ____ Warm ____ Cool
      Turgor: ____ WNL ____ Poor
      Edema: ____ No ____Yes/Description/location _____
      Lesions: ____ None ____ Yes/Description/location _____
      Bruises: ____ None ____ Yes/Description/location _____
      Reddened: ____ No ____ Yes/Description/location _____
      Pruritus: ____ No ____ Yes/Description/location _____
      Tubes: Specify _____
      Changes_____None. If yes; description/location
    MOUTH:
      Gums: ____ WNL ____ White plaque ____ Lesions ____ Other _____
      Teeth: ____ WNL ____ Other _____
    ABDOMEN:
      Bowel Sounds: ____ Present ____ Absent

4. NEURO/SENSORY
    Pupils ____ Equal ____ Unequal
      Left: ____ mm
      Right: ____ mm
    Reactive to light:
      Left: ____ Yes ____ No/Specify _____
      Right: ____ Yes ____ No/Specify _____
    Eyes: ____ Clear ____ Draining ____ Reddened ____ Other _____

5. MUSCULAR-SKELETAL
    Range of Motion: ____ Full ____ Other _____
    Balance and Gait: ____ Steady ____ Unsteady
    Hand Grasps: ____ Equal ____ Strong ____ Weakness/Paralysis (__ Right __Left)
    Leg Muscles: ____ Equal ____ Strong ____ Weakness/Paralysis (__ Right __Left)

DISCHARGE PLANNING
Lives: Alone ____ With _____ No known residence _____
Intended Destination Post Discharge: ____ Home ____ Undetermined ____ Other ____
Previous Utilization of Community Resources:
    ____ Home care/Hospice ____ Adult day care ____ Church groups ____ Other _____
    ___Meals on Wheels ___Homemaker/Home health aide ___Community support group
Post-discharge Transportation:
    ____ Car ____ Ambulance ____ Bus/Taxi
    ____ Unable to determine at this time
Anticipated Financial Assistance Post-discharge?: ____ No ____ Yes _____
Anticipated Problems with Self-care Post-discharge?: ___No ____ Yes _____
Assistive Devices Needed Post-discharge?: ____ No ____ Yes _____
Referrals: (record date)
    Discharge Coordinator _____ Home Health _____
    Social Service _____ V.N.A. _____
Other Comments: _____
_____

SIGNATURE/TITLE _____ DATE _____

FIGURE 2.1
continued.

- They provide goals/outcome criteria for reviewing and evaluating care.
- They direct specific interventions for the client, family, and other nursing staff members to implement.

To direct and evaluate nursing care effectively, the care plan should include the following:

- Diagnostic statements (collaborative problems or nursing diagnoses)
- Goals (outcome criteria) or nursing goals
- Nursing orders or interventions
- Evaluation (status of diagnosis and client progress)

Diagnostic Statements

Diagnostic statements can be either collaborative problems or nursing diagnoses. Refer to Chapter 1, The Bifocal Clinical Practice Model, for information on these two types of diagnostic statements.

Goals/Outcome Criteria

Client goals, or outcome criteria, are statements that describe a measurable behavior of the client or family, denoting a favorable status (changed or maintained) after delivery of nursing care (Alfaro, 2002). They serve as standards for measuring the care plan's effectiveness. *Goals/outcome criteria for nursing diagnoses should represent favorable statuses that the client can achieve or maintain through nursing-prescribed (independent) interventions* (Carpenito, 1992; Carpenito-Moyet, 2008). If the client is not achieving goals, the nurse must reevaluate the diagnosis and revise the goals and the plan or collaborate with a physician.

When the nurse collaborates with the physician, the diagnosis is a collaborative problem, not a nursing diagnosis. For example, if a client with a collaborative problem of Potential Complication: Dysrhythmia experiences premature ventricular contractions, the nurse would not change the nursing care plan, but would instead, initiate physician-prescribed interventions. Collaborative problems should not have client goals (outcome criteria). *Any goals or outcome criteria written for collaborative problems would need to represent the criteria for evaluating both nursing and medical care. Physiologic stability is the overall goal for collaborative problems. Such measures are represented through nursing goals.*

Nursing Interventions

As written in Chapter 1, there are two types of nursing interventions: nurse-prescribed and physician-prescribed. Care plans should contain nurse-prescribed interventions. *Care plans should not contain directions for nurses regarding delegated (physician-prescribed) treatments. Instead, nurses enter physicians' orders on care and treatment records, Kardexes, and medication administration records.* For this reason, the care plans presented in Unit II list only nurse-prescribed (independent) interventions. At the end of the Collaborative Problems section in each care plan, a section titled Related Physician-Prescribed Interventions provides these interventions as additional information. This chapter later explains the relationship of standards of care, physician-prescribed interventions, and critical pathways.

In the care plans, the interventions listed under nursing diagnoses generally consist of these types (Alfaro-LeFevre, 2002):

- Performing activities for the client or assisting the client with activities
- Performing nursing assessments to identify new problems and to determine the status of existing problems
- Teaching the client to help him or her gain new knowledge about health or the management of a disorder
- Counseling the client to make decisions about his or her own health care
- Consulting with other health care professionals
- Performing specific actions to remove, reduce, or resolve health problems

In contrast, the interventions listed under collaborative problems focus primarily on the following:

- Monitoring for physiologic instability
- Consulting with a physician to obtain appropriate interventions
- Performing specific actions to manage and to reduce the severity of the event
- Explaining the problem and the rationale for actions

Care Planning Systems

Standards of Care

Standards of care are detailed guidelines that represent the predicted care indicated in a specific situation. Standards of care should represent the care that nurses are responsible for providing, not an ideal level of care. *The nurse cannot hope to address all or even most of the problems that a client may have. Rather, the nurse must select those problems that are the most serious or most important to the client.* Ideal standards that are un-realistic only frustrate nurses and hold them legally accountable for care that they cannot provide. Nurses must create realistic standards based on client acuity, length of stay, and available resources.

A care planning system can contain three levels of directions:

• Level I—Generic Unit Standards of Care
• Level II—Diagnostic Cluster or Single Diagnosis Guidelines
• Level III—Addendum Care Plans

Level I Standards of Care predict the generic care that all or most individuals or families in a unit will need. Examples of generic unit standards of care are medical, surgical, oncologic, pediatric, postpartum, operating room, emergency room, mental health unit, rehabilitation unit, and newborn nursery. Figure 2.2 presents a diagnostic cluster for most hospitalized adults. The Generic Medical Care Plan at the beginning of Section 1 and the Generic Surgery Care Plan at the beginning of Section 2 are Level I standards. Because they apply to all clients, nurses do not need to write the nursing diagnoses or collaborative problems associated with the generic standard of care on an individual client's care plan. Instead, institutional policy can specify that the generic standard will be implemented for all clients. Documentation of the generic standard is discussed later in this chapter.

Level II guideline care plans contain a diagnostic cluster or a single nursing diagnosis or collaborative problem. A diagnostic cluster is a set of nursing diagnoses and collaborative problems that have been pre-dicted to be present and of high priority for a given population. Unit II contains Level II care plans orga-

---

Collaborative Problems
Potential Complication: Cardiovascular
Potential Complication: Respiratory

Nursing Diagnoses
Anxiety related to unfamiliar environment, routines, diagnostic tests and treatments, and loss of control
Risk for Injury related to unfamiliar environment and physi-cal/mental limitations secondary to condition, medications, therapies, and diagnostic test
Risk for Infection related to increased microorganisms in envi-ronment, the risk of person-to-person transmission, and inva-sive tests and therapies
Self-Care Deficit related to sensory, cognitive, mobility, endurance, or motivation problems
Risk for Imbalanced Nutrition: Less Than Body Requirements related to decreased appetite secondary to treatments, fatigue, environment, changes in usual diet, and increased protein/vitamin requirements for healing
Risk for Constipation related to change in fluid/food intake, rou-tine and activity level, effects of medications, and emotional stress
Disturbed Sleep Pattern related to unfamiliar or noisy environ-ment, change in bedtime ritual, emotional stress, and change in circadian rhythm
Risk for Spiritual Distress related to separation from religious support system, lack of privacy, or inability to practice spiritual rituals
Interrupted Family Processes related to disruption of routines, change in role responsibilities, and fatigue associated with increased workload and visiting hour requirements

FIGURE 2.2
Level I diagnostic cluster for hospitalized adults.

nized using diagnostic clusters. Those diagnoses indicated as primary have been reported to be managed by nurses 75%–100% of the time. Those diagnoses that are indicated to be important are managed 50%–74% of the time. Refer to the description of the Validation Study, p. x. Examples of Level II single-diagnosis standards are High Risk for Impaired Skin Integrity, High Risk for Violence, and PC: Fluid/Electrolyte Imbalances.

Although standards of care do not have to be part of the client's record, the record should specify what standards have been selected for the client. The problem list serves this purpose. The problem list represents the priority set of nursing diagnoses and collaborative problems for an individual client. Figure 2.3 presents a sample problem list. Next to each diagnosis, the nurse would indicate where the directions for the care can be found—on a standardized form or on the addendum plan. The nurse can use the last column to indicate client progress.

Priority Set of Diagnoses

Nurses cannot address all or even most of the nursing diagnoses and collaborative problems in clients and families. Priority diagnoses are those nursing diagnoses and collaborative problems for which nursing resources will be directed toward goal achievement. They take precedence over other nursing diagnoses/collaborative problems that

Nursing Problem List/Care Plan

Nursing Diagnosis/Collaborative Problem	Status	Standard	Addendum	Evaluation of Progress				

Status Code: A = Active   R = Resolved   RO = Ruled-out
Evaluation Code: S = Stable   I = Improved   *W = Worsened   *U = Unchanged   P = Progressing   *NP = Not Progressing

Addendum Care Plan

NSG DX/COLL PROB	CLIENT/NURSING GOALS	DATE/INITIALS	INTERVENTIONS

Initials/Signature			
1.	3.	5.	7.
2.	4.	6.	8.

FIGURE 2.3
Nursing problem list and care plan.

may be important but not priorities (Carpenito, 1995). In acute care settings, priority diagnoses are those nursing diagnoses or collaborative problems that

1. Are associated with the primary medical or surgical condition
2. If not managed now will deter progress or negatively affect functional status

Important but nonpriority nursing diagnoses or collaborative problems need to be referred to the client for management after discharge. A referral to a community resource may be indicated. For example, the nurse can refer a woman with peripheral vascular disease who wants to quit smoking to a smoking cessation program in the community.

The problem list in Figure 2.4 illustrates three priority diagnoses in addition to those on the Post-Operative Standard of Care.

Addendum Care Plans

An addendum care plan represents additional interventions to be provided for the client. Nurses can add these specific interventions to a Level II guideline care plan or may associate them with additional priority nursing diagnoses or collaborative problems not included on the standardized plan.

FIGURE 2.4
Sample problem list and addendum care plan.

The initial care of most hospitalized clients can be directed responsibly using standards of care. With subsequent nurse–client interactions, specific data may warrant specific addendum additions to the client's care plan to ensure holistic, empathic nursing care. Figure 2.4 presents a problem list and addendum care plan for a client recovering from gastric surgery. In addition to the diagnostic cluster in the postoperative standard of care, this client has three addendum diagnoses. High Risk for Impaired Skin Integrity is being managed with interventions from a standard for this diagnosis. Documentation will be completed at each shift on the flow record. Impaired Swallowing is being treated with generic interventions and with addendum intervention specifying foods that this client can tolerate. The last diagnosis, Impaired Physical Mobility, involves only addendum interventions prescribed to increase the client's motivation and to promote correct ambulation techniques.

Critical Pathways

The concept of critical pathways has been a well-known management tool for many years in such disciplines as economics and engineering, in which they are organized as a timeline grid to monitor the progress of a project. Critical pathways in nursing were developed at the New England Medical Center in 1985 by Kathleen Bower and Karen Zander. Since then, numerous versions of critical pathways have been developed in hundreds of facilities under various names such as CareMap, critical paths, Collaborative Action Track, and Milestone Action Plans.

Critical pathways "are based on the process of anticipating and describing *in advance* the care clients, within the specific case types, require and then comparing the actual status of the client to that anticipated" (Bower, 1993). They are developed on selected client populations with the participation of the disciplines involved in the care. Each discipline is asked to outline the usual anticipated care requirements and the outcomes (Bower, 1993). So, before creating a critical pathway, nurses must identify their standard of care for the population. A standard of care for a population should include

1. The priority set of nursing diagnoses and collaborative problems predicted to need nursing interventions during the expected length of stay
2. Realistic, achievable outcomes
3. Realistic, pertinent interventions

Critical pathways are multidisciplinary; standards of care may or may not be. Nursing diagnoses and collaborative problems are excellent language for other disciplines such as respiratory therapy, physical therapy, social service, nutritional therapy, and so on. After the standard of care is established for nursing, it could be passed on to other disciplines for addition of interventions specific to them (Carpenito, 1995). Figure 2.5 illustrates a section from a multidisciplinary care plan for a client with a fractured hip.

The additional physician orders for the client usually are not indicated on the standard of care, because the problems in the standard are nursing diagnoses and collaborative problems. Physician standard orders are reflected on the critical pathway. After nursing and other disciplines have completed the standard of care, the critical pathway can be formulated.

FIGURE 2.5
Sample multidisciplinary care plan for a client after a total hip replacement. (Carpenito, L. J. [2004]. *Nursing diagnosis: Application to clinical practice* [10th ed.]. Philadelphia: Lippincott Williams & Wilkins.)

Nursing Diagnosis: *Impaired Physical Mobility related to pain, stiffness, fatigue, restrictive equipment, and prescribed activity restrictions.*

Goal: *The client will increase activity to a level consistent with abilities*

Interventions:

PT
1. Establish an exercise program tailored to the client's ability.
2. Implement exercises at regular intervals.

PT/Nsg
3. Teach body mechanics and transfer techniques.

PT/Nsg
4. Encourage independence.
5. Teach and supervise use of ambulatory aids.

Critical Pathway Format

Critical pathways can be developed for client populations using the medical diagnosis, the surgical or diagnostic procedure, or a therapy such as ventilator dependent or chemotherapy (Bower, 1993). The critical pathway outlines the anticipated care requirements and the outcomes to achieve within a pre-established timeframe.

The outcomes identified on a critical pathway can be those linked to collaborative problems and nursing diagnoses identified for the population. Another approach is to identify the discharge criteria for the population. In either case, the client is evaluated daily for progress. Figure 2.6 represents a CareMap from the Center for Case Management, which illustrates problem statements linked with outcomes. The lower portion of the CareMap describes the staff tasks on a timeline.

Linking Standards of Care to Critical Paths

The care plans in this book represent care for a population. As a result of the validation work described on p. xiii, the nursing diagnoses and collaborative problems treated frequently by nurses have been established. These findings will assist nurses in establishing the standard from which critical pathways are derived.

The remainder of this section will outline the creation of a standard of care and critical pathway from the care plan for an individual undergoing a hip replacement. Table 2.1 illustrates the critical pathway derived from the standard of care. On the basis of the findings of the validation study, only those nursing diagnoses and collaborative problems reported to be monitored for or treated more than 75% of the time are included on the standard. In addition, outcomes that are achievable during the expected length of stay and interventions to achieve these outcomes are illustrated online.

Care Plans and Critical Paths

As discussed earlier, critical pathways offer an at-a-glance timeline to evaluate the progress of a client in a population. Critical pathways frequently do not accommodate additional nursing diagnoses or collaborative problems (addendum diagnoses) that are present and need nursing interventions. These addendum diagnoses can delay client progress if not addressed. For example, a woman scheduled for a hip replacement also has diabetes mellitus. This would necessitate monitoring for the collaborative problem, "PC: Hypo/Hyperglycemia." How will the nurse communicate this problem to other nurses with a critical path? One option is to write this additional problem under the problem list in the critical path and to insert the monitoring of blood glucose levels under the assessment section. This would work if the interventions were brief, such as "monitor blood glucose levels." However, what if this woman is also confused before surgery? This would necessitate the addition of Disturbed Thought Processes to the problem list. The interventions for this addendum diagnosis are not brief. A problem list/care plan can provide the solution. Figure 2.7 illustrates a problem list/care plan for this woman. A detailed explanation of problem lists can be found online.

Documentation and Evaluation

Care plans represent documentation of the nursing care planned for a client. They also reflect the status of a diagnosis: active, resolved, or ruled out. The documentation of care delivered and the client's status or response after care are recorded on specific forms, including:

• Graphic records
• Flow records
• Progress notes
• Teaching records
• Discharge planning/summary

The nurse is responsible for evaluating a client's status and progress to outcome achievement daily. Evaluation of the client's status and progress is different for collaborative problems versus nursing diagnoses. For nursing diagnoses, the nurse will:

(text continues on page 23)

CareMap™: Congestive Heart Failure

Problem	Day 1 ER 1–4 hours	Day 1 Floor Telemetry or CCU 6–24 hours	Day 2 Floor	Day 3 Floor	Day 4 Floor	Day 5 Floor	Day 6 Floor
Location			Benchmark Quality Criteria				
1) Alteration in gas exchange/perfusion and fluid balance due to decreased cardiac output, excess fluid volume	Reduced pain from admission or pain free Uses pain scale O₂ sat. improved over admission baseline on O₂ therapy	Respirations equal to or less than on admission	O₂ sat = 90 Resp 20–22 Vital signs stable Crackles at lung bases Mild shortness of breath with activity	Does not require O₂ Vital signs stable Crackles at base Respirations 20–22 Mild shortness of breath with activity	Does not require O₂ (O₂ sat on room air 90%) Vital signs stable Crackles at base Respirations 20–22 Completes activities with no increase in respirations No edema	Can lie in bed at baseline position Chest X-ray clear or at baseline	No dyspnea
2) Potential for shock	No signs/symptoms of shock	No signs/symptoms of shock	No signs/symptoms of shock	No signs/symptoms of shock Normal lab values	No signs/symptoms of shock	No signs/symptoms of shock	No signs/symptoms of shock
3) Potential for consequences of immobility and decreased activity: skin breakdown, DVT	No redness at pressure points No falls	No redness at pressure points No falls	Tolerates chair, washing, eating, and toileting	Has bowel movement Up in room and bathroom with assist	Up ad lib for short periods	Activity increased to level used at home without shortness of breath	Activity increased to level used at home without shortness of breath
4) Alteration in nutritional intake due to nausea and vomiting, labored		No c/o nausea No vomiting Taking liquids as offered	Eating solids Takes in 50% each meal	Taking 50% each meal	Taking 50% each meal Weight 2 lbs. from patient's normal baseline	Taking 75% each meal	Taking 75% each meal
5) Potential for arrhythmias due to decreased cardiac output: decreased irritable foci, valve problems, decreased gas exchange	No evidence of life-threatening dysrhythmias	Normal sinus rhythm with benign ectopy	Potassium (WNL) Benign or no arrhythmias	Digoxin level DNL Benign or no arrhythmias	Digoxin level WNL Benign or no arrhythmias	Digoxin level WNL Benign or no arrhythmias	Digoxin level WNL Benign or no arrhythmias
6) Patient/family response to future treatment and hospitalization	Patient/family expressing concerns Following directions of staff	Patient/family expressing concerns Following directions of staff	Patient/family expressing concerns Following directions of staff	States reasons for and cooperates with rest periods Patient begins to assess own knowledge and ability to care for CHF at home	Patient decides if he/she wants discussion with physician about advanced directives	States plan for 1–2 days postdischarge as to meds., diet, activity, follow-up appointments Expresses reaction to having CHF	Repeats plans States signs and symptoms to notify physician/ER Signs discharge consent
7) Individual problem:							

FIGURE 2.6

Sample CareMap. (*From the Center for Case Management, South Natick, MA. CareMap is a registered trademark of the Center for Case Management; used with permission.*)

(continued on page 20)

Staff Tasks							
Assessments/Consults	Vital signs q 15 min Nursing assessments focus on lung sounds, edema, color, skin integrity, jugular vein distention Cardiac monitor Arterial line if needed Swan Ganz Intake and output	Vital signs q 15 min–1 hr Repeat nursing assessments Cardiac monitor Arterial line Swan Ganz Daily weight Intake and output	Vital signs q 4 hrs Repeat nursing assessments D/C cardiac monitor 24 hr D/C arterial and Swan Ganz Daily weight Intake and output	Vital signs q 6 hrs Repeat nursing assessments Daily weight Intake and output	Vital signs q 6 hrs Repeat nursing assessments Daily weight Intake and output Nutrition consult	Vital signs q 6 hrs Repeat Nursing assessments Daily weight Intake and output	Vital signs q 6 hrs Repeat Nursing assessments Daily weight Intake and output
Specimens/Tests	Consider TSH studies Chest X-ray EKG CPK q 8 hr x 3 ABG if pulse Ox: (range) Lytes, Na, K, Cl, CO_2, Glucose, BUN, Creatinine Digoxin: (range)	B/G	Evaluate for ECHO Lytes, BUN, Creatinine			Chest X-ray Lytes, BUN, Creatinine	
Treatments	O_2 or intubate IV or Heparin lock	O_2 IV or Heparin lock	IV or Heparin lock	DC pulse Ox if stable D/C IV or Heparin lock			
Medications	Evaluate for Digoxin Nitrodrip or paste Diuretics IV Evaluate for antiemetics Evaluate for antiarrhythmics	Evaluate for Digoxin Nitrodrip or paste Diuretics IV Evaluate for pre-load/afterload reducers K supplements	D/C Nitrodrip or paste Diuretics IV or PO K supplements Stool softeners Evaluate for nicotine patch	Change to PO Digoxin PO diuretics K supplements Stool softeners Nicotine patch if consent	PO diuretics K supplement Stool softeners Nicotine patch if consent	PO diuretics K supplement Stool softeners Nicotine patch if consent	PO diuretics K supplement Stool softeners Nicotine patch if consent
Nutrition	None	Clear liquids	Cardiac, low-salt diet	Cardiac, low-salt diet	Cardiac, low-salt diet	Cardiac, low-salt diet	
Safety/Activity	Commode Bedrest with head elevated Reposition patient q 2 hrs Bedrails up Call light available	Commode Bedrest with head elevated Dangle Reposition patient q 2 hrs Enforce rest periods Bedrails up Call light available	Commode Enforce rest periods Chair with assist 1/2 hr with feet elevated Bedrails up Call light available	Commode Enforce rest periods Chair x 3 Bedrails up Call light available	Bathroom privileges Chair x 3 Bedrails up Call light available	Ambulate in hall x 2 Up ad lib between rest periods Bedrails up Call light available	Encourage ADLs that approximate activities at home Bedrails up Call light available
Teaching	Explain procedures Teach chest pain scale and importance of reporting	Explain course, need for energy conservation Orient to unit and routine	Clarify CHF Dx and future teaching needs Orient to unit and routine Schedule rest periods Begin medication teaching	Importance of weighing self every day Provide smoking cessation information Review energy conservation schedule	Cardiac rehab level as indicated by consult Provide smoking cessation support Dietary teaching	Review CHF education material with patient	Reinforce CHF teaching
Transfer/Discharge Coordination	Assess home situation: notify significant other If no arrhythmias or chest pain, transfer to floor Otherwise transfer to ICU	Screen for discharge needs Transfer to floor	Consider Home Health Care referral		Evaluate needs for diet and anti-smoking classes Physician offers discussion opportunities for advanced directives	Appointment and arrangement for follow-up care with Home Health Care nurses Contact VNA	Reinforce follow-up appointments

FIGURE 2.6
continued.

TABLE 2.1   Critical Pathways for a Client Undergoing a Total Hip Replacement

Nursing Diagnosis/ Collaborative Problem	Intermediate Goals							Outcomes
	Day 1	Day 2	Day 3	Day 4	Day 5	Day 6	Day 7	Day 8
Potential complication: Fat emboli Compartmental syndrome Hemorrhage Joint displacement Sepsis Thrombosis	Nurse will manage and minimize vascular and joint complications.	→	→	→	→	→	→	State signs and symptoms that must be reported to a health care professional.
High Risk for Infection		Will exhibit wound healing free of infection	→	→	→	→	→	Demonstrate healing with evidence of intact, approximated wound edges or granulation tissue
Impaired Physical Mobility	Will relate the purpose of strengthening exercises	Will do strengthening exercises	→	Will demonstrate use of assistive device	→	→	→	Regain mobility while adhering to weight-bearing restrictions using an assistive device
Pain	Will report satisfactory pain relief	→	Will report a lessening of pain	Will report relief from PO medications	→	→	→	Report progressive reduction of pain and an increase in activity
High Risk for Injury	Will identify factors that increase risk of injury; will describe appropriate safety measures	→	→	→	→	→	→	Describe risk factors for injury in home
High Risk for Impaired Skin Integrity	Will demonstrate skin integrity free of pressure ulcers	→	→	→	→	→	→	Demonstrate skin integrity free of pressure ulcers
High Risk for Ineffective Therapeutic Regimen Management	Will communicate questions and concerns	→	→	→	→	Demonstrate skills needed for activities of daily living (ADLs)	→	Describe activity restrictions Describe a plan for resuming ADLs

(continued on page 22)

TABLE 2.1   Critical Pathways for a Client Undergoing a Total Hip Replacement (continued)

Timeline	OR Day	POD #1	POD #2	POD #3	POD #4	POD #5	POD #6	POD #7	POD #8
Consults		OT PT Home Care							
Test	Post-op x-ray Hct; SMA6 PT/PIT	→	→	→	PT/PIT	→	→	→	
Treatments	Hemovac drain IV	→	D/C Hemovac	→	D/C IV D/C dressing	→	→	→	D/C Staples
Medication	Antibiotic pre-op	Antibiotic IM pain meds. Anticoagulant	PO pain meds.	→	Anticoagulant	→	→	→	Prescription D/C anticoagulant
Diet	As ordered	→	→	→	As ordered	→	→	→	
Activity	Bedrest with abduction pillow; maintain alignment	OOB/chair	Weight bear as tolerated; transfer/assist Ambulate/walker	→	Weight bear as tolerated; transfer/assist Ambulate/walker	Crutches Independent with walker	Stairs with assist	→	→
Assessments	Post-op assessments	Assess Ace wrap Monitor neurovascular status Monitor tissue integrity	→	→	Turn q 2 hrs Monitor incision Monitor neurovascular status Monitor tissue integrity	→	→	→	
Teaching	S/S neurovascular compromise; reinforce activity and safety measures	Post-op exercises	→	→	Evaluate Pt/S.O. understanding	→	→	→	Written instructions
Discharge Planning			Social work prn Home care prn	→					Written instructions

NURSING DIAGNOSIS/ COLLABORATIVE PROBLEM	STATUS	STANDARD	ADDENDUM	EVALUATION OF PROGRESS						
Total Hip Replacement	A	√								
PC: Hypo/Hyperglycemia	A	√								
Disturbed Thought Processes RT effects of dementia	A	√	√							

STATUS CODE: A = Active   R = Resolved   RO = Ruled-out
EVALUATION CODE: S = Stable,   I = Improved,   *W = Worsened, U = Unchanged
                            *NP = Not Progressing,   P = Progressing

Reviewed With Client/Family ___9/23___ , _____, _____, (Date)

ADDENDUM CARE PLAN

Nsg Dx/Coll Prob	Client/Nursing Goals	Date/Initials	Interventions
Dis thought process	Agitated episodes will diminish	LJC 9/23	1–7 STANDARD
			8. focus on decreasing fear
			9. encourage to share fears

Initials/Signature 1. LJC/ *LJ Carpenito RN*	3	5.	7.
2.	4.	6	8.

FIGURE 2.7
Nursing problem list/care plan.

• Assess the client's status.
• Compare this response to the outcome criteria.
• Conclude if the client is progressing to outcome achievement.

The nurse can record this evaluation on a flow record as

7 AM–3 PM
Comfort

Acute Comfort   Report satisfaction relief from measures or on a progress note as
Sub. The medication relieved my pain well. It is easier to move and cough.
Eval. Pain controlled; continue plan.

Not all nursing diagnoses require a progress note to record evaluation. A well-designed flow record can be used.

For collaborative problems, the nurse will:

• Collect selected data.
• Compare the data to the established norms.
• Judge if the data are within an acceptable range.

The nurse can record the assessment data for collaborative problems on flow records. Progress notes can be used if the findings are significant, followed by the nursing management of the situation. The last column of Figure 2.3 represents the place where the nurse can document client progress for each diagnosis on the problem list. The frequency of this documentation will be determined by the institution (e.g., q 24 h). If a client has not improved or has worsened an I* or N* is used. In addition, a progress note is required to record the nursing actions undertaken.

So, the evaluation for nursing diagnoses is focused on progress to achievement of client outcome, whereas the evaluation for collaborative problems is focused on the client's condition compared with established norms.

Discharge Planning

Discharge planning is a systematic process of appraisal, preparation, and coordination done to facilitate provision of health care and social services before and after discharge. Discharge planning can be categorized as standard or addendum.

Standard discharge planning includes the teaching deemed necessary based on the client's specific medical or surgical condition. The standard of care usually can address the content to be taught under two nursing diagnoses: Risk for Ineffective Management of Therapeutic Regimen, and Risk for Impaired Home Maintenance Management. Standard discharge planning is the responsibility of the professional nurse caring for the client or family.

Addendum discharge planning requires coordinated and collaborative action among health care providers within the institution and in the community at large. Multidisciplinary actions may be indicated. A discharge coordinator or a case manager should coordinate this type of discharge planning.

I. Planning (initiate on admission)

Lives alone _____ With _____ No known residence _____

Intended destination after discharge:

   Home _____ Other _____ Undetermined _____

Anticipated caregiver: Self _____ Other _____

Prehospital functioning ability
- Home management: Independent / Assistance needed / Dependent
- Cooking: Independent / Assistance needed / Dependent
- Shopping: Independent / Assistance needed / Dependent
- Self-care: Independent / Assistance needed / Dependent

Anticipated financial assistance post discharge?   No _____   Yes _____

Anticipated problems with self-care post discharge?   No _____   Yes _____

Assistive devices needed post discharge?   No _____   Yes _____

Referrals: (record date)

   Discharge coordinator _____   Home health _____

   Social service _____   Other _____

II. Discharge Criteria and Instructions

1. Nutrition:

   _____ Explain diet to be followed upon discharge.

   Diet _____

   _____

   Restrictions _____

2. Medications:

   _____ State correct dose, time, special precautions, and side effects of medications

Name/Dose	Time(s)	Special instructions (in addition to those on container)

3. Activity

   _____ State activity restrictions

   _____ Demonstrate prescribed exercises

   _____ Demonstrate correct use of appliances/assistive devices

   ☐ Resume normal activity
   ☐ Sponge bath only   ☐ Tub bath   ☐ Shower

   ☐ Restricted activity for _____ (length of time)
     ☐ No lifting   ☐ No climbing stairs   ☐ No driving

   ☐ No sexual activity   ☐ Other _____

   _____

   _____

4. Special instructions

   _____ Correctly describe or demonstrate the prescribed treatment

   _____ State signs and symptoms that necessitate reporting

FIGURE 2.8
Discharge planning and summary record.

Staff nurses usually do not have the time or resources available for addendum discharge planning. However it is the staff nurse who refers high-risk clients or families to the discharge coordinator.

The goal of discharge planning is to identify the specific needs for maintaining or achieving maximum function after discharge. The discharge needs of clients and families can result in two types of nursing actions:

• Teaching the client or family how to manage the situation at home
• Referring the client or family to support services (e.g., community nurses, physical therapists, or self-help groups) for assistance with management at home

All unresolved outcome criteria on the problem list require either teaching for self-management or referrals before discharge.

Discharge planning should begin at admission. After the admission assessment, the nurse must analyze the data to identify if the client or family needs addendum discharge planning and referrals. Figure 2.8 presents questions that can help the nurse identify high-risk clients and families. These questions can be placed either as a section at the end of the admission assessment form, as illustrated in Figure 2.1, or as a section on a combined discharge planning and summary record as in Figure 2.8. High-risk clients and families require a referral to the discharge coordinator at admission.

Certain events that may not be predicted on admission also necessitate referral to a discharge coordinator. Some examples follow:

• Newly diagnosed chronic disease; terminal illness
• Prolonged recuperation after illness or surgery
• Complex home care regimens
• Insufficient or no health insurance
• Emotional instability

Symptoms to report: _____
_____
_____

Other: _____
_____
_____

_____ Describe follow-up care and available community resources
☐ Appointment with _____ Date _____ Time _____
☐ Patient/Family to make appointment in _____ days/weeks
☐ Referral to _____
☐ Records sent with patient (list) _____
_____

III. Discharge Summary
Discharge criteria met?   Yes _____   No _____
Action taken if discharge criteria not met: _____
_____
_____
_____

Discharged to _____ Date _____ Time _____
Mode of transportation _____
Accompanied by _____
Personal effects/Valuables sent home?   Yes _____   No _____
   List _____
Medications sent home from pharmacy?   Yes _____   No _____
Other comments _____
_____
_____
_____
Discharge nurse's signature _____

FIGURE 2.8
continued.

Discharge Summary

The Joint Commission on Accreditation of Healthcare Organizations (JCAHO) recommends that a discharge summary represent instructions given, referrals, client status, and the client's understanding of the instructions. The nurse can use progress notes to record this information; however, a more efficient system for recording the discharge summary can be designed. This record could be adapted with specific outcomes related to the medical or surgical condition. For example, a preprinted discharge summary record for a postoperative client could include these items:

• The client will correctly describe wound care measures.
• The client will state signs and symptoms that must be reported to a health care professional: fever, chills, redness or drainage of wound, and increasing pain.

A systematic, efficient discharge planning program can promote continuity of care by identifying a client's discharge needs early. Early identification of discharge needs also may help to eliminate unnecessary hospital days and unnecessary readmissions.

Summary

The development of an efficient, professional nursing documentation system is possible within the scope of existing standards of practice. The elimination of repetitive narrative charting on progress notes can reduce the total time spent in charting and produce a more accurate and useful representation of professional practice and client or family response. A streamlined documentation system that integrates the nursing process from admission to discharge with the designated charting requirements also presents the nurse with an optimum defense in the event of litigation proceedings and legal challenges.

3 11 STEPS TO CARE PLANNING

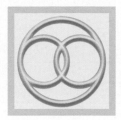

Care plans have one primary purpose: to provide directions for the nursing staff for a particular client. For students and nurses inexperienced in caring for a client with a particular condition or after a certain surgical procedure, these directions (care plan) need to be detailed. For nurses experienced in caring for people with a particular condition or after a certain surgical procedure, these directions (care plan) will be limited to only those specific interventions that are different for this particular client.

For example, a client who has diabetes mellitus is having abdominal surgery. An inexperienced nurse or student will need to refer to the generic care plan for a surgical client and an additional section on hypo/hyperglycemia (low or high blood glucose). An experienced nurse will not need to read a care plan for abdominal surgery but will need to know that the client also has diabetes and will need blood glucose monitoring. In hospitals and other health care agencies, general care plans for certain conditions or surgical procedures are usually in a computer or pre-printed to use as a reference. Other problems that are not on the general care plan are added individually.

Author's note: Some hospitals have problem lists for each client. This would list problems associated with general surgery and an additional problem of hyper/hypoglycemia.

Step 1: Assessment

If you interview your assigned client before you write your care plan, complete your assessment using the form recommended by your faculty. If you need to write a care plan before you can interview the client, go to Step 2. After you complete your assessment, circle all information that points to client strengths. Write all the strengths on an index card.

Author's note: Strengths are factors that will help the client recover, cope with stressors, and progress to his or her original health prior to hospitalization, illness, or surgery. Examples of strengths include:

- Positive spiritual framework
- Positive support system
- Ability to perform self-care
- No eating difficulties
- Effective sleep habits
- Alert, good memory
- Financial stability
- Relaxed most of the time

Highlight all information that points to client strengths. Write all the strengths on the back of the index card.

Author's note: Risk factors are situations, personal characteristics, disabilities, or medical conditions that can hinder the client's ability to heal, cope with stressors, and progress to his or her original health prior to hospitalization, illness, or surgery. Examples of risk factors include:

- Obesity
- Fatigue
- Limited ability to speak or understand English
- Memory problems
- Hearing problems
- Self-care problems before hospitalization
- Difficulty walking
- Financial problems
- Tobacco use

- Alcohol problem
- Moderate to high anxiety most of the time
- Frail, elderly
- Presence of chronic diseases
  Arthritis   Depression
  Diabetes mellitus   Cardiac disorder
  HIV   Pulmonary disease
  Multiple sclerosis

Step 2: Same Day Assessment

If you have not completed a screening assessment of your assigned client, determine the following as soon as you can by asking the client, family, or nurse assigned to your client.

- Before hospitalization:
  - Could the client perform self-care?
  - Did the client need assistance?
  - Could the client walk unassisted?
  - Did the client have memory problems?
  - Did the client have hearing problems?
  - Did the client smoke cigarettes?
- What conditions or diseases does the client have that make him or her more vulnerable to:
  - Falling
  - Infection
  - Nutrition/fluid imbalances
  - Pressure ulcers
  - Severe or panic anxiety
  - Physiological instability (e.g., electrolytes, blood glucose, blood pressure, respiratory function, healing problems)
- When you meet the assigned client, determine if any of the following risk factors are present:
  - Obesity
  - Impaired ability to speak/understand English
  - Communication difficulties
  - High anxiety

Write significant data on the index card. Go to Step 3.

Author's note: In some nursing programs, students do not have the opportunity to see or assess their assigned client prior to the clinical day. Therefore they must assess the client on their first clinical day.

Step 3: Create Your Initial Care Plan

Why is your client in the hospital? Go to the index in this book and look up the medical condition or surgical procedure. If you find the condition or surgical procedure, go to Step 4.

If the condition your client is hospitalized for is not in the index, refer to the generic medical care plan at the beginning of Section 1. If your client had surgery, refer to the generic surgical or ambulatory care plan at the beginning of Section 2.

Step 4: Additional Problems

If the medical condition or risk factor puts your client at high risk for a physiological complication such as electrolyte imbalances or increased intracranial pressure or for nursing diagnoses such as Impaired Skin Integrity, Risk for Infection Transmission, or Self-Care Deficit, go to the individual indexes for collaborative problems and/or nursing diagnoses. You will find the problem or nursing diagnoses there. Go to Step 5.

Author's note: These individual indexes provide numerous options when your assigned client has risk factors and medical conditions in addition to the primary reason he or she is hospitalized.

Step 5: Review Standard Plan

- Review each section of the care plan. Review your client's risk factors on your index card.
- Review the collaborative problems listed. These are the physiological complications that you need to monitor. Do not delete any because they all relate to the condition or procedure that your client has had. You will need to add how often you should take vital signs, record intake and output, change dressings, etc. Ask the nurse you are assigned with for these times or review the Kardex, which may also have the time frames.
- Review each intervention for collaborative problems. Are any interventions unsafe or contraindicated for your client? For example, if your client has edema and renal problems, the fluid requirements may be too high for him or her.

Author's note: Review the collaborative problems on the standard plan. *Also* review all additional collaborative problems that you found in the separate index that relate to your assigned client.

Step 6: Review the Nursing Diagnoses on the Standard Plan

Review each nursing diagnosis on the plan.

- Does it apply to your assigned client?
- Does your client have any risk factors (see your index card) that could make this diagnosis worse?

An example on the Generic Medical Care Plan is, *Risk for Injury related to unfamiliar environment and physical or mental limitations secondary to condition, medication, therapies, or diagnostic tests.*
     Now look at the list of risk factors for your assigned client. Can any of the factors listed contribute to the client sustaining an injury? For example, is he or she having problems walking or seeing? Is he or she experiencing dizziness?
     If your client has an unstable gait related to peripheral vascular disease (PVD), you would add the following to the diagnosis: *Risk for Injury related to unfamiliar environment and unstable gait secondary to PVD.*

Author's note: If you know your client has PVD, but you do not know how this can affect functioning, look up the diagnosis in this book (or another textbook) and review what problems PVD causes. Examples include unstable gait, poor circulation to the legs, and risk for injury.

Interventions

Review the intervention for each nursing diagnosis:

- Are they relevant for your client?
- Will you have time to provide them?
- Are any interventions not appropriate or contraindicated for your assigned client?
- Can you add any specific interventions?
- Do you need to modify any interventions because of risk factors (see index card)?

Author's note: Remember that you cannot individualize a care plan for a client until you spend time with him or her, but you can add and delete any inappropriate interventions based on your preclinical knowledge of this client (e.g., medical diagnosis, coexisting medical conditions).

Goals/Outcome Criteria

Review the goals listed for the nursing diagnosis:

- Are they pertinent to your client?
- Can the client demonstrate achievement of the goal on the day you provide care?
- Do you need more time?

     Delete goals that are inappropriate for your client. If the client will need more time to meet the goal, add "by discharge." If the client can accomplish the goal by a certain day, write "by (insert date)" after the goal.

Hint: Faculty and references may have different words to describe goals. Ask your faculty which terminology they use.

Using the same diagnosis, *Risk for Injury related to unfamiliar environment and physical or mental limitations secondary to the condition, therapies, and diagnostic tests*, consider this goal:

The client will not sustain an injury.

Indicators

• Identify factors that increase risk of injury.
• Describe appropriate safety measures.

If it is realistic for your client to achieve all the goals on the day of your care, you should add the date to all of them. If your client is confused, you can add the date to the main goal, but you would delete all the indicators because the client is confused. Or you could modify the goal by writing:

Family member will identify factors that increase the client's risk of injury.

Author's note: Consult with clinical faculty to assure this is acceptable.

Step 7: Prepare the Care Plan (Written or Printed)

You can prepare the care plan by:

• Typing a care plan from this book into your word processor then deleting or adding specifics for your client (use another color for additions/deletions)
• Photocopying a care plan from this book then adding or deleting specifics for your client
• Writing the care plan

Author's note: Ask your faculty person what options are acceptable. Using different colors or fonts allows him or her to clearly see your analysis. Be prepared to provide rationales for why you added or deleted items.

Step 8: Initial Care Plan Completed

Now that you have a care plan of the collaborative problems and nursing diagnoses, which are associated with the primary condition for which your client was admitted? If your assigned client is a healthy adult undergoing surgery or was admitted for an acute medical problem and you have not assessed any significant risk factors in Step 1, you have completed the initial care plan. Go to Step 10.

Step 9: Additional Risk Factors

If your client has risk factors (on the index card) that you identified in Steps 1 and 2, evaluate if these risk factors make your assigned client more vulnerable to develop a problem. The following questions can help to determine if the client or family has additional diagnoses that need nursing interventions:

• Are additional collaborative problems associated with coexisting medical conditions that require monitoring (e.g., hypoglycemia)?
• Are there additional nursing diagnoses that, if not managed or prevented now, will deter recovery or affect the client's functional status (e.g., High Risk for Constipation)?
• What problems does the client perceive as priority?
• What nursing diagnoses are important but treatment for them can be delayed without compromising functional status?

You can address nursing diagnoses not on the priority list by referring the client for assistance after discharge (e.g., counseling, weight loss program).

Author's note: Priority identification is a very important but difficult concept. Because of shortened hospital stays and because many clients have several chronic diseases at once, nurses cannot address all nursing diagnoses for every client. Nurses must focus on those for which the client would be harmed or not make progress if they were not addressed. Ask your clinical faculty to review your list. Be prepared to provide rationales for your selections.

Step 10: Evaluate the Status of Your Client (After You Provide Care)

Collaborative Problems

Review the nursing goals for the collaborative problems:

- Assess the client's status.
- Compare the data to established norms (indicators).
- Judge if the data fall within acceptable ranges.
- Conclude if the client is stable, improved, unimproved, or worse.

Is your client stable or improved?

- If yes, continue to monitor the client and to provide interventions indicated.
- If not, has there been a dramatic change (e.g., elevated blood pressure, decreased urinary output)? Have you notified the physician or advanced practice nurse? Have you increased your monitoring of the client?

Communicate your evaluations of the status of collaborative problems to your clinical faculty and to the nurse assigned to your client.

Nursing Diagnosis

Review the goals or outcome criteria for each nursing diagnosis. Did the client demonstrate or state the activity defined in the goal? If yes, then communicate (document) the achievement on your plan. If not and the client needs more time, change the target date. If time is not the issue, evaluate why the client did not achieve the goal. Was the goal:

- Not realistic because of other priorities
- Not acceptable to the client

Author's note: Ask your clinical faculty where to document evaluation of goal achievement.

Step 11: Document the Care on the Agency's Forms, Flow Records, and Progress Notes

Author's note: Ask your clinical faculty person where you should document the client evaluation after you have provided care.

4 THE ILL ADULT: ISSUES AND RESPONSES

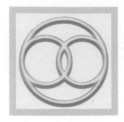

Illness, trauma, hospitalization, diagnostic studies, and treatments can precipitate various client responses. Depending on the situation, the client's individual personality, and other factors, these responses may include:

- Fear
- Anxiety
- Anger
- Denial
- Grief
- Apathy
- Confusion
- Hopelessness
- Loss of control

The nurse, as the primary presence 24 hours a day, and as the practitioner of the science and art of nursing, represents the optimal health care provider for an ill client and his or her support persons (family members or significant others).

According to Henderson and Nite (1960), "Nursing is primarily assisting individuals (sick or well) with those activities contributing to health or its recovery (or to a peaceful death) that they perform unaided when they have the necessary strength, will, or knowledge." Nursing also helps clients carry out prescribed therapy and become independent of assistance as soon as possible (Henderson & Nite, 1960).

Stress and Adaptation

According to Hoskins (2000), "Stress is a state produced by a change in the environment that is perceived as challenging, threatening or damaging to the person's dynamic equilibrium." Lazarus and Folkman (1980) have developed a theory of stress that focuses on the interaction or transaction between the person and the external environment. Lazarus and Monat (1977) describe coping as the psychological and behavioral activities done to master, tolerate, or minimize external or internal demands and conflicts. According to Miller (1999), individuals "who have a rigid set or narrow range of coping skills are at more risk for impaired coping because different types of coping strategies are effective in different situations."

Every person has a concept of self that encompasses feelings about self-worth, attractiveness, lovability, and capabilities. Everyone also has implicit or explicit goals. Illness, other disruptions to health, and associated treatments can negatively affect a person's self-concept and ability to achieve goals. These negative effects are losses, which precipitate grieving. The extent of a person's grief response is directly related to the extent of interference in goal-directed activity and the significance of the goal.

Coping Strategies

Adaptive and effective coping strategies produce these results (Visotsky, 1961):

- Distress is kept at or returned to a manageable level.
- Hope is maintained or renewed.
- Positive self-esteem is maintained or restored.
- Cooperative relationships are maintained.

Cohen and Lazarus (1983) have described five modes of coping:

- Information-seeking
- Direct action
- Inhibition of actions

- Intrapsychic processes
- Turning to others for support.

Table 4.1 presents examples of these five modes.

Information-Seeking

A person attempting to cope with a disturbing or unfamiliar situation often seeks out knowledge to help in managing the situation. Many nurses assume that a client always needs to know as much information as possible about his or her condition and treatments. In reality, according to Burckhardt (1987), "sometimes little attention is paid to whether the client is seeking information and, if so, what information is most valuable." Burckhardt goes on to state that some clients may need to be allowed *not* to acquire information. However, if a client's lack of information for self-care is seen as detrimental, the nurse must continue to supervise the client or initiate a referral so that the client can be supervised.

In today's health care delivery system, interaction time between nurses and clients has been reduced as a direct result of shorter hospital stays. To facilitate the coping strategy of information-seeking despite decreased interaction time, the nurse can provide the client and family with opportunities to acquire information in the following ways:

- By creating and distributing printed material
- By developing audio or visual programs
- By providing information on community groups or commercial products that provide relevant information
- By directing them to call the unit with questions

Direct Action

This coping strategy incorporates any change or effort (except cognitive) that a person does to manage a situation. For example, having an ample supply of work- or leisure-related items when traveling by air or waiting for an appointment can help to reduce the frustration associated with delays. Initiation of a regular exercise program is another example of direct action.

Inhibition of Action

Effective coping commonly requires avoiding or limiting certain situations or actions that are problematic or triggers for injury. This strategy can sometimes cause problems. A person has to weigh the advantages and

TABLE 4.1 Emotion-Focused Behaviors Versus Problem-Focused Behaviors

	Description	Advantages/Disadvantages
Emotion-Focused Behaviors		
Intrapsychic processes		
Minimization	Reduces the seriousness of the event or problem	Provides time for appraisal and adjustment
Projection, displacement, suppression of anger	Directs anger to a less threatening person or object	Suppressed anger may increase stress
Anticipatory preparation	Rehearsal of possible consequences of behavior in stressful situations	Provides opportunity to prepare for worst; becomes dysfunctional when it produces unmanageable stress
Attribution	Finds personal meaning in the problem situation (e.g., religious faith)	Offers consolation, becomes dysfunctional when self-responsibility is lost
Problem-Focused Behaviors		
Goal setting	Setting time limitations on behaviors	May increase stress if unrealistic
Information-seeking	Learning all about the problem	Reinforces self-control
Direct action or mastery	Learning new skills	Facilitates self-esteem by providing control
Help-seeking	Sharing feelings with others for support	Provides an emotional release and comfort; if excessive, may alienate others
Inhibition of action	Eliminating an action	May increase stress if action is valued

disadvantages of each action. In some cases, coping that protects or enhances physical health but compromises self-esteem can have more detrimental effects. For example, a person with Parkinson's disease may be safer using a wheelchair rather than a walker; however, if embarrassment and loss of control result from wheelchair use, the outcome may be decreased mobility and social isolation. As another example, a recovering alcoholic may have to change his usual "Friday night out with the boys, drinking."

Sometimes, well-intentioned family members may inhibit the actions of the ill person without evaluating the other losses that coexist with the loss of these actions. For example, prohibiting an elderly woman from continuing to host Thanksgiving dinner may damage her self-esteem and reduce her perception of her purpose in life. Instead, it may be more constructive to allow her to supervise the meal preparation.

Intrapsychic Processes

The coping strategies involved in intrapsychic processes represent attempts to manage a stressful situation through the cognitive activities of defense mechanism, such as denial, avoidance, or rationalization; or of stress reduction strategies such as thought-stopping or relaxation.

These coping activities provide the person with much-needed control over the emotions of fear and anxiety. Although some health care professionals view defense mechanisms as pathologic, in most cases these mechanisms are actually constructive. If, however, the person does not use any other coping strategy (i.e., information-seeking, direct action, or support-seeking), then defense mechanisms may produce unsatisfactory or destructive outcomes. If a person delays dealing with a situation or retreats, this may be seen as maladaptive when actually it may give the person a reprieve for internal readjustment.

For example, anger is often perceived as negative. Anger can, however, energize behavior, assist with expression of negative feelings, and help the person to defend against a threat. The nurse must proceed cautiously when determining how much time a client or family needs for internal readjustment. Reduced lengths of stay often propel nurses to push clients faster than their coping abilities can adapt. Again, it may be more constructive to provide clients and families with community resources that they can contact after internal readjustment has been achieved.

Turning to Others

This coping response involves a client's social network and social support. *Social network* is defined as the structural interrelationship of the client's family, friends, neighbors, coworkers, and others who provide support; *social support* is the psychological and tangible aid provided by the social network. House (1981) has defined four basic types of social support:

- Emotional (communicates concern and trust, listens)
- Appraisal (communicates respect and self-worth)
- Informational (communicates information for problem-solving)
- Instrumental (provides tangible assistance [e.g., money, food] help with chores)

The nurse assesses and evaluates the client's perception that he or she received enough support, and the extent to which the client can return support to others—a quality known as *reciprocity*. Reciprocity is crucial to balanced, healthy relationships. According to Tilden and Weinert (1987), "ill persons, unlike healthy people, who can terminate relationships that fail to satisfy their needs, often are locked into unsatisfactory relationships." In an ill client, impaired ability to reciprocate often leads to feelings of depression, dependency, and low self-esteem. Moreover, caregiver burnout can result from "one-way giving," particularly when caring for a chronically ill person (Tilden & Weinert, 1987). The nurse may be able to help a client identify effective ways of reciprocating. For example, an ill client may not be able to cook but can offer to peel or chop vegetables.

Coping With Chronic Illness

Chronic illness is the number one health problem in the United States. More than 30 million Americans have chronic disabilities, and over 15 million have limited ability for independent self-care. In American culture, the ability to be productive is a highly-valued trait. Vitality, productivity, and success often are linked; thus chronic illness assaults a person's core values.

According to Burckhardt (1987), "persons with chronic illness face permanent changes in life style, threats to dignity and self-esteem, disruption of normal life-transitions, and decreasing resources." The nurse must assist an ill client's family in recognizing and agreeing on how chronic illness has affected the family system and its individual members. Open dialogue about the influences of the chronic illness may help to preserve family relationships. Failure to acknowledge the effects and changes likely will lead to destruction and dissolution of the family system.

Social supports can buffer stress and reduce adverse health effects (Broadhead, Kaplan, & James, 1983). Unfortunately, chronic illness can negatively influence social supports and networks.

As discussed earlier, chronic illness presents a unique and often frustrating challenge for clients, support networks, and health care professionals. Responses to the losses associated with the experience of illness and its aftermath can include denial, anger, fear, anxiety, guilt, and sadness.

Denial

To cope with a difficult situation, sometimes a person disavows or minimizes the seriousness of the situation and the feelings connected to it. In many cases, denial is a useful and healthy way to deal with a problematic situation, because it provides the time needed to regain and maintain emotional equilibrium. However, denial can be harmful if it leads to detrimental outcomes (e.g., refusal of appropriate treatment for depression, continued abuse of alcohol).

Anger

Anger can be an appropriate response to an unacceptable situation. Unfortunately, direct expressions of anger are usually considered inappropriate and commonly evoke feelings of guilt afterward. But a person who habitually suppresses angry feelings cultivates hostility. *As a result of the person's inability or unwillingness to express anger, conflicts remain unresolved; unresolved conflicts can lead to depression.*

Nurses, like others, typically are uncomfortable with clients' expressions of anger. However, anger may be a productive response for a client in a vulnerable position. A person typically expresses anger to those he or she deems least likely to retaliate or to be least important; thus, nurses are often the target of the anger of clients or their families (just as nurses may use peers or family as targets for their anger at hospital administration or the "system"). A nurse may deal with an angry client by avoiding him or her. In most persons, this avoidance is commonly seen as a benign response; for a nurse, however, avoidance is a malignant response, because it results in reducing or withholding nursing care.

To deal effectively with an angry client, the nurse must first examine her or his own feelings about and responses to angry behavior. Did the nurse witness anger as a child? Was she or he allowed to express anger as a child? Next, the nurse should examine the client's or family's anger by asking her- or himself these questions:

• What could be the source(s) of the anger? Loss of control? Fear? Embarrassment?
• Is this the client's or family's usual response to stress?
• Is the anger serving a useful purpose?

When intervening with an angry client, the nurse may find it productive to give the client a direct message that he or she has a right to be angry (if appropriate), but that screaming, verbal abuse, obscene language, and physical violence are not acceptable. Helping a client express anger without alienation is a difficult but productive strategy. Communicating the message that "if I were in your position or situation, I would be angry too; however, screaming at me will not reduce your anger or contribute to finding satisfying options" validates that the client has a right to feel anger but not to express it in a hurtful manner.

Anxiety

Anxiety is a state in which a person experiences feelings of uneasiness or apprehension and activation of the autonomic nervous system in response to a vague, nonspecific threat. Anxiety differs from fear in that an anxious person cannot identify the threat, whereas a fearful person can. Anxiety can occur without fear; however, fear usually does not occur without anxiety (Carpenito-Moyet, 2004).

Feelings of uneasiness, dread, and inadequacy accompany anxiety. The response to a threat may range from mild anxiety to panic. The four degrees of anxiety—mild, moderate, severe, and panic—are differentiated in Box 4.1. Mild anxiety has been described as normal anxiety, moderate anxiety as chronic anxiety, and severe anxiety as acute anxiety. Mild anxiety is necessary for a person to function and respond effectively to the environment and events.

BOX 4.1 TYPES OF ANXIETY

Mild Anxiety
• Heightened perception and attention; alertness
• Ability to deal with problems
• Ability to integrate past, present, and future experiences
• Sleeplessness

Moderate Anxiety
• Slightly narrowed perception; selective inattention that can be directed
• Slight difficulty concentrating; learning requires more effort
• Voice/pitch changes, tremors, shakiness
• Increased respiratory and heart rates

Severe Anxiety
• Distorted perception; focus on scattered details; inability to attend to more even when instructed
• Severely impaired learning; high distractibility and inability to concentrate
• Hyperventilation, tachycardia, headache, dizziness, nausea
• Complete self-absorption

Panic
• Irrational reasoning; focuses on blown-up detail
• Inability to learn
• Inability to function; usually increased motor activity or unpredictable responses to minor stimuli; communication not understandable
• Feelings of impending doom (dyspnea, dizziness/faintness, palpitations, trembling, choking, paresthesia, hot/cold flashes, sweating)

(Carpenito-Moyet, L. J. [2008]. *Nursing diagnosis: Application to clinical practice* [12th ed.]. Philadelphia: Lippincott Williams & Wilkins)

Management of Therapeutic Regimen

Successful management of the therapeutic regimen requires a person to initiate one or more activities or life style changes (Bandura, 1982). These activities can be as simple as blood pressure monitoring or as complex as home dialysis. Activities or life style changes treat, prevent, or monitor problems. Box 4.2 illustrates examples of activities for each of the three types.

Bandura (1982) described self-efficacy theory as an individual's evaluation of his or her capabilities to manage stressful situations or to change behaviors to manage the situation. Successful management depends on outcome expectancy and self-efficacy expectancy. Outcome expectancy is the belief that a behavior change will improve the situation. Self-efficacy is the belief that one can make the behavior change (Bandura, 1982).

Individuals with a history of coping successfully in a similar situation have higher self-efficacy than those who were unsuccessful. In addition to a history of successful coping, three other factors that promote positive self-efficacy are:

• Witnessing others successfully coping
• Others believing that the individual can successfully cope or manage
• Not experiencing high autonomic arousal in response to the situation

BOX 4.2 EXAMPLES OF ACTIVITIES TO MANAGE THERAPEUTIC REGIMEN

Treatment	Preventive	Monitoring
Wound care	Balanced diet	Blood pressure
Medications	Exercise program	Foot assessment
Range-of-motion exercises	Dental hygiene	Urine testing
Low-salt diet		

BOX 4.3 INTERVENTIONS TO PROMOTE POSITIVE SELF-EFFICACY

1. Explore with client(s) past successful management of problems.
2. Emphasize past successful coping.
3. Tell stories of other "successes."
4. If appropriate, encourage opportunities to witness others successfully coping in a similar situation.
5. Encourage participation in self-help groups.
6. If high autonomic response (e.g., rapid pulse, diaphoresis) is reducing feeling of confidence, teach short-term anxiety interrupters (Grainger, 1990).
   a. Look up.
   b. Control breathing.
   c. Lower shoulders.
   d. Slow thoughts.
   e. Alter voice.
   f. Give self directions (out loud if possible).
   g. Exercise.
   h. "Scruff your face"—change facial expression.
   i. Change perspective: imagine watching the situation from a distance.

(Carpenito-Moyet, L. J. [2008]. *Nursing diagnosis: Application to clinical practice* [12th ed.]. Philadelphia: Lippincott Williams & Wilkins)

Addressing the preceding three factors, nurses can initiate related interventions to promote positive self-efficacy. Box 4.3 illustrates interventions to promote positive self-efficacy.

Summary

Like other stressors that affect lives and life events, illness, trauma, and hospitalization have the potential to leave the involved parties (clients and families or significant others) disorganized and devastated. However, they may also provide an opportunity for increased growth and cohesiveness. The nurse can be instrumental in directing clients and families to paths of mutual support and individual autonomy.

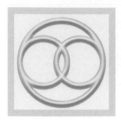

5 RESPONSE TO THE SURGICAL EXPERIENCE

A planned trauma, surgery evokes a range of physiologic and psychologic responses in a client that are based on personal and unique past experiences, coping patterns, strengths, and limitations. Most clients and their families view any surgery, regardless of its complexity, as a major event, and they react with some degree of anxiety and fear.

Perioperative nursing *is the term used to describe the nursing responsibilities associated with the preoperative, intraoperative, postanesthesia recovery, and postoperative surgical phases.* Throughout the perioperative period, the nurse applies the nursing process to identify the client's positive functioning, altered functioning, and potential for altered functioning. The nursing responsibilities for each phase focus on specific actual or potential health problems.

Preoperative Assessment

The nursing history and physical assessment of a preoperative client focus on present status and the potential for complications. Because all clients receive a nursing assessment on admission, these criteria can be integrated into the general nursing interview (see Figure 2.1, Nursing Admission Database).

In addition to the general data collected on admission, the nurse caring for a client in any phase of the perioperative period completes focus assessments—acquisition of selected or specific data as determined by the nurse and the client or family, or as directed by the client's condition. The nurse who assesses a new postoperative client's condition (e.g., vital signs, incision, hydration, comfort) is performing a focus assessment. Preoperative focus assessments involve evaluating certain factors that can influence the client's risk for intraoperative or postoperative complications:

- Client's understanding of events, ability to communicate
- Alcohol use, substance abuse
- Acute or chronic conditions
- Latex allergy
- Client's previous surgical experience
- Nutritional status
- Fluid and electrolyte status
- Risk for infection (e.g., obesity, compromised immune system)
- Emotional status

Communication, Cognitive, Mobility Status

Preoperatively, the nurse must assess the client's ability to process information and to communicate questions and needs. Assessment of preoperative mobility or communication limitations can help the nurse determine if specific strategies are needed intraoperatively.

Understanding Events

The surgeon is responsible for explaining the nature of the operation, any alternative options, the expected results, and the possible complications. The surgeon obtains two consents—one for the procedure and another for the anesthesia. The nurse is responsible for determining the client's understanding of the information and notifying the surgeon if more information is needed for a valid informed consent.

Acute or Chronic Condition

To compensate for the effects of surgical trauma and anesthesia, the human body needs optimal respiratory, circulatory, cardiac, renal, hepatic, and hematopoietic functions. Any condition that interferes with any of these systems' functions (e.g., diabetes mellitus, congestive heart failure, chronic obstructive pulmonary disease, anemia, cirrhosis, renal failure, lupus erythematosus, substance abuse [alcohol or drugs]) compromises recovery. In addition to preexisting medical conditions, advanced age, obesity, and alcohol abuse also make a client more vulnerable to complications, as outlined in Table 5.1.

TABLE 5.1 Intraoperative and Postoperative Implications of Preexisting Compromised Functions

Condition	Associated Compromised Functions	Intraoperative Implications	Postoperative Implications
Advanced age	↑ Arterial thickening	Cardiac failure———————————→	
	↑ Peripheral resistance————————————————→		Thrombosis
	↓ Ability to increase cardiac output	Hypotension/shock———————————→	
	↓ Lung capacity	Hypoxia	Pneumonia, atelectasis
	↑ Residual volume	Electrolyte imbalances———————→	
	↓ Cough reflex———————————————————→		Respiratory infection
	↓ Renal blood flow	Shock	
	↓ Glomerular filtration	Impaired ability to excrete anesthetics———→	
	Enlarged prostate———————————————————→		Urinary retention
	↓ Gastric motility———————————————————→		Paralytic ileus, constipation
	↑ Bone resorption	Fractures———————————————→	
	Impaired ability to regulate temperature	Hypothermia	Hypo/hyperthermia
	↓ Sound transmission	Difficulty hearing———————————→	
	↓ Lens elasticity———————————————————→		Risk for falls
	↓ Hepatic function	↓ Excretion of medications = ↑ toxicity	Impaired protein synthesis ↓ phagocytosis
Obesity	Excess of adipose tissue (vascularity)	Larger incision	Delayed healing
		Prolonged anesthesia time	Dehiscence/evisceration
	Impaired mobility	↑ Risk of injury	Thrombosis
	↓ Efficiency of respiratory muscles	Hypoventilation	Respiratory infection
	↓ Gastric emptying time———————————————→		Aspiration, pneumonia
Alcoholism	↓ Hepatic function	↓ Excretion of medications = ↑ toxicity	Malnourishment
	↓ Phagocytosis→		Delayed healing
	Impaired protein synthesis	Cross-tolerance to anesthetics	Cross-tolerance to analgesics
	↓ Adrenocortical response———————————————→		Withdrawal symptoms

Latex Allergy

The increased incidence of latex allergies from 1988 to 1992 and the report of 1000 systematic allergic reactions to latex, with 15 deaths, necessitates identification of persons at high risk. Box 5.1 outlines the assessment. *High-risk individuals should be placed under latex precaution protocol (e.g., latex-free vials, syringes, gloves, ID bracelets, etc.).*

Previous Surgical Experience

The nurse must ask the client and family specific questions regarding past surgical experiences. The information obtained is used to promote comfort (physical and psychologic) and to prevent serious complications.

To detect a possible predisposition to malignant hyperthermia, the nurse should ask, "Has a doctor or a nurse ever mentioned to you or a family member that you had difficulty with anesthesia—excessive somnolence, vomiting, allergic reaction, or hyperthermia?" and "Has a family member experienced difficulty with anesthesia?" Malignant hyperthermia—a life-threatening syndrome occurring during surgery—predominantly in apparently healthy children and young adults—is associated with a hereditary predisposition and the use of muscle relaxants and inhalation anesthetics. Incidence was previously 80%, but now has been reduced to 10%.

Nutritional Status

The client's preoperative nutritional status directly influences his or her response to surgical trauma and anesthesia. After any major wound from either trauma or surgery, the body must build and repair tissue and protect itself from infection. To facilitate these processes, the client must increase protein–carbohydrate intake sufficiently to prevent negative nitrogen balance, hypoalbuminemia, and weight loss. Malnourished

> ## BOX 5.1   CASE FINDING: HIGH-RISK INDIVIDUAL FOR LATEX SENSITIVITY
>
> ### Allergic History
> Asthma, eczema, hay fever, food allergy (especially banana, avocado, potato, and tomato)
>
> ### Surgical History
> Multiple surgeries, multiple urinary catheterizations, urticaria, angioedema or respiratory distress during surgery, reactions during dental or radiological procedures
>
> ### Occupational History
> Latex exposure, work-related symptoms of cutaneous dermatitis, eczema, and urticaria, upper respiratory symptoms, rhinorrhea, pruritus, sneezing, or lower respiratory symptoms, cough, wheezing, shortness of breath
>
> Local or systemic symptoms with the use of household gloves, balloons, condoms, diaphragms, or touching poinsettia plants
>
> Gender—75% are female

(From Jackson, D. [1995], Latex allergy and anaphylaxis: What to do. *Journal of Intravenous Nursing*, 18; 33–52; and Williams, G. D. C. [1997]. Preoperative assessment and health history interview, *Nursing Clinics of North America; 32*[2]; 395–416.)

states result from inadequate intake, compromised metabolic function, or increased metabolic demands. Healthy clients can tolerate short periods of negative nitrogen balance postoperatively, but clients who are malnourished before surgery are at high risk for infections, sepsis, and evisceration (Summer & Ebbert, 1992). Preoperatively the nurse should identify those clients who are malnourished and those who are at higher risk for postoperative nutritional compromise. The nurse can then consult with the nutritionist and the physician for preoperative treatment to correct nutritional deficits.

Fluid and Electrolyte Status

A client with a fluid and electrolyte imbalance is prone to complications of shock, hypotension, hypoxia, and dysrhythmias, both intraoperatively and postoperatively. Fluid volume fluctuations result from decreased fluid intake or abnormal fluid loss, both of which occur in surgical trauma. Adults with no preexisting fluid and electrolyte problem usually can compensate for the losses associated with surgery. However, clients of advanced age and those with cirrhosis, cancer, chronic obstructive pulmonary disease, diabetes mellitus, renal disorders, adrenal or thyroid dysfunction, cardiovascular disorders, or those on corticosteroid therapy may be unable to compensate.

Infection Risk

Skin is the first line of defense in the prevention of infection. Because surgery reduces this defense, all surgical clients are theoretically at risk for infections. Routine nursing interventions prevent contamination of the wound and, if healthy, the client's defenses will prevent infection. Any factor that delays healing will increase the risk for infection. The following factors have been identified as contributing to delayed wound healing: malnourishment, diabetes mellitus, fever, dry wound surface, steroids, anemia, radiation, and chemotherapy. Nursing interventions focus on factors that can be improved, such as nutritional status, glucose control, hydration, and smoking reduction (temporary).

Emotional Status

A client's, family's, and significant other's responses to anticipated surgery depend on:

- Past experiences
- Usual coping strategies
- Significance of the surgery
- Support system (quality and availability)

Most clients anticipating surgery experience anxiety and fear. The uncertainties of surgery produce anxiety; anticipated pain, incisions, and immobility can produce fear. Anxiety has been classified as mild, moderate, severe, and panic (see Box 4.1 for more information).

Anxiety can be differentiated into *state anxiety* and *trait anxiety*. *State anxiety* is the response to a stressful situation; *trait anxiety* refers to the variable interpretations persons make of threatening situations. It is expected that clients and their families would have state anxiety. To help assuage this anxiety, the nurse should explore with the client and family their fears and concerns. Besides identifying sources of anxiety, the nurse should also assess possible avenues of support or comfort by asking questions such as "What would provide you with more comfort before surgery?" and "What do you usually do when you are under stress?"

Moderate anxiety is expected before surgery. Usually clients with moderate anxiety are willing to share their concerns. *Clients who demonstrate panic anxiety or verbalize that they will die in the operating room present a serious situation clinically. When faced with such a client, the nurse should consult with the physician, who may want to consider postponing surgery.*

A client who is suffering tends to respond positively to a nurse who accepts his or her response. For example, explaining that fear before surgery is normal to a client experiencing fear usually is comforting; sharing with a grieving family that you understand their loss does not eliminate the loss but does convey support. The ability to communicate effectively does not come automatically; it is a planned and learned art involving practice and caring.

Preoperative Nursing Record

Figure 5.1 presents a preoperative assessment/care plan that the nurse completes before surgery or, if this is not possible, on the morning of surgery. This form can also be used in a same-day surgical setting. This record helps the nurse to collect essential preoperative data. Section I outlines specific areas concerning medical and surgical history, informed consent, and laboratory or diagnostic studies. Section II is a combination of assessment and plan of care. Content areas relating to present status and risk factors are specified in the left-hand column. If the data indicate no anticipated problems or identify no specific risk factors, they are recorded in the assessment column only. If the data present a problem or a risk factor for a potential problem, they are recorded under the diagnosis/plan column and the diagnostic statement is checked, as are the contributing or risk factors. If the nurse has identified additional contributing or risk factors, they can be written in. The diagnoses identified on this form are both nursing diagnoses and collaborative problems.

Each nursing diagnosis or collaborative problem identified has corresponding standards of care that specifically direct the nurse to reduce or eliminate, monitor, or report the problem. These standards of care are in addition to the generic standards of care that have been identified by the American Association of Operating Room Nurses. Under this standard, the only documentation required is if an unusual response is observed (item 13).

Policies that require nurses to copy from standards of care further reduce nurse–client interaction time. Copy from a printed sheet does not produce an individualized plan; rather, it would be more prudent to require that only specific interactions be handwritten. Space is provided on the assessment form under each diagnosis so the nurse can add any additional interventions beyond the standard when indicated. Figure 5.2 illustrates some additional interventions added for a client by the nurse prior to surgery. Any additional interventions provided by the nurse but not identified preoperatively should be recorded on the progress or nurse's notes, not on the care plan. Remember that a care plan is written only if another nurse will be responsible for providing the care; a nurse should not write a care plan just for her- or himself to follow.

If the nurse has not identified any specific diagnoses, she or he places a checkmark before this statement at the end of the form:

Problems requiring addendum nursing interventions are not present at this time. Follow standard of care for perioperative nursing care.

The nurse completing the preoperative section then signs in the space indicated. When a nurse cannot visit all postoperative clients, she or he should select certain clients according to preoperative assessment findings, with clients having problems or risk factors validated before surgery receiving top priority. During the postoperative visit, the nurse assesses whether the interventions provided have prevented or reduced the problems.

The Postanesthesia Recovery Period

Surgical trauma and anesthesia disrupt all major body system functions, but most clients have the compensatory capability to restore homeostasis. However, certain clients are at greater risk for ineffective compensation for the adverse effects of surgery and anesthesia on cardiac, circulatory, respiratory, and other functions. During the immediate postoperative period, a client is extremely vulnerable to physiologic complications resulting from the effects of

Section I Peroperative Phase

Date _____

Diagnosis _____
_____

Surgeon _____
Procedure scheduled and date_____
Age_____ Weight _____ Height _____
I.D. Band on   Yes_____ No_____
H & P done   Yes_____ No_____
Medical clearance   Yes_____ No_____
Pre-op instruction done   Bedside_____ Group_____
Consent signed
    Scheduled procedure   Yes_____ No_____
    Blood   Yes_____ No_____
    Other   Yes_____ No_____
    (specify)_____
    _____ Chart incomplete   _____Patient not available for visit

Lab/Diagnostic Studies

	Normal	Abnormal	No Results	Not Ordered
Hct				
HgB				
K				
Na				
PT/PTT				
Calcium				
RPR				
HIV				
Cultures				
Glucose				
Chest X-ray				
EKG				
Type and cross units				
Urinalysis				
Other				

Medical Problems and Surgical History

Previous surgical experience?   Yes_____ No_____
    Specify:_____
Past problems with anesthesia?   Individual   Yes_____No_____Unknown_____
                      Family   Yes_____ No_____ Unknown_____
Existing medical problems: (check)
_____Diabetes   _____Cardiac disease   _____Arthritis
_____Hypertension   _____Cancer   _____Respiratory
_____Hematologic   _____Hepatic   _____AIDS
_____Seizures   _____CVA   _____Renal
_____Other _____

Section II Peroperative Nursing Record

ASSESSMENT	DIAGNOSIS/PLAN
I. Ability to Communicate Verbal ☐ Appropriate Language spoken ☐ English ☐ Spanish ☐ Other (specify)_____ Hearing ☐ Appropriate	Impaired Verbal Communication related to ☐ Inability to speak secondary to (specify)_____ ☐ Inability to communicate in English Impaired communication related to ☐ Deafness ☐ Impaired hearing ☐ Diminished level of consciousness

FIGURE 5.1
Preoperative nursing
assessment/care plan.

anesthetics on respiratory and circulatory function. Throughout the client's stay in the postanesthesia recovery room (PAR), the nurse should monitor the client at least every 15–20 minutes.

Level I standards of care should include the nursing diagnoses and collaborative problems present in most clients in the PAR. Box 5.2 lists the collaborative problems and nursing diagnoses commonly seen in postsurgical clients in PAR. The nurse should record assessments and usual interventions on the PAR flow record. Unusual data or events will be recorded on the progress note.

Level II standards in the PAR would refer to additional standard care needed after a specific surgery (e.g., mastectomy). Level II standards could also address a single diagnosis. For example, if the preoperative assessment indicates that a client recovering from a hip-pinning operation has a nursing diagnosis of Disturbed Thought Processes related to unknown etiology (as manifested by repetitive questions of "Where am I?" or "Why am I here?"), the PAR nurse would continually need to orient the client to the environment and to the reasons for the hip pain. The standardized care plan for Disturbed Thought Processes would contain the usual nursing interventions. Interventions for specific nursing diagnoses should be recorded, as should the client's status.

ASSESSMENT	DIAGNOSIS/PLAN
II. Risks for Injury	
1. Level of consciousness ☐ Alert	High Risk for Injury related to ☐ Confusion ☐ Drowsiness ☐ Nonresponsive state
2. Weight _____ Height _____ ☐ Within normal limits (WNL) within 15% of ideal wt.	High Risk for Injury: Fall related to ☐ Obesity > 15%
3. Allergies (latex, chemicals, tape, meds) ☐ None reported	☐ Drug allergy (specify) _____
4. Therapeutic devices ☐ None present	☐ IV, Foley, drains, casts (circle or specify)

5. Skin integrity
☐ Prescence of lesions/edema
    ☐ None
    ☐ Deferred
	Impaired Skin Integrity related to
	
	☐ Lesions ☐ Edema
	(specify size and location) _____

☐ Allergies (refer to 3) ☐ None reported	High Risk for Impaired Skin Integrity related to ☐ Allergy to metal, chemicals, cleansers, adhesives, latex (circle or specify) _____
☐ Weight ☐ Within 15% of ideal weight	☐ Cachexia ☐ Obesity
☐ Circulatory status ☐ WNL	Anxiety related to ☐ Lack of understanding of (specify) _____

6. Understanding of surgical experience
☐ Satisfactory
☐ Unable to evaluate
	Anxiety/fear:
	☐ Moderate ⎫
	☐ Severe ⎬ related to impending surgical experience and:
	    ☐ First surgical experience
	    ☐ History of negative surgical experience (own, relative, specify)

7. Emotional status ☐ Anxiety ☐ Mild	☐ Specify _____
8. Risk for hemorrhage ☐ History of hematologic disorder ☐ None reported	Potential Complication: Hemorrhage ☐ History of hematologic disorder (specify) _____
☐ Presence of medications that increase risk ☐ None	☐ Aspirin or NSAID therapy ☐ Anticoagulants ☐ None
9. History of: ☐ Substance use:	Potential Complication: Cardiac, Hepatic, Respiratory, Hemorrhage

☐ Alcohol use
    ☐ None reported
	☐ Alcohol use
	    Drinks day/wk

☐ Smoking
    ☐ None reported
    ☐ <1/2 pk/day
	☐ pk/day

☐ Street drugs ☐ None reported	☐ (Specify)
☐ Anesthesia problems (individual, family) ☐ None reported	Support System ☐ Unavailable ☐ No support system
10. Support system ☐ Available identity: _____ ☐ Can be notified at no. _____	☐ (Specify) ☐ Problems requiring addendum nursing interventions are not present at this time. Follow standard of care for perioperative nursing care.
11. Other problems ☐ None identified	_____RN

FIGURE 5.1 continued.

Figure 5.3 illustrates how the nurse can record nursing diagnoses and collaborative problems that frequently occur in the PAR, and Figure 5.4 presents a nursing record form for documenting the client's status and nursing interventions in the PAR.

Before discharge or transfer from the PAR to the nursing unit, the client must meet preestablished criteria. The criteria used in many PAR discharge protocols include:

- Ability to turn head
- Extubated with clear airway
- Conscious, easily awakened
- Vital signs stable (blood pressure within 20 mm Hg of client's baseline)
- Dry, intact dressing
- Urine output at least 5 mL/kg/h
- Ability to swallow and retain fluids
- Patent, functioning drains, tubes, and intravenous lines
- Anesthesiologist's approval for discharge (Ebbert & Summer, 1992)

Exceptions for these discharge criteria can be made if the transfer is to the intensive care unit or if the surgeon or anesthesiologist has evaluated the client and approved discharge.

ASSESSMENT	DIAGNOSIS/PLAN
I. Ability to Communicate Verbal ☒ Appropriate	Impaired Verbal Communication related to ☐ Inability to speak secondary to (specify) _____ ☐ Inability to communicate in English
Language spoken ☒ English ☐ Spanish ☐ Other (specify) _____	
Hearing ☐ Appropriate	Impaired communication related to ☐ Deafness ☒ Impaired hearing ☐ Diminished level of consciousness *Speak into left ear.* _____
II. Risks for Injury 1. Level of consciousness ☒ Alert	Potential for Injury related to ☐ Confusion ☐ Drowsiness ☐ Nonresponsive state
2. Weight __140__ Height __5'6"__ ☒ Within normal limits (WNL) within 15% of ideal wt.	Potential for Injury: Fall related to ☐ Obesity > 15%
3. Allergies ☒ None reported	☐ Drug allergy (specify) _____
4. Therapeutic devices ☐ None present	☒ ⓘⓥ Foley, drains, casts (circle or specify) _____
5. Skin integrity Presence of lesions/edema ☒ None ☐ Deferred	Impaired Skin Integrity related to ☐ Lesions ☐ Edema (specify size and location) _____
Allergies (refer to 3) ☒ None reported	Potential Impaired Skin Integrity related to ☐ Allergy to metal, chemicals, cleansers, adhesives (circle or specify) _____
Weight ☐ within 15% of ideal weight	☐ Cachexia ☐ Obesity

FIGURE 5.2
Preoperative nursing record.

Same-Day Surgery, Same-Day Admission

In same-day surgery (also known as outpatient or ambulatory surgery), the client is admitted the morning of surgery and discharged when stable later that day to recover at home. In same-day admissions, the client is admitted the morning of surgery and will stay in the hospital and not be discharged the same day. *For this reason, departments of nursing and selected nursing areas must have systems in place to address the nursing process efficiently, even when client contact time is limited. A nurse's accountability for assessment, diagnosis, planning, implementation, and evaluation does not diminish merely because the client is not hospitalized the day before surgery.* As discussed earlier, there are several options available (video, telephone, interview, and group classes). If

---

BOX 5.2 PREDICTIVE COLLABORATIVE PROBLEMS AND NURSING DIAGNOSES FOR POST–GENERAL SURGERY CLIENTS IN THE POSTANESTHESIA RECOVERY ROOM

Collaborative Problems

Potential Complication: Respiratory
Potential Complication: Hypo/hypervolemia
Potential Complication: Hemorrhage
Potential Complication: Cardiac

Nursing Diagnoses

Risk for Aspiration related to somnolence and increased secretions secondary to intubation
Anxiety related to acute pain secondary to surgical trauma to tissue and nerves
Risk for Injury related to somnolence secondary to anesthesia
Risk for Hypothermia related to exposure to cool OR temperature

High Risk for Aspiration related to: □ Anesthesia   □ Surgery
Data: □ Airway in place   □ Uncuffed ET   □ Deflated ET Cuff
Intervention: □ Close observation   □ Removal of airway/ET tube   □ Position on side: □ (L)   □ (R)
Evaluation: □ Pulse oximeter readings   □ ABGs   □ Lung Sounds   □ Chest   RN: _____

PC: Cardiac □ Dysrhythmia   □ COPD/CHF   □ Hyper/Hypotension
Data: □ ECG monitor   □ Swan-Ganz   □ Dyspnea   □ Tachycardia   □ Bradycardia
             □ Hypotension   □ Hypertension   □ Abnormal lung sounds
Intervention: □ Adjust IV rate □ Analgesic given □ HOB → □ Notify MD   □ Trendelenberg
Evaluation: □ BP > 90 systolic □ Stable cardiac rhythm/rate   □ Pre- and post-op SPO$_2$ within 2–3 percentage points
             RN: _____

FIGURE 5.3
Documentation example for postanesthesia care unit. (*Developed by Cecilia A. Cathey, RN, and nursing staff in PACU, St. Cloud Hospital, St. Cloud, Minnesota; reprinted with permission.*)

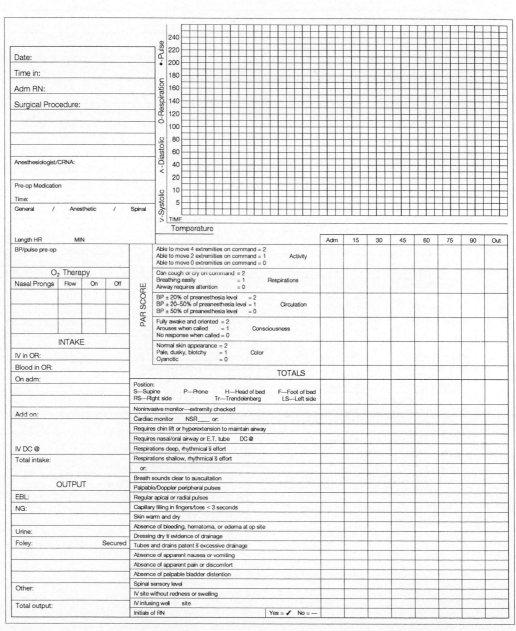

FIGURE 5.4
Sample PAR nursing record.

(continued on page 46)

Initials	Signatures		Time		Initials

Laboratory Reports:

Allergies:

Isolation required: _____ Yes _____ No

Care classification:
I-Requires one RN for
50% of stay (1:2)   II-Requires one RN for
† 50% of stay (1:1)   III-Requires † one RN for
50% of stay (2:1)

☐ Emergency after hours

Anesthesiologist:

Medications

Discharge: Yes = ✓   No = —

Discharge criteria met: _____
Instructed to deep breath/cough: _____
Instructed to stay in bed and call for assistance: _____
Instructed to call for pain/nausea medication: _____
Instructed on food/fluid intake: _____
Appears to understand: _____
Family member/friend present: _____
Special instructions: _____
_____

Side rails up: _____ Bed in low position: _____
Call light within range: _____
Dentures: _____
Vital signs on arrival to unit: _____
_____
Transferred to care of: _____

Time: _____ PACU Nurse: _____
Signature receiving nurse: _____

FIGURE 5.4
continued.

assessment has been conducted by telephone or mail, the nurse must still assess certain areas on the morning of surgery. Figure 5.5 presents a short-stay nursing record. On this record, Section I includes the areas to be assessed before surgery; Section II is designated for postoperative care and status documentation. The nurse should also complete a preoperative diagnosis summary record (Fig. 5.6). This summary record can also be used for clients coming from in-house units. All this information should be communicated to the operating room/PAR staff.

Because another shift will not care for a same-day surgery client, writing an individualized care plan is unnecessary. Instead, care plans in short-stay units can be standardized. Appendix III presents a generic Level I standard of care for same-day surgical clients. The nurse documents delivery of care primarily on a flow record. If the client has additional diagnoses or interventions to address, the nurse records these addendum diagnoses or interventions as a progress note, not as part of a care plan. Discharge planning should be addressed in the standardized care plan under the diagnosis Risk for Ineffective Therapeutic Regimen Management.

Section I: Preoperative

Date: ____________

Time of Arrival on Unit: ____________ A.M. P.M.

Via: ☐ Ambulatory ☐ Wheelchair ☐ Stretcher

Accompanied by: ☐ Member of family ☐ Friend ☐ Unaccompanied

Name and phone number of person driving client home
Name: ____________
Phone no.: ____________
Waiting room: ______ Yes ______ No

Patient Has?

	No	Yes
Hearing aid	☐	☐
Eye glasses	☐	☐
Contact lenses	☐	☐
Artificial eye	☐	☐
Prosthesis	☐	☐
Wig or hair piece	☐	☐

Dentures
None ☐
Partial ☐
Upper ☐
Lower ☐
Denture cup ☐
Removed ☐

Medical Problems and Surgical History

Previous surgical experience? Yes______ No ______
Specify: ____________

Past problems with anesthesia? Individual Yes______ No ______
Family Yes______ No ______

Existing medical problems: (Circle)
____ Diabetes ____ Cardiac disease ____ Arthritis ____ Seizures ____ Pregnancy
____ Hypertension ____ Cancer ____ Respiratory ____ CVA
____ Hematologic ____ Liver ____ AIDS ____ Renal
____ Other ____________

Allergies (tape, chemicals, latex, meds) ____________

☐ No known allergies

Medications (Include time of last dose.) ____________

Vital signs: Temperature ________ Respiration ________
BP ________ Pulse ________ Height ________ Weight ________ Actual/Reported

Diet:
Last solid food ________ A.M. P.M.
Last liquids ________ A.M. P.M.

Skin:

	No	Yes	
Rash	☐	☐	______
Bruises	☐	☐	______
Cuts	☐	☐	______
Scars	☐	☐	______
Lesions	☐	☐	______
Other	☐	☐	______

Abnormal lab work ____ No ____ Yes Called to ____________

Abnormal X-ray results ____ No ____ Yes Called to ____________

Pre-op teaching done ____ Video ____ Printed ____ Bedside
Operative permit signed ____ Yes ____ No
Identification band on ____ Yes ____ No
PAT studies done ____ Yes ____ No
H & P done ____ Yes ____ No

Time	Premedication given	Site	By

FIGURE 5.5
Same-day surgery nursing record.

(continued on page 47)

NOTES:

_____
_____
_____
_____
_____

_____ R.N.
Signature of Admitting Nurse

Section II: Postoperative

Graphic Chart

Name: _____

Time: _____

260													
240													
RESP o 220													
200													
180													
PULSE. 160													
140													
120													
DIAS ^ 100													
80													
60													
SYST v 40													
20													
TEMP													
URINE													
STOOLS													

Date _____ Time _____ A.M. P.M.

Operation _____

Dressings _____

Other _____

Medications given:

Time	Medication	Site	By

Nourishment _____
Amt _____
Tolerated _____ Yes _____ No

Activity tolerated
_____ HOB 60° _____ Time
_____ Dangle _____ Time
_____ OOB chair _____ Time

Section III: Discharge Summary

Discharge Status:

BP _____ Pulse _____ Respiration _____ Temperature _____
IV D/c'd: Time _____ Amt absorbed _____
Voided _____ Yes _____ No
Dressing intact/dry _____ Yes _____ No
Pain tolerable _____ Yes _____ No
Prescriptions given _____ No _____ Yes List: _____
General instruction sheets given _____ Client _____ Other _____
_____ Instruction sheet given _____ Client _____ Other _____
Instructed to call for appointment _____ Yes _____ No
Accompanied by _____ Family _____ Friend _____ Unaccompanied in taxi

Notes: (Unusual events, interactions)

_____
_____
_____
_____

Discharged by _____ R.N.

FIGURE 5.5
continued.

ASSESSMENT	DIAGNOSIS/PLAN
Impaired Communication related to ☐ Deafness ☐ Impaired hearing ☐ Diminished level of consciousness ☐ Inability to speak secondary to (specify) _____ ☐ Inability to communicate in English	Potential Complication: Hemorrhage ☐ History of hematologic disorder (specify) _____ ☐ Aspirin therapy ☐ Anticoagulants ☐ None

High Risk for Infection Transmission related to
☐ HIV positive
☐ Hepatitis: Type _____
☐ Other _____
	Potential Complication: Cardiac, Hepatic, Respiratory, Hemorrhage
	☐ Alcohol use
	   ___ Drinks day/wk
	☐ Smoking
	   ___ pk/day
	☐ Street drugs (specify) _____

High Risk for Injury related to ☐ Confusion ☐ Drowsiness ☐ Nonresponsive state ☐ Obesity > 15% ☐ IV, Foley, drains, casts (circle or specify) _____	Support System ☐ Unavailable ☐ No support system (Specify) _____
Impaired Skin Integrity related to ☐ Lesions ☐ Edema (specify size and location) _____	Allergies ☐ None reported ☐ Unable to determine ☐ List: _____
High Risk for Impaired Skin Integrity related to ☐ Allergy to metal, chemicals, cleansers, adhesives, latex (circle or specify) _____ ☐ Cachexia ☐ Obesity ☐ ↓Circulation secondary to (specify) _____	Other Significant Data/Comments _____ _____ _____ _____ _____ _____ _____
Anxiety related to ☐ Lack of understanding of (specify) _____	

Anxiety/Fear:
☐ Moderate
☐ Severe
  ☐ First surgical experience
  ☐ History of negative surgical experience (own, relative, specify)
  _____
☐ Specify _____
	☐ Problems requiring addendum nursing interventions are not present at
	this time. Follow standard of care for perioperative nursing care.
	
	                                      R.N.

FIGURE 5.6
Preoperative diagnosis summary record.

Summary

Surgery produces both expected and unexpected responses in clients. Through vigilant assessment, the nurse identifies those clients at high risk for complications and those who are responding negatively to the surgical experience.

Because many events occur in a short time span for a surgical client, documentation in the perioperative phases must be concise but specific. The described documentation reflects the use of the nursing process by the nurse preoperatively and postoperatively, with attention to professional standards and efficiency.

6 REDUCING MORAL DISTRESS IN NURSES

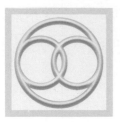

Moral Distress is a new nursing diagnosis approved by NANDA-I in 2006. This newly accepted NANDA-I nursing diagnosis has application in all settings where nurses practice. In its present version it applies only to nurses, not clients or families. The literature to support this diagnosis, when submitted, focused primarily on moral distress in nursing. Box 6.1 presents the New NANDA-I Nursing Diagnosis—Moral Distress.

If moral distress occurs in a client or family, this author suggests a referral to a professional expert in this area (e.g., counselor, therapist, nurse, spiritual advisor). This chapter presents Moral Distress as a Standard of Practice for the Department of Nursing. Strategies are outlined for addressing moral distress for individual unit nurses.

Moral Distress: The Concept

Nurses are in a unique position to advocate for the client and family and assist in decision-making because they are closely integrated with them during care-giving and because they do not benefit financially from treatment decisions. Nurses experience conflicts when attempting to balance authority, responsibility, and duty to the client and family (Corley, Elwisk, Gorman, & Clor, 2001). Often, nurses have more responsibility than authority (Corley et al., 2001). Nurses have to respond to dual authorities—physicians who write client orders and administrators who employ them (Corley et al., 2001). Kramer (1974) found that new graduates reported psychologic disequilibrium, discomfort, and distress when they found that the values they learned in school were difficult, if not impossible, to apply to the real world.

Coping behaviors of nurses with moral distress are conscious and unconscious (Wilkinson, 1987–1988). Unconscious behaviors focus on:

• The immoral actions of others, rather than their own
• The powerful constraints preventing their moral actions
• That their care of the person was not negatively affected

Conscious behaviors were:

• Avoidance of the client
• Leaving the unit, the institution, or nursing altogether

Nurses report constraints to follow one's moral actions as external and internal (Wilkinson, 1987–1988):

• External
  • Physicians
  • Fear of lawsuits
  • Unsupportive nursing administrators, agency administration
  • Policies
• Internal
  • Fear of losing their jobs
  • Self-doubts
  • Futility of past actions
  • Socialization to follow orders
  • Lack of courage

In the United States, fewer than 1 out of every 5 deaths involve hospitalization with the use of the intensive care unit (Angus et al., 2004). The distinction between critical illness and terminal illness is not clear (Elpern, Covert, & Kleinpell, 2005). Dying while receiving aggressive interventions to extend life produces confusion, conflicts, and distress in caregivers, clients, and families (Elpern et al., 2005). In 2001, Corley et al. reported that 15% of the nurses studied related that they had left a job because of moral distress. In 2005, Corley et al. reported this percentage to be greater than 25.5%. Elpern, Covert, and

BOX 6.1 MORAL DISTRESS

Definition

Moral Distress: the state in which an individual experiences psychological disequilibrium, physical discomforts, anxiety and/or anguish that results when a person makes a moral decision but does not follow through with the moral behavior.

Defining Characteristics: Major

Expresses anguish over difficulty acting on one's moral choice

Defining Characteristics: Minor

Feelings of:
- Powerlessness
- Anxiety
- Guilt
- Fear
- Frustration
- Anger
- Avoidance

Related Factors

The following factors do not cause moral distress in every nurse. For example, if a nurse does not support terminating ventilators on a client, then she or he would not experience moral distress if a terminally ill client was kept on a ventilator. Moral Distress results from a nurse not acting on her or his own moral beliefs and then suffering because of her or his inaction.

- End of Life Decisions
  - Related to providing treatments which were perceived as futile for hopelessly ill persons (e.g., blood transfusions, chemotherapy, organ transplants, mechanical ventilation)
  - Related to conflicting attitudes toward advanced directives
  - Related to participation in life-saving actions when they only prolong dying
- Treatment Decisions
  - Related to the client's or family's refusal of treatments deemed appropriate by the health care team
  - Related to inability of the family to make the decision to stop ventilator treatment on a hopelessly ill client
  - Related to a family's wishes to continue life support even though it is not in the best interest of the client
  - Related to performing a procedure that increases the client's suffering
  - Related to providing care that does not relieve the client's suffering
  - Related to conflicts between wanting to disclose poor medical practice and wanting to maintain trust in the physician
- Professional Conflicts
  - Related to insufficient resources for care (e.g., time, staff)
  - Related to failure to be included in the decision-making process
  - Related to more emphasis on technical skills and tasks than on relationships and caring
- Cultural Conflicts
  - Related to health care decisions made for women by male family members
  - Related to cultural conflicts with the American health care system

Kleinpell (2005), using the Moral Distress Scale (Corley et al., 2001), reported the following situations with the highest levels of moral distress:

- Continuing to participate in the care for a hopelessly ill person who is being sustained on a ventilator, when no one will make a decision to "pull the plug."
- Following a family's wishes to continue life support even though it is not in the best interest of the client.
- Initiating extensive life-saving actions when it only prolongs death.
- Following the family's wishes for the client's care when the nurse does not agree with them, but does so because the hospital administration fears a lawsuit.
- Carrying out the physician's orders for unnecessary tests and treatments for terminally ill clients.

• Providing care that does not relieve the client's suffering because the physician fears increasing doses of pain medication will cause death (Elpern et al., 2005, p. 526).

In 2005, Corley et al. reported unsafe staffing as the highest source of moral distress.

Strategies to Prevent Moral Distress

Strategy	Rationale
Explore moral work and action: • Educate yourself about moral distress. (Refer to articles on reference list.) • Share your stories of moral distress. Elicit stories from coworkers. • Read stories of moral action. Refer to Gordon's *Life Support: Three Nurses on the Front Lines* and Kritek's *Reflections on Healing: A Central Construct* on reference list.	Stories can help nurses identify strengths, insights, shared distress, and options for moral actions (Tiedje, 2000). Nurses responded positively when they were asked to discuss their feelings regarding moral issues (Elpern, et al., 2005).
Investigate how morally problematic clinical situations are managed in the institution. If an ethics committee exists, determine its mission and procedures.	Organizational practices that support open discussions of client care issues and problems with ethical and moral implications contribute to perceptions of an ethical climate for clinicians (Olson, 1998).
Do not try to avoid moral distress.	Responding to moral distress is viewed as negative (Hanna, 2004). It can also be viewed "as a life challenge that develops moral character for those who manage it well" (Hanna, 2004, p. 77).
Initiate dialogue with client and family, if possible. Explore their perception of the situation. Pose questions (e.g., What options do you have in this situation?). Elicit feelings about the present situation. Gently explore their end-of-life decisions.	Direct but gentle inquiries and discussions can assist the client/family to examine the situation clearly and the implications of treatment options and decisions.
If indicated, explain "no code" status. Explain the focus of palliative care that replaces aggressive care.	Often, family think that "NO CODE" status means no care. Palliative care focuses on comfort during the dying process.
Dialogue with unit colleagues about the situation that causes you moral distress.	Elpern et al. (2005) found that nurses were relieved that their personal distress was shared and that they were not unique in their feelings.
Enlist a colleague as a coach, or engage as a coach for a coworker.	A coach is a person who can listen, guide, and provide feedback throughout the process (Tiedje, 2000).
Initially, start your approach to address low-risk, morally unsatisfactory clinical situations and evaluate the risks before taking action. Be realistic.	Moral action takes courage. Risk-taking is a skill that can be learned.
Engage in open communication with other involved professional colleagues. Start your conversation with your concern; for example, "I am not comfortable with . . . ," "The family is asking/questioning/feeling . . . ," "Mr. . . . is asking/questioning/feeling . . ."	Each professional has rights and duties and conflict may be resolved through open communication, sharing of feelings and values (Caswell, 1993). Non-threatening language can reduce embarrassment and blaming.
Dialogue with other professionals (e.g., chaplain, manager, social worker, ethics committee).	Nurses can be assisted in moral work with support from others in the organization.
Incorporate health promotion and stress reduction in your life style.	Healthy life styles can reduce stress and increase energy levels for moral work.

Summary

Moral Distress in nursing affects not just the nurse but also the individual and the loved ones they care for. Protecting dignity is acknowledgement of humanity in people alive or deceased, rather than treating them as objects or allowing others to bypass their humanity because of their agendas (Haddock, 1996). When people are helpless or unconscious, preserving their dignity is of utmost priority for nurses (Mairis, 1994).

Clinical Nursing
Care Plans

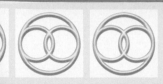

Unit 2 comprises care plans for 77 clinical situations. The 43 care plans in Section 1 focus on persons experiencing medical conditions; the 22 care plans in Section 2 discuss people experiencing surgery; and the 12 care plans in Section 3 address people undergoing diagnostic studies or therapeutic procedures. These care plans represent the nursing diagnoses and collaborative problems known to occur frequently in these clinical situations and to be of major importance. Data collected about a specific client must confirm the diagnosis.

Components of Each Care Plan

Definition

Each care plan begins with a description of the clinical situation. This information highlights certain aspects of the condition or situation or summarizes a knowledge base for the reader.

Time Frame

A client's response to certain situations or conditions can vary depending on when the event occurs in the health–illness continuum. For example, a client with newly diagnosed diabetes mellitus will have different responses from a client with an exacerbation of the same disease. Therefore, each care plan designates a time frame. The focus of the care plans in this book is the initial diagnosis. The nurse can also use the care plan if a client is readmitted for the same condition; however, the nurse will need to reevaluate the client and his or her needs.

Diagnostic Cluster

A diagnostic cluster represents a set of collaborative problems and nursing diagnoses anticipated and of key significance in a selected clinical situation. Clients, of course, can experience many collaborative problems and nursing diagnoses. The diagnostic cluster represents those with high predictability. As discussed previously under the validation project section, this edition contains the results of a multi-site validation project. Nurses were asked to identify which nursing diagnoses and collaborative problems are treated most frequently. These findings are reported in the care plans of the 70 conditions studied. However, the client may have additional nursing diagnoses or collaborative problems not listed in the diagnostic cluster for a given situation. Therefore, these diagnostic clusters serve to assist the nurse in creating the initial care plan. As the nurse interacts with and assesses the client, he or she can add more specific diagnoses, goals, and interventions.

In addition, collaborative problems and nursing diagnoses not detailed in a care plan are listed under the heading "Refer to." These are included in the diagnostic cluster to give the nurse a complete picture of clinical care.

Discharge Criteria

Discharge criteria are the client or family behaviors desired to maintain or to achieve maximum functioning after discharge. The discharge needs of clients and families can necessitate two types of nursing actions: teaching the client and family to manage the situation at home, and referring the client and family to agencies for assistance with continuing care and management at home. The discharge criteria cited in each care plan represent those that a staff nurse can usually achieve with a client or family during a typical length of stay.

Many of the care plans use the nursing diagnosis "High Risk for Ineffective Therapeutic Regimen Management related to insufficient knowledge of _____" or "High Risk for Impaired Home Maintenance related to _____." These two diagnoses apply to a client or family at risk for problems after discharge. The plan of care for these diagnoses aims to prevent them. For these two diagnoses, then, the discharge criteria also represent the goals. In other words, the goals—measurable behaviors that represent a favorable status—are for the client to meet the discharge criteria. Therefore, no goals are cited for these two diagnoses. The nurse is referred instead to the discharge criteria.

Collaborative Problems

Each care plan describes and discusses nursing care for one or more physiologic complications that the nurse jointly treats with medicine. These collaborative problems have both physician- and nursing-prescribed interventions associated with them. The independent nursing interventions consist of monitoring the client for the onset of the complication or for an occurring complication's status. Other independent nursing interventions may include positioning, activity restrictions, etc. Keep in mind that collaborative problems are not physiologic nursing diagnoses. Physiologic nursing diagnoses that nurses independently treat are listed in the care plan as nursing diagnoses, e.g., Impaired Skin Integrity.

You will note that collaborative problems do not have client goals. Client goals are not useful in assisting the nurse to evaluate the effectiveness of nursing interventions for collaborative problems. For example, consider the collaborative problem "Potential Complication: Increased Intracranial Pressure." Appropriate goals might be as follows: The client will be alert and oriented, and the pupils will be equal and react to light accommodation. If the client's sensorium changes and the pupils respond sluggishly to light, will these data accurately evaluate the effectiveness of nursing care? The answer, of course, is no. The data evaluate the client's clinical status, which is the result of many factors.

Goals are used to assist the nurse in evaluating whether to continue, revise, or discontinue the care plan. The goals in the above example clearly do not serve this purpose. They set forth monitoring criteria that the nurse can add to the care plan as established norms for evaluating the client's condition (e.g., normal range for urine output, blood pressure, serum potassium). These are clearly not *client* goals. Certain nursing goals will serve to evaluate the effectiveness of nursing actions for collaborative problems, because nurses are accountable for detecting early changes in physiologic status and managing these episodes. Thus, collaborative problems on the care plans in Unit 2 will have associated *nursing* goals. Refer to Chapter 1 of this book and to Chapter 2 in Carpenito (2003) for a more thorough discussion of collaborative problems.

Related Physician-Prescribed Interventions

This section is provided as reference material. It outlines physician-prescribed interventions for the specific condition or situation. These interventions have established systems for delivery and communication (e.g., physician order forms). Physician-prescribed interventions do not treat nursing diagnoses. Along with nursing-prescribed interventions, they do treat collaborative problems.

Nursing Diagnoses

Each care plan has at least two actual or high-risk nursing diagnoses. Keep in mind that the nurse should have validation for the diagnosis before initiating the care plan. Appropriate major signs and symptoms validate actual nursing diagnoses. Appropriate risk factors validate high-risk nursing diagnoses.

Goals

The goals outlined for each nursing diagnosis consist of measurable behaviors of the client or family that represent a favorable status. Goals are from the Nursing Outcomes Classification (NOC), and interventions from the Nursing Interventions Classification (NIC) developed at the University of Iowa. These have been included for use in electronic systems, if desired. Because a high-risk nursing diagnosis represents a situation that a nurse can prevent, the goals for that diagnosis represent a health status that the nurse will aim to maintain, thereby preventing the situation. The following is an example of a high-risk nursing diagnosis and its corresponding goal:

High Risk for Impaired Skin Integrity related to immobility
Goal: The client will demonstrate continued intact tissue.

If the goals are associated with an *actual* nursing diagnosis, they represent a behavior or status that the nurse will assist the client to achieve. The following is an example of an actual nursing diagnosis and its corresponding goal:

Impaired Skin Integrity related to immobility
Goal: The client will demonstrate evidence of granulation tissue.

Rationales

A supporting rationale is presented for each nursing intervention for both collaborative problems and nursing diagnoses. The rationale explains why the intervention is appropriate and why it will produce the desired response. Rationales may be scientific principles derived from the natural, physical, and behavioral sciences, or they may be drawn from the humanities and nursing research. The rationales for client teaching interventions also include why the teaching is needed and why the specific content is taught.

Some topics in nursing are well studied, whereas others have had little or no research. Whenever possible, references no older than five years are used. A reference that is five or more years old is used because it is a classic or represents the most recent source on the subject.

Documentation

Each nursing diagnosis or collaborative problem section ends with a list of where and how the nurse will most appropriately document the care given. For some diagnoses, responsible documentation is recorded on a flow record (e.g., vital signs or urine output). For others, the nurse records a progress note. Teaching can be recorded on a teaching flow record or on a discharge summary record. The department of nursing determines policies for documentation. This section can serve to assist departments of nursing in formulating their documentation policies. It is unnecessary to record a progress or nursing note for every diagnosis on the care plan. Flow records can be used to document such routine or standard care as repetitive assessment results and even interventions.

Addendum Diagnoses

Frequently the nurse will identify and validate the presence of a high-risk or actual diagnosis that is not included in the given care plan for the situation or diagnostic cluster. The nurse can refer to the index of nursing diagnoses and collaborative problems in the back of this book for information about the identified diagnosis. For example, Mr. Jamie has had a myocardial infarction: the nurse initiates the care plan for an individual experiencing an MI. In addition, Mr. Jamie is immobile. The nurse can find "Disuse Syndrome" in the index and retrieve the information about that diagnosis. Then, the diagnosis, goals, and interventions can be added as additional or addendum diagnoses.

Medical Conditions

Generic Medical Care Plan for the Hospitalized Adult Client

This care plan (Level I) presents nursing diagnoses and collaborative problems that commonly apply to clients (and their significant others) undergoing hospitalization for any medical disorder. Nursing diagnoses and collaborative problems specific to a disorder are presented in the care plan (Level II) for that disorder.

■■■■■■ DIAGNOSTIC CLUSTER

Collaborative Problems

PC: Cardiovascular Dysfunction
PC: Respiratory Insufficiency

Nursing Diagnoses

Anxiety related to unfamiliar environment, routines, diagnostic tests, treatments, and loss of control

Risk for Injury related to unfamiliar environment and physical and mental limitations secondary to condition, medications, therapies, and diagnostic tests

Risk for Infection related to increased microorganisms in environment, risk of person-to-person transmission, and invasive tests and therapies

(Specify) Self-Care Deficit related to sensory, cognitive, mobility, endurance, or motivation problems

Risk for Imbalanced Nutrition: Less Than Body Requirements related to decreased appetite secondary to treatments, fatigue, environment, and changes in usual diet, and to increased protein and vitamin requirements for healing

Risk for Constipation related to change in fluid and food intake, routine, and activity level; effects of medications; and emotional stress

Risk for Impaired Skin Integrity related to prolonged pressure on tissues associated with decreased mobility, increased fragility of the skin associated with dependent edema, decreased tissue perfusion, malnutrition, and urinary/fecal incontinence

Disturbed Sleep Pattern related to unfamiliar, noisy environment, change in bedtime ritual, emotional stress, and change in circadian rhythm

Risk for Spiritual Distress related to separation from religious support system, lack of privacy, or inability to practice spiritual rituals

Interrupted Family Processes related to disruption of routines, change in role responsibilities, and fatigue associated with increased workload and visiting hour requirements

Risk for Compromised Human Dignity related to multiple factors (intrusions, unfamiliar procedures and personnel, loss of privacy) associated with hospitalization

Risk for Ineffective Therapeutic Regimen Management related to complexity and cost of therapeutic regimen, complexity of health care system, shortened length of stay, insufficient knowledge of treatment, and barriers to comprehension secondary to language barriers, cognitive deficits, hearing and/or visual impairment, anxiety and lack of motivation

Discharge Criteria

Specific discharge criteria vary depending on the client's condition. Generally, all diagnoses in the above diagnostic cluster should be resolved before discharge.

Collaborative Problems

PC: Cardiovascular Dysfunction

PC: Respiratory Insufficiency

Nursing Goal

The nurse will detect early signs and symptoms of (a) cardiovascular dysfunction, and (b) respiratory insufficiency, and will intervene collaboratively to stabilize the client.

Indicators

- Calm, alert, oriented (a, b)
- Respiration 16–20 breaths/min, relaxed and rhythmic (b)
- Breath sounds present all lobes, no rales or wheezing (b)
- Pulse 60–100 beats/min (a, b)
- BP >90/60, <140/90 mmHg (a, b)
- Capillary refill <3 seconds; skin warm and dry (a, b)
- Peripheral pulses full, equal (a)
- Temperature 98.5–99°F (a, b)

Interventions	Rationales
1. Monitor cardiovascular status:	1. Physiologic mechanisms governing cardiovascular function are very sensitive to any change in body function, making changes in cardiovascular status important clinical indicators.
a. Radial pulse (rate and rhythm)	a. Pulse monitoring provides data to detect cardiac dysrhythmia, blood volume changes, and circulatory impairment.
b. Apical pulse (rate and rhythm)	b. Apical pulse monitoring is indicated if the client's peripheral pulses are irregular, weak, or extremely rapid.
c. Blood pressure	c. Blood pressure represents the force that the blood exerts against the arterial walls. Hypertension (systolic pressure >140 mmHg, diastolic pressure >85 mmHg) may indicate increased peripheral resistance, cardiac output, blood volume, or blood viscosity. Hypotension can result from significant blood or fluid loss, decreased cardiac output, and certain medications.
d. Skin (color, temperature, moisture) and temperature	d. Skin assessment provides information evaluating circulation, body temperature, and hydration status.
e. Pulse oximetry	e. Pulse oximetry is a noninvasive method (probe sensor on fingertip) for continuous monitoring of oxygen saturation of hemoglobin.
2. Monitor respiratory status: a. Rate b. Rhythm c. Breath sounds	2. Respiratory assessment provides essential data for evaluating the effectiveness of breathing and detecting adventitious or abnormal sounds, which may indicate airway moisture, narrowing, or obstruction.

 Related Physician-Prescribed Interventions

Dependent on the underlying pathology

Documentation

Flow records
Pulse rate and rhythm

Blood pressure
Respiratory assessment
Progress notes
Abnormal findings
Interventions

Nursing Diagnoses

Anxiety Related to Unfamiliar Environment, Routines, Diagnostic Tests, Treatments, and Loss of Control

NOC Anxiety Control, Coping, Impulse Control

Goal

The client will communicate feelings regarding the condition and hospitalization.

Indicators

• Verbalize, if asked, what to expect regarding routines and procedures.
• Explain restrictions.

NIC Anxiety Reduction, Impulse Control Training, Anticipatory Guidance

Interventions	Rationales
1. Introduce yourself and other members of the health care team, and orient the client to the room (e.g., bed controls, call bell, bathroom).	1. A smooth, professional admission process and warm introduction can put a client at ease and set a positive tone for his or her hospital stay.
2. Explain hospital policies and routines: a. Visiting hours b. Mealtimes and availability of snacks c. Vital-sign monitoring d. Availability of newspapers e. Television rental and operation f. Storage of valuables g. Telephone use h. Smoking policy i. Policy for off-unit trips 3. Determine the client's knowledge of his or her condition, its prognosis, and treatment measures. Reinforce and supplement the physician's explanations as necessary.	2,3. Providing accurate information can help decrease the client's anxiety associated with the unknown and unfamiliar.
4. Explain any scheduled diagnostic tests, covering the following: a. Description b. Purpose c. Pretest routines d. Who will perform the procedure and where e. Expected sensations f. Posttest routines g. Availability of results	4–6. Teaching the client about tests and treatment measures can help decrease his or her fear and anxiety associated with the unknown, and improve his or her sense of control over the situation.

(continued on page 65)

Interventions	Rationales

5. Discuss all prescribed medications:
  a. Name and type
  b. Purpose
  c. Dosage
  d. Special precautions
  e. Side effects
 	
6. Explain any prescribed diet:
  a. Purpose
  b. Duration
  c. Allowed and prohibited foods	

7. Provide the client with opportunities to make decisions about his or her care whenever possible.	7. Participating in decision-making can help give a client a sense of control, which enhances his or her coping ability. Perception of loss of control can result in a sense of powerlessness, then hopelessness.
8. Provide reassurance and comfort. Spend time with the client, encourage him or her to share feelings and concerns, listen attentively, and convey empathy and understanding.	8. Providing emotional support and encouraging sharing may help a client clarify and verbalize his or her fears, allowing the nurse to get realistic feedback and reassurance.
9. Correct any misconceptions and inaccurate information the client may express.	9. A common contributing factor to fear and anxiety is incomplete or inaccurate information; providing adequate, accurate information can help allay client fears.
10. Allow the client's support people to share their fears and concerns, and encourage them in providing meaningful and productive support.	10. Supporting the client's support people can enhance their ability to help the client.

Documentation

Progress notes
   Unusual responses or situations
Multidisciplinary client education record
   Client's knowledge/information provided related to diagnosis, treatment, and hospital routine

Risk for Injury Related to Unfamiliar Environment and Physical or Mental Limitations Secondary to the Condition, Medications, Therapies, and Diagnostic Tests

NOC Risk Control, Safety Status: Falls Occurrence

Goal

The client will not injure him- or herself during hospital stay.

Indicators

- Identify factors that increase risk of injury.
- Describe appropriate safety measures.

NIC Fall Prevention, Environmental Management: Safety, Health Education, Surveillance: Safety, Risk Identification

Interventions	Rationales
1. Orient the client to his or her environment (e.g., location of bathroom, bed controls, call bell). Leave a light on in the bathroom at night.	1. Orientation helps provide familiarity; a light at night helps the client find his or her way safely.
2. Instruct the client to wear slippers with nonskid soles and to avoid newly washed floors.	2. These precautions can help prevent foot injuries and falls from slipping.
3. Teach him or her to keep the bed in the low position with side rails up at night.	3. The low position makes it easier for the client to get in and out of bed.
4. Make sure that the telephone, eyeglasses, and frequently used personal belongings are within easy reach.	4. Keeping objects at hand helps prevent falls from overreaching and overextending.
5. Instruct the client to request assistance whenever needed.	5. Getting needed help with ambulation and other activities reduces a client's risk of injury.
6. Explain the hospital's smoking policy.	6. The hospital is a nonsmoking institution.
7. For an uncooperative, high-risk client, consult with the physician for a 24-hour sitter or restraints, as indicated.	7. In some cases, extra measures are necessary to ensure a client's safety and prevent injury to him or her and others.

Documentation

Progress notes
Multidisciplinary client education record
Client teaching
Response to teaching

Risk for Infection Related to Increased Microorganisms in the Environment, Risk of Person-to-Person Transmission, and Invasive Tests or Therapies

NOC Infection Status, Wound Healing: Primary Intention, Immune Status

Goal

The client will describe or demonstrate appropriate precautions to prevent infection.

NIC Infection Control, Wound Care, Incision Site Care, Health Education

Interventions	Rationales
1. Teach the client to wash his or her hands regularly, especially before meals and after toileting.	1. Proper hand washing deters the spread of microorganisms.
2. Teach the client to avoid coughing, sneezing, or breathing on others, and to use disposable tissues.	2. These techniques help prevent transmission of infection through airborne droplets.
3. Follow institutional policies for IV and indwelling urinary catheter insertion and care.	3. Proper insertion and care reduce the risk of inflammation and infection.

(continued on page 67)

Interventions	Rationales
4. Teach a client undergoing IV therapy not to bump or disturb the IV catheterization site.	4. Movement of the device can cause tissue trauma and possible inflammation.
5. Teach a client with an indwelling catheter in place to do the following: a. Avoid pressure on the catheter. b. Wipe from front to back after a bowel movement.	5. Catheter movement can cause tissue trauma, predisposing to inflammation. Feces can readily contaminate an indwelling catheter.
6. Instruct the client to watch for and report immediately any signs and symptoms of inflammation: a. Redness or pain at the catheter insertion site b. Bladder spasms and cloudy urine (for a client with an indwelling urinary catheter) c. Feelings of warmth and malaise	6. Nosocomial infections occur in 5–6% of all hospitalized clients. Early detection enables prompt intervention to prevent serious complications and a prolonged hospital stay.

Documentation

Flow records
   Catheter and insertion site care
Progress notes
   Abnormal findings
Multidisciplinary client education record

(Specify) Self-Care Deficit Related to Sensory, Cognitive, Mobility, Endurance, or Motivational Problems

NOC See Self-Care: Bathing, Self-Care: Hygiene, Self-Care: Eating, Self-Care: Dressing, Self-Care: Toileting, and/or Self-Care: Instrumental Activities of Daily Living for NOC

Goal

The client will perform self-care activities (feeding, toileting, dressing, grooming, bathing), with assistance as needed.

Indicators

• Demonstrate optimal hygiene after care is provided.
• Describe restrictions or precautions needed.

NIC See Feeding, Bathing, Dressing, and/or Instrumental Self-Care Deficit for NIC

Interventions	Rationales
1. Promote the client's maximum involvement in self-feeding: a. Determine the client's favorite foods and provide them, when possible.	1–4. Enhancing a client's self-care abilities can increase his or her sense of control and independence, promoting overall well-being.

(continued on page 68)

Interventions	Rationales

b. As feasible, arrange for meals to be served in a pleasant, relaxed, and familiar setting without too many distractions.

c. Ensure good oral hygiene before and after meals.

d. Encourage the client to wear his or her dentures and eyeglasses when eating, as appropriate.

e. Have the client sit upright in a chair at a table, if possible. If not, position him or her as close to upright as he or she can be.

f. Provide some social contact during meals.

g. Encourage a client who has trouble handling utensils to eat "finger foods" (e.g., bread, sandwiches, fruit, nuts).

h. Provide needed adaptive devices for eating, such as a plate guard, suction device under the plate or bowl, padded-handle utensils, wrist or hand splints with clamp, and special drinking cup.

i. Assist with meal setup as needed—open containers, napkins and condiment packages, cut meat, and butter bread.

j. Arrange foods so the client can eat them easily.

2. Promote the client's maximum involvement in bathing.
   a. Encourage and help set up a regular bathing schedule.
   b. Keep the bathroom and bath water warm.
   c. Ensure privacy.
   d. Provide needed adaptive equipment, such as bath board, tub chair or stool, washing mitts, and hand-held shower spray.
   e. Make sure the call bell is within easy reach of a client who is bathing alone.

3. Promote or provide assistance with grooming and dressing:
   a. Deodorant application
   b. Cosmetic application
   c. Hair care: shampooing and styling
   d. Shaving and beard care
   e. Nail and foot care

4. Promote the client's maximum involvement in toileting activities.
   a. Evaluate his or her ability to move to and use the toilet unassisted.
   b. Provide assistance and supervision only as needed.
   c. Provide needed adaptive devices (e.g., commode chair, spill-proof urinal, fracture bedpan, raised toilet seat, support rails).
   d. Whenever possible, encourage a regular elimination routine using the toilet and avoiding a bedpan or urinal.

Documentation

Flow records
Assistance needed for self-care

Risk for Imbalanced Nutrition: Less Than Body Requirements Related to Decreased Appetite Secondary to Treatments, Fatigue, Environment, and Changes in Usual Diet, and to Increased Protein and Vitamin Requirements for Healing

NOC Nutritional Status, Teaching: Nutrition

Goal

The client will ingest daily nutritional requirements in accordance with activity level, metabolic needs, and restrictions.

Indicators

- Relate the importance of good nutrition.
- Relate restrictions, if any.

NIC Nutrition Management, Nutritional Monitoring

Interventions	Rationales
1. Explain the need for adequate consumption of carbohydrates, fats, protein, vitamins, minerals, and fluids.	1. During illness, good nutrition can reduce the risk of complications and speed up recovery.
2. Consult with a nutritionist to establish appropriate daily caloric and food type requirements for the client.	2. Consultation can help ensure a diet that provides optimal caloric and nutrient intake.
3. Discuss with the client possible causes of his or her decreased appetite.	3. Factors such as pain, fatigue, analgesic use, and immobility can contribute to anorexia. Identifying a possible cause enables interventions to eliminate or minimize it.
4. Encourage the client to rest before meals.	4. Fatigue further reduces an anorexic client's desire and ability to eat.
5. Offer frequent small meals instead of a few large ones.	5. Even distribution of total daily caloric intake throughout the day helps prevent gastric distention, possibly increasing appetite.
6. Restrict liquids with meals and avoid fluids one hour before and after meals.	6. These fluid restrictions help prevent gastric distention.
7. Encourage and help the client to maintain good oral hygiene.	7. Poor oral hygiene leads to bad odor and taste, which can diminish appetite.
8. Arrange to have high-calorie and high-protein foods served at the times that the client usually feels most like eating.	8. This measure increases the likelihood of the client's consuming adequate calories and protein.
9. Take steps to promote appetite: a. Determine the client's food preferences and arrange to have those foods provided, as appropriate. b. Eliminate any offensive odors and sights from the eating area. c. Control any pain or nausea before meals. d. Encourage the client's family and/or support persons to bring allowed foods from home, if possible. e. Provide a relaxed atmosphere and some socialization during meals.	9. These measures can improve appetite and lead to increased intake.

(continued on page 70)

Interventions	Rationales
10. Give the client printed materials outlining a nutritious diet that includes the following: a. High intake of complex carbohydrates and fiber b. Decreased intake of sugar, simple carbohydrates, salt, cholesterol, total fat, and saturated fats c. Moderate use of alcohol d. Proper caloric intake to maintain ideal weight e. Approximately 10 cups of water daily, unless contraindicated	10. Today, diet planning focuses on avoiding nutritional excesses. Reducing fats, salt, and sugar can reduce the risk of heart disease, diabetes, certain cancers, and hypertension.

Documentation

Flow records
  Dietary intake
  Daily weight
Multidisciplinary client education record
  Diet instruction
  Use of assistive devices

Risk for Constipation Related to Change in Fluid or Food Intake, Routine, or Activity Level; Effects of Medications; and Emotional Stress

NOC Bowel Elimination, Hydration, Symptom Control

Goal

The client will maintain prehospitalization bowel patterns.

Indicators

• State the importance of fluids, fiber, and activity.
• Report difficulty promptly.

NIC Bowel Management, Fluid management, Constipation/Impaction Management

Interventions	Rationales
1. Auscultate bowel sounds.	1. Bowel sounds indicate the nature of peristaltic activity.
2. Implement measures to eat a balanced diet that promotes regular elimination: a. Encourage increased intake of high-fiber foods, such as fresh fruit with skin, bran, nuts and seeds, whole-grain breads and cereals, cooked fruits and vegetables, and fruit juices. (Note: If the client's diet is low in fiber, introduce fiber slowly to reduce irritation to the bowel.) b. Discuss the client's dietary preferences and plan diet modifications to accommodate them, whenever possible. c. Encourage the client to eat approximately 800 grams of fruits and vegetables—the equivalent of about four pieces of fresh fruit and a large salad—daily to promote regular bowel movements.	2. A well-balanced high-fiber diet stimulates peristalsis and regular elimination.

(continued on page 71)

Interventions	Rationales
3. Promote adequate daily fluid intake: a. Encourage intake of at least 2 liters (8 to 10 glasses) per day, unless contraindicated. b. Identify and accommodate fluid preferences, whenever possible. c. Set up a schedule for regular fluid intake.	3. Adequate fluid intake helps maintain proper stool consistency in the bowel and aids regular elimination.
4. Establish a regular routine for elimination: a. Identify the client's usual elimination pattern before the onset of constipation. b. Review the client's daily routine to find an optimal time for elimination, and schedule adequate time. c. Suggest that the client attempt defecation about one hour following meals; instruct him or her to remain on the toilet for a sufficient length of time.	4. Devising an elimination routine based on the body's natural circadian rhythms can help stimulate regular defecation.
5. Attempt to simulate the client's home environment for elimination: a. Have the client use the toilet rather than a bedpan or commode, if possible. Offer a bedpan or commode only when necessary. b. Assist the client into proper position on the toilet, bedpan, or commode, as necessary. c. Provide privacy during elimination attempts—close the bathroom door or draw curtains around the bed, play the television or radio to mask sounds, use a room deodorizer. d. Provide adequate comfort, reading material as a diversion, and a call bell for safety reasons.	5. A sense of normalcy and familiarity can help reduce embarrassment and promote relaxation, which may aid defecation.
6. Teach the client to assume an optimal position on the toilet or commode (sitting upright, leaning forward slightly) or bedpan (head of bed elevated to put the client in high Fowler's position or at permitted elevation); assist him or her in assuming this position as necessary.	6. Proper positioning takes full advantage of abdominal muscle action and the force of gravity to promote defecation.
7. Explain how physical activity affects daily elimination. Encourage and, as necessary, assist with regular ambulation, unless contraindicated.	7. Regular physical activity aids elimination by improving abdominal muscle tone and stimulating appetite and peristalsis.

Documentation

Flow records
  Bowel movements
  Bowel sounds
Multidisciplinary client education record
  Instructions for obtaining regular elimination pattern

Risk for Impaired Skin Integrity Related to Prolonged Pressure on Tissues Associated with Decreased Mobility, Increased Fragility of the Skin Associated with Dependent Edema, Decreased Tissue Perfusion, Malnutrition, Urinary/Fecal Incontinence

NOC Tissue Integrity: Skin and Mucous Membranes

Goal

The client will maintain present intact skin/tissue.

Indicators

- No redness (erythema)
- Relate risk factors to skin/tissue trauma.

NIC Pressure Management, Pressure Ulcer Care, Skin Surveillance, Positioning

Interventions	Rationales

1. Skin assessment
  a. *Assessment.* All clients will be assessed upon admission for risk factors that predispose to skin breakdown. These risk factors include, but are not limited to, the following:
  • Altered level of consciousness
  • Poor nutrition/hydration
  • Impaired mobility
  • Impaired sensation (paralysis)
  • Incontinence
  • Multisystem failure
  • Steroid or immunosuppressive therapy
  • Age over 65
  b. *Inspection.* Upon admission, bony prominences and skin folds will be inspected for evidence of redness or skin breakdown.
  c. *Documentation.* Within 8 hours of admission, document the following information on the skin section of the Nursing Admission History:
  • Indicate by checking appropriate boxes whether the client is at risk for skin breakdown and the risk factors present.
  • Describe existing areas of breakdown and indicate their location on the body.
	1. To prevent pressure ulcers, individuals at risk must be identified so that risk factors can be reduced through intervention.

2. Prevention protocol
  a. Pressure relief
  • Change client's position when in bed at least every two hours around the clock. Use large and small shifts of weight.
  • Post position change schedule ("turn clock") at bedside.
  • Utilize prevention mode on specialty beds.
  • Use foam with cushion in chair; no donuts.
  b. Limit shearing forces/friction
  • Keep the head of the bed at or below 30 degrees whenever possible.
  • Avoid dragging the client in bed. Use lift sheet or overhead trapeze.
  • Use elbow protectors. Remove to inspect at every shift.
  • Apply transparent film dressing (Tegaderm) over bony prominences, as appropriate.
	2.
	  • The critical time period for tissue changes due to pressure is between 1 and 2 hours, after which irreversible changes can occur.
	  • The "turn clock" alerts the nurse to recommended position changes and appropriate time intervals for turning.
	  • The risk of developing a pressure ulcer can be diminished by reducing the mechanical loading on the tissue. This can be accomplished by using pressure-reducing devices. Donuts are known to cause venous congestion and edema. A study of at-risk clients found that ring cushions are more likely to cause pressure ulcers than prevent them. The donut relieves pressure in one area but increases pressure in the surrounding areas.
	  • Clinically, shear is exerted on the body when the head of the bed is elevated. In this position, the skin and superficial fascia remain fixed against the bed linens while the deep fascia and skeleton slide down toward the foot of the bed. As a result of shear, blood vessels in the sacral area are likely to become twisted and distorted and tissue may become ischemic and necrotic (Porth, 2005).

(continued on page 73)

Interventions	Rationales
	• Friction injuries to the skin occur when it moves across a coarse surface such as bed linens. Most friction injuries can be avoided by using appropriate techniques when moving individuals so that their skin is never dragged across the bed linens. • Voluntary and involuntary movements by the individuals themselves can lead to friction injuries, especially on elbows and heels. Any agent that eliminates this contact or decreases the friction between the skin and the bed linens will reduce the potential for injury.

3. Nutritional assessment
• Monitor intake and consider consultation with physician/dietary if the client:
  • Eats less than 50% of meals for 3 or more days
  • Is NPO or on a clear liquid diet for 5 days
  • Has a serum albumin of <3.5
• Place on intake and output. If intake is less than 2000 mL/24 hours, force fluids unless contraindicated.
• Record actual weight on admission and weekly thereafter.
• Request multivitamin/mineral supplement and/or dietary supplements (Burnshakes, Ensure) if indicated.
• Assess lab values:
  • CBC
  • Albumin
  • Hemoglobin/hematocrit
	3. Nutritional deficit is a known risk factor for the development of pressure ulcers. Poor general nutrition is frequently associated with loss of weight and muscle atrophy. The reduction in subcutaneous tissue and muscle reduces the mechanical padding between the skin and the underlying bony prominences, thus increasing susceptibility to pressure ulcers. Poor nutrition also leads to decreased resistance to infection and interferes with wound healing.

4. Skin care • Inspect skin at least daily during bath for reddened areas or breakdown. Check bony prominences for redness with each position change. • Keep skin clean and dry. Gently apply moisturizers such as Eucerin, Lubriderm, or Sween Cream, as needed. • Avoid massage over bony prominences.	4. Skin inspection is fundamental to any plan for preventing pressure ulcers. Skin inspection provides the information essential for designing interventions to reduce risk and for evaluating the outcomes of those interventions. • For maximum skin vitality, metabolic wastes and environmental contaminants that accumulate on the skin should be removed frequently. It is prudent to treat clinical signs and symptoms of dry skin with a topical moisturizer. • There is research evidence to suggest that massage over bony prominences may be harmful.
5. Incontinence care • Assess the cause of incontinence: History of incontinence Change in medications Antibiotic therapy Client disoriented at night • Check client for incontinence every 1 to 2 hours. • Take client to bathroom or offer bedpan every 2 hours while awake and at bedtime • If diapers are used, check every 2 hours and prn for wetness. • If plastic protectors are used, place inside lift sheet, never in direct contact with the client's skin. • Cleanse perineal area after each incontinent episode, followed by the application of a moisture barrier ointment (Desitin, Vaseline, A & D Ointment, Baza.)	5. • Moist skin due to incontinence leads to maceration, which can make the skin more susceptible to injury. Moisture from urine or fecal incontinence also reduces the resistance of the skin to bacteria. Bacteria and toxins in the stool increase the risk of skin breakdown. • Plastic pads hold moisture next to the skin. They are not absorbent and serve only as "bed protectors." Never use plastic pads unless they are covered with smooth linen to absorb moisture. • A moisture barrier is a petrolatum-based ointment that repels urine and fecal material and moisturizes the skin to assist in healing reddened, irritated areas resulting from incontinence.

Documentation

Flow record
    Turning and repositioning
    Skin assessment

Disturbed Sleep Pattern Related to an Unfamiliar, Noisy Environment, a Change in Bedtime Ritual, Emotional Stress, and a Change in Circadian Rhythm

 NOC Rest, Sleep, Well-Being

Goal

The client will report a satisfactory balance of rest and activity.

Indicators

• Complete at least four sleep cycles (100 min) undisturbed.
• State factors that increase or decrease the quality of sleep.

NIC Energy Management, Sleep Enhancement, Environmental Management

Interventions	Rationales
1. Discuss the reasons for differing individual sleep requirements, including age, life style, activity level, and other possible factors.	1. Although many believe that a person needs 8 hours of sleep each night, no scientific evidence supports this. Individual sleep requirements vary greatly. Generally, a person who can relax and rest easily requires less sleep to feel refreshed. With age, total sleep time usually decreases (especially Stage IV sleep) and Stage I sleep increases.

2. Institute measures to promote relaxation:
  a. Maintain a dark, quiet environment.
  b. Allow the client to choose pillows, linens, and covers, as appropriate.
	2. Sleep is difficult without relaxation. The unfamiliar hospital environment can hinder relaxation.

3. Schedule procedures to minimize the times you need to wake the client at night. If possible, plan for at least two-hour periods of uninterrupted sleep.	3. In order to feel rested, a person usually must complete an entire sleep cycle (70 to 100 min) four or five times a night.
4. Explain the need to avoid sedative and hypnotic drugs.	4. These medications begin to lose their effectiveness after a week of use, requiring increased dosages and leading to the risk of dependence.
5. Assist with usual bedtime routines as necessary, such as personal hygiene, snack, or music for relaxation.	5. A familiar bedtime ritual may promote relaxation and sleep.

6. Teach the client sleep-promoting measures:
  a. Eating a high-protein snack (such as cheese or milk) before bedtime
  b. Avoiding caffeine
  c. Attempting to sleep only when feeling sleepy
  d. Trying to maintain consistent nightly sleep habits
	6. These practices may help promote sleep.
	  a. Digested protein produces tryptophan, which has a sedative effect.
	  b. Caffeine stimulates metabolism and deters relaxation.
	  c. Frustration may result if the client attempts to sleep when not sleepy or relaxed.
	  d. Irregular sleeping patterns can disrupt normal circadian rhythms, possibly leading to sleep difficulties.

7. Explain the importance of regular exercise in promoting good sleep.	7. Regular exercise not only increases endurance and enhances the ability to tolerate psychological stress, but also promotes relaxation.

Documentation

Progress notes
Reports of unsatisfactory sleep

Risk for Spiritual Distress Related to Separation from Religious Support System, Lack of Privacy, or Inability to Practice Spiritual Rituals

NOC Hope, Spiritual Well-Being

Goal

The client will maintain usual spiritual practices not detrimental to health.

Indicators

• Ask for assistance as needed.
• Relate support from staff as needed.

NIC Spiritual Growth Facilitation, Hope Instillation, Active Listening, Presence, Emotional Support, Spiritual Support

Interventions	Rationales
1. Explore whether the client desires to engage in an allowable religious or spiritual practice or ritual. If so, provide opportunities for him or her to do so.	1. For a client who places a high value on prayer or other spiritual practices, these practices can provide meaning and purpose and can be a source of comfort and strength.
2. Express your understanding and acceptance of the importance of the client's religious or spiritual beliefs and practices.	2. Conveying a nonjudgmental attitude may help reduce the client's uneasiness about expressing his or her belief and practices.
3. Provide privacy and quiet for spiritual rituals, as the client desires and as practicable.	3. Privacy and quiet provide an environment that enables reflection and contemplation.
4. If you wish, offer to pray with the client or read from a religious text.	4. The nurse—even one who does not subscribe to the same religious beliefs or values as the client—can still help that client meet his or her spiritual needs.
5. Offer to contact a religious leader or hospital clergy to arrange for a visit. Explain available services (e.g., hospital chapel, Bible).	5. These measures can help the client maintain spiritual ties and practice important rituals.
6. Explore whether any usual hospital practices conflict with the client's beliefs (e.g., diet, hygiene, treatments). If so, try to accommodate the client's beliefs to the extent that policy and safety allow.	6. Many religions prohibit certain behaviors; complying with restrictions may be an important part of the client's worship.

Documentation

Progress notes
Spiritual concerns

Interrupted Family Processes Related to Disruption of Routines, Changes in Role Responsibilities, and Fatigue Associated with Increased Workload, and Visiting Hour Requirements

NOC Family Coping, Family Normalization, Family Environment: Internal, Parenting

Goal

The client and family members will verbalize feelings regarding the diagnosis and hospitalization.

Indicators

• Identify signs of family dysfunction.
• Identify appropriate resources to seek when needed.

NIC Family Involvement Promotion, Coping Enhancement, Family Integrity Promotion, Family Therapy, Counseling, Referral

Interventions	Rationales
1. Approach the family and attempt to create a private and supportive environment.	1. Approaching a family communicates a sense of caring and concern.
2. Provide accurate information using simple terms.	2. Moderate or high anxiety impairs the ability to process information. Simple explanations impart useful information most effectively.
3. Explore the family members' perceptions of the situation.	3. Evaluating family members' understanding can help identify any learning needs they may have.
4. Assess their current emotional response—guilt, anger, blame, grief—to the stresses of hospitalization.	4. A family member's response to another member's illness is influenced by the extent to which the illness interferes with his or her goal-directed activity, the significance of the goal interfered with, and the quality of the relationship.
5. Observe the dynamics of client–family interaction during visitations. Evaluate the following: a. Apparent desire for visit b. Effects of visit c. Interactions d. Physical contact	5. These observations provide information regarding family roles and interrelationships and the quality of support family members provide for each other.
6. Determine whether the family's current coping mechanism is effective.	6. Illness of a family member may necessitate significant role changes, putting a family at high risk for maladaptation.
7. Promote family strengths: a. Involve family members in caring for the client. b. Acknowledge their assistance. c. Encourage a sense of humor and perspective.	7. These measures may help maintain an existing family structure, allowing it to function as a supportive unit.
8. As appropriate, assist the family in reorganizing roles at home, resetting priorities, and reallocating responsibilities.	8. Reordering priorities may help reduce stress and maintain family integrity.
9. Warn family members to be prepared for signs of depression, anxiety, anger, and dependency in the client and other family members.	9. Anticipatory guidance can alert family members to impending problems, enabling intervention to prevent the problems from occurring.

(continued on page 77)

Interventions	Rationales
10. Encourage and help the family to call on their social network (friends, relatives, church members) for support.	10. Adequate support can eliminate or minimize family members' feelings that they must "go it alone."
11. Emphasize the need for family members to address their own physical and psychological needs. To provide time for this, suggest measures such as: a. Taking a break and having someone else visit the client for a change b. Calling the unit for a status report rather than traveling to the hospital every day	11. A family member who ignores his or her own needs for sleep, relaxation, or nutrition and changes his or her usual health practices for the worse impairs his or her own effectiveness as a support person.
12. If the family becomes overwhelmed, help them prioritize their duties and problems and act accordingly.	12. Prioritizing can help a family under stress focus on and problem-solve situations requiring immediate attention.
13. At the appropriate time, have family members list perceived problems and concerns. Then, develop a plan of action to address each item.	13. Addressing each problem separately allows the family to identify resources and reduce feelings of being overwhelmed.
14. Encourage the family to continue their usual method of decision-making, including the client when appropriate.	14. Joint decision-making reduces the client's feelings of dependency and reinforces the availability of continued support.
15. As possible, adjust visiting hours to accommodate family schedules.	15. This measure may help promote regular visitation, which can help maintain family integrity.
16. Identify any dysfunctional coping mechanisms: a. Substance abuse b. Continued denial c. Exploitation of one or more family members d. Separation or avoidance e. Assess for domestic abuse/violence • *Any person who has been physically, emotionally, or sexually abused by an intimate partner or former intimate partner.* • *Involves infliction or threat of infliction of any bodily injury; harmful physical contact; the destruction of property or threat thereof as a method of coercion, control, revenge, or punishment.* • Subcategories of domestic abuse/violence Physical Sexual Harassment Intimidation of a dependent Interference with personal liberty or willful deprivation • High risk indicators for suspected abuse: Should you notice any of the following indicators in combination with each other, it may warrant a referral to either the Medical Social Work Department (clients admitted to medical units) or Crisis Intervention. *Physical indicators:* • Physician's exam reveals that the client has injuries the spouse/intimate partner/client had not divulged	16. Families with a history of unsuccessful coping may need additional resources. Families with unresolved conflicts prior to a member's hospitalization are at high risk.

(continued on page 78)

Interventions	Rationales
• Too many "unexplained" injuries or explanations inconsistent with injuries • Over time, explanations for injuries become inconsistent • Prolonged interval between trauma or illness and presentation for medical care • Conflicting or implausible accounts regarding injuries or incidents • History of MD shopping or ER shopping *Social indicators:* • Age Young (chronologically or developmentally) Older • Spouse/intimate partner is forced by circumstances to care for client who is unwanted • Spouse/intimate partner inappropriately will not allow you to interview the client alone despite explanation • Client/spouse/intimate partner socially isolated or alienated • Client/spouse/intimate partner demonstrates poor self-image • Financial difficulties • Client claims to have been abused *Behavioral indicators:* • Client/spouse/intimate partner presents vague explanation regarding injuries with implausible stories • Client/spouse/intimate partner is very evasive in providing explanations • Client has difficulty maintaining eye contact and appears shameful about injuries • Client appears very fearful, possibly trembling • Client expresses ambivalence regarding relationship with spouse/intimate partner • Client quickly blames himself/herself for injuries • Client is very passive or withdrawn • Spouse/intimate partner appears "overprotective" • Client appears fearful of spouse/intimate partner Refer for counseling if necessary.	
17. Direct the family to community agencies and other sources of emotional and financial assistance, as needed.	17. Additional resources may be needed to help with management at home.
18. As appropriate, explore whether the client and family have discussed end-of-life decisions; if not, encourage them to do so.	18. Intense stress is experienced when families and health care providers are faced with decisions regarding either initiation or discontinuation of life-support systems or other medical interventions that prolong life (e.g., nasogastric tube feeding). If the client's wishes are unknown, additional conflicts may arise, especially if the family disagrees with decisions made by the health care providers, or vice versa.

(continued on page 79)

Interventions	Rationales
19. When appropriate, instruct the client or family members to provide the following information: a. Person to contact in the event of emergency b. Person whom the client trusts with personal decisions c. Decision whether to maintain life support if the client were to become mentally incompetent d. Any preference for dying at home or in the hospital e. Desire to sign a living will f. Decision on organ donation g. Funeral arrangements; burial, cremation	19. During an episode of acute illness, these discussions may not be appropriate. Clients and families should be encouraged to discuss their directions to be used to guide future clinical decisions, and their decisions should be documented. One copy should be given to the person designated as the decision-maker in the event the client becomes incapacitated or incompetent, with another copy retained in a safe deposit box and one copy on the chart.

Documentation

Progress notes
    Interactions with family
Assessment of family functioning
End-of-life decisions, if known
    Advance directive in chart

Risk for Compromised Human Dignity Related to Multiple Factors (Intrusions, Unfamiliar Environment and Personnel, Loss of Privacy) Associated With Hospitalization

NOC Abuse Protection, Comfort Level, Knowledge: Illness Care, Self-Esteem, Dignified Dying, Spiritual Well-Being, Information Processing

Goal

The individual will report respectful and considerate care.

Indicators

- Respect for privacy
- Consideration of emotions
- Asked for permission
- Given options
- Minimization of body part exposure

NIC Patient Rights Protection, Anticipatory Guidance, Counseling, Emotional Support, Preparatory Sensory Information, Family Support, Humor, Mutual Goal Setting, Teaching: Procedure/Treatment, Touch

Interventions	Rationales
1. Determine if the agency/hospital has a policy for prevention of compromised human dignity (Note: This type of policy or standard may be titled differently [e.g., Mission Statement]).	1. Agency policies can assist the nurse when problematic situations occur. However, the moral obligation to protect and defend the dignity of clients and their families does not depend on the existence (or lack) of a policy.
2. Review the policy. Does it include (Walsh & Kowanko, 2002): • Protection of privacy and private space • Acquiring the client's and family's permission for planned care, treatments and procedures	2. This type of policy can project the philosophy and culture of moral and respectful care of the institution among its personnel.

(continued on page 80)

Interventions	Rationales
• Providing adequate time for the client and family to make decisions regarding the planned care, treatments and procedures • Advocating for the client • Clear guidelines regarding the number of personnel (e.g., students, nurses, physicians [residents, interns]) that can be present when confidential and/or stressful information is discussed, or when procedures that leave a client exposed need to be done.	
3. Minimize exposure of the client's body with the use of drapes. Ensure that the client is not exposed to the gaze of others whose presence is not needed for the procedure.	3. Individuals have reported being physically exposed as their central source of humiliation and indignity (Walsh & Kowanko, 2002).
4. Provide care to each client and family as you would expect or demand for your family, partner, child, friend, or colleague.	4. Setting this personal standard can spur you to defend the dignity of a client/family, especially when they do not belong to the same socio-economic group as you.
5. When performing a procedure, engage the client in conversation. Act like the situation is matter-of-fact for you, to reduce embarrassment. In awkward situations, talk to the client even if she or he is unresponsive. Use humor if appropriate.	5. Clients have reported that in unavoidable, embarrassing situations (e.g., bowel or bladder accident), a nurse who was matter-of-fact and who made them feel at ease with small talk or humor made the situation better (Walsh & Kowanko, 2002).
6. Explain the procedure to the client. During painful or embarrassing procedures, show that you understand and accept how the client feels.	6. Clients reported they did not like being rushed and needed time to understand the upcoming procedure.
7. Determine if unnecessary personnel are present before a vulnerable or stressful event is initiated (e.g., code as painful procedure, embarrassing) and advise them that they are not needed at this time.	7. Protecting dignity and privacy always includes unconscious or deceased clients (Mairis, 1994).
8. Allow the client an opportunity to share his or her feelings after a difficult situation. Maintain privacy of client's information and emotional responses.	8. Allowing the client to share their feelings can help them maintain or regain dignity. Recognition of the client as a living, thinking, and experiencing human being enhances dignity (Walsh & Kowanko, 2002).
9. Be a role model and an advocate for the preservation of the client's dignity after death.	9. Role-modeling considerate and respectful care can lead others to a heightened awareness and encourage them to emulate this care themselves.
10. Discuss with involved personnel any incident that was disrespectful to the client or his or her family and report repetitive incidents or any incident that is a violation of client's dignity to the appropriate personnel. 11. Engage in dialogue with client and family regarding their thoughts on the present plan of care and decisions that may need explanation.	10,11. Professionals have a responsibility to practice ethical and moral care and to address situations and personnel that compromise human dignity.
12. When extreme measures are planned or are being provided for a client which are futile, refer to Moral Distress. 13. "Practice expecting that honoring and protecting the dignity of individual/groups is not a value but a way of being." (Sodenberg et al, 1998)	12,13. "Extreme measures, when futile, are an infringement of the basic respect for the dignity innate in being a person" (Walsh & Kowanko, 2002 p.146).

Documentation

Care plan
  Specify preferences

Risk for Ineffective Therapeutic Regimen Management Related to Complexity and Cost of Therapeutic Regimen, Complexity of Health Care System, Insufficient Knowledge of Treatment, and Barriers to Comprehension Secondary to Language Barriers, Cognitive Deficits, Hearing and/or Visual Impairment, Anxiety, and Lack of Motivation

NOC Compliance Behavior, Knowledge: Treatment Regimen, Participation in Health Care Decisions, Treatment Behavior: Illness or Injury

Goal

The client or primary care giver will describe disease process, causes, and factors contributing to symptoms, and the regimen for disease or symptom control.

Indicators

* Relate the intent to practice health behaviors needed or desired for recovery from illness/symptom management and prevention of recurrence or complications.
* Describe signs and symptoms that need reporting.

NIC Anticipatory Guidance, Learning Facilitation, Risk Identification, Health Education, Teaching: Procedure/Treatment, Health System Guidance

Interventions	Rationales
1. Determine the client's knowledge of his or her condition, prognosis, and treatment measures. Reinforce and supplement the physician's explanations as necessary.	1. Assessing the client's level of knowledge will assist in the development of an individualized learning program. Providing accurate information can decrease the client's anxiety associated with the unknown and unfamiliar.
2. Identify factors that influence learning.	2. The client's ability to learn will be affected by a number of variables that need to be considered. Denial of illness, lack of financial resources, and depression may affect the client's ability and motivation to learn. Cognitive changes associated with this might influence the client's ability to learn new information.
3. Provide the client and family with information about how to utilize the health care system (billing and payment, making appointments, follow-up care, resources available, etc.).	3. Information on how to "work the system" will help the client and family feel more comfortable and more in control of client's health care. This will positively influence compliance with the health care regimen.

4. Explain and discuss with client and family/caregiver (when possible):
  a. Disease process
  b. Treatment regimen (medications, diet, procedures, exercises, equipment use)
  c. Rationale for regimen
  d. Side effects of regimen
	4. Depending on client's physical and cognitive limitations, it may be necessary to provide the family/caregiver with the necessary information for managing the treatment regimen. In order to assist the client with postdischarge care, the client needs information about the disease process, treatment regimen, symptoms of complications, etc., as well as resources available for assistance.

(continued on page 82)

Interventions	Rationales
e. Lifestyle changes needed f. Follow-up care needed g. Signs or symptoms of complications h. Resources and support available i. Home environment alterations needed	
5. Promote a positive attitude and active participation of the client and family. 　a. Solicit expression of feelings, concerns, and questions from client and family. 　b. Encourage client and family to seek information and make informed decisions. 　c. Explain responsibilities of client/family and how these can be assumed.	5. Active participation in the treatment regimen helps the client and family feel more in control of the illness, which enhances the effective management of the therapeutic regimen.
6. Ensure that a client with visual and/or hearing impairments has glasses and a hearing aid available and uses them during teaching sessions. Provide adequate lighting and a quiet place for teaching sessions. Provide written teaching materials in the client's first language when possible.	6. Vision and hearing aids, adequate lighting, written materials in client's primary language, etc., will help to compensate for barriers to learning. Decreasing external stimuli will assist the client to correctly perceive what is being said.
7. Explain that changes in lifestyle and needed learning will take time to integrate. 　a. Provide printed material (in client's primary language when possible). 　b. Explain whom to contact with questions. 　c. Identify referrals or community services needed for follow-up.	7. Explaining that changes are expected to take time to integrate will provide reassurance for the client that he or she does not have to make changes all at once. Support and reassurance will assist the client with compliance. Providing information about available resources also helps the client to feel supported in his or her efforts.

Documentation

Progress notes
　Specific discharge needs and plans
Discharge instructions
　Referrals made
Multidisciplinary client education record
　Client and family teaching about disease, plan of treatment, referrals, etc.

CARDIOVASCULAR AND PERIPHERAL VASCULAR DISORDERS

Heart Failure

Heart failure (HF) is defined as a clinical syndrome characterized by specific symptoms (dyspnea and fatigue) in the medical history, and by signs (edema, rales) on the physical examination.

HF is a syndrome that occurs when there is a structural or functional impairment in the ability of the heart to fill with or eject blood. HF can present in a myriad of ways, from minimal symptoms to those that are totally debilitating. These symptoms include fatigue, exercise intolerance, shortness of breath, breathing difficulty, retention, pulmonary congestion, and peripheral edema.

There are four recognizable stages of HF: The first two stages, A and B, are early precursors to HF; they allow for earlier intervention and prevention of HF. Clients at these stages of HF have risk factors such as arteriosclerotic heart disease (ASHD), coronary artery disease (CAD), hypertension, or diabetes. In stage A clients do not have impaired left ventricular function (LVF). In stage B clients are usually mildly symptomatic and show evidence of LVF decline. There may also be hypertrophy from cardiac remodeling.

Stage C clients have past symptoms and demonstrable structural heart disease. Stage D clients require significant interventions and have refractory HF. They are candidates for serious end-of-life discussion and planning (American Heart Association, 2005, Guideline Update for the Diagnosis and Management of Chronic Heart Failure in the Adult).

HF is primarily a condition of the elderly; thus, the widely recognized "aging of the population" also contributes to the increasing incidence of HF. The incidence of HF approaches 10 per 1,000 population after age 65, and approximately 80% of clients hospitalized with HF are more than 65 years old. HF is the most common Medicare diagnosis-related group (i.e., hospital discharge diagnosis), and more Medicare dollars are spent for the diagnosis and treatment of HF than for any other diagnosis. The total estimated direct and indirect costs for HF in 2005 were approximately $27.9 billion. In the United States, approximately $2.9 billion annually is spent on drugs for the treatment of HF (American Heart Association, 2005).

 Time Frame
- Initial diagnosis (nonintensive care unit or intensive care unit)
- Exacerbation of chronic condition

■■■■■ DIAGNOSTIC CLUSTER

Collaborative Problems	Refer to
▲ PC: Hypoxia	
△ PC: Deep Vein Thrombosis	Acute Coronary Syndrome
△ PC: Cardiogenic Shock	Acute Coronary Syndrome
✳ PC: Dysrhythmias	
✳ PC: Multiple Organ Failure	
PC: Hepatic Insufficiency	Cirrhosis

Nursing Diagnoses	Refer to
▲ Activity Intolerance related to insufficient oxygen for activities of daily living	Chronic Obstructive Pulmonary Disease
▲ Anxiety related to breathlessness	Chronic Obstructive Pulmonary Disease

(continued on page 84)

Nursing Diagnoses	Refer to
△ Imbalanced Nutrition: Less Than Body Requirements related to nausea; anorexia secondary to venous congestion of gastrointestinal tract, and fatigue	Chronic Obstructive Pulmonary Disease
△ Impaired Peripheral Tissue Perfusion related to venous congestion secondary to right-side heart failure	Cirrhosis
△ Disturbed Sleep Pattern related to nocturnal dyspnea and inability to assume usual sleep position	Chronic Obstructive Pulmonary Disease
△ Powerlessness related to progressive nature of condition	Chronic Obstructive Pulmonary Disease
△ High Risk for Ineffective Therapeutic Regimen Management related to lack of knowledge of low-salt diet, drug therapy (diuretic, digitalis, vasodilators), activity program, signs and symptoms of complications	
✳ High Risk for Impaired Skin Integrity related to edema and decreased tissue perfusion	Deep Vein Thrombosis

▲ This diagnosis was reported to be monitored for or managed frequently (75%–100%).
△ This diagnosis was reported to be monitored for or managed often (50%–74%).
✳ This diagnosis was not included in the validation study.

Discharge Criteria

Before discharge, the client or family will

1. Describe the rationales for prescribed treatments.
2. Demonstrate the ability to count pulse rate correctly.
3. State the causes of symptoms and describe their management.
4. State the signs and symptoms that must be reported to a health care professional.

Collaborative Problems

Potential Complication: Hypoxia

Nursing Goal

The nurse will detect early signs of hypoxia and collaboratively intervene to stabilize the client.

Indicators

- Serum pH 7.35–7.45
- Serum PCO_2 35–45 mmHg
- Regular pulse rate and rhythm (60–100 beats/min)
- Respiration 16–20 breaths/min
- Blood pressure <140/90, >90/60 mmHg
- Urine output >5 mL/kg/h

Interventions	Rationales

1. Monitor for signs and symptoms of hypoxia:
  a. Increased and irregular pulse rate
  b. Increased respiratory rate
  c. Decreased urine output (<5 mL/kg/h)
  d. Changes in mentation, restlessness
  e. Cool, moist, cyanotic, mottled skin
  f. Decreased capillary refill time
	1. Decreased cardiac output leads to insufficient oxygenated blood to meet the tissues' metabolic needs. Decreased circulating volume/cardiac output can cause hypoperfusion of the kidneys and decreased tissue perfusion with a compensatory response of decreased circulation to the extremities and increased pulse and respiratory rates. Changes in mentation may result from cerebral hypoperfusion. Vasoconstriction and venous congestion in dependent areas (e.g., limbs) produce changes in skin and pulses.

2. Use a pulse oximeter.	2. The pulse oximeter is an accurate, noninvasive monitor of oxygen concentrations.

3. Monitor for signs and symptoms of acute pulmonary edema:
  a. Severe dyspnea with use of accessory muscles
  b. Tachycardia
  c. Adventitious breath sounds
  d. Persistent cough
  e. Productive cough with frothy sputum
  f. Cyanosis
  g. Diaphoresis
	3. Circulatory overload can result from the reduced size of the pulmonary vascular bed. Hypoxia causes increased capillary permeability that, in turn, causes fluid to enter pulmonary tissue, producing the signs and symptoms of pulmonary edema.

4. Cautiously administer intravenous (IV) fluids. Consult with the physician if the ordered rate plus the PO intake exceeds 2–2.5 L/24 h. Be sure to include additional IV fluids (e.g., antibiotics) when calculating the hourly allocation.	4. Failure to regulate IV fluids carefully can cause circulatory overload.
5. Assist the client with measures to conserve strength, such as resting before and after activities (e.g., meals).	5. Adequate rest reduces oxygen consumption and decreases the risk of hypoxia.

 ### Related Physician-Prescribed Interventions

Medications. Digitalis glycosides, diuretics, potassium supplements, vasodilators, morphine, angiotensin-converting enzyme (ACE) inhibitors, sympathomimetics, anticoagulants, nitrates, sedatives, aspirin (low-dose), beta blockers

Intravenous Therapy. Nonsaline solutions with replacement electrolytes (minimal volume)

Laboratory Studies. Urinalysis; complete blood count (CBC); electrolytes (including magnesium and calcium); renal panel; blood urea nitrogen (BUN); creatinine; liver function studies; serum glutamic-oxaloacetic transaminase (SGOT); lactate dehydrogenase (LDH); coagulation studies; arterial blood gas analysis; β-type natriuretic peptide (BNP); lipid count; thyroid panel (especially TSH [thyroid-stimulating hormone]); screen for hemochromatosis; screen for human immunodeficiency virus (HIV) is recommended by some health care providers

Diagnostic Studies. The focus will be on identifying and measuring cardiac structure and function: left ventricular size and pumping ability; ejection fraction (EF); cardiac output (CO); chest x-ray; electrocardiogram (ECG); hemodynamic monitoring; transthoracic echocardiography; radionuclide ventriculography; cardiac catheterization; PAP monitoring; nuclear imaging scan; exercise stress testing

Therapies. Emergency protocols (cardiac shock, dysrhythmias); fluid restrictions; sodium-restricted diet; oxygen via cannula/mask; intra-aortic balloon pump; fluid removal by hemodialysis; continuous renal replacement therapy (CRRT) or ultrafiltration; inotropic therapy; pacemaker insertion (in selected cases); rehabilitation therapy; anti-embolism stockings

Documentation

Flow records
  Vital signs

Intake and output
Assessment data
Pulse oximeter
Progress notes
Change in physiologic status
Interventions
Client response to interventions

Nursing Diagnoses

High Risk for Ineffective Therapeutic Regimen Management Related to Insufficient Knowledge of Low-Salt Diet, Activity Program, Drug Therapy (Diuretics, Digitalis, Vasodilators), and Signs and Symptoms of Complications

NOC Compliance Behavior, Knowledge: Treatment Regimen, Participation in Health Care Decisions, Treatment Behavior: Illness or Injury

Goal

The goals for this diagnosis represent those associated with discharge planning. Refer to the discharge criteria.

NIC Anticipatory Guidance, Risk Identification, Health Education, Learning Facilitation

Interventions	Rationales
1. Teach the client and family about HF and its causes.	1. Teaching reinforces the need to comply with prescribed treatments (diet, activity, and medications).
2. Explain the importance of nonpharmacologic interventions: a. Relaxation strategies b. Self-monitoring c. Exercise training	2. Outcome studies have shown multimodal nonpharmacologic therapy to significantly improve functional capacity, body weight, and mood (Sullivan & Hawthorne, 1996).
3. Explain the need to adhere to a low-sodium (<2 gm a day) and fluid-restricted (2 liters a day) diet, as prescribed. Consult with a nutritionist, as necessary.	3. Excess sodium intake increases fluid retention, which in turn increases vascular volume and cardiac workload.
4. Explain the actions of prescribed medications, particularly digitalis preparations, vasodilators, and diuretics. Digitalis increases the heart's stroke volume, which reduces congestion and diastolic pressure. Diuretics decrease the reabsorption of electrolytes, particularly sodium, thus promoting water loss. Vasodilators reduce preload and afterload, thus improving cardiac performance.	4. Such explanations can help increase client compliance and reduce errors in self-administration.
5. Teach the client how to measure his or her pulse rate.	5. Pulse-taking can detect an irregular rhythm or a high (>120) or low (<60) rate, which may indicate a drug side effect or disease complication.
6. Teach the client to weigh him- or herself daily and to report a gain of three or more pounds.	6. Daily weights can help to detect fluid retention early, enabling prompt treatment to prevent pulmonary congestion.

(continued on page 87)

Interventions	Rationales
7. Explain the need to increase activity gradually, and to rest if dyspnea and fatigue occur.	7. Regular exercise, such as walking, can improve circulation and increase cardiac stroke volume and cardiac output. Dyspnea and fatigue indicate hypoxemia resulting from overexertion.
8. Explain the effects of smoking and obesity on cardiac function. Refer the client to appropriate services.	8. Nicotine is a powerful vasoconstrictor. Obesity causes compression of vessels, leading to peripheral resistance, which increases cardiac workload.
9. Instruct the client and family to report the following signs and symptoms to a health care professional: a. Loss of appetite b. Visual disturbances c. Shortness of breath d. Persistent cough e. Edema in the ankles and feet f. Muscle weakness or cramping g. Chest pain h. Increased fatigue	9. Early detection and prompt intervention can reduce the risk of severe drug side effects or worsening HF. a,b. These are common side effects of digitalis. c,d. These indicate worsening HF. e. Edema indicates circulatory overload secondary to decreased cardiac output. f. These may indicate hypokalemia secondary to increased potassium excretion from diuretic therapy. g,h. These indicate worsening HF.
10. Provide information about or initiate referrals to community resources (e.g., American Heart Association, home health agencies).	10. They may provide the client and family with needed assistance in home management and self-care.

Documentation

Discharge summary record
    Client teaching
    Outcome achievement or status
    Referrals, if indicated

Deep Venous Thrombosis

Deep vein thrombosis (DVT) is a clot in the deep veins of the legs or pelvis. Predisposing causes are Virchow's triad (venous stasis, hypercoagulability, and endothelial injury, with inflammation to the vessel lining), antithrombin III deficiency, protein S and protein C deficiency, dysfibrinogenemia, thrombocytosis, systemic lupus erythematosus, and polycythemia vera (Byrne, 2002). Risk factors include prolonged immobility especially while sitting (such as a prolonged airline flight or driving), debilitating chronic disease (e.g., cancer, HF), pelvic or lower-extremity surgery, obesity, oral contraceptive use, varicose veins (Byrne, 2002), recent fractures, and hormone use. An estimated one in 10 episodes of DVT are related to central venous catheters.

 Time Frame
Initial diagnosis
Recurrent acute episodes

■■■■■ DIAGNOSTIC CLUSTER

Collaborative Problems

▲ PC: Pulmonary Embolism
▲ PC: Chronic Leg Edema

Nursing Diagnoses	Refer to
▲ Acute pain related to Impaired Circulation	
▲ High Risk for Impaired Skin Integrity related to chronic ankle edema	
△ High Risk for Ineffective Therapeutic Regimen Management related to lack of knowledge of prevention of recurrence of deep vein thrombosis and signs and symptoms of complications	
△ High Risk for Ineffective Respiratory Function related to immobility	Immobility or Unconsciousness
△ High Risk for Constipation related to decreased peristalsis secondary to immobility	Immobility or Unconsciousness

▲ This diagnosis was reported to be monitored for or managed frequently (75%–100%).
△ This diagnosis was reported to be monitored for or managed often (50%–74%)

Related Care Plan

Anticoagulant Therapy

Discharge Criteria

Before discharge, the client or family will:

1. Identify factors that contribute to recurrence of thrombosis.
2. Relate the signs and symptoms that must be reported to a health care professional.
3. Verbalize intent to implement life style changes.

Collaborative Problems

Potential Complication: Pulmonary Embolism

Potential Complication: Chronic Leg Edema

Nursing Goal

The nurse will detect early signs/symptoms of pulmonary embolism and vascular alterations and collaboratively manage to stabilize the client.

Indicators

- No chest pain
- Respiration 16–20 breaths/min
- Clear breath sounds
- Heart rate 60–100 beats/min
- Temperature 98–99.5°F
- Normal sinus rhythm

Interventions	Rationales
1. Monitor respiratory function.	1. Assessment should establish a baseline for subsequent comparisons to detect any changes.
2. If the client is on anticoagulant therapy, monitor prothrombin time (PT) according to the international normalized ratio (INR), activated partial thromboplastin time (aPTT), and platelets.	2. Anticoagulant therapy can cause thrombocytopenia. PT and aPTT values greater than two times normal (control) can produce bleeding and hemorrhage.
3. Instruct the client to maintain strict bed rest with legs elevated above the heart.	3. The recumbent position promotes venous drainage.
4. Explain the rationale for anticoagulant therapy and for immobilization.	4. The client's understanding of the need for treatments may improve compliance.
5. Avoid massaging the affected extremity.	5. Massage may dislodge the clot.
6. Instruct the client to report (and save) any pink-tinged sputum.	6. Blood-tinged sputum may indicate pulmonary bleeding.
7. Monitor for signs and symptoms of pulmonary embolism (Eftychiou, 1996): a. Symptoms • Dyspnea • Pleuritic chest pain • Anxiety/apprehension • Cough • Hemoptysis • Diaphoresis b. Signs • Tachypnea (>16 breaths/min) • Tachycardia (>100 beats/min) • Fever (>99.5°F) • Dropping SPO_2 • Crackles, wheezes, ↓breath sounds • Accentuated S_2 and P_2 heart sounds • Thrombophlebitis	7. a,b. The clot causes obstruction with increased resistance to pulmonary blood flow, which can progress to right ventricular failure. These effects produce hypoxia with a tachypnea response. The local obstruction produces an inflammatory response (e.g., cough, fever, pain, diaphoresis).
8. Instruct the client to immediately report any change in breathing or sudden feelings of apprehension.	8. Early reporting enables prompt evaluation and treatment.
9. Monitor leg edema, pain, and inflammation. Measure leg circumference 10 cm below and above the knee. Report any increases immediately.	9. These measures help to track the progression of the clot and inflammation.
10. If you suspect an increase in the thrombosis, consult the physician or nurse practitioner for a venous Doppler examination done by the vascular laboratory.	10. Propagation of a thrombosis from the calf to the thigh increases the risk of a pulmonary embolus; Doppler exam can detect thrombosis propagation.
11. Prepare the client for embolectomy or insertion of a vena cava filter if thrombosis continues to propagate during heparin therapy.	11. Occasionally a venous thrombosis continues to propagate despite heparin therapy, for instance, if a malignancy alters the clotting mechanism. The only way to prevent the clot from traversing the vena cava to the lungs is to provide a mechanical barrier such as a vena cava filter.
12. Refer to Anticoagulant care plan. If elastic support stockings are ordered, remove and reapply them every eight hours. Inspect the client's skin during changes.	12. Compression stockings promote venous return and reduce chronic leg edema (Byrne, 2002).

Related Physician-Prescribed Interventions

OTHER INTERVENTIONS: Vena cava filter, Embolectomy.
Medications. Warfarin, analgesics, antipyretics, heparin, unfractionated heparin (UH), or fractionated heparin (also known as low molecular weight heparin), clopidogrel bisulfate (Plavix©)
Intravenous Therapy. Continuous or intermittent intravenous
Laboratory Studies. CBC, cardiac isoenzymes, INR, arterial blood gases, PT/aPPT, SMA7, D-dimmer
Diagnostic Studies. Duplex ultrasound, noninvasive vascular studies (Doppler, oscillometry, plethysmography), ventilation/perfusion (V/Q scan), contrast venography, chest x-ray, ECG, spiral CT
Therapies. Graduated or sequential compression/decompression stockings, elastic support hose, moist heat

Documentation

Flow records
    Position in bed and activity restrictions
    Leg measurements and changes in measurement, color, or pain
Progress notes
    Client teaching

Nursing Diagnoses

Acute Pain Related to Impaired Circulation

NOC Comfort Level, Pain Control

Goal

The client will report a decrease in pain after pain relief measures.

Indicators

- Report factors that increase pain.
- Demonstrates a relaxed mode.

NIC Pain Management, Medication Management, Emotional Support, Teaching: Individual

Interventions	Rationales
1. Elevate the affected leg higher than the heart.	1. Venous pain usually is aggravated with leg in the dependent position and is slightly relieved with the leg elevated to promote venous return.

2. Explain the need to avoid
  a. Aspirin
  b. Medications containing aspirin (e.g., Bismuth, Pepto-Bismol, Alka-Seltzer, and some cold and allergy remedies)
  c. Nonsteroidal anti-inflammatory medications (e.g., Advil, Midol, Motrin, Indocin, and Feldene)
	2. These products interfere with plasma platelet coagulation.

3. Refer to the General Surgery care plan, Appendix II, for additional interventions for pain.	

Documentation

Medication administration record
    Type, route, dosage of all medications
Progress notes
    Response to pain relief measures

High Risk for Impaired Skin Integrity Related to Chronic Ankle Edema

NOC Tissue Integrity: Skin and Mucous Membranes

Goal

The client will demonstrate intact skin integrity.

Indicators

- Explain rationale for interventions.
- Demonstrate no erythema, blanching, or ulceration.

NIC Pressure Management, Pressure Ulcer Care, Skin Surveillance, Positioning

Interventions	Rationales
1. Teach the client about the vulnerability of the skin on the ankles to the effects of chronic venous insufficiency.	1. Postphlebitic syndrome, caused by incompetent valves in deep veins, results in edema, altered pigmentation, and stasis dermatitis.
2. Teach the client to avoid situations that impede leg circulation (e.g., sitting for long periods).	2. Impeded leg circulation can cause recurrence of DVT.
3. Teach the client to perform leg exercises every hour, when possible.	3. Leg exercises promote the muscle pumping effect on the deep veins, which improves venous return.
4. If ankle edema occurs, encourage the use of elastic stockings for support.	4. Elastic stockings reduce venous pooling by exerting an even pressure over the leg, and increase flow to deeper veins by reducing the caliber of the superficial veins.
5. Teach the client to immediately report any ankle injury or lesion.	5. Decreased circulation can cause a minor injury to become serious.
6. Instruct the client to report history of thrombosis at all future hospitalizations.	6. A high-risk client should alert nursing and medical staff so preventive measures can be initiated.

Documentation

Flow record
    Present condition of ankles
    Client teaching
    Client's response to teaching

High Risk for Ineffective Therapeutic Regimen Management Related to Lack of Knowledge of Prevention of Recurrence of Deep Vein Thrombosis and Signs and Symptoms of Complications

NOC Compliance Behavior, Knowledge: Treatment Regimen,
Participation in Health Care Decisions,
Treatment Behavior: Illness or Injury

Goal

The goals for this diagnosis represent those associated with discharge planning. Refer to the discharge criteria.

NIC Anticipatory Guidance, Risk Identification,
Health Education, Learning Facilitation

Interventions	Rationales
1. Explain relevant venous anatomy and physiology, including: a. Leg vein anatomy b. Function of venous valves c. Importance of muscle pumping action 2. Teach the pathophysiology of DVT, including: a. Effect of thrombosis on valves b. Hydrostatic pressure in venous system c. Pressure transmitted to capillary system d. Pressure in subcutaneous tissue	1,2. This teaching helps reinforce the need to comply with instructions (restrictions, exercises).
3. Teach preventive measures: a. Initiating a regular exercise program (e.g., walking or swimming) b. Avoiding immobility c. Elevating the legs whenever possible d. Using nonconstricting elastic support stockings (*Note:* These stockings should be checked by a health care professional to ensure proper fit.) e. Using extra means of support if exposed to additional risk (e.g., ace wraps or compression pump if prolonged immobility is necessary)	3. These measures can help to prevent subsequent episodes of DVT. a. Exercise increases muscle tone and promotes the pumping effect in the veins. b. Immobility increases venous stasis. c. Elevation reduces venous pooling and promotes venous return. d. The use of over-the-counter support stockings is controversial; improperly fitted stockings may produce a tourniquet effect. e. External elastic compression or a compression pump can provide the external pressure during a long period of immobility and helps to prevent venous pooling.
4. If the client is being discharged on anticoagulant therapy, refer to the Anticoagulant Therapy care plan for more information.	4. Low-dose heparin therapy has been shown to be of value by preventing DVT in clients for whom it is not contraindicated.
5. Explain the need to do the following: a. Maintain a fluid intake of 2500 mL a day, unless contraindicated. b. Stop smoking. c. Maintain ideal weight. d. Avoid garters, girdles, and over-the-counter (OTC) knee-high stockings.	5. These practices help to decrease risk of recurrence. a. Adequate hydration prevents increased blood viscosity. b. Nicotine is a potent vasoconstrictor. c. Obesity increases compression of vessels and causes hypercoagulability. d. Garters, girdles, and knee-high stockings constrict vessels, causing venous pooling.
6. Teach the client and family to watch for and promptly report these symptoms: a. Diminished sensation in legs or feet b. Coldness or bluish color in legs or feet c. Increased swelling or pain in legs or feet d. Sudden chest pain or dyspnea	6. Early detection enables prompt intervention to prevent serious complications. a,b,c. These changes in the legs and feet may point to an extension of the clot with resulting compromised circulation and inflammation. d. Sudden chest pain or dyspnea may indicate a pulmonary embolism.

(continued on page 93)

Interventions	Rationales
7. Instruct the client and family to advise health care providers of the client's history of deep vein thrombosis (DVT) (e.g., before surgery).	7. Clients with previous DVT are at four times greater risk for developing new DVT (Porth, 2002).

8. Explain postthrombotic syndrome, including:
  a. Pain, fatigue
  b. Heaviness in leg
  c. Pigmentation
  d. Spider veins
  e. Ulceration
  f. Edema of the leg(s)
	8. Postthrombotic syndrome refers to persistent symptoms after the acute episode (e.g., edema). These symptoms can persist for years.

Documentation

Discharge summary record
>   Client teaching
>   Outcome achievement or status

Hypertension

The Joint National Committee on Detection, Evaluation, and Treatment of High Blood Pressure (JNC, 2002) has introduced a new classification that includes the term "prehypertension." Additionally, Stage 2 and Stage 3 hypertension are combined into a single category—Stage 2.

Blood pressure for adults 18 years of age and older:

Optimal:	Systolic <120 mmHg	Diastolic ≤80 mmHg

PREHYPERTENSION

Normal	Systolic: 120–129 mmHg	Diastolic: 80–84 mmHg
Borderline	Systolic 130–139 mmHg	Diastolic: 85–89 mmHg

HYPERTENSION ≥140/90 mmHg

Stage 1:	Systolic 140–159 mmHg	Diastolic: 90–99 mmHg
Stage 2:	Systolic ≥160 mmHg	Diastolic: ≥100 mmHg

Hypertension is the major cause of coronary heart disease, cerebrovascular accident, and renal failure. The increasing prevalence of hypertension is cause for concern for all. The risk of systolic hypertension rises dramatically after age 50, representing the most common form of hypertension (JNC, 2002, p. 14). Sustained hypertension and accompanying increased peripheral resistance cause a disruption in the vascular endothelium, forcing plasma and lipoproteins into the vessel's intimal and subintimal layers and causing plaque formation (atherosclerosis). Increased pressure also causes hyperplasia of smooth muscle, which scars the intima and results in thickened vessels with narrowed lumina. Elevated systemic blood pressure increases the work of the left ventricle, leading to hypertrophy and increased myocardial oxygen demand.

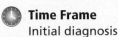 **Time Frame**
Initial diagnosis

■■■■■■ DIAGNOSTIC CLUSTER*

Collaborative Problems

PC: Vascular Insufficiency

Nursing Diagnoses

High Risk for Noncompliance related to negative side effects of prescribed therapy versus the belief that treatment is not needed without the presence of symptoms

High Risk for Ineffective Therapeutic Regimen Management related to lack of knowledge of condition, diet restrictions, medications, risk factors, and follow-up care

*This medical condition was not included in the validation study.

Discharge Criteria

Before discharge, the client will

1. Demonstrate blood pressure self-measurement.
2. Identify risk factors for hypertension.
3. Explain the action, dosage, side effects, and precautions for all prescribed medications.
4. Verbalize dietary factors associated with hypertension.
5. Relate an intent to comply with life style changes and prescriptions postdischarge.
6. Describe the signs and symptoms that must be reported to a health care professional.
7. Articulate commonly identified goals for blood pressure.

Collaborative Problems

Potential Complication: Vascular Insufficiency

Nursing Goal

The nurse will detect early signs and symptoms of vascular insufficiency and collaboratively intervene to stabilize client.

Indicators

- No new visual defects
- Oriented
- Equal strength upper/lower extremities
- Serum protein

Interventions	Rationales
1. Monitor for evidence of tissue ischemia:	1. Hypertension adversely affects the entire cardiovascular system. Chronic increases in perfusion pressure result in hypertrophy of vascular smooth muscle and increased collagen concentration. These changes reduce the lumen size of the blood vessels, changes the vessels' shape, and gives rise to cyclospasm of the vessel cells. The results are plaque formation from increased adherence of monocytes to the endothelium. The increase in the wall-to-lumen ratio in the arteries causes greater vessel resistance and a reduced ability to dilate in response to increased metabolic need for oxygen (Porth, 2005).

(continued on page 93)

Interventions	Rationales
a. Visual defects including blurring, spots, and loss of visual acuity	a. Evidence of blood vessel damage in the retina indicates similar damage elsewhere in the vascular system
b. Cerebrovascular deficits • Orientation or memory deficits • Weakness • Paralysis • Mobility, speech, or sensory deficits	b. In the brain, sustained hypertension causes progressive cerebral arteriosclerosis and ischemia. Interruption of cerebral blood supply caused by cerebral artery occlusion or rupture results in sensory and motor deficits.
c. Renal insufficiency • Decreased serum protein level • Sustained elevated urine specific gravity • Elevated urine sodium levels • Sustained insufficient urine output (<30 mL/h) • Increased BUN, serum creatinine, potassium, phosphorus, and ammonia levels; decreased creatinine clearance	c. With decreased blood supply to the nephrons, the kidney loses some ability to concentrate and form normal urine (Porth, 2005). • Further structural abnormalities may cause the vessels to become more permeable and allow leakage of protein into the renal tubules. • Decreased ability of the renal tubules to reabsorb electrolytes causes increased urine sodium levels and increased urine specific gravity. • Decreased glomerular filtration rate eventually causes insufficient urine output and stimulates renin production, which results in increased blood pressure in an attempt to increase blood flow to the kidneys. • Decreased renal function impairs the excretion of urea and creatinine in the urine, thus elevating BUN and creatinine levels.
d. Cardiac insufficiency • Substernal discomfort	d. Microvascular coronary atherosclerotic plaques or vasospasm reduce the caliber of vessel and its ability to oxygenate tissue (Porth, 2005).

 ## Related Physician-Prescribed Interventions

Medications. Diuretics, calcium-channel blockers, beta-adrenergic inhibitors, adrenergic inhibitors, angiotensin II receptor blockers, vasodilators, angiotensin-converting enzyme inhibitors, lipid-lowering agents. Thiazide-type diuretics have been the basis of antihypertensive therapy in most outcome trials (Patsy et al., 1997). In these trials, including the recently published *Antihypertensive and Lipid Lowering Treatment to Prevent Heart Attack Trial* (ALLHAT, 2002), diuretics have been virtually unsurpassed in preventing the cardiovascular complications of hypertension. The exception is the Second Australian National Blood Pressure trial, which reported slightly better outcomes in White men with a regimen that began with an angiotensin converting enzyme inhibitor (ACE) compared to one starting with a diuretic (Wing et al., 2003). Diuretics enhance the antihypertensive efficacy of multi-drug regimens, can be useful in achieving BP control, and are more affordable than other antihypertensive agents.

Intravenous Therapy. Not indicated

Laboratory Studies. Hemoglobin/hematocrit, serum cholesterol, triglycerides; thyroid studies; urinalysis, BUN/creatinine clearance; 24-h urine for vanillylmandelic acid (VMA), catecholamine; aldosterone (serum, urine); uric acid; serum glucose/fasting; urine steroids; serum potassium, calcium. Routine laboratory tests recommended before initiating therapy include an electrocardiogram; urinalysis; blood glucose and hematocrit; serum potassium, creatinine (or the corresponding estimated glomerular filtration rate [GFR]), and calcium (http://www.hdcn.com/calcf/gfr.htm); and a lipid profile, after 9- to 12-hour fast, that includes high-density lipoprotein cholesterol and low-density lipoprotein cholesterol, and triglycerides. Optional tests include measurement of urinary albumin excretion or albumin/creatinine ratio.

Diagnostic Studies. ECG, chest x-ray, renal scan

Therapies. Sodium-restricted diet, decreased fat diet

Documentation

Graphic/flow record
    Vital signs
    Intake and output
    Laboratory values
Progress notes
    Status of client
    Unusual events
    Changes in behavior

Nursing Diagnoses

High Risk for Noncompliance Related to Negative Side Effects of Prescribed Therapy Versus the Belief that Treatment is not Needed Without the Presence of Symptoms

NOC Adherence Behavior, Compliance Behavior, Symptom Control, Treatment Behavior: Illness or Injury

Goal

The client will

1. Verbalize feelings related to following the prescribed regimen.
2. Identify sources of support for assisting with compliance.
3. Verbalize the potential complications of noncompliance.

NIC Health Education, Self-Modification Assistance, Self-Responsibility Facilitation, Coping Enhancement, Decision-Making Support, Health System Guidance, Mutual Goal Setting, Teaching: Disease Process

Interventions	Rationales

1. Identify any factors that may predict client noncompliance, such as:
  a. Lack of knowledge
  b. Noncompliance in the hospital
  c. Failure to perceive the seriousness or chronicity of hypertension
  d. Belief that the condition will go away
  e. Belief that the condition is hopeless
	1. Motivation improves when clients have positive experiences with and trust in their clinicians. Empathy builds trust and is a potent motivator (Barrier & Jensen, 2003). Client attitudes are greatly influenced by cultural differences, beliefs, and previous experiences with the health care system (Betancourt, Carrillo, & Green, 1999). These attitudes must be understood if the clinician is to build trust and increase communication with clients and families (http://www.hdcn.com/calcf/gfr.htm).

2. Emphasize to the client the potentially life-threatening consequences of noncompliance. (Refer to Collaborative Problems for more information.)	2. This emphasis may encourage the client to comply with treatment by pointing out the seriousness of hypertension.
3. Point out that blood pressure elevation typically produces no symptoms.	3. Absence of symptoms often encourages noncompliance.
4. Discuss the likely effects of a future stroke, renal failure, or coronary disease on significant others (spouse, children, grandchildren)	4. This discussion may encourage compliance by emphasizing the potential impact of the client's hypertension on his or her significant others.

(continued on page 97)

Interventions	Rationales
5. Include the client's significant others in teaching sessions whenever possible.	5. Significant others also should understand the possible consequences of noncompliance; this encourages them to assist the client to comply with treatment (Miller et al., 1992).
6. Emphasize to the client that, ultimately, it is his or her choice whether or not to comply with the treatment plan.	6. Helping the client to understand that he or she is responsible for compliance may enhance the client's sense of control and self-determination, which may help to improve compliance.
7. Instruct the client to check or have someone else check his or her blood pressure at least once a week and to keep an accurate record of readings.	7. Weekly blood pressure readings are needed to evaluate the client's response to treatments and life style changes.
8. Explain the possible side effects of antihypertensive medications (e.g., impotence, decreased libido, vertigo); instruct the client to consult the physician for alternative medications should these side effects occur.	8. A client who experiences these side effects may be tempted to discontinue medication therapy on their own.
9. If the cost of antihypertensive medications is a burden for the client, consult with social services.	9. The client may require financial assistance to prevent noncompliance due to financial reasons.

Documentation

Discharge summary record
  Client teaching
  Response to interventions

High Risk for Ineffective Therapeutic Regimen Management Related to Lack of Knowledge of Condition, Diet Restrictions, Medications, Risk Factors, and Follow-up Care

NOC Compliance Behavior, Knowledge: Treatment Regimen, Participation in Health Care Decisions, Treatment Behavior: Illness or Injury

Goal

The goals for this diagnosis represent those associated with discharge planning. Refer to the discharge criteria.

NIC Anticipatory Guidance, Risk Identification, Health Education, Learning Facilitation

Interventions	Rationales

1. Discuss blood pressure concepts using terminology the client and significant other(s) can understand:
  a. Normal values (target/goals). The clinician and the client must agree upon BP goals. A client-centered strategy to achieve the goal and an estimation of the time needed to reach that goal are important (Boulware et al., 2001).
  b. Effects of sustained high blood pressure on the brain, heart, kidneys, and eyes
  c. Control versus cure
	1. Risk of stroke rises directly with a person's blood pressure (both systolic and diastolic). The reported decline in strokes coincides with the aggressive treatment and effective control of hypertension during the past several years (American Heart Association, 1989).

(continued on page 98)

Interventions	Rationales
2. Teach the client blood pressure self-measurement, or teach significant other(s) how to measure the client's blood pressure.	2. Self-monitoring is more convenient and may improve compliance.
3. Discuss life style modifications that can reduce hypertension.	3. Adoption of healthy life styles by all persons is critical for the prevention of high BP and is an indispensable part of the management of those with hypertension. Major life style modifications shown to lower BP include weight reduction in those individuals who are overweight or obese (The Trials of Hypertension Prevention Collaborative Research Group, 1997; He, Whelton, Appel, Charleston, & Klag, 2000); adoption of the Dietary Approaches to Stop Hypertension (DASH) eating plan (Sacks et al., 2001), which is rich in potassium and calcium (Vollmer et al., 2001); dietary sodium reduction (Chobanian & Hill, 2000; Sacks et al., 2001; Vollmer et al., 2001); physical activity (Kelley & Kelley, 2000; Whelton, Chin, Xin, & He, 2002), and moderation of alcohol consumption (See table 5 in Xin et al., 2001.)
	Life style modifications reduce BP, enhance antihypertensive drug efficacy, and decrease cardiovascular risk. For example, a 1600 mg sodium DASH eating plan has effects similar to single drug therapy (Sacks et al., 2001). Combinations of two (or more) life style modifications can achieve even better results.
a. Achieve weight loss to within 10% of ideal weight.	a. Obesity (BMI >30 kg/m²) is an increasingly prevalent risk factor for the development of hypertension and cardiovascular disease. The Adult Treatment Panel III guideline (Pickering, 1996) for cholesterol management defines the metabolic syndrome as the presence of three or more of the following conditions: abdominal obesity (waist circumference >40 inches in men or >35 inches in women), glucose intolerance (fasting glucose >110 mg/dL), BP >130/85 mmHg, high triglycerides (>150 mg/dL), or low HDL (<40 mg/dL in men or <50 mg/dL in women) (National Cholesterol Education Program, 2002).
b. Limit alcohol intake daily (2 oz liquor, 8 oz wine, or 24 oz beer).	b. Alcohol is a vasodilator causing rebound vasoconstriction that has been associated with increased blood pressure.
c. Engage in regular exercise (30–45 min) three to five times a week.	c. Regular exercise increases peripheral blood flow and muscle and cardiac efficiency. The results are a more effective cardiovascular system (NHBPE, 1997).
d. Reduce sodium intake to 4.6 g of sodium chloride.	d. Sodium controls water distribution throughout the body. An increase in sodium causes an increase in water, thus increasing circulating volume and raising blood pressure.
e. Stop smoking.	e. Tobacco acts as a vasoconstrictor, which raises blood pressure.
f. Reduce saturated fat and cholesterol to <30% of dietary intake.	f. A high-fat diet contributes to plaque formation and narrowing vessels.
g. Ensure the daily allowance of calcium, potassium, and magnesium in diet.	g. These elements maintain the cardiovascular and muscular systems.
4. Provide the client or significant other(s) with medication guidelines and drug information cards for all prescribed medications. Explain the following: a. Dosage b. Action c. Side effects d. Precautions	4. This teaching conveys to the client which side effects should be reported and precautions that should be taken.

(continued on page 99)

Interventions	Rationales

5. Alert the client and significant other(s) to OTC medications that are contraindicated, such as:
  a. High-sodium medications (Maalox, Bromoseltzer, Rolaids)
  b. Decongestants (e.g., Vicks Formula 44)
 	
  c. Laxatives (e.g., Phospho-soda)
  d. Diet pills
	5. OTC medications commonly are viewed as harmless, when in fact many can cause complications.
	  a. High-sodium content medications promote water retention.
	  b. Decongestants act as vasoconstrictors that raise blood pressure.
	  c. Some laxatives contain high levels of sodium.
	  d. *Diet pills have been linked to and associated with pulmonary hypertension.*

6. Stress the importance of follow-up care.	6. Follow-up care can help to detect complications.

7. Teach the client and significant other(s) to report these symptoms:
  a. Headaches, especially on awakening
  b. Chest pain
  c. Shortness of breath
  d. Weight gain or edema
  e. Changes in vision
  f. Frequent nosebleeds
  g. Side effects of medications
	7. These signs and symptoms may indicate elevated blood pressure or other cardiovascular complications.

Documentation

Discharge summary record
   Status of goal attainment
   Status at discharge
   Discharge instructions
   Referrals

Acute Coronary Syndrome

Acute Coronary Syndrome (ACS) is the umbrella term that encompasses myocardial ischemia, unstable angina, and all types of myocardial infarction: Q-Wave, non Q-Wave, ST segment elevation myocardial infarction, and those without ST wave elevations, non-ST segment elevation myocardial infarction. Myocardial infarction (MI) is the death of myocardial tissue resulting from impaired myocardial coronary blood flow. The cause of inadequate blood flow most commonly is the narrowing or occlusion of the coronary artery resulting from atherosclerosis, or decreased coronary blood flow from shock or hemorrhage. Diminished ability to bind oxygen to the hemoglobin can also result in an MI.

 Time Frame
Initial diagnosis
Post intensive care
Recurrent episodes

▪▪▪▪▪ DIAGNOSTIC CLUSTER

Collaborative Problems

▲ PC: Dysrhythmias
▲ PC: Cardiogenic Shock

(continued on page 100)

▲ PC: Heart Failure
▲ PC: Thromboembolism
▲ PC: Recurrent Acute Coronary Syndrome
✳ PC: Pericarditis
✳ PC: Pericardial Tamponade/Rupture
✳ PC: Structural Defects
✳ PC: Extension of Infarct

Nursing Diagnoses

▲ Anxiety/Fear (individual, family) related to unfamiliar situation status, unpredictable nature of condition, negative effect on life style, fear of death, possible sexual dysfunction

▲ Pain related to cardiac tissue ischemia or inflammation

▲ Activity Intolerance related to insufficient oxygenation for activities of daily living (ADLs) secondary to cardiac tissue ischemia, prolonged immobility, narcotics or medications

△ Grieving related to actual or perceived losses secondary to cardiac condition

△ High Risk for Ineffective Therapeutic Regimen Management related to lack of knowledge of hospital routines, procedures, equipment, treatments, conditions, medications, diet, activity progression, signs and symptoms of complications, reduction of risks, follow-up care, community resources

▲ This diagnosis was reported to be monitored for or managed frequently (75%–100%).
△ This diagnosis was reported to be monitored for or managed often (50%–74%).
✳ This diagnosis was not included in the validation study.

Discharge Criteria

Before discharge, the client or family will

1. State the cause of cardiac pain and the rationales for medication therapy and activity and dietary restrictions.
2. Demonstrate accuracy in taking pulse.
3. Identify modifiable personal risk factors.
4. Describe at-home activity restrictions.
5. Describe self-administration of daily and PRN medications.
6. Describe signs and symptoms that must be reported to a health care professional.
7. Verbalize the follow-up care needed and the community resources available.
8. Describe appropriate actions to take in the event of problems.

Collaborative Problems

Potential Complication: Dysrhythmias

Potential Complication: Cardiogenic Shock

Potential Complication: Heart Failure

Potential Complication: Thromboembolism

Potential Complication: Recurrent ACS

Potential Complication: Pericarditis

Potential Complication: Pericardial Tamponade/Rupture

Potential Complication: Structural Defects

Nursing Goal

The nurse will detect early signs and symptoms of cardiac and vascular alterations and collaboratively intervene to stabilize the client.

Indicators

- Oxygen saturation >95% (pulse oximeter)
- Normal sinus rhythm
- No life-threatening dysrhythmias
- No chest pain
- Pulse: regular rhythm, rate 60–100 beats/min
- Respiration 16–20 breaths/min
- Blood pressure: Systolic <120 mmHg, Diastolic <85 mmHg
- Urine output >5 mL/kg/h
- Serum pH 7.35–7.45
- Serum PCO_2 35–45 mmHg

Interventions	Rationales
1. Per protocol, initiate pharmacologic reperfusion therapy (e.g., thrombolytics).	1. These agents restore full blood flow through the blocked artery.
2. Maintain continuous EKG, blood pressure, and pulse oximetry monitoring; report changes.	2. Continuous monitoring allows for early detection of complications.
3. Administer medications, as indicated, and continue to monitor for side effects. Consult pharmaceutical reference for specifics.	3. Multiple classes of medications (e.g., nitrates, beta blockers, analgesics) are used.
4. Monitor for signs and symptoms of dysrhythmias: a. Abnormal rate, rhythm b. Palpitations, syncope c. Hemodynamic compromise (e.g., hypotension) d. Cardiac emergencies (arrest, ventricular fibrillation)	4. Myocardial ischemia results from reduced oxygen to myocardial tissue. Ischemic tissue is electrically unstable, causing dysrhythmias, such as premature ventricular contractions, that can lead to ventricular fibrillation and death. Dysrhythmias can result from reperfusion of ischemic tissue secondary to thrombolytics.
5. Maintain oxygen therapy, as prescribed. Evaluate pulse oximeter readings.	5. Supplemental oxygen therapy increases the circulating oxygen available to myocardial tissue. Pulse oximeter readings should be >95%. Exceptions may be necessary for those with Chronic Obstructive Pulmonary Disease.
6. Monitor for signs and symptoms of cardiogenic shock: a. Tachycardia b. Urine output <30 mL/h c. Restlessness, agitation, change in mentation d. Tachypnea e. Diminished peripheral pulses f. Cool, pale, or cyanotic skin g. Mean arterial pressure <60 mmHg h. Cardiac index <2.0 L i. Increased systemic vascular resistance j. Failure to maintain adequate Stroke Volume/Stroke Volume Variation (SV/SVV)	6. Cardiogenic shock results most often from loss of viable myocardium and impaired contractility. This manifests as decreased stroke volume and cardiac output. The compensatory response to decreased circulatory volume aims to increase blood oxygen levels by increasing heart and respiratory rates, and to decrease circulation to extremities (marked by decreased pulses and cool skin). Diminished oxygen to the brain causes changes in mentation.

(continued on page 102)

Interventions	Rationales
7. Monitor for signs and symptoms of HF and decreased cardiac output: a. Gradual increase in heart rate b. Increased shortness of breath c. Adventitious breath sounds d. Decreased systolic blood pressure e. Presence of or increase in S_3 or S_4 gallop f. Peripheral edema g. Distended neck veins h. Elevation in BNP (β-type natriuretic peptide)	7. Myocardial ischemia causes HF. Ischemia reduces the ability of the left ventricle to eject blood, thus decreasing cardiac output and increasing pulmonary vascular congestion. Fluid enters pulmonary tissue, causing rales, productive cough, cyanosis, and possibly signs and symptoms of respiratory distress.
8. Monitor for signs and symptoms of thromboembolism: a. Diminished or no peripheral pulses, decreased Ankle Brachial index b. Unusual warmth/redness or cyanosis/coolness c. Leg pain localized to calf area d. Sudden severe chest pain, increased dyspnea e. Positive Homans' sign f. Claudication	8. Prolonged bed rest, increased blood viscosity and coagulability, and decreased cardiac output contribute to thrombus formation. a. Insufficient circulation causes pain and diminished peripheral pulse. b. Unusual warmth and redness point to inflammation; coolness and cyanosis indicate vascular obstruction. c. Leg pain results from tissue hypoxia. d. Obstruction to pulmonary circulation causes sudden chest pain and dyspnea. e. In a positive Homans' sign, dorsiflexion of the foot causes pain as a result of insufficient circulation. f. Pain with walking is caused by insufficient circulation.
9. Monitor for signs and symptoms of pericarditis: a. Chest pain influenced by change in respiration or position b. Pericardial rub. c. Temperature elevation >101°F d. Diffuse ST segment electrocardiogram (ECG) changes	9. Pericarditis is inflammation of the pericardial sac. Damage to the epicardium causes it to become rough, which tends to irritate and inflame the pericardium.
10. Monitor for signs and symptoms of pericardial tamponade/cardiac rupture: a. Hypotension b. Distended neck veins c. Tachycardia d. Pulsus paradoxus e. Equalization of cardiac pressures f. Narrowed pulse pressure g. Muffled heart tones h. Electrical alternans	10. Cardiac tamponade results from accumulation of fluid in the pericardial space, causing impaired cardiac function and decreased cardiac output. Cardiac rupture occurs most often from three to 10 days after MI, resulting from leukocyte scavenger cells removing necrotic debris, which thins the myocardial wall. The onset is sudden, with bleeding into the pericardial sac.
11. Monitor for signs and symptoms of structural defects: a. Severe chest pain b. Syncope c. Hypotension d. New loud holosystolic murmur e. CHF f. Left-to-right shunt	11. Ventricular aneurysm, ventricular septal defect, and papillary muscle rupture all result from ischemia or necrosis to the structures.
12. Monitor for signs and symptoms of recurrent MI: a. Classic symptoms: Sudden, severe chest pain with nausea/vomiting and diaphoresis; pain may or may not radiate. ACS can occur without pain and without change in EKG. b. Increased dyspnea c. Increased ST elevation and abnormal Q waves on ECG	12. These signs and symptoms indicate myocardial tissue deterioration with increasing hypoxia.
13. Apply below-knee antiembolic stockings. 14. Progressive activity after chest pain is controlled; involve client in cardiac rehabilitation.	13,14. These measures actively promote venous return.

Related Physician-Prescribed Interventions

Medications. Vasodilators, antianginals, antidysrhythmics, beta-blockers, Calcium channel blockers, stool softeners, angiotensin-converting enzyme (ACE) inhibitors, anticoagulants, analgesics, diuretics, sedatives/hypnotics, thrombolytics, GP IIa IIIb inhibitors, inotropic therapy (selected cases), nitrates, aspirin, antiplatelets

Intravenous Therapy. IV access for medication administration, IV access for blood sampling, arterial access for ABGs and blood pressure monitoring, sheath access for coronary interventions

Laboratory Studies. Arterial blood gas analysis, electrolytes, cholesterol, white blood count, tri-glycerides, sedimentation rate, coagulation studies, chemistry profile, creatinine kinase, MB isoenzyme, troponin I, troponin T, myoglobin, CK-MB isoforms

Diagnostic Studies. ECG, stress test, chest x-ray film, cardiac catheterization, echocardiogram, digital subtraction angiography, nuclear imaging studies, thallium scans, magnetic resonance imaging, thoracic electrical bioimpedance (IEB), SvO_2 monitoring, hemodynamic monitoring, Stroke Volume (SV) and Stoke Volume Variations (SVV), Cardiac Output (CO) and Cardiac Index (CI), Systemic Vascular Resistance (SVR), Central Venous Pressure (CVP)

Therapies. Oxygen via cannula; (in selected cases) pacemakers, transcutaneous, transvenous, and permanent single or dual chamber; therapeutic diet (low-salt, low-saturated fats, low-cholesterol); cardiac rehabilitation program; pulse oximetry

Interventional Therapies. Percutaneous transluminal coronary angioplasty, intracoronary stents, atherectomy, intra-aortic balloon pump.

Documentation

Graphic/flow record
  Vital signs
  Intake and output
  Rhythm strips
Progress notes
  Status of client
  Unusual events

Nursing Diagnoses

Anxiety/Fear (individual, family) Related to Unfamiliar Situation, Unpredictable Nature of Condition, Fear of Death, Negative Effects on Life Style, or Possible Sexual Dysfunctions

 Anxiety Level, Coping, Impulse Control

Goal

The client or family will relate increased psychological and physiologic comfort.

Indicators

- Verbalize fears related to the disorder.
- Share concerns about the disorder's effects on normal functioning, role responsibilities, and life style.
- Use at least one relaxation technique.

 Anxiety Reduction, Impulse Control Training, Anticipatory Guidance

Interventions	Rationales

1. Assist the client to reduce anxiety:
   a. Provide reassurance and comfort.
   b. Convey understanding and empathy. Do not avoid questions.
   c. Encourage the client to verbalize any fears and concerns regarding MI and its treatment.
   d. Identify and support effective coping mechanisms.
	1. An anxious client has a narrowed perceptual field and a diminished ability to learn. He or she may experience symptoms caused by increased muscle tension and disrupted sleep patterns. Anxiety tends to feed on itself, trapping the client in a spiral of increasing anxiety, tension, and emotional and physical pain.

(continued on page 104)

Interventions	Rationales
2. Assess the client's anxiety level. Plan teaching when level is low or moderate.	2. Some fears are based on inaccuracies; accurate information can relieve them. A client with severe or panic anxiety does not retain learning.
3. Encourage family and friends to verbalize fears and concerns.	3. Verbalization allows sharing and provides the nurse with an opportunity to correct misconceptions.
4. Provide the client and family valid reassurance; reinforce positive coping behavior.	4. Praising effective coping can reinforce future positive coping responses.
5. Encourage the client to use relaxation techniques, such as guided imagery and relaxation breathing.	5. These techniques enhance the client's sense of control over her or his body's responses to stress.
6. Contact the physician immediately if the client's anxiety is at severe or panic level. Sedate if necessary.	6. Severe anxiety interferes with learning and compliance and also increases heart rate.
7. Refer also to the nursing diagnosis Anxiety in the Generic Care Plan, for general assessment and interventions.	

Documentation

Progress notes
Present emotional status
Response to interventions
Teaching sheets

Pain Related to Cardiac Tissue Ischemia or Inflammation

NOC Comfort Level, Pain Control

Goal

The client will report satisfactory control of chest pain within an appropriate time frame.

Indicators

* Report pain relief after pain relief measures.
* Demonstrate a relaxed mode.

NIC Pain Management, Medication Management, Emotional Support, Teaching: Individual, Heat/Cold Application, Simple Massage

Interventions	Rationales
1. Instruct the client to immediately report any pain episode.	1. Less pain medication generally is required if administered early. Acute intervention can prevent further ischemia or injury.
2. Administer nitrates and oxygen or analgesics, per physician order. Document administration and degree of relief the client experiences.	2. Severe, persistent pain unrelieved by analgesics may indicate impending or extending infarction.

(continued on page 105)

Interventions	Rationales
3. Instruct the client to rest during a pain episode.	3. Activity increases oxygen demand, which can exacerbate cardiac pain.
4. Reduce environmental distractions as much as possible.	4. Environmental stimulation can increase heart rate and may exacerbate myocardial tissue hypoxia, which increases pain.
5. After acute pain passes, explain its cause and possible precipitating factors (physical and emotional).	5. Calm explanation may reduce the client's stress associated with fear of the unknown.
6. Obtain and evaluate a 12-lead ECG and rhythm strip during pain episodes. If IMMEDIATELY available, do so before nitrates administration. Notify the physician.	6. Cardiac monitoring may help to differentiate variant angina from extension of the infarction.
7. Explain and assist with alternative pain relief measures: a. Positioning b. Distraction (activities, breathing exercises) c. Massage d. Relaxation exercises	7. These measures can help to prevent painful stimuli from reaching higher brain centers by replacing the painful stimuli with another stimulus. Relaxation reduces muscle tension, decreases heart rate, may improve stroke volume, and enhances the client's sense of control over the pain.

Documentation

Graphic/flow record
Medication administration
Progress notes
Unsatisfactory pain relief
Status of pain

Activity Intolerance Related to Insufficient Oxygenation for ADLs Secondary to Cardiac Tissue Ischemia, Prolonged Immobility, Narcotics or Medications

NOC Activity Tolerance

Goal

The client will progress activity to (specify level of activity desired).

Indicators

- Identify factors that increase cardiac workload.
- Demonstrate cardiac tolerance (marked by stable pulse, respiration, and blood pressure) to activity increases.
- Identify methods to reduce activity intolerance.

NIC Activity Therapy, Energy Management, Exercise Promotion, Sleep Enhancement, Mutual Goal Setting

Interventions	Rationales
1. Increase the client's activity each shift, as indicated: a. Allow the client's legs to dangle first while supporting him or her from the side. b. Gradually increase the progression of activities. c. Allow the client to set her or his rate of ambulation. Provide adequate rest periods.	1. Gradual activity progression, directed by the client's tolerance, enhances physiologic functioning and reduces cardiac tissue hypoxia.

(continued on page 106)

Interventions	Rationales
d. Set an increased ambulation distance goal for each shift, as agreed upon with the client. e. Increase activity when pain is at a minimum or after pain relief measures take effect. f. Increase the client's self-care activities from partial to complete self-care, as indicated.	
2. Monitor vital signs: • Before ambulation • During ambulation • Immediately after activity • If pulse rate is 20–30 beats above the baseline at the end of ambulation, monitor vital signs at one-, two-, and three-minute checks.	2. Tolerance to increased activity depends on the client's ability to adapt to the accompanying physiologic requirements. Adaptation requires optimal cardiovascular, pulmonary, neurologic, and musculoskeletal function. The expected immediate physiologic responses to activity include: • Increased pulse rate and strength • Increased systolic blood pressure • Increased respiratory rate and depth After three minutes, pulse should return to within 10 beats/min of the client's resting pulse rate.
3. Assess for abnormal responses to increased activity: a. Tachycardia (20–30 beats above baseline) b. Decreased or no change in systolic blood pressure c. Excessive increase or decrease in respiratory rate d. Failure of pulse to return to near-resting rate within three minutes after activity e. Confusion, vertigo, uncoordinated movements f. Chest pain g. Change in rhythm/ECG pattern h. Dizziness/syncope	3. Abnormal responses indicate intolerance to increased activity.
4. Plan adequate rest periods according to the client's daily schedule.	4. Rest provides the body with intervals of low energy expenditure.
5. Identify and acknowledge the client's progress.	5. Providing incentives can promote a positive attitude and decrease frustration associated with dependency.
6. Take steps to increase the quality and quantity of the client's sleep and rest periods. Make provisions for at least two hours of uninterrupted sleep at night.	6. A person must complete an entire sleep cycle (70–100 min) to feel rested.
7. Instruct the client how to monitor his or her physiologic response to activities postdischarge.	7. This self-monitoring can detect early signs and symptoms of hypoxia.
8. Teach the client how to conserve energy during ADLs, at work, and during recreational activities: a. Explain the need for rest periods both before and after certain activities. b. Instruct the client to stop an activity if fatigue or other signs of cardiac hypoxia occur. c. Instruct the client to consult with the physician or nurse practitioner before increasing activity after discharge.	8. Energy conservation prevents oxygen requirements from exceeding a level that the heart can meet.

Documentation

Graphic/flow record
Vital signs
Ambulation (time, amount)
Progress notes (Teaching sheets)
Abnormal or unexpected response to increased activity

Grieving Related to Actual or Perceived Losses Secondary to Cardiac Condition

NOC Coping, Family Coping, Grief Resolution, Psychosocial Adjustment: Life Change

Goals

The client will express his or her grief freely

Indicators

- Describe the meaning of loss.
- Report an intent to discuss feelings with significant others.

NIC Family Support, Grief Work Facilitation, Coping Enhancement, Anticipatory Guidance, Emotional Support

Interventions	Rationales

1. Provide client opportunities to express feelings:
  a. Discuss the loss openly.
  b. Explain that grief is a normal reaction to a loss.
  c. Explore the client's perception of the loss.
	1. Frequent contact by the nurse indicates acceptance and may facilitate trust. Open communication can help the client work through the grieving process.

2. Encourage the client to use coping strategies that have helped in the past.	2. This strategy helps the client to refocus on problem-solving and enhances his or her sense of control.

3. Promote grief work—the adaptive process of mourning—with each response.
  a. Denial:
    • Explain the presence of denial in the client or a family member to the other members.
    • Do not push the person to move past denial without emotional readiness.
  b. Isolation:
    • Convey acceptance by allowing expressions of grief.
    • Encourage open, honest communication to promote sharing.
    • Reinforce the person's sense of self-worth by allowing privacy when desired.
    • Encourage a gradual return to social activities (e.g., support groups, church activities, etc.).
  c. Depression:
    • Reinforce the person's sense of self-esteem.
    • Identify the level of depression and tailor your approach accordingly.
    • Use empathetic sharing; acknowledge the grief (e.g., "It must be very difficult for you.").
    • Identify any signs of suicidal ideation or behavior (e.g., frequent statements of intent, revealed plan).
  d. Anger:
    • Encourage verbalization of anger.
    • Explain to other family members that the person's anger is an attempt to control his or her environment more closely because of the inability to control the loss.
  e. Guilt:
    • Acknowledge the person's expressed self-view.
    • Encourage the person to focus on positive aspects.
    • Avoid arguing with the person about what she or he should have done differently.
	3. Responses to grief vary. To intervene appropriately, the nurse must recognize and accept each client's individual response.

(continued on page 108)

Interventions	Rationales
f. Fear: • Focus on the present reality, and maintain a safe and secure environment. • Help the person to explore reasons for his or her fears. g. Rejection: • Reassure the person by explaining that this response is normal. • Explain this response to other family members. h. Hysteria: • Reduce environmental stressors (e.g., limit staff, minimize external noise). • Provide a safe, private area to display grief in client's own fashion.	
4. Promote family cohesiveness: a. Support the family at its level of functioning. b. Encourage family members to evaluate their feelings and to support one another.	4. A grieving person often isolates him- or herself physically and especially emotionally. Repression of feelings interferes with family relationships.

Documentation

Progress notes
Present emotional status
Teaching Sheets
Interventions
Client's and family's response to interventions

High Risk for Ineffective Therapeutic Regimen Management Related to Lack of Knowledge of Condition, Hospital Routines (Procedures, Equipment), Treatments, Medications, Diet, Activity Progression, Signs and Symptoms of Complications, Reduction of Risks, Follow-Up Care, and Community Resources

NOC Compliance Behavior, Knowledge: Treatment Regimen, Participation in Health Care Decisions, Treatment Behavior: Illness or Injury

Goal

The goals for this diagnosis represent those associated with discharge planning. Refer to the discharge criteria.

NIC Anticipatory Guidance, Risk Identification, Health Education, Self-Modification Assistance, Learning Facilitation

Interventions	Rationales
1. Explain the pathophysiology of MI using teaching aids appropriate for client's educational level (e.g., pictures, models, written materials).	1. Such explanations reinforce the need to comply with instructions on diet, exercise, and other aspects of the treatment regimen.

(continued on page 109)

Interventions	Rationales
2. Explain risk factors for MI that can be eliminated or modified:	2. Focusing on controllable factors can reduce the client's feelings of powerlessness.
a. Obesity	a. Obesity increases peripheral resistance and cardiac workload. Fifty percent of coronary artery disease in women is attributed to overweight (American Heart Association, 2005). Refer to the obesity care plan.
b. Tobacco use	b. Smoking unfavorably alters lipid levels. It impairs oxygen transport while increasing oxygen demand (Porth, 2007).
c. Diet high in fat or sodium	c. A high-fat diet contributes to plaque formation in the arteries; excessive sodium intake increases water retention.
d. Sedentary life style	d. A sedentary life style leads to poor collateral circulation and predisposes the client to other risk factors.
e. Excessive alcohol intake	e. Alcohol is a potent vasodilator; subsequent vasoconstriction increases cardiac workload.
f. Hypertension	f. Hypertension with increased peripheral resistance damages the arterial intima, which contributes to arteriosclerosis.
g. Oral contraceptives	g. Oral contraceptives alter blood coagulation, platelet function, and fibrinolytic activity, thereby affecting the integrity of the endothelium.
h. Diabetes	h. Elevated glucose levels damage the arterial intima.
3. Teach the client the importance of stress management through relaxation techniques and regular, appropriate exercise.	3. Although the exact effect of stress on CAD is unclear, release of catecholamines elevates systolic blood pressure, increases cardiac workload, induces lipolysis, and promotes platelet clumping (Porth, 2005).
4. Teach the client how to assess radial pulse and instruct her or him to report any of the following: a. Dyspnea b. Chest pain unrelieved by nitroglycerin c. Unexplained weight gain or edema d. Unusual weakness, fatigue e. Irregular pulse or any unusual change	4. These signs and symptoms may indicate myocardial ischemia and vascular congestion (edema) secondary to decreased cardiac output.
5. Instruct the client to report side effects of prescribed medications which may include diuretics, digitalis, beta-adrenergic blocking agents, ACE inhibitors, or aspirin.	5. Recognizing and promptly reporting medication side effects can help to prevent serious complications (e.g., hypokalemia, hypotension).
6. Reinforce the physician's explanation for the prescribed therapeutic diet. Consult with a dietitian, if indicated.	6. Repetitive explanations may help to improve compliance with the therapeutic diet as well as promote understanding.
7. Explain the need for activity restrictions and how activity should progress gradually. Instruct the client to a. Increase activity gradually. b. Avoid isometric exercises and lifting objects weighing more than 30 lbs. c. Avoid jogging, heavy exercise, and sports until the physician advises otherwise. d. Consult with the physician on when to resume work, driving, sexual activity, recreational activities, and travel. e. Take frequent 15- to 20-min rest periods, four to six times a day for one to two months. f. Perform activities at a moderate, comfortable pace; if fatigue occurs, stop and rest for 15 minutes, then continue.	7. Increasing activity gradually allows cardiac tissue to heal and accommodate increased demands. Overexertion increases oxygen consumption and cardiac workload.

(continued on page 110)

Interventions	Rationales

8. When the physician allows the client to resume sexual activity, teach the client to do the following:
  a. Avoid sexual activity in extremes of temperature, immediately after meals (wait two hours), when intoxicated, when fatigued, with an unfamiliar partner or in an unfamiliar environment, and with anal stimulation.
  b. Rest before and after engaging in sexual activity (mornings are the best time)
  c. Terminate sexual activity if chest pain or dyspnea occurs.
  d. Take nitroglycerin before sexual activity, if prescribed.
  e. Use usual positions, unless they increase exertion.
  f. Consult with the physician before using any erectile dysfunction medications (e.g., Viagra, Cialis, Levitra).
	8. To meet the increased myocardial oxygen demands resulting from sexual activity, the client should avoid all situations that cause vasoconstriction and vasodilation, which lead to anal stimulation and decrease heart rate.

9. Reinforce the necessity of follow-up care.	9. Proper follow-up is essential to evaluate if and when progression of activities is advisable.
10. Provide information on community resources such as the American Heart Association, self-help groups, counseling, and cardiac rehabilitation groups.	10. Such resources can provide additional support, information, and follow-up assistance which the client and family may need postdischarge.

Documentation

Discharge summary record
Discharge instructions
Follow-up instructions
   Status at discharge (pain, activity, wound)
   Achievement of goals (individual or family)

Peripheral Arterial Disease (Atherosclerosis)

Atherosclerosis obliterans, a progressive disease, is the leading cause of obstructive arterial disease of the extremities in people older than 30 years. At least 95% of arterial occlusive disease is atherosclerotic in origin.

The World Health Organization describes *atherosclerosis as "a variable combination of changes in the intima of arteries, consisting of the focal accumulation of lipids, complex carbohydrates, blood and blood products, fibrous tissue, and calcium deposits and associated with medial changes."* It is characterized by specific changes in the arterial wall as well as the development of an intraluminal plaque. Atherosclerosis can lead to myocardial infarction, renal hypertension, stroke, and amputation.

The known risk factors for atherosclerosis include hyperlipidemia, smoking history, hypertension, diabetes mellitus, and a family history of strokes or heart attacks, especially at an early age. Altering modifiable risk factors has been shown to reduce significantly the chances of progressing to the morbid consequences of this disease. Teaching the risk factors and modifying behaviors that reduce risk factors are important components of nursing interventions for atherosclerotic disease.

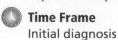

Time Frame
Initial diagnosis

▪▪▪▪▪ DIAGNOSTIC CLUSTER*

Collaborative Problems

PC: Stroke
PC: Ischemic Ulcers
PC: Acute Arterial Thrombosis
PC: Hypertension (refer to Hypertension)

Nursing Diagnoses

Activity Intolerance related to claudication

High Risk for Injury related to effects of orthostatic hypotension

High Risk for Ineffective Therapeutic Regimen Management related to lack of knowledge of condition, management of claudication, risk factors, foot care, and treatment plan

*This medical condition was not included in the validation study.

Discharge Criteria

Before discharge, the client or family will

1. List common risk factors for atherosclerosis.
2. State specific activities to manage claudication.
3. Describe principles and steps of proper foot care.
4. Describe any life style changes indicated (e.g., cessation of smoking, low-fat diet, regular exercise program).
5. State goal to reduce low-density lipoprotein (LDL) cholesterol to less than 100 optimal, 100–129 near optimal/above optimal (NCEP, 3rd Report ATP III).
6. Relate the signs and symptoms that must be reported to a health care professional.
7. Identify community resources available for assistance.

Collaborative Problems

Potential Complication: Stroke
Potential Complication: Ischemic Ulcers
Potential Complication: Acute Arterial Thrombosis

Nursing Goal

The nurse will detect early signs/symptoms of cardiovascular complications and collaboratively intervene to stabilize the client.

Indicators

- BP >90/60, <140/90 mmHg
- Oriented and alert
- Palpable peripheral pulses
- Warm, dry skin
- Intact motor/sensation of extremities
- Ankle-brachial index (difference between the blood pressure of the arm to the ankle. If the ankle pressure is 50% or less than the arm, indicates impaired circulation.)
- Claudication, sudden onset or progressive deterioration.

Interventions	Rationales
1. Teach the client about the signs and symptoms of transient ischemic attack (TIA) and the importance of reporting to the physician if they occur. a. Dizziness, loss of balance, or fainting b. Changes in sensation or motor control in arms or legs c. Numbness in face d. Speech changes e. Visual changes or loss of vision f. Temporary loss of memory	1. The risk of stroke increases in clients who have had a TIA. Disruption of cerebral circulation can result in motor or sensory deficits.
2. Assess for ischemic ulcers in extremities. Report ulcers or darkened spots of skin to the physician.	2. Atherosclerosis causing arterial stenosis and subsequent decreased tissue perfusion interferes with and may prevent healing of skin ulcers. Darkened spots of skin distal to arterial stenosis may indicate tissue infarctions related to ischemia.
3. Reinforce teaching of foot care. (Refer to the nursing diagnosis High Risk for Ineffective Management of Therapeutic Regimen for more information.)	3. Protection from skin loss may preserve tissue by preventing access to infective agents.
4. Monitor peripheral circulation (pulses, sensation, skin color). Report any changes immediately.	4. In acute arterial thrombosis, loss of sensation distal to the thrombosis occurs first with accompanying ischemic pain. This may be followed by a decrease in motor function.

 Related Physician-Prescribed Interventions

Specific interventions also depend on how atherosclerosis affects circulation and renal, cerebral, and cardiac functions.

Refer to specific care plan (e.g., Hypertension, Renal Failure) for more information.

Medications. Vasodilators, adrenergic blocking agents

Intravenous Therapy. Not indicated

Laboratory Studies. Cholesterol levels (LDL/HDL), homocystine levels, triglyccridcs

Diagnostic Studies. Duplex ultrasound, pulse volume recording, magnetic resonance angiography (MRA), angiography, oscillometry, exercise test

Therapies. Angioplasty (selected), stenting, endarterectomy, bypass, pentoxifylline, aspirin, lipid-lowering agents, antiplatelet agents, hemoglobin/hematocrit, plethysmography, low-salt diet, diet designed to decrease saturated fats and lower cholesterol

Documentation

Flow record
  Assessment results
Progress notes
  Changes in condition

Nursing Diagnoses

Activity Intolerance Related to Claudication

NOC Activity Tolerance

Goal

The client will progress activity to (specify level of activity desired).

Indicators

- Identify activities that cause claudication.
- State why pain occurs with activity.
- Develop a plan to increase activity and decrease claudication.

NIC Activity Tolerance, Energy Management, Exercise Promotion, Sleep Enhancement, Mutual Goal Setting

Interventions	Rationales
1. Teach the client about the physiology of blood supply in relation to activity and the pathophysiology of claudication.	1. The client's understanding of the condition may promote compliance with restrictions and the exercise program.
2. Reassure the client that activity does not harm the claudicating tissue.	2. The client may be tempted to discontinue activity when pain occurs in an attempt to avoid further injury.

3. Plan activities to include a scheduled ambulation time:
  a. Institute a daily walking regimen of at least 30 minutes.
  b. Teach client to "walk into" the pain, to pause when claudication occurs, and then to continue as soon as discomfort disappears.
  c. Start slowly.
  d. Emphasize that the *action* of walking is important, not the speed or distance.
	3. A regimented exercise program can help develop collateral blood flow and ameliorate claudication.

4. Have the client keep a continuous written record of actual activities and distances. Review it to evaluate his or her progress.	4. Self-reports of activity have low reliability.

5. Provide information on antiplatelet medications, as prescribed. Explain the following:
  a. Drug action
  b. The drug does not reduce the need for other activities to reduce risk factors.
  c. An immediate effect should not be expected because it takes from four to six weeks of therapy to determine effectiveness.
	5. These medications reportedly improve red blood cell flexibility, decrease platelet aggregation, and improve vascular vasodilatation.

Documentation

Discharge summary record
  Client teaching
  Outcome achievement or status
  Referrals

High Risk for Injury Related to Effects of Orthostatic Hypotension

NOC Risk Control, Safety Status: Falls Occurrence

Goal

The client will relate fewer episodes of dizziness.

Indicators

- State the relationship of blood pressure changes to symptoms.
- State activities that cause orthostatic hypotension.
- Plan activities to reduce symptoms of orthostatic hypotension.

NIC   Fall Prevention, Environmental Management:
Safety, Health Education, Surveillance:
Safety, Risk Identification

Interventions	Rationales
1. Teach the client about the nature of orthostatic hypotension and its probable causes. Explain that the change to an upright position normally causes a decrease in venous return and cardiac output (caused by venous pooling) of 500 mL to 1 liter of blood in the legs. The corresponding drop in blood pressure stimulates baroreceptors, causing venous and arterial constriction and an increase in heart rate through increased sympathetic activity.	1. Understanding orthostatic hypotension may help the client to modify behavior to reduce the frequency and severity of episodes.
2. If brachial pressures between the arms differ, explain the need to use one arm consistently for blood pressure measurement.	2. Use of the arm with the higher pressure gives a more accurate assessment of the mean blood pressure.
3. Instruct the client to avoid prolonged bed rest, and to rise in stages from the supine to the standing position—first with one leg dependent, then the other.	3. Prolonged bed rest increases venous pooling. Gradual position change allows the body to compensate for venous pooling.
4. Teach the client to maintain adequate hydration especially in summer months or in hot, dry climates.	4. Adequate hydration is necessary to prevent decreased circulating volume.
5. Refer to a physician if you suspect that a prescribed medication may be responsible for the symptoms.	5. Certain medications (e.g., vasodilators and antihistamines) can precipitate orthostatic hypotension.
6. Teach to prevent postprandial hypotension (Miller, 2004): a. Take hypertensive medications after meals. b. Eat small, frequent meals. c. Remain seated or lie down after meals. d. Avoid excessive alcohol intake.	6. Studies have shown a blood pressure reduction of 20 mmHg within one hour of eating the morning or noon meal in healthy, older adults. This is thought to be due to impaired baroreflex compensatory response to splanchnic blood pooling during digestion (Miller, 2004).
7. Instruct the client to avoid hot baths or showers.	7. External heat may dilate the superficial vessels sufficiently to shunt blood from the brain, causing neurologic symptoms.
8. If a pressure (40–50 mmHg) support garment (waist-high stocking) is prescribed, teach the client how to use it properly. Instruct the client to put on the garment early in the day and to avoid sitting while wearing it.	8. This device reduces venous pooling by applying constant pressure over the leg surface. Elastic compression garments are easier to put on in the morning, before gravity causes increased edema. Bending at the groin and the knee causes garment constriction and increases pressure.
9. Teach the client to sleep with pillows under the head.	9. Decreasing the contrast between the supine and upright positions helps to decrease the amount of intravascular fluid shift with position changes.

Documentation

Progress notes
Episodes of vertigo
Client teaching and response
Application of support garment

High Risk for Ineffective Therapeutic Regimen Management Related to Lack of Knowledge of Condition, Management of Claudication, Risk Factors, Foot Care, and Treatment Plan

NOC Compliance Behavior, Knowledge: Treatment Regimen, Participation in Health Care Decisions, Treatment Behavior: Illness or Injury

Goal

The outcome criteria for this diagnosis represent those associated with discharge planning. Refer to the discharge criteria.

NIC Anticipatory Guidance, Risk Identification, Health Education, Learning Facilitation

Interventions	Rationales
1. Explain atherosclerosis and its effects on cardiac, circulatory, renal, and neurologic functions.	1. Health education offers clients some control over the direction of their disease.
2. Briefly explain the relationship of certain risk factors to the development of atherosclerosis: a. Smoking • Vasoconstriction • Decreased blood oxygenation • Elevated blood pressure • Increased lipidemia • Increased platelet aggregation b. Hypertension • Constant trauma of pressure causes vessel lining damage, which promotes plaque formation and narrowing. c. Hyperlipidemia • Promotes atherosclerosis d. Sedentary life style • Decreases muscle tone and strength • Decreases circulation e. Excess weight (>10% of ideal) • Fatty tissue increases peripheral resistance. • Fatty tissue is less vascular.	2. a. The effects of nicotine on the cardiovascular system contribute to coronary artery disease, stroke, hypertension, and peripheral vascular disease. b. Changes in arterial walls increase the incidence of stroke and coronary artery disease (Porth, 2005). c. High circulating lipids increase the risk of coronary heart disease, peripheral vascular disease, and stroke. d. Lack of exercise inhibits the pumping action of muscles that enhance circulation. With peripheral vascular disease, exercise promotes collateral circulation. e. Overweight increases cardiac work load, thus causing hypertension.
3. Encourage the client to share feelings, concerns, and understanding of risk factors, disease process, and effects on life.	3. This dialogue will provide data to assist with goal setting.
4. Assist the client to select life style behaviors that he or she chooses to change (Burch, 1991). a. Avoid multiple changes. b. Consider personal abilities, resources, and overall health. c. Be realistic and optimistic.	4. An older client may have life style patterns of inactivity, smoking, and high-fat diet.
5. Assist the client to set goal(s) and the steps to achieve them (e.g., will walk 30 minutes daily.) a. Will walk 10 minutes daily. b. Will walk 10 minutes daily and 20 minutes three times a week. c. Will walk 20 minutes daily. d. Will walk two minutes daily and 30 minutes three times a week.	5. Attaining short-term goals can foster motivation to continue the process.

(continued on page 116)

Interventions	Rationales
6. Suggest a method to self-monitor progress (e.g., graph, checklist).	6. A structured monitoring system increases client involvement beyond the goal-setting stage.
7. Provide specific information to achieve selected goals (e.g., self-help programs, referrals, techniques).	7. The educational program should not overload the client.
8. If appropriate, refer to Obesity Care Plan for additional interventions in weight loss and exercise.	
9. Explain the risks that atherosclerotic disease poses to the feet: a. Diabetes-related peripheral neuropathy and micro-vascular disease b. Pressure ulcers	9. Understanding may encourage compliance with necessary life style changes. a. Diabetes accelerates the atherosclerotic process. Diabetic neuropathy prevents the client from feeling ischemic or injured areas. b. Healing of open lesions requires approximately 10 times the blood supply necessary to keep live tissue intact.
10. Teach foot care measures. a. Daily inspection • Use a mirror. • Look for corns, calluses, bunions, scratches, redness, and blisters. • If vision is poor, have a family member or other person inspect the feet. b. Daily washing • Use warm, not hot, water (check the water temperature with the hand or elbow before immersing feet). • Avoid prolonged soaking. • Dry well, especially between the toes. c. Proper foot hygiene • Clip nails straight across; use an emery board to smooth edges. • Avoid using any chemicals on corns or calluses. • Avoid using antiseptics, such as iodine. • If feet are dry, apply a thin coat of lotion. Avoid getting lotion between the toes.	10. a. Daily foot care can reduce tissue damage and helps to prevent or detect early further injury and infection. b. • This will prevent burning in sensitive tissue. • This can macerate tissue. • They can cause an injury that will not heal. • These can damage healthy tissue.
11. Teach the client to a. Avoid hot water bottles and heating pads. b. Wear wool socks to warm the feet at night. c. Wear warm foot covering before going out in cold weather (wool socks and lined boots). d. Avoid walking barefoot.	11. These precautions help to reduce the risk of injury.
12. Instruct the client to wear well-fitting leather shoes (may require shoes made with extra depth), to always wear socks with the shoes, to avoid sandals with straps between the toes, and to inspect the insides of the shoes daily for worn areas, protruding nails, or other objects.	12. Well-fitting shoes help to prevent injury to skin and underlying tissue.
13. Teach the client to a. Wear socks that fit well. b. Avoid socks with elastic bands. c. Avoid sock garters. d. Avoid crossing the legs.	13. Tight garments and certain leg positions constrict the leg vessels, which further reduces circulation.

(continued on page 117)

Interventions	Rationales
14. Emphasize the importance of visiting a podiatrist for nail/callus/corn care if the client has poor vision or any difficulty with self-care.	14. The client may require assistance with foot care to ensure adequate care and prevent self-inflicted injuries.
15. Explain that if the client cannot inspect his or her feet, he or she should arrange for another person to inspect them regularly.	15. Daily inspection helps to ensure early detection of skin or tissue damage.
16. Identify available community resources.	16. They can assist with weight loss, smoking cessation, diet, and exercise programs.

Documentation

Discharge summary record
    Client teaching
    Outcome achievement or status
    Referrals when indicated

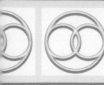

RESPIRATORY DISORDERS

 ## Asthma

Asthma is a chronic disorder of airway inflammation and bronchial hyperactivity characterized symptomatically by cough, chest tightness, shortness of breath, increased sputum production, and wheezing as a result of decreased airflow. In 2001, almost 31 million people had been diagnosed with asthma at some time. The prevalence is greater in children than in adults, and in boys than in girls, but greater in women than in men, and is the primary chronic childhood illness (Polgar Bailey, 2008). Exposure to common aeroallergens (e.g., animal dander, tobacco smoke, dust, molds) can trigger an acute episode up to 24 hours after exposure (Sims, 2006). Additional triggers include emotional and hormonal changes, cold temperatures, certain exercise activities, and viral or occupational exposures (Porth, 2005).

Many people ignore the seriousness of this disease. Frequent hospitalizations result from disregarding the warning signs of impending asthma attacks and noncompliance with the therapeutic regimen. Status asthmaticus refers to a severe case of asthma that does not respond to conventional treatment. This life-threatening situation requires prompt action.

⏱ Time Frame
Acute episode

■■■■■ DIAGNOSTIC CLUSTER

Collaborative Problems

▲ PC: Hypoxemia
△ PC: Acute Respiratory Failure
△ PC: Status Asthmaticus

Nursing Diagnoses	Refer to
▲ Ineffective Airway Clearance related to increased mucus production, tenacious secretions, and bronchospasm	
△ High Risk for Ineffective Therapeutic Regimen Management related to lack of knowledge of condition, treatment, prevention of infection, breathing exercises, risk factors, and signs and symptoms of impending attack	
△ Anxiety related to breathlessness and fear of suffocation	Chronic Obstructive Pulmonary Disease
✳ Powerlessness related to feeling of loss of control and restrictions that this condition places on life style	Chronic Obstructive Pulmonary Disease
✳ High Risk for Ineffective Breathing Pattern related to increased work of breathing, hypoxemia, agitation, and impending respiratory failure	Mechanical Ventilation

▲ This diagnosis was reported to be monitored for or managed frequently (75%–100%).
△ This diagnosis was reported to be monitored for or managed often (50%–74%).
✳ This diagnosis was not included in the validation study.

Collaborative Problems

Potential Complication: Hypoxemia
Potential Complication: Respiratory Failure
Potential Complication: Status Asthmaticus

Nursing Goal

The nurse will detect early signs/symptoms of hypoxemia and respiratory failure and collaboratively intervene to stabilize client.

Indicators

- Serum pH 7.35–7.45
- Serum PCO_2 35–45 mmHg
- Pulse: regular rhythm, rate 60–100 beats/min
- Blood pressure: >90/60, <140–90 mmHg
- Urine output >5 mL/kg/h
- Alert, oriented
- No abnormal breath sounds
- Oxygen saturation >95% (pulse oximetry)

Interventions	Rationales
1. Obtain a thorough history from either the client or family (medications and frequency of short-acting β_2 agonist use).	1. History-taking is an essential factor in the treatment of asthma. Points to focus on are: What triggered the event? What methods have been used to alleviate the symptoms? Did they work? What medications are generally prescribed? What stimulants exacerbate the asthma? How long did the client wait before seeking treatment?
2. Monitor for signs and symptoms of acid–base imbalance: a. Initially pH >7.45, PCO_2 <35 mmHg (alkalemia); look for decompensation: pH <7.35, PCO_2 >45 mmHg (acidemia)	2. a. Acid–base analysis helps to evaluate gas exchange in the lungs. Anxiety and air hunger will lead to an increase in the respiratory rate. In severe cases, a decreased PO_2 will lead to hypoxemia. Respiratory alkalosis will be exhibited. In status asthmaticus the client will tire and air trapping will worsen. Acid–base results will return to baseline, which is an ominous sign. The PCO_2 will then rise quickly. Respiratory acidosis and failure will result. Intubation will be required (Porth, 2005).
b. Increased/decreased blood pressure c. Monitor intake and output d. Cool, pale, cyanotic skin	b,c,d. First the client will have an elevated blood pressure resulting from anxiety and feelings of air hunger. As the client's condition and air trapping worsen, pressure in the thoracic cavity will increase, which decreases venous return. Thus the client will then exhibit a decrease in blood pressure and the signs and symptoms of decreased cardiac output.
e. Tachypnea and dyspnea at rest. Respiratory rate >20 breaths/min.	e. The client experiences dyspnea because of narrowed passages and air trapping related to bronchospasms (Porth, 2005).
f. Evaluate overall appearance	f. The client, often sitting while leaning forward, may appear anxious, diaphoretic, and restless. He or she may appear to be gulping air. Also, an increased anteroposterior diameter and a lowered diaphragm will be noted because of hyperinflation of the lungs. As breathing becomes more labored, use of shoulder, neck, and intercostal muscles will be evident.

(continued on page 120)

Interventions	Rationales
g. Abnormal breath sounds	g. Auscultation of the chest is often misleading. Initially, wheezing may be heard throughout all lung fields during both phases of respiration. As airflow becomes restricted because of severe obstruction and mucus secretion, breath sounds become diminished or absent. This is a sign of impending respiratory failure.
h. Cough	h. For some clients with asthma, cough may be their only symptom. Spasmodic contractions of the bronchi produce the cough.
i. Changes in mental status	i. The client is often anxious and restless. However, changes in mentation reflect changes in oxygenation. Confusion, agitation, and lethargy are signs of imminent respiratory failure.
3. Administer O_2 via nasal cannula.	3. Hypoxemia is common due to ventilation/perfusion disturbances. Air trapping and increased respiratory rate impede gas exchange. PO_2 <60 mmHg requires supplemental oxygen. Administration of O_2 via nasal cannula is preferred to reduce the client's feelings of suffocation. In severe cases, however, intubation and mechanical ventilation may be required.
4. Administer intravenous hydration.	4. Excess mucus production is common. Adequate hydration prevents dehydration and enhances clearance of secretions. Daily fluid intake of two to four liters is recommended.
5. Obtain sputum specimen.	5. Sputum is generally clear, mucoid, or white during exacerbation of asthma. Discoloration of sputum can be indicative of infection. Administration of antihistamines and decongestants is common to decrease mucus production.
6. Monitor for GI reflux	6. GI reflux commonly triggers bronchospasm, even during sleep (Porth, 2005).
7. Assess pulmonary function.	7. Examining pulmonary function aids in determining the degree of destruction and responsiveness to treatment. Forced expiratory volume (FEV-1) measures the force of exhaled air. An FEV-1 <1000 mL or 25% of the client's normal predicted value indicates a severe obstruction. Pulsus paradoxus (a decrease in the systolic blood pressure of 12 mmHg during inspiration) is associated with breathing and is assessed to determine responsiveness to treatment. A decrease in pulsus paradoxus reflects favorable responsiveness to treatment.
8. Identify and eliminate stimulants.	8. Irritants such as smoke, pollen, and dusts may exacerbate asthma. Avoidance of environmental stimulants should be stressed.
9. Administer sedatives, as ordered.	9. Clients are often anxious, which intensifies the situation. Sedatives aid in minimizing anxiety and decreasing the respiratory rate. A decreased respiratory rate increases exhalation, enhancing gas exchange and correcting respiratory alkalosis.
10. Monitor for status asthmaticus: • Labored breathing • Prolonged exhalation • Engorged neck veins • Wheezing	10. Status asthmaticus does not respond to conventional therapy. As status asthmaticus worsens, the $PaCO_2$ increases and pH falls. The extent of wheezing does not indicate the severity of the attack (Porth, 2005).

(continued on page 121)

Interventions	Rationales
11. Evaluate level of hypoxia with arterial blood gases and (PCO₂, PaO₂, pH, SaO₂) pulse oximetry.	11. During an acute episode, the PaO_2 and serum pH will decrease. Blood gases will show respiratory alkalosis in the early stages of an asthma attack, and then move toward a neutral pH. As the episode intensifies in severity, blood gases will confirm respiratory acidosis, paralleling the rising $PaCO_2$. An electrocardiogram may show dysrhythmias, or ischemia (Sims, 2006)
12. Initiate treatment: a. O₂ low-flow humidified oxygen with Venturi mask or nasal catheter b. Nebulizer treatment with albuterol c. Intravenous fluids d. Corticosteroids e. Possible mechanical ventilation	12. Ventilation perfusion abnormality results in hypoxemia and respiratory alkalosis, followed by respiratory acidosis (Porth, 2005). a. Oxygen therapy is needed to treat dyspnea, cyanosis, and hypoxemia. b. The nebulizer disperses a bronchodilator into microscopic particles that reach the lungs with inhalations. c. Fluid intake is critical to prevent dehydration and to facilitate expectoration by liquefying the secretions d. Corticosteroids may be administered parenterally to reduce inflammation of the airways. e. Respiratory acidosis is tiring; mechanical ventilation may be required. (Refer to Care Plan for Mechanical Ventilation, if needed.)
13. Provide a quiet environment and eliminate environmental respiratory irritants (flowers, perfumes, cleaning agent odors, tobacco smoke [direct or on clothes]).	13. Irritants will aggravate an already compromised respiratory status.
14. Monitor for medication side effects.	14. Many side effects of asthma medications are treatable by altering the regime, thereby increasing compliance.

Related Physician-Prescribed Interventions

Medications. β₂ agonists (short- or long-acting; inhaled or oral), anticholinergics, glucosteroids (inhaled, oral, intravenous in acute stages), cromolyn sodium (nonsteroidal anti-inflammatory drug), antimicrobials, sympathomimetics, sedatives, theophylline (rarely) (Sims, 2006), leukotriene synthesis inhibitors and receptor antagonists, anti-IgE antibody therapy, phosphodiesterase (PDE) inhibitors.

The drugs utilized are dependent on the indication: albuterol, a short-acting β₂ agonist, is used for acute episodes, but long-acting β₂ agonists, such as salmeterol, are prescribed for disease maintenance.

Intravenous Therapy. 2–4 L/day

Laboratory Studies. Arterial blood gas analysis, sputum culture, electrolytes, serum IgE levels, complete blood count (CBC) with differential

Diagnostic Studies. Pulmonary function tests, chest x-rays, electrocardiogram, allergy skin testing, incentive spirometry, x-ray or MRI of sinuses

Therapies. Oxygen therapies, high-flow nebulizers, chest physiotherapy

Nursing Diagnoses

Ineffective Airway Clearance Related to Increased Mucus Production, Tenacious Secretions, and Bronchospasm

NOC Aspiration Control, Respiratory Status: Airway Patency

Goal

The client will no longer aspirate.

Indicators

- Assume comfortable position that facilitates increased air exchange.
- Demonstrate effective coughing.
- Relate strategies to decrease tenacious secretions.

 NIC Cough Enhancement, Airway Suctioning, Positioning, Energy Management

Interventions	Rationales

1. Instruct the client on the proper method of controlled coughing:
  a. Breathe deeply and slowly while sitting up as high as possible.
  b. Use diaphragmatic breathing.
  c. Hold the breath for three to five seconds, then slowly exhale as much as possible through the mouth (the lower rib cage and abdomen should sink).
  d. Take a second breath, hold, and cough from the chest (not from the back of the mouth or throat) using two short, forceful coughs.
  e. Demonstrate pursed-lip breathing.
	1. Uncontrolled coughing is tiring and ineffective, leading to frustration.
	  a. Sitting high shifts the abdominal organs away from the lungs, enabling greater expansion.
	  b. Diaphragmatic breathing reduces the respiratory rate and increases alveolar ventilation.
	  c,d. Increasing the air volume in the lungs promotes expulsion of secretions.
	
	  e. Pursed-lip breathing prolongs exhalation and decreases air trapping.

2. Teach the client measures to reduce the viscosity of secretions:
  a. Maintain adequate hydration: Increase fluid intake two to four liters a day, if not contraindicated by decreased cardiac output or renal disease.
  b. Maintain adequate humidity of inspired air.
  c. Avoid environmental stimulants.
	2. Thick secretions are difficult to expectorate and can cause mucus plugs, which can lead to atelectasis.

3. Auscultate the lungs before and after treatment.	3. This assessment helps to evaluate treatment effectiveness.
4. Encourage or provide good mouth care.	4. Good oral hygiene promotes a sense of well-being and prevents mouth odor.

Documentation

Progress notes
  Effectiveness of cough
  Description of sputum
  Lung assessment
  Quality and workload of respirations

High Risk for Ineffective Therapeutic Regimen Management Related to Lack of Knowledge of Condition, Treatment, Prevention of Infection, Breathing Exercises, Risk Factors, and Signs and Symptoms of Impending Attack

NOC Compliance Behavior, Knowledge: Treatment Regimen, Participation in Health Care Decisions, Treatment Behavior: Illness or Injury

Goal

The goals for this diagnosis represent those associated with discharge planning. Refer to discharge criteria.

NIC Anticipatory Guidance, Risk Identification, Health Education,
Learning Facilitation

Interventions	Rationales
1. Help the client to formulate and accept realistic short- and long-term goals.	1. This may help the client to realize his or her control over life and make choices to improve his or her quality of life.
2. Teach the client about the diagnosis and treatment regimen.	2. Understanding may help to encourage compliance and participation in self-care.
3. Teach the client measures to manage asthma and prevent hospitalization:. a. Eat a well-balanced diet. b. Have sufficient rest. c. Increase activities gradually. d. Avoid exposure to: • Smoke • Dust • Severe air pollution • Extremely cold or warm temperatures	3. a,b,c. These practices promote overall good health and increase the resistance to infection. d. Exposure to these respiratory irritants can cause bronchospasm and increase mucus production. Smoking destroys the ciliary cleansing mechanism of the respiratory tract. Heat raises the body temperature and increases the body's oxygen requirements, possibly exacerbating the symptoms.
4. Teach and have the client demonstrate breathing exercises: a. Use incentive spirometer. b. Assume a leaning-forward position. c. Use pursed-lip breathing.	4. Clients experiencing asthma frequently become anxious and assume an ineffective breathing pattern. Decreasing labored breathing through positioning and effective breathing patterns may reduce asthmatic episodes and prevent hospitalization. a. Incentive spirometry encourages deep, sustained inspiratory efforts. b. Leaning forward enhances diaphragmatic excursions and diminishes the use of accessory muscles. c. Pursed-lip breathing prolongs exhalation, which prevents air trapping and air gulping.
5. Explain the hazards of infection and ways to reduce the risk: a. Avoid contact with infected persons. b. Receive immunization against influenza and bacterial pneumonia, if indicated. c. Take antibiotics, if prescribed. d. Adhere to medications and hydration schedule.	5. a. Upper respiratory infections can cause airway narrowing and inflammation. b. Influenza vaccines will decrease the likelihood of contracting the flu, or decrease the severity of the occurrence. Clients with asthma should receive the inactivated form only (Bailey, 2008). c. In addition to infection, yellow or green sputum may also be due to eosinophil peroxidase, which enhances destruction of bacteria (Bailey, 2008). d. Compliance with these regimes improves outcomes.
6. Instruct the client to report: a. Change in sputum characteristics or failure of sputum to return to usual color after three days of antibiotic therapy b. Elevated body temperature c. Increase in cough, weakness, or shortness of breath d. Weight gain or swelling in ankles and feet	6. Upper respiratory infections (URI) are associated with asthma. Viral infections are the most common culprit. It is thought that the URI causes inflammation of the bronchial tree, leading to bronchoconstriction and air trapping. a. Sputum changes may indicate an infection or resistance of the infective organism to the prescribed antibiotic. b. Circulating pathogens stimulate the hypothalamus to elevate body temperature. c. Hypoxia is chronic; exacerbations must be detected early to prevent complications. In addition to infection, yellow or green sputum may also be due to eosinophil peroxidase which enhances destruction of bacteria (Bailey, 2008). d. These signs may indicate fluid retention secondary to pulmonary arterial hypertension and decreased cardiac output.

(continued on page 124)

Interventions	Rationales
7. The client should seek medical attention if asthma is not relieved after using method outlined in the client therapeutic regimen.	7. Unrelieved symptoms of asthma may lead to status asthmaticus. It is documented that clients with asthma repeatedly ignore the warning signs and seek medical attention only when the condition becomes life-threatening.
8. Teach and observe proper use of a hand-held inhaler and nebulizer. a. For inhalers: • Shake canister. • Blow out air. • Put inhaler to mouth, release medication, and breathe in deeply. • Hold breath for 10 seconds; then exhale slowly. • Wait one minute, then repeat. • Rinse mouth if using a corticosteroid inhaler. • Add a spacer if needed. b. For nebulizer: • Follow directions for assembly. • Using mouthpiece or mask, slowly take deep breaths and exhale. • When mist is gone, stop treatment.	8. Accurate instructions can help to prevent medication overdose. Improper use of inhalers has been outlined as an antecedent of asthma. Clients tend to overuse inhalers, which leads to inhaler ineffectiveness.
9. Develop an exercise routine.	9. Exercise increases the client's stamina. Warn the client that improper exercise may also trigger asthma. Instruct the client to avoid exercising in extremely hot or cold weather. Wearing a paper mask may reduce the sensitivity to stimulants. Emphasize the importance of a cool-down period. Suggest swimming and exercising indoors to avoid exposure to stimulants.
10. Enlist the client to create a management plan: a. Instruct the client to keep a diary of peak flows for at least seven days (every morning and at bedtime). b. If β-antagonist inhaler is needed, measure peak flow before and after using, and document. c. Determine the client's personal best peak flow. d. Calculate zones for management: • Green: 80%–100% of personal best • Yellow: 50%–80% of personal best • Red: <50% of personal best e. Instruct the client what to do in response to peak flow in yellow: • $β_2$-Antagonist inhaler: Call primary care provider (PCP) if response is incomplete. • Instruct the client to contact PCP if the peak flow <70% of baseline (yellow zone; Bailey, 2008) • Instruct the client to treat a peak flow <60% of baseline (yellow zone) as a severe attack (Sims, 2006) f. Instruct the client to go to emergency room if response to initial therapy or if peak flow is <50% of baseline (red zone).	10. Individuals are taught the warning signs and seek medical attention when the condition becomes life-threatening.
11. Instruct the client to reduce irritants at home: a. Eliminate smoking and smoke on clothes around the affected person. b. Remove carpets from the bedroom. c. Avoid pets at home (at least keep them out of bedroom).	11. These are known triggers.

(continued on page 125)

Interventions	Rationales
d. Vacuum and dust regularly when affected person is not present. e. Avoid people with colds and perfume. f. Reduce exposure to high ozone levels and high humidity. g. Eliminate insects and mold in home. h. Avoid food containing metabisulfate preservatives (e.g., beer, wine, deli meats). i. Caution client about use of aspirin, nonsteroidal anti-inflammatory drugs, and ophthalmic β-antagonists.	
12. Instruct the client on the use of inhalers: a. Use controller medications (oral, inhalers) every day (e.g., inhaled steroids, leukotriene-receptor antagonists). b. Use quick-relief or rescuer inhaler, as needed. c. Instruct the client to call primary health care provider if using the rescuer inhaler more than twice a week, or awakening with symptoms of asthma more than twice a month.	12. a,b. Proper use of inhalers will promote control. c. Asthma is not under control; a reevaluation is needed.

Documentation

Discharge summary record
    Client teaching
    Outcome achievement or status
    Referrals if indicated

Chronic Obstructive Pulmonary Disease

Chronic obstructive pulmonary disease (COPD) refers to a group of disorders that cause airway obstruction, including chronic bronchitis, emphysema, bronchiectasis, and asthma. More than 14 million Americans have COPD, most commonly caused by cigarette smoking. COPD is now the fourth leading cause of death (Porth, 2005) and the second leading cause of disability in the United States (Boardman, 2008).

Chronic bronchitis and bronchiectasis are characterized by excessive bronchial mucus production and cough caused by chronic inflammation of the bronchioles and hypertrophy and hyperplasia of the mucous glands. In emphysema, airway obstruction is caused by hyperinflation of the alveoli, loss of lung tissue elasticity, and narrowing of small airways. Asthma is characterized by narrowing of the bronchial airways.

COPD most commonly results from chronic irritation by chemical irritants (industrial, tobacco), air pollution, or recurrent respiratory tract infections. Acute exacerbations are usually due to infection or exposure to allergens and pollutants.

Effective education has been proven recently to have a profound role in the decrease in patient morbidity, due to the resultant behavior modification (Boardman, 2008). Clients and families who understand the disease process and the rationales for the interventions more readily recognize the signs of COPD and are able to more effectively implement appropriate therapies and achieve optimal health. This is particularly true of formal exercise programs.

 Time Frame
Acute episode (nonintensive care)

■■■■■ **DIAGNOSTIC CLUSTER**

Collaborative Problems

▲ PC: Hypoxemia
▲ PC: Right-Sided Heart Failure

Nursing Diagnoses

▲ Ineffective Airway Clearance related to excessive and tenacious secretions

▲ Activity Intolerance related to fatigue and inadequate oxygenation for activities

▲ Anxiety related to breathlessness and fear of suffocation

△ Powerlessness related to feelings of loss of control and life style restrictions

△ Disturbed Sleep Pattern related to cough, inability to assume recumbent position, environmental stimuli

△ High Risk for Imbalanced Nutrition: Less Than Body Requirements related to anorexia secondary to dyspnea, halitosis, and fatigue (refer to Pressure Ulcers)

▲ High Risk for Ineffective Therapeutic Regimen Management related to lack of knowledge of condition, treatments, prevention of infection, breathing exercises, risk factors, signs and symptoms of complications

▲ This diagnosis was reported to be monitored for or managed frequently (75%–100%).
△ This diagnosis was reported to be monitored for or managed often (50%–74%).

Discharge Criteria

Before discharge, the client or family will

1. Identify long- and short-term goals to modify risk factors (e.g., diet, smoking, exercise).
2. Identify adjustments needed to maintain self-care.
3. State how to prevent further pulmonary deterioration.
4. State signs and symptoms that must be reported to a health care professional.
5. Identify community resources that can provide assistance with home management.

Collaborative Problems

Potential Complication: Hypoxemia

Potential Complication: Right-Sided Heart Failure

Nursing Goal

The nurse will detect early signs/symptoms of hypoxia and heart failure and collaboratively intervene to stabilize the client.

Indicators

- Serum pH 7.35–7.45
- Serum PCO_2 35–45 mmHg
- Pulse: regular rhythm and rate 60–100 beats/min
- Respiration 16–20 breaths/min
- Blood pressure <140/90, >90/60 mmHg
- Urine output >30 mL/h

Interventions	Rationales
1. Monitor for signs of acid–base imbalance: a. Arterial blood gas (ABG) analysis: pH <7.35 and PCO_2 >46 mmHg	1. a. ABG analysis helps to evaluate gas exchange in the lungs. In mild to moderate COPD, the client may have a normal $PaCO_2$ level because of chemoreceptors in the medulla responding to increased $PaCO_2$ by increasing ventilation. In severe COPD, the client cannot sustain this increased ventilation and the $PaCO_2$ value increases.
b. Increased and irregular pulse c. Increased respiratory rate, followed by decreased rate	b,c. Respiratory acidosis develops due to excessive CO_2 retention. The client with respiratory acidosis from chronic disease at first increases heart rate and respiration in an attempt to compensate for decreased oxygenation. After a while, the client breathes more slowly and with prolonged expiration. Eventually, the client's respiratory center may stop responding to the higher CO_2 levels, and breathing may stop abruptly.
d. Changes in mentation e. Decreased urine output (<30 mL/h) f. Cool, pale, or cyanotic skin	d. Changes in mentation result from cerebral tissue hypoxia. e,f. The compensatory response to decreased circulatory oxygen is to increase blood oxygen by increasing heart and respiratory rates and to decrease circulation to the kidneys and to the extremities (marked by decreased pulse and skin changes).
2. Administer low-flow (2 L/min) oxygen, as needed, through a cannula.	2. This measure increases circulating oxygen levels. Higher flow rates increase carbon dioxide retention. The use of a cannula rather than a mask reduces the client's fears of suffocation.
3. Obtain a sputum sample for culture and sensitivity.	3. Sputum culture and sensitivity determine if an infection is contributing to the symptoms.
4. Eliminate smoke and strong odors in the client's room.	4. Irritants to the respiratory tract can exacerbate the symptoms.
5. Monitor electrocardiogram (ECG) for dysrhythmias secondary to altered arterial blood gases (ABGs).	5. ABG alterations may precipitate cardiac dysrhythmias.
6. Monitor for signs of right-sided heart failure: a. Elevated diastolic pressure b. Distended neck veins c. Peripheral edema d. Elevated central venous pressure (CVP)	6. The combination of arterial hypoxemia and respiratory acidosis acts locally as a strong vasoconstrictor of pulmonary vessels. This leads to pulmonary arterial hypertension, increased right ventricular systolic pressure, and, eventually, right ventricular hypertrophy and failure.
7. Refer to the Heart Failure care plan for additional interventions if right-sided failure occurs.	
8. Refer to thoracotomy if surgery is planned.	

 Related Physician-Prescribed Interventions

Medications. Methylxanthines (IV), anticholinergics (inhaled), bronchodilators (inhaled), adrenergics, corticosteroids (oral, inhaled, IV), antimicrobials, sympathomimetics (inhaled), mucoactives, antitussives (nonnarcotic)

Intravenous Therapy. Variable, depending on mode of medication administration

Laboratory Studies. ABG analysis, electrolytes, serum albumin, liver function studies, sputum culture, complete blood count (CBC) with differential

Diagnostic Studies. Chest x-ray film, pulmonary function tests, bronchography, stress test

Therapies. Intermittent positive-pressure breathing (IPPB), chest physiotherapy, low oxygen through a cannula, ultrasonic nebulizer

Documentation

Flow record
   Vital signs
   Intake and output
   Assessment data
Progress notes
   Change in status
   Interventions
   Client's response to interventions

Nursing Diagnoses

Ineffective Airway Clearance Related to Excessive and Tenacious Secretions

NOC Aspiration Control, Respiratory Status: Airway Patency

Goal

The client will no longer aspirate.

Indicators

• Demonstrate effective coughing and increased air exchange in lungs.
• Relate strategies to decrease tenacious secretions.

NIC Cough Enhancement, Airway Suctioning, Positioning, Energy Management

Interventions	Rationales
1. Instruct the client on the proper method of controlled coughing: a. Breathe deeply and slowly while sitting up as high as possible. b. Use diaphragmatic breathing. c. Hold the breath for three to five seconds, then slowly exhale as much as possible through the mouth (the lower rib cage and abdomen should sink in the process). d. Take a second breath, hold, and cough from the chest (not from the back of the mouth or throat) using two short, forceful coughs.	1. Uncontrolled coughing is tiring and ineffective, leading to frustration. a. Sitting high shifts the abdominal organs away from the lungs, enabling greater expansion. b. Diaphragmatic breathing reduces the respiratory rate and increases alveolar ventilation. c,d. Increasing the volume of air in lungs promotes expulsion of secretions.
2. Teach the client measures to reduce the viscosity of secretions: a. Maintain adequate hydration; increase fluid intake to two to three quarts a day, if not contraindicated by decreased cardiac output or renal disease. b. Maintain adequate humidity of inspired air.	2. a,b. Thick secretions are difficult to expectorate and can cause mucus plugs, which can lead to atelectasis.
3. Auscultate the lungs before and after the client coughs.	3. This assessment helps to evaluate the effectiveness of the client's cough effort.
4. Encourage or provide good mouth care after coughing.	4. Good oral hygiene promotes a sense of well-being and prevents mouth odor.

Documentation

Progress notes
  Effectiveness of cough
  Description of sputum

Activity Intolerance Related to Fatigue and Inadequate Oxygenation for Activities

NOC Activity Tolerance

Goal

The client will progress activity to (specify level of activity).

Indicators

• Demonstrate methods of effective coughing, breathing, and conserving energy.
• Identify a realistic activity level to achieve or maintain.

NIC Activity Tolerance, Energy Management, Exercise Promotion, Sleep Enhancement, Mutual Goal Setting

Interventions	Rationales

1. Explain activities and factors that increase oxygen demand:
   a. Smoking
   b. Extremes in temperature
   c. Excessive weight
   d. Stress
	1.
	a,b,c,d. Smoking, extremes in temperature, and stress cause vasoconstriction, which increases cardiac workload and oxygen requirements. Excess weight increases peripheral resistance, which also increases cardiac workload.

2. Provide the client with ideas for conserving energy:
   a. Sit whenever possible when performing ADLs (e.g., on a stool when showering).
   b. Pace activities throughout the day.
   c. Schedule adequate rest periods.
   d. Alternate easy and hard tasks throughout the day.
	2.
	a,b,c,d. Excessive energy expenditure can be prevented by pacing activities and allowing sufficient time to recuperate between activities.

3. Gradually increase the client's daily activities as tolerance increases.	3. Sustained moderate breathlessness from supervised exercise improves accessory muscle strength and respiratory function.
4. Teach the client effective breathing techniques, such as diaphragmatic and pursed-lip breathing.	4. Diaphragmatic breathing deters the shallow, rapid, inefficient breathing that usually accompanies COPD. Pursed-lip breathing slows expiration, keeps alveoli inflated longer, and provides some control over dyspnea.
5. Teach the client the importance of supporting arm weight.	5. When arms are not supported, the respiratory muscles are required to perform dual roles: increase respirations and stabilize the chest wall in support of arm weight and activity (Bauldoff, Hoffman, Sciurba, & Zullo, 1996).
6. Teach the client how to increase unsupported arm endurance with lower-extremity exercises performed during exhalation.	6. Increasing endurance will improve metabolic function of trained extremity and respiratory muscles and reduced dyspnea with longer endurance limits (Bauldoff et al., 1996).
7. Maintain supplemental oxygen therapy, as needed.	7. Supplemental oxygen increases circulating oxygen levels and improves activity tolerance.
8. Provide emotional support and encouragement.	8. Fear of breathlessness may impede increased activity.

(continued on page 130)

Interventions	Rationales

9. After activity, assess for abnormal responses to increased activity:
  a. Decreased pulse rate
  b. Decreased or unchanged systolic blood pressure
  c. Excessively increased or decreased respiratory rate
  d. Failure of pulse to return to near resting rate within three minutes after activity
  e. Confusion, vertigo, uncoordinated movements
	9.
	a,b,c,d,e. Intolerance to activity can be assessed by evaluating cardiac, circulatory, and respiratory statuses.

10. Plan adequate rest periods according to the client's daily schedule.	10. Rest periods allow the body a period of low energy expenditure, which increases activity tolerance.

11. Evaluate client's nutritional status.
 	
12. Explain the effects of malnutrition:
 	
  a. Higher mortality
 	
  b. Depressed immune system
 	
  c. Decreased muscle strength of diaphragm and chest wall
 	
  d. Decreased surfactant production
	11,12. The increased work of breathing causes decreased appetite and intake. Increased carbohydrate (CHO) intake increases CO_2 production. Decreased intake causes an energy deficit. Energy deficit causes malnutrition and muscle wasting, which decreases diaphragm and muscle strength.
	  a. While planned weight loss usually lowers mortality rates, unintentional weight losses increase mortality rates (Wong & Ciliska, 2003).
	  b. Clients, particularly the elderly, have a greater risk of infection when faced with unintended weight loss (Huffman, 2002).
	  c. These effects will reduce inspiratory and expiratory volumes and the ability to cough effectively (Hunter & King, 2001).
	  d. Lining the epithelium, surfactants decrease surface tension, opening the alveolus, promoting gas exchange, and decreasing the workload of breathing (Davies, 2002).

13. Assess for problems associated with eating:
  a. Breathing competing with eating
  b. Abdominal gas
  c. Grocery shopping
  d. Meal preparation
	13.
	a,b,c,d. Identification of barriers to proper nutrition can prevent or reduce malnutrition.

14. Teach strategies to increase nutritional status:
  a. Eat a diet high in lipid/proteins and low in carbohydrates.
  b. Avoid foods high in calories.
  c. Prepare meals in advance.
  d. Sit at table when preparing food.
  e. Have a large fluid intake (2000–2500 mL) daily.
 	
  f. Avoid milk, chocolates, and other foods that increase the viscosity of saliva.
  g. Avoid caffeine and alcohol.
  h. Reduce amount of liquids at meals.
 	
  i. Avoid dry and hot foods.
  j. Eat four to six small meals daily.
	14.
	  a. CHO digestion produces more carbon dioxide. Protein is essential for healing.
	  b. They offer the client little benefit.
	  c. Client can rest before warming meal.
	  d. Sitting reduces energy expenditure.
	  e. This reduces viscosity of secretions and choking sensations.
	  f. Secretions that can be expectorated will lessen anorexia.
	  g. These act as diuretics.
	  h. This will reduce bloating and volume of material in stomach.
	  i. These irritate throat and stimulate coughing.
	  j. These irritate throat and stimulate coughing.

Documentation

Progress notes
  Activity level
    Physiologic response to activity (vital signs)

Anxiety Related to Breathlessness and Fear of Suffocation

NOC Anxiety Self-Control, Coping, Impulse Self-Control

Goal

The client will verbalize increased psychological and physiologic comfort.

Indicators

- Verbalize feelings of anxiety.
- Demonstrate breathing techniques to decrease dyspnea.

NIC Anxiety Reduction, Impulse Control Training, Anticipatory Guidance

Interventions	Rationales
1. Provide a quiet, calm environment when the client is experiencing breathlessness.	1. Reducing external stimuli promotes relaxation.
2. Do not leave the client alone during periods of acute breathlessness.	2. The client needs reassurance that help is available if needed.
3. Acknowledge the client's fear and give positive reinforcement for efforts. Acknowledge when dyspnea is worse than usual.	3. Fear triggers dyspnea and dyspnea increases fear. Clients report a nurse's acknowledgment of their fear assuaged their fear and alleviated their breathing difficulty.
4. Acknowledge feelings of helplessness. Avoid suggesting "take control" or "relax."	4. Feelings of helplessness and hopelessness can seriously impair a client's ability to comply with his or her plan of care, and may actually increase his or her disability (Sirey, Raue, & Alexopoulos, 2007).
5. Provide assistance with all tasks during acute episodes of dyspnea.	5. The client will not be capable of performing his or her usual activities.
6. During acute episodes, do not discuss preventive measures.	6. Teaching is warranted when the client is less dyspneic.
7. Demonstrate breathing techniques and have the client imitate the technique with the nurse.	7. Role modeling breathing techniques for the client to imitate will reduce the need to spend energy in concentration.
8. During nonacute episodes, teach relaxation techniques (e.g., tapes, guided imagery).	8. Relaxation techniques have been shown to decrease anxiety, dyspnea, and airway obstruction.
9. During periods of acute breathlessness, do the following: a. Open curtains and doors. b. Eliminate unnecessary equipment. c. Limit visitors. d. Eliminate smoke and odors.	9. These measures may help reduce feelings of suffocation.
10. Encourage the client to use breathing techniques especially during times of increased anxiety. Coach the client through the breathing exercises.	10. Concentrating on diaphragmatic or pursed-lip breathing slows the respiratory rate and gives the client a sense of control.

Documentation

Progress notes
    Acute anxiety episodes
    Interventions
    Client's response to interventions

Powerlessness Related to Feelings of Loss of Control and Life Style Restrictions

NOC Depression Self-Control, Health Beliefs: Perceived Control, Participation in Health Care Decisions

Goal

The client will verbalize ability to influence situations and outcomes.

Indicators

- Identify personal strengths.
- Identify factors that he or she can control.

NIC Mood Management, Teaching: Individual, Decision-Making Support, Self-Responsibility Facilitation, Health System Guidance, Spiritual Support

Interventions	Rationales
1. Explore the effects of the condition on: a. Client's occupation b. Leisure and recreational activities c. Role responsibilities d. Relationships	1. Illness can negatively affect the client's self-concept and ability to achieve goals. Specifically in COPD, dyspnea can interfere with the client's ability to work and play.
2. Determine the client's usual response to problems.	2. To plan effective interventions, the nurse must determine if the client usually seeks to change his or her own behaviors to control problems, or if she or he expects others or external factors to control problems.
3. Allow the client to share his or her losses. a. Life style b. Independence c. Roles	3. These changes in self-perception play a key role in health outcomes. The client's self-image helps to formulate a strategy to cope with his or her disease (Ninot et al., 2002).
4. Help the client to identify personal strengths and assets.	4. Clients with chronic illness need to be assisted not to see themselves as helpless victims. Clients with a sense of hope, self-control, direction, purpose, and identity are better able to meet the challenges of their disease.
5. Assist in identifying energy patterns and in scheduling activities around these patterns.	5. A review of the client's daily schedule can help the nurse and client to plan activities that promote feelings of self-worth and dignity and to schedule appropriate rest periods to prevent exhaustion.
6. Discuss the need to accept help from others and to delegate some tasks.	6. The client may need assistance to prevent exhaustion and hypoxia.
7. Help the client to seek support from other sources (e.g., self-help groups, support groups).	7. The client may benefit from opportunities to share similar experiences and solve problems with others in the same situation.
8. Encourage the client to make decisions that might increase her or his ability to cope.	8. By fostering self-care decisions, clients gain control of their health care and potentially enhance the quality of their lives, especially in older adults (Leenerts, Teel, & Pendelton, 2002).

(continued on page 133)

Interventions	Rationales
9. Help the client to establish a goal, determine alternatives, and select the best course of action.	9. Setting realistic goals can increase motivation and hope.
10. For clients with severe disease, avoid emphasizing what caused their disease (e.g., smoking).	10. Research has shown that 75% of clients with COPD do not think about the cause of their illness. Clients who do not engage in causal thinking may be in denial. This denial may produce a feeling of control, enabling them to be more functional. Contemplating causes may produce feelings of powerlessness, depression, and decreased functional status (Weaver & Narsavage, 1992).

Documentation

Progress notes
   Interactions with the client

Disturbed Sleep Pattern Related to Cough, Inability to Assume Recumbent Position, Environmental Stimuli

NOC Rest, Sleep, Well-Being

Goals

The client will report a satisfactory balance of rest and activity.

Indicators

- Describe factors that inhibit sleep.
- Identify techniques to induce sleep.

NIC Energy Management, Sleep Enhancement, Environmental Management

Interventions	Rationales
1. Explain the sleep cycle and its significance: a. Stage I: Transitional stage between wakefulness and sleep (5% of total sleep) b. Stage II: Asleep but easily aroused (50%–55% of total sleep) c. Stage III: Deeper sleep; arousal is more difficult (10% of total sleep) d. Stage IV: Deepest sleep; metabolism and brain waves slow (10% of total sleep)	1. A person typically goes through four or five complete sleep cycles each night. If the person awakens during a sleep cycle, he or she may not feel rested in the morning.
2. Discuss individual differences in sleep requirements based on these factors: a. Age b. Activity level c. Life style d. Stress level	2. The usual recommendation of eight hours of sleep every night actually has no scientific basis. A person who can relax and rest easily requires less sleep to feel refreshed. With aging, total sleep time generally decreases, especially Stage IV sleep, and Stage I sleep time increases.

(continued on page 134)

Interventions	Rationales
3. Promote relaxation: a. Provide a dark, quiet environment. b. Allow choices regarding pillows, linens, covers. c. Provide comforting bedtime rituals as necessary. d. Ensure good room ventilation. e. Close the room door if the client desires.	3. Sleep is difficult until relaxation is attained. The hospital environment can impair relaxation.
4. Plan procedures to limit sleep disturbances. Allow the client at least 2-hour segments of uninterrupted sleep.	4. Clients must be permitted to complete all cycles of sleep to allow for cellular growth and tissue repair, as well as the release of growth hormones. It takes approximately 90–120 min to complete a full sleep cycle (Nagel et al., 2003).
5. Explain why hypnotics or sedatives should be avoided.	5. These medications lose their effectiveness after a week; increasing dosages carries the risk of dependence.
6. If desired, elevate the head of the bed on 10-inch blocks or use a gatch with pillows under the arms.	6. This can enhance relaxation and sleep by giving the lungs more room for expansion by reducing upward pressure of abdominal organs.
7. Take measures to control coughing: a. Avoid giving the client cold or hot liquids at bedtime. b. Consult the physician for antitussives, if indicated.	
8. Teach the client measures to promote sleep: a. Eat a high-protein snack before bedtime (e.g., cheese, milk). b. Avoid caffeine. c. Attempt to sleep only when feeling sleepy. d. If sleeping difficulty occurs, leave the bedroom and engage in a quiet activity, such as reading, in another room. e. Try to maintain the same sleep habits seven days a week.	8. These measures help to prevent cough stimulation and disruption of sleep. a. Digested protein produces tryptophan, which has a sedating effect. b. Caffeine stimulates metabolism and deters relaxation. c. Frustration increases if sleep is attempted when not sleepy or relaxed. d. The bedroom should be reserved specifically for sleep. e. Irregular retiring and arising patterns can disrupt the biological clock, which exacerbates sleep difficulties.
9. Assist with usual bedtime routine (e.g., personal hygiene, snack, music).	9. Following a familiar bedtime routine may help to promote relaxation and aid sleep.

Documentation

Progress notes
Sleep patterns (amount, awakenings)
Client's evaluation of sleep quantity and quality

High Risk for Ineffective Therapeutic Regimen Management Related to Lack of Knowledge of Condition, Treatments, Prevention of Infection, Breathing Exercises, Risk Factors, Signs and Symptoms of Complications

NOC Compliance Behavior, Knowledge: Treatment Regimen, Participation in Health Care Decisions, Treatment Behavior: Illness or Injury

Goal

The goals for this diagnosis represent those associated with discharge planning. Refer to the discharge criteria.

NIC Anticipatory Guidance, Learning Facilitation, Risk Management, Health Education, Teaching: Procedure/Treatment, Health System Guidance

Interventions	Rationales
1. Help the client to formulate and accept realistic short- and long-term goals.	1. This may help the client to realize that he or she has much control over his or her life and can make choices to improve quality of life.
2. Teach the client about the diagnosis and the treatment regimen.	2. Understanding may help to encourage compliance and participation in self-care.
3. Teach the client measures to help control dyspnea and infections: a. Eat a well-balanced diet. b. Take sufficient rest periods. c. Gradually increase activity. d. Increase fluids, unless contraindicated. e. Avoid exposure to: • Smoke • Dust • Severe air pollution (rush hour traffic) • Extremely cold or warm temperatures	3. a. Weight loss and, specifically, malnutrition decrease the client's ability to exercise, and increases fatigue, dyspnea, and the likelihood of respiratory infections (Porth, 2005). b,c,d. These practices promote overall good health and increase resistance to infection. e. Exposure to these respiratory irritants can cause bronchospasm and increased mucus production. Smoking destroys the ciliary cleansing mechanism of the respiratory tract. Heat raises body temperature and increases the body's oxygen requirements, possibly exacerbating the symptoms.
4. Teach and have the client demonstrate breathing exercises (Pederson, 1992): a. Incentive spirometer b. Diaphragm exercise: Place fingers on the lower ribs; inhale, pushing out against light pressure of fingers. c. Lung apex exercise: Apply light pressure just below the clavicle as you inhale. While exhaling, apply pressure to the sternum with the heel of your hand. d. Posterior lung exercise: Lie on your side, and have someone else place both hands over your lower thorax and apply pressure as you exhale. e. Lateral lower rib area exercise: Exhale completely, then have another person apply pressure to the lower rib cage area with both hands as you inhale. During exhalation, tighten the abdomen as the other person again applies pressure.	4. A client with COPD typically breathes shallowly from the upper chest. Breathing exercises increase alveolar ventilation and reduce respiratory rate. a. Incentive spirometry encourages deep, sustained inspiratory efforts. b. Expanding and contracting the diaphragm muscle can help to strengthen it. c. Counterpressure forces the client to breathe harder, which strengthens muscles and aerates lung apexes. d. Adequate fluids will liquefy secretion. e. Breathing against counterpressure strengthens respiratory muscles. Complete exhalation promotes maximum expansion of the rib cage.
5. Teach and evaluate the technique of postural drainage: a. Assume a dependent position to drain the involved lung area, using pillows or a reclining chair. b. Cough and expectorate secretions while in the dependent position. c. Hold the position for 10–15 min.	5. The force of gravity helps to loosen and drain secretions.

(continued on page 136)

Interventions	Rationales
6. Advise the client not to perform breathing exercises shortly before or after eating.	6. The exertion associated with breathing exercises may reduce appetite. Performing the exercises after eating may cause vomiting.
7. Explain the hazards of infection and ways to reduce the risk: a. Avoid contact with infected persons. b. Receive immunization against influenza and bacterial pneumonia. c. Take antibiotics as prescribed if sputum becomes yellow or green. d. Adhere to chest physiotherapy, medications, and hydration schedule. e. Cleanse all equipment well.	7. A client with COPD is prone to infection due to inadequate primary defenses (i.e., decreased ciliary action and stasis of secretions). Minor respiratory infections can cause serious problems in a client with COPD. Chronic debilitation and retention of secretions (which provide a medium for microorganism growth) put the client at high risk for complications.
8. Instruct the client to report: a. Change in sputum characteristics or failure of sputum to return to usual color after three days of antibiotic therapy b. Elevated temperature c. Increase in cough, weakness, or shortness of breath d. Increased confusion or drowsiness e. Weight loss f. Weight gain or swelling in ankles and feet	8. a. Sputum changes may indicate an infection or resistance of the infective organism to the prescribed antibiotic. b. Circulating pathogens stimulate the hypothalamus to elevate body temperature. c. Hypoxia is chronic; exacerbations must be detected early to prevent complications. d. Cerebral hypoxia can produce confusion or drowsiness. e. Inadequate intake can result from dyspnea, fatigue, medication side effects, and anorexia secondary to hypoxia and sputum production. f. These signs may indicate fluid retention secondary to pulmonary arterial hypertension and decreased cardiac output.
9. Teach and observe use of a hand-held nebulizer or metered-dose inhaler and oxygen therapy. a. Hand washing b. Assembling equipment, supplies c. Using correct dose of medication d. Correct positioning e. Proper cleaning of equipment after use	9. Accurate instructions can help to prevent medication overdose or infections, and increase effectiveness of treatments.
10. Teach the client methods to conserve energy. See the nursing diagnosis Fatigue in the Inflammatory Joint Disease care plan for more information.	10. Energy conservation helps prevent exhaustion and exacerbation of hypoxia.
11. Consult with a primary care provider for possible referral to physical therapy for strength and endurance training.	11. Evidence suggests 15–20 rehabilitation sessions that include exercise, breathing techniques, and physical therapy reduce anxiety more effectively than the same amount of counseling (Boardman, 2008). This outcome, coupled with their improved strength and endurance, affords the client the ability to increase both their ADLs and quality of life.
12. Explain the effects of smoking on the progression of the disease and mortality. Explain the benefits of quitting.	12. The mortality rate for 60-year-old smokers with chronic bronchitis is four times higher than for 60-year-old non-smokers with asthma.

(continued on page 137)

Interventions	Rationales

13. Discuss various available methods to quit smoking
  • Individual/group counseling
  • Self-help materials (written, audio, video)
  • Nicotine replacement therapy (transdermal patch, gum, spray)
  • Bupropion (Zyban)
	13. Each of these modalities has varying degrees of effectiveness. Clients should be encouraged to continue trying different therapies until they succeed (Sheahan, 2002). Comprehensive smoking cessation guidelines are available at http://www.surgeongeneral.gov/tobacco.

14. Provide information about or initiate referrals to community resources such as the American Lung Association, self-help groups, Meals-on-Wheels, and home health agencies.	14. These resources can provide the client needed assistance with home management and self-care.

Documentation

Discharge summary record
    Client teaching
    Outcome achievement or status
    Referrals, if indicated

Pneumonia

Pneumonia is the seventh leading cause of death in the United States, and the most common cause of death from any infectious disease. This lower respiratory tract infection may cause general malaise, fever, cough, or abnormal chest radiograph results, as well as dyspnea, increased sputum production, hemoptysis, or hypoxia (Harvey & Whelan, 2008).

    An inflammatory process of the lung parenchyma, usually in the bronchioles and alveolar sacs, pneumonia can be caused by bacteria, viruses, fungi, parasites, chemical inhalation, aspiration of gastric contents, or fluid accumulation in lung bases. One-fourth to one-third of clients hospitalized with pneumococcal pneumonia develop bacteremia. About 50% of all pneumococcal pneumonias occur in people older than 60 years (King & Pippin, 1997).

 Time Frame
Acute episode

◼◼◼◼◼ DIAGNOSTIC CLUSTER

Collaborative Problems

▲ PC: Respiratory Insufficiency
▲ PC: Septic Shock
▲ PC: Paralytic Ileus

(continued on page 138)

Nursing Diagnoses	Refer to
▲ Activity Intolerance related to insufficient oxygenation for ADLs	COPD
▲ Ineffective Airway Clearance related to pain, increased tracheobronchial secretions, and fatigue	COPD
△ High Risk for Impaired Oral Mucous Membrane related to mouth breathing, frequent expectorations, and decreased fluid intake secondary to malaise	
△ High Risk for Imbalanced Nutrition: Less Than Body Requirements related to anorexia, dyspnea, and abdominal distention secondary to air swallowing	Cirrhosis
△ High Risk for Ineffective Therapeutic Regimen Management related to lack of knowledge of condition, infection transmission, prevention of recurrence, diet, signs and symptoms of recurrence, and follow-up care	

▲ This diagnosis was reported to be monitored for or managed frequently (75%–100%).
△ This diagnosis was reported to be monitored for or managed often (50%–74%).

Discharge Criteria

Before discharge, the client or family will

1. Describe how to prevent infection transmission.
2. Describe rest and nutritional requirements.
3. Describe methods to reduce the risk of recurrence.
4. State signs and symptoms that must be reported to a health care professional.

Collaborative Problems

Potential Complication: Respiratory Insufficiency

Potential Complication: Septic Shock

Potential Complication: Paralytic Ileus

Nursing Goal

The nurse will detect early signs/symptoms of hypoxia and septic shock and collaboratively intervene to stabilize client.

Indicators

- Temperature 98–99.5°F
- Pulse regular rhythm rate 60–100 beats/min
- Blood pressure >90/60, <140/90 mmHg
- Urine output >5 mL/kg/h
- Bowel sounds detected
- Alert

Interventions	Rationales
1. Closely monitor high-risk individuals: • Age >65 • Unstable vital signs (heart rate >140 beats/min, systolic BP <90 mmHg, respiratory rate >30 breaths/min) • Altered mental status • PO_2 <60 mmHg • Severe underlying disease [COPD, diabetes mellitus (DM), liver disease, heart failure, renal failure] • Immunocompromised state (HIV, cancer, history of corticosteroid use) • Mechanically ventilated individuals • Severe electrolyte, hematologic, or metabolic abnormality	1. These factors further compromise hypoxemia and increase mortality rates (King & Pippin, 1997).
2. Monitor for signs and symptoms of hyperthermia: a. Fever of 103°F or above b. Chills c. Tachycardia d. Signs of shock: restlessness or lethargy, confusion, decreased systolic blood pressure	2. Bacteria can act as a pyrogen by raising the hypothalamic thermostat through the production of endogenous pyrogens, which may mediate through prostaglandins. Chills can occur when the temperature setpoint of the hypothalamus changes rapidly. High fever increases metabolic needs and oxygen consumption. The impaired respiratory system cannot compensate and tissue hypoxia results (Porth, 2005).
3. Provide cooling measures (e.g., reduced clothing and bed linen, tepid baths, increased fluids, hypothermia blanket).	3. Reduced body temperature is necessary to lower metabolic rate and reduce oxygen consumption.
4. Obtain sputum for Gram stain and cultures and blood cultures.	4. Cultures help to identify specific causative organisms and sensitive or resistant antibiotics.
5. Monitor respiratory status and assess for signs and symptoms of hypoxia. a. Increased respiratory rate (tachypnea) b. Fever, chills (sudden or insidious) c. Productive (pink, rusty, purulent, green, yellow, or white sputum [Dillon, 2007]) or nonproductive cough (Harvey & Whelan, 2008) d. Diminished or absent breath sounds e. Crackles, rhonchi, bronchial breath sounds, positive bronchophony, increased tactile fremitus, and/or dullness on percussion (Dillon, 2007) f. Pleuritic pain g. Tachycardia h. Marked dyspnea i. Cyanosis j. Hemoptysis	5. Tracheobronchial inflammation, impaired alveolar capillary membrane function, edema, fever, and increased sputum production disrupt respiratory function and alter the blood's oxygen-carrying capacity. Reduced chest wall compliance in older adults also affects the quality of respiratory effort. In older adults, tachypnea >26 respirations/min is one of the earliest signs of pneumonia and often occurs three to four days before a confirmed diagnosis. Delirium or mental status changes are often seen early in pneumonia in older clients. Sputum specimens often are contaminated with oropharyngeal secretions and may not identify the causative organism. Specimens that have more than 25 polymorphonuclear leukocytes and less than 10 squamous epithelial cells per low-power field are considered to be adequate specimens.
6. Monitor for signs and symptoms of septic shock: a. Subnormal body temperature b. Hypotension c. Decreased level of consciousness d. Weak, rapid pulse e. Rapid, shallow respirations f. Cold, clammy skin g. Oliguria h. Pallor or flushing	6. Sepsis may develop in a client with pneumonia if treatment is delayed or if the causative organism is very virulent and drug resistant. An older client has an increased risk of other complicating illnesses and may exhibit only subtle signs of sepsis.

(continued on page 140)

Interventions	Rationales

7. Monitor for signs and symptoms of paralytic ileus:
  a. Initially, visible peristaltic waves
  b. No bowel movements
  c. No bowel sounds
  d. Intermittent colicky pain
  e. Abdominal rigidity and distention
  f. Nausea and vomiting
	7. Paralytic ileus can result from anorexia and decreased food intake or from increased insensible fluid loss related to hyperthermia and hyperventilation. Abdominal distention is aggravated by "air hunger"—mouth breathing resulting from hypoxia.

8. Administer cough suppressants or expectorants, as ordered by the physician.	8. Dry, hacking cough interferes with sleep and saps energy. Cough suppressants should be used judiciously, however, because complete depression of the cough reflex can cause atelectasis by preventing the movement of tracheobronchial secretions.
9. Initiate antibiotics as prescribed. Consult pharmacological reference for specifics.	9. Current pharmacological references provide information regarding action, administration, cautions, and side effects.
10. Maintain oxygen therapy, as prescribed, and monitor its effectiveness.	10. Oxygen therapy may help to prevent restlessness if the client is becoming dyspneic, and also may help to prevent pulmonary edema. Because the client is no longer gasping for air, the risk of abdominal distention is decreased. Frequent ABG analysis is essential to detect depressed ventilatory drive.
11. Provide respiratory physiotherapy (e.g., percussion, postural drainage) to move thick, tenacious secretions along the tracheobronchial trees.	11. Exudate in the alveoli and bronchospasms caused by an increase in bronchopulmonary secretions can decrease ventilatory effort and impair gas exchange.

 ## Related Physician-Prescribed Interventions

Medications. Antimicrobials, analgesics (nonnarcotic), bronchodilators, mucolytics, expectorants
Intravenous Therapy. Supplemental as needed
Laboratory Studies. ABG analysis, serologic tests, sputum cultures/Gram stain, sedimentation rate, complete blood count, electrolytes, thoracentesis
Diagnostic Studies. Chest x-ray film (Note: False negative results may be caused by dehydration and neutropenia [Harvey & Wheelan, 2008]), pulse oximeter, protected specimen brush (PSB), bronchoalveolar lavage (BAL)
Therapies. Continuous positive airway pressure (CPAP), ultrasonic nebulizer, oxygen via cannula

Documentation

Medication administration record
    Type, dosage, routes of all medications
Flow record
    Vital signs
    Assessments
Progress notes
    Cooling measures employed
    Effects on temperature

Nursing Diagnoses

High Risk for Impaired Oral Mucous Membrane Related to Mouth Breathing, Frequent Expectorations, and Decreased Fluid Intake Secondary to Malaise

NOC Oral Tissue Integrity

Goal

The client will exhibit intact, moist oral mucous membranes.

Indicators

• Describe factors that increase oral injury.
• Relate the techniques of optimal oral hygiene.

NIC Oral Health Restoration, Oral Health Maintenance

Interventions	Rationales
1. Discuss importance of frequent oral hygiene.	1. Oral hygiene removes microorganisms that increase the risk of infection.
2. Encourage frequent rinsing of the mouth with water; discourage mouth breathing.	2. Dry oral mucosa causes discomfort and increases the risk of breakdown and infection. Mouth breathing causes loss of oral moisture.
3. Teach the client to avoid lemon-glycerin swabs and mouthwashes containing alcohol.	3. These agents dry mucous membranes.
4. Monitor hydration status: a. Oral intake b. Parenteral therapy c. Intake and output d. Urine specific gravity	4. Proper hydration must be maintained to liquefy secretions and prevent drying of oral mucosa.
5. If the mouth or lips are sore, instruct the client to avoid acidic and very hot or cold foods.	5. These foods can irritate oral mucosa.
6. Encourage the client to avoid alcohol and tobacco use.	6. Alcohol and tobacco can irritate oral mucosa.
7. Encourage the client to lubricate the lips every two hours or as needed.	7. Proper lip care replaces moisture and reduces cracking.

Documentation

Flow record
    Oral Assessment
    Oral care
Discharge summary record
    Client teaching

High Risk for Ineffective Therapeutic Regimen Management Related to Lack of Knowledge of Condition, Infection Transmission, Prevention of Recurrence, Diet, Signs and Symptoms of Recurrence, and Follow-up Care

NOC Compliance Behavior, Knowledge: Treatment Regimen, Participation in Health Care Decisions, Treatment Behavior: Illness or Injury

Goal

The goals for this diagnosis represent those associated with discharge planning. Refer to the discharge criteria.

NIC Anticipatory Guidance, Risk Identification, Learning Facilitation, Health Education

Interventions	Rationales
1. Explain the pathophysiology of pneumonia using teaching aids (e.g., illustrations, models) appropriate for the client's or family's educational level.	1. Understanding the disease process and its possible complications may encourage the client's compliance with the therapeutic regimen.

2. Explain measures to prevent the spread of infection:
  a. Cover the nose and mouth when sneezing or coughing.
  b. Dispose of used tissues in a paper bag; when the bag is half-full, close it securely and place it in a larger disposal unit.
  c. Wash hands frequently.
	2. Although pneumococcal pneumonia is not highly communicable, the client should refrain from visiting with persons predisposed to pneumonia during the acute phase (e.g., elderly or seriously ill persons, those with sickle cell disease, postsurgical clients, or persons with chronic respiratory disease).

3. Explain measures to prevent recurrence:
 	
  a. Complete the entire course of prescribed antibiotic therapy and report any side effects.
 	
  b. Keep scheduled, follow-up medical appointments.
	3. A client with pneumonia commonly has an underlying chronic disease; impaired host defenses increase the risk of recurrence.
	  a. If there is no response to treatment within 24 to 48 hours, a reevaluation should be initiated. Possibly there has been an inaccurate diagnosis, the causative organism is resistant to prescribed antibiotic, or dosage has to be adjusted. More invasive techniques for obtaining respiratory secretions for culture may be required. The possibility of infection in the pleural space or the presence of an obstructive lesion, particularly in smokers, should be considered (LaForce, 1992). Because most clients notice a decrease in symptoms after 72 hours of treatment, they sometimes do not recognize the importance of continuing the antibiotic as prescribed. The course of medication is usually seven to 14 days, but may be as long as 21 days, depending on severity of illness, presence of underlying disease, and client response. Antibiotics should be continued until completed and a follow-up x-ray film confirms that infection has subsided.
	  b. Even though clinical signs may be absent, particularly in older clients, a chest x-ray film is necessary to confirm absence of pneumonia. This also allows further evaluation, as some clients with lung cancer initially present with pneumonia. In older clients, initial chest x-rays may indicate progression of the pneumonia; however, this is usually a reflection of better hydration. The follow-up x-ray films take longer to show resolution, often showing opacities far beyond 14 weeks. In younger clients, complete resolution is usually seen in four to eight weeks (Marrie, 1992).

(continued on page 143)

Interventions	Rationales
c. Continue deep breathing exercises for six to eight weeks during the convalescent period.	c. Deep breathing increases alveolar expansion and thus facilitates movement of secretions from the tracheobronchial tree with coughing. Routine planned deep breathing and coughing sessions increase vital capacity and pulmonary compliance. Sometimes dry cough occurs with chest wall pain related to myalgias of the intercostal muscles, so increased efforts must be made to encourage regular lung expansion. A pillow may be used to splint the chest wall while coughing.
d. Plan morning and afternoon rest periods.	d. Increased metabolism results from hyperthermia and from the body's defense mechanisms for fighting infection. More energy is expended as the lungs work harder to perfuse the body tissues adequately. These factors result in increased physical fatigue.
e. Obtain influenza and pneumococcal immunizations if the client has a chronic respiratory condition, is elderly, or is immunosuppressed.	e. Because bacterial pneumonia may occur as a complication of influenza, yearly influenza immunization is recommended for at-risk groups. Those individuals are (1) adults with chronic disorders of the pulmonary or cardiovascular systems; (2) residents of nursing homes or other chronic care facilities that house individuals with chronic medical conditions; (3) persons aged 65 or older; and (4) adults requiring regular medical follow-up or hospitalization during the previous year because of chronic metabolic diseases, renal dysfunction, hemoglobinopathies, or immunosuppression. The currently used pneumococcal vaccine (Pneumovax) confers a very high rate of immunity because it contains 23 of the most common pneumococcal organisms that protect against types that cause 85% of bacteremia infections. Current studies identify if more than one pneumococcal immunization is necessary. Current recommendations are that individuals who are at high risk for sepsis-related complications such as asplenics or those who are nephrotic or immunosuppressed should be vaccinated every six years (Arcangelo & Peterson, 2005). Otherwise, Pneumovax should be administered only on a one-time basis.
4. Encourage adequate hydration with intake of 3000 mL/day, if not contraindicated.	4. Insensible fluid losses from hyperthermia and productive cough predispose the client to dehydration, particularly an elderly client.
5. Encourage adequate, nutritious food intake and use of high-protein supplements, if necessary.	5. Increased metabolism raises the client's calorie requirements; however, dyspnea and anorexia sometimes prevent adequate caloric intake. High-protein supplements provide increased calories and fluids if anorexia and fatigue from eating interfere with food intake.
6. Encourage the client to avoid smoking.	6. Chronic smoking destroys the tracheobronchial ciliary action, the lungs' first defense against infection. It also inhibits alveolar macrophage function and irritates the bronchial mucosa.
7. Instruct the client and family to report any signs or symptoms after initiation of treatment (e.g., thickening of respiratory secretions, return or persistence of fever, increased chest pain, malaise).	7. Pneumonia may be resistant to the prescribed antibiotic, or secondary infection with organisms not susceptible to prescribed antibiotic may have occurred.

(continued on page 144)

Interventions	Rationales
8. Position the client to minimize aspiration.	8. Approximately 50% of healthy individuals aspirate during sleep with minimal problems. In recently hospitalized individuals, there is increased chance of oropharyngeal colonization. Hydrochloric acid protects against pneumonia from aspiration; however, antacids, by changing the pH of the stomach contents, increase the risk of nosocomial pneumonia. Sucralfate and other agents that do not alter normal gastric pH reduce the risk of nosocomial pneumonia with aspiration. Individuals at increased risk for aspiration are those with impaired pulmonary defenses, such as those on O_2 therapy, steroids, antibiotics, and tracheal suctioning, as well as those suffering from alcoholism and diabetes. Also, individuals receiving tube feedings, even in the jejunum, and receiving sedatives, are at risk.
9. Encourage the client to avoid factors that lower resistance to pneumonia (e.g., overexertion, chilling, and excessive alcohol intake) particularly during the convalescent period.	9. A client who has had one episode of pneumonia is at increased risk for recurrence. Any upper respiratory infection may lead to bacterial invasion in the lower respiratory tract.

Documentation

Graphic/flow record
    Discharge instructions
    Follow-up instructions
Progress notes
    Status at discharge
    Outcome achievement or status
For a Care map on pneumonia, visit http://thePoint.lww.com

Cirrhosis

A set of changes in liver tissue characterized by the nodular regeneration of parenchymal cells and scar tissue formation, cirrhosis is divided into three types: (1) Laennec's portal cirrhosis, which results from chronic alcohol toxicity and the accompanying malnutrition; (2) postnecrotic cirrhosis, which involves scar tissue resulting from viral hepatitis, primarily Types B and C; and (3) biliary cirrhosis, in which scarring results from chronic biliary obstruction. In all types, the fibrosis or scarring interferes with normal liver function and portal blood flow. Impaired portal blood flow causes venous congestion in the spleen and gastrointestinal (GI) tract.

 Time Frame
Initial diagnosis
Recurrent acute episodes

■■■■■■ DIAGNOSTIC CLUSTER

Collaborative Problems

▲ PC: Hemorrhage
▲ PC: Medication Toxicity (opiates, short-acting barbiturates, major tranquilizers)
△ PC: Metabolic Disorders
△ PC: Portal Systemic Encephalopathy
△ PC: Renal Insufficiency

Nursing Diagnoses	Refer to
▲ Imbalanced Nutrition: Less Than Body Requirements related to anorexia, impaired protein, fat, glucose metabolism, and impaired storage of vitamins (A, C, K, D, E)	
▲ Impaired Comfort related to pruritus secondary to accumulation of bilirubin pigment and bile salts	
▲ Excess Fluid Volume related to portal hypertension, lowered plasma colloidal osmotic pressure, and sodium retention	
▲ Pain related to liver enlargement and ascites (Pancreatitis)	
▲ High Risk for Ineffective Therapeutic Regimen Management related to lack of knowledge of pharmacologic contraindications, nutritional requirements, signs and symptoms of complications, and risks of alcohol ingestion	
▲ Diarrhea related to excessive secretion of fats in stool secondary to liver dysfunction	Pancreatitis
▲ High Risk for Infection related to leukopenia secondary to enlarged, overactive spleen and hypoproteinemia	Leukemia

▲ This diagnosis was reported to be monitored for or managed frequently (75%–100%).
△ This diagnosis was reported to be monitored for or managed often (50%–74%).

Discharge Criteria

Before discharge, the client or family will

1. Describe the causes of cirrhosis.
2. Describe activity restrictions, nutritional requirements, and the need for alcohol abstinence.
3. State actions that reduce anorexia, edema, and pruritus at home.
4. State the signs and symptoms that must be reported to a health care professional.

Collaborative Problems

Potential Complication: Hemorrhage

Potential Complication: Metabolic Disorders

Potential Complication: Portal Systemic Encephalopathy

Potential Complication: Medication Toxicity

Potential Complication: Renal Insufficiency

Nursing Goal

The nurse will monitor to detect early signs/symptoms of (a) hemorrhage, (b) metabolic disorders, (c) encephalopathy, (d) renal insufficiency, and (e) medication toxicities, and collaboratively intervene to stabilize the client.

Indicators

- BP >90/60, <140/90 mmHg (a, b, c, d)
- Heart rate 60–100 beats/min (a, b, c, d)
- Respiration 16–20 breaths/min (a, b, c, d)
- Hemoglobin (a)
  - Male 14–18 g/dL
  - Female 12–16 g/dL
- Hematocrit (a)
  - Male 42%–52%
  - Female 37%–47%
- Stools negative occult blood (a)
- Prothrombin time 11–12.5 seconds (a)
- Electrolytes within normal range (b)
- Serum pH 7.35–7.45 (a, b, c)
- Serum PCO_2 35–45 mmHg (b, c)
- Oxygen saturation >95% (pulse oximeter) (a, b, c)
- Alert, oriented (a, b, c)
- Urine output >5 mL/kg/h (a, b, d)
- Urine specific gravity 1.005–1.030 (b, d)
- Sodium 135–145 mEq/L (b, d)
- Creatinine 0.7–1.4 mg/dL (b, d)
- Albumin 3.5–5.0 m/U/mL (b, d)
- Prealbumin 16–40 m/U/mL (b, d)
- Blood urea nitrogen 5–25 mg/dL

Interventions	Rationales
1. Monitor for hemorrhage by assessing the following: a. Vital signs b. Hematocrit and hemoglobin c. Stools, for occult blood d. Prothrombin time	1. The liver has a central role in hemostasis. Decreased platelet count results from impaired production of new platelets from the bone marrow. Decreased clearance of old platelets by the reticuloendothelial system also results. In addition, the synthesis of coagulation factors (II, V, VII,

(continued on page 147)

Interventions	Rationales
	IX, and X) is impaired, resulting in bleeding. Most frequent site is upper GI tract. Other sites are nasopharynx, lungs, retroperitoneum, kidneys, and intracranial and skin puncture sites.

2. Monitor for bleeding from esophageal varices:
  a. Hematemesis (vomiting blood)
  b. Melena (black, sticky stools)
	2. One-third of clients with cirrhosis and varices experience bleeding. Varices are dilated tortuous veins in the lower esophagus. Portal hypertension caused by obstruction of the portal venous system results in increased pressure on the vessels in the esophagus, making them fragile (Porth, 2007).

3. Teach the client to report unusual bleeding (e.g., in the mouth after brushing teeth) and ecchymotic areas.	3. Mucous membranes are more prone to injury because of their great surface vascularity.

4. Monitor for signs and symptoms of (refer to index under each electrolyte for specific signs and symptoms):
  a. Hypoglycemia
 	
  b. Hyponatremia
 	
  c. Hypokalemia
 	
  d. Hypocalcemia
 	
  e. Hypomagnesemia
 	
  f. Hypophosphatemia
	4.
	
	  a. Hypoglycemia is caused by loss of glycogen stores in the liver from damaged cells, and decreased serum concentrations of glucose, insulin, and growth hormones.
	  b. Reduced capacity of kidneys to excrete water results in dilutional hyponatremia.
	  c. Potassium losses are from vomiting, nasogastric suctioning, diuretics, or excessive renal losses.
	  d. Hypomagnesemia or pancreatitis can decrease calcium levels.
	  e. The loss of potassium ions causes the proportional loss of magnesium ions.
	  f. Increased phosphate loss, transcellular shifts, and decreased phosphate intake contribute to hypophosphatemia.

5. Monitor for acid–base disturbances.	5. Hepatocellular necrosis can result in accumulation of organic anions resulting in metabolic acidosis. Persons with ascites often have metabolic alkalosis from increased bicarbonate levels resulting from increased sodium/hydrogen exchange in distal tubule (Porth, 2005).

6. Monitor for portal systemic encephalopathy by assessing the following:
  a. General behavior
  b. Orientation to time and place
  c. Speech patterns
	6. Profound liver failure results in accumulation of ammonia and other identical toxic metabolites in the blood. The blood–brain barrier permeability increases, and both toxins and plasma proteins leak from capillaries to the extracellular space, causing cerebral edema.

7. Assess for side effects of medications. 8. Avoid administering medications that can impair liver function (e.g., narcotics, sedatives, tranquilizers, lipid-lowering agents, hypoglycemic agents).	7,8. Liver dysfunction results in decreased metabolism of certain medications, which increases the risk of toxicity from high drug blood levels. Some drugs increase liver dysfunction.

9. Monitor for renal failure by assessing the following:
  a. Intake and output
  b. Urine specific gravity
  c. Laboratory values: serum sodium, creatinine, prealbumin
	9. Obstructed hepatic blood flow results in decreased blood to the kidneys, which impairs glomerular filtration and leads to fluid retention and decreased urinary output.

10. Monitor for hypertension.	10. Fluid retention and overload can cause hypertension.

(continued on page 148)

Interventions	Rationales

11. Teach the client and family to report signs and symptoms of complications:
  a. Increased abdominal girth
 	
  b. Rapid weight loss or gain
 	
  c. Bleeding
 	
  d. Tremors
 	
  e. Confusion
	11. Early detection allows prompt intervention to help prevent progression of complications.
	  a. Increased abdominal girth may indicate worsening portal hypertension.
	  b. Rapid weight loss points to negative nitrogen balance; rapid weight gain points to fluid retention.
	  c. Bleeding indicates decreased prothrombin time and clotting factors.
	  d. Tremors result from impaired neurotransmission due to failure of the liver to detoxify enzymes that act as false neurotransmitters.
	  e. Confusion results from cerebral hypoxia caused by high serum ammonia levels due to the liver's impaired ability to convert ammonia to urea.

 Related Physician-Prescribed Interventions

Medications. Vitamin/mineral supplement, lactulose, digestive enzymes, potassium-sparing diuretics, vasodilators, electrolyte replacements

Intravenous Therapy. Hyperalimentation

Laboratory Studies. Blood urea nitrogen (BUN); serum bilirubin, albumin, prealbumin; serum ammonia; serum glutamic-oxaloacetic transaminase (SGOT), serum glutamic-pyruvic transaminase, lactate dehydrogenase (LDH); serum glucose; electrolytes; urine urobilinogen; alkaline phosphatase; aspartate aminotransferase (AST); IgA, IgG; alanine aminotransferase (ALT); CBC; prothrombin time

Diagnostic Studies. Liver scan, percutaneous transhepatic cholangiography, liver biopsy, chest x-ray film, esophagogastroduodenoscopy, upper GI series, CT scan, MRI

Therapies. Diet (high-calorie, low-fat, moderate-protein, low-salt); oxygen via cannula; fluid restrictions; paracentesis; enteral feedings

Documentation

Flow records
  Weight
  Vital signs
  Stools for occult blood
  Abdominal girth
  Urine specific gravity
  Intake and output
Progress notes
  Evidence of bleeding
  Evidence of tremors or confusion

Nursing Diagnoses

Imbalanced Nutrition: Less Than Body Requirements Related to Anorexia, Impaired Protein, Fat, and Glucose Metabolism, and Impaired Storage of Vitamins (A, C, K, D, E)

 Nutritional Status, Knowledge: Diet

Goal

1. The client will describe the reasons for nutritional problems.
2. The client will relate which foods are high in protein and calories.
3. The client will gain weight (specify amount) without increased edema.
4. The client will explain the rationale for sodium restrictions.

NIC Nutrition Management, Nutrition Monitoring

Interventions	Rationales
1. Discuss the causes of anorexia, dyspepsia, and nausea. Explain that obstructed hepatic blood flow causes GI vascular congestion (which results in gastritis and diarrhea or constipation), and that impaired liver function causes metabolic disturbances (fluid, electrolyte, glucose metabolism), resulting in anorexia and fatigue.	1. Helping the client understand the condition can reduce anxiety and may help improve compliance.
2. Teach and assist the client to rest before meals.	2. Fatigue further decreases the desire to eat.
3. Offer frequent small feedings (six per day plus snacks).	3. Increased intra-abdominal pressure from ascites compresses the GI tract and reduces its capacity.
4. Restrict liquids with meals and avoid fluids 1 one hour before and after meals.	4. Fluids can overdistend the stomach, decreasing appetite and intake.
5. Maintain good oral hygiene (brush teeth, rinse mouth) before and after ingestion of food.	5. Accumulation of food particles in the mouth can contribute to foul odors and taste that diminish appetite.
6. Arrange to have foods with the highest protein/calorie content served at the time the client feels most like eating.	6. This increases the likelihood of the client consuming adequate amounts of protein and calories.
7. Teach the client measures to reduce nausea: a. If possible, avoid the smell of food preparation, and try eating cold foods that have fewer odors. b. Loosen clothing when eating. c. Sit in fresh air when eating. d. Avoid lying down flat for at least 2 hours after eating. (A client who must rest should sit or recline so their head is at least 4 inches higher than their feet.)	7. Venous congestion in the GI tract predisposes the client to nausea.
8. Limit high-fat foods and fluids.	8. Impaired bile flow results in malabsorption of fats.
9. Explain the need to increase intake of foods high in the following elements: a. Vitamin B_{12} (eggs, chicken, shellfish) b. Folic acid (green leafy vegetables, whole grains, meat) c. Thiamine (legumes, beans, oranges) d. Iron (organ meats, dried fruit, green vegetables, whole grains)	9. Vitamin intake must be increased to compensate for decreased metabolism and vitamin storage due to liver tissue damage.
10. Teach the client the need to take water-soluble forms of fat-soluble vitamins (A, D, and E).	10. Impaired bile flow interferes with absorption of fat-soluble vitamins.
11. Explain the risks of alcohol ingestion.	11. Alcohol is toxic to the liver and decreases appetite, contributing to inadequate intake.
12. Consult with the physician if the client does not consume sufficient nutrients.	12. High-protein supplements, total parenteral nutrition, or tube feedings may be needed.

Documentation

Flow records
Weight
Intake (type, amount)
Abdominal girth

Impaired Comfort Related to Pruritus Secondary to Accumulation of Bilirubin Pigment and Bile Salts

NOC Symptom Control

Goal

The client will verbalize decreased pruritus.

Indicators

• Describe factors that increase pruritus.
• Describe factors that improve pruritus.

NIC Pruritus Management, Fever Treatment, Environmental Management: Comfort

Interventions	Rationales

1. Maintain hygiene without causing dry skin:
  a. Give frequent baths using cool water and mild soap (castile, lanolin) or a soap substitute.
  b. Blot skin dry; do not rub.
	1. Dryness increases skin sensitivity by stimulating nerve endings.

2. Prevent excessive warmth by maintaining cool room temperatures and low humidity, using light covers with a bed cradle, and avoiding overdressing.	2. Excessive warmth aggravates pruritus by increasing sensitivity through vasodilation.
3. Advise against scratching; explain the scratch-itch-scratch cycle. Instruct the client to apply firm pressure to pruritic areas instead of scratching.	3. Scratching stimulates histamine release, which produces more pruritus.
4. Consult with the physician for a pharmacologic treatment (e.g., antihistamines, antipruritic lotions), if necessary.	4. If pruritus is unrelieved or if the skin is excoriated from scratching, topical or systemic medications are indicated.
5. Keep room cool and with humidity at 30%–40%.	5. Coolness will reduce vasodilation, and humidity will reduce dryness.

Documentation

Progress notes
Unrelieved pruritus
Excoriated skin

Excess Fluid Volume Related to Portal Hypertension, Lowered Plasma Colloidal Osmotic Pressure, and Sodium Retention

NOC Electrolyte Balance, Fluid Balance, Hydration

Goal

1. The client will relate actions that decrease fluid retention.
2. The client will list foods high in sodium.

NIC Electrolyte Management, Fluid Management, Fluid Monitoring, Skin Surveillance

Interventions	Rationales

1. Assess the client's diet for inadequate protein or excessive sodium intake.
 	
2. Encourage the client to decrease salt intake. Teach the client to take the following actions:
  a. Read food labels for sodium content.
  b. Avoid convenience foods, canned foods, and frozen foods.
  c. Cook without salt, and use spices (e.g., lemon, basil, tarragon, mint) to add flavor.
  d. Use vinegar instead of salt to flavor soups, stews, etc. (e.g., 2–3 teaspoons of vinegar to 4–6 quarts of soup, according to taste).
	1,2. Decreased renal flow results in increased aldosterone and antidiuretic hormone secretion, causing water and sodium retention and potassium excretion.

3. Ascertain with the physician if the client may use a salt substitute. Avoid substitutes containing ammonium.	3. Ammonium elevates serum ammonia levels and may contribute to hepatic coma.

4. Take measures to protect edematous skin from injury:
  a. Inspect the skin for redness and blanching.
  b. Reduce pressure on skin (e.g., pad chairs and footstools).
  c. Prevent dry skin by using soap sparingly, rinsing off soap completely, and using a lotion to moisten skin.
	4. Edematous skin is taut and easily injured. Dry skin is more vulnerable to breakdown and injury.

Documentation

Progress notes
Presence of edema

High Risk for Ineffective Therapeutic Regimen Management Related to Lack of Knowledge of Pharmacologic Contraindications, Nutritional Requirements, Signs and Symptoms of Complications, and Risks of Alcohol Ingestion

NOC Compliance Behavior, Knowledge: Treatment Regimen, Participation in Health Care Decisions, Treatment Behavior: Illness or Injury

Goal

The goals for this diagnosis represent those associated with discharge planning. Refer to the discharge criteria.

NIC Anticipatory Guidance, Risk Identification, Health Education, Learning Facilitation

Interventions	Rationales
1. Teach the client or family about the condition and its causes and treatments.	1. This teaching reinforces the need to comply with the therapeutic regimen, including diet and activity restrictions.
2. Explain portal system encephalopathy to the family. Teach them to observe for and report any confusion, tremors, night wandering, or personality changes.	2. Family members typically first note the development of encephalopathy.

(continued on page 152)

Interventions	Rationales
3. Explain the need for adequate rest and avoidance of strenuous activity.	3. As the liver repairs itself, physical activity depletes the body of the energy needed for healing. Adequate rest is needed to prevent relapse.
4. Explain the need for a diet high in protein and calories and low in salt. (Refer to the nursing diagnosis Altered Nutrition in the index for specific interventions.)	4. Protein and caloric requirements are greater when tissue is healing.
5. Explain the hazards of certain medications, including narcotics, sedatives, tranquilizers, and ammonia products.	5. Impaired liver function slows the metabolism of some drugs, causing levels to accumulate and increasing toxicity.
6. Teach the client or family to watch for and report signs and symptoms of complications: a. Bleeding (gums, stools) b. Hypokalemia (muscle cramps, nausea, vomiting) c. Confusion, altered speech patterns, fluctuating moods, and personality changes d. Increasing severity of symptoms e. Rapid weight loss or gain	6. Progressive liver failure affects hematopoietic function and electrolyte and fluid balance, causing potentially serious complications that require prompt intervention. a. Bleeding indicates decreased platelets and clotting factors. b. Hypokalemia results from overproduction of aldosterone, which causes sodium and water retention and potassium excretion. c. Confusion and altered speech patterns result from cerebral hypoxia because of high serum ammonia levels caused by the liver's impaired ability to convert ammonia to urea. d. Exacerbation of symptoms indicates progressive liver damage. e. Rapid weight loss points to negative nitrogen balance; weight gain, points to fluid retention.
7. Explain the need to avoid alcohol.	7. Alcohol increases hepatic irritation and may interfere with recovery.
8. Stress the importance of follow-up care and laboratory studies.	8. Timely follow-up enables evaluation of liver function and early detection of relapse or recurrence.

Documentation

Flow records
    Client teaching
    Referrals when indicated
Progress notes
    Unachieved outcomes

Diabetes Mellitus

Diabetes mellitus is a chronic disease of abnormal metabolism requiring lifelong treatment with diet, exercise, and medication. One in 14 Americans has diabetes and another 40% are at risk for developing the disease. There are three clinical subclasses of diabetes: type 1, type 2, and other types (gestational diabetes, glucose intolerance, and secondary diabetes). The diagnosis of diabetes is can be made in one of three ways: based on two fasting plasma glucose measurements greater than or equal to 126 mg/dL; a plasma glucose >200 mg/dL two hours after an oral glucose tolerance test; or symptoms of diabetes—polyuria, polydipsia, unexplained weight loss—and a causal plasma glucose of >200 mg/dL (American Diabetes Association [ADA], 2006).

There are three clinical subclasses of diabetes: type 1, type 2, and other types (gestational diabetes, glucose intolerance, and secondary diabetes). Although the etiology, clinical course, and treatment differ, the common denominator of all types is glucose intolerance. Type 1 diabetes is characterized by acute onset. Clients with type 1 diabetes account for 10% of known cases in the United States. Type 2 affects 90% of people with diabetes and has an insidious onset. Usual clients are older, obese, and usually have a family history of the disease. Diabetes affects all body systems, because clients are susceptible to its chronic complications, specifically retinopathy, nephropathy, neuropathy, and vascular disease (ADA, 2006).

▪▪▪▪▪ DIAGNOSTIC CLUSTER

Collaborative Problems

▲ PC: Diabetic Ketoacidosis (DKA)
▲ PC: Hypoglycemia
▲ PC: Infections
▲ PC: Vascular Disease
▲ PC: Neuropathy
▲ PC: Hyperglycemic, Hyperosmolar, Nonketotic Coma (HHNK)
▲ PC: Retinopathy
▲ PC: Nephropathy

Nursing Diagnoses

▲ Imbalanced Nutrition: More Than Body Requirements related to intake in excess of activity expenditures, lack of knowledge, or ineffective coping

△ Risk for Ineffective Management of Therapeutic Regimen related to insufficient knowledge of diabetes, self-monitoring of blood glucose, medications, ADA exchange, diet, hypoglycemia, weight control, sick day care, exercise, foot care, signs and symptoms of complications, and the need for comprehensive diabetes outpatient education

▲ This diagnosis was reported to be monitored for or managed frequently (75%–100%).
△ This diagnosis was reported to be monitored for or managed often (50%–74%).

Discharge Criteria

Before discharge, the client or family will

1. Define diabetes as a chronic disease requiring lifelong treatment with food, exercise, and usually, medications for control.
2. Consult with a dietitian for an individualized ADA meal plan.
3. State the relationship of food and exercise to blood glucose (BG) and hemoglobin A_{Ic} levels.
4. State the effects of weight loss on BG control with type 2 diabetes.
5. Describe self-care measures that may prevent or decrease progression of chronic complications (microvascular, macrovascular, neuropathy).
6. State the value of monitoring BG and a plan to obtain supplies and begin testing BG.
7. Explain the importance of foot care and regular assessments.
8. Agree to attend comprehensive outpatient diabetes education programs.
9. Agree to home care referral for diabetes education and self-care management.

For Clients Requiring Medications

Oral Agents

1. State name, dose, action, and time to take diabetes medications.
2. State risk of hypoglycemia with delayed meals or increased activities.

3. State signs, symptoms, and treatment of hypoglycemia.
4. State intent to wear diabetes identification.
5. Describe self-care measures during illness.

Insulin

1. Demonstrate technique for insulin administration.
2. State brand, type, onset, peak, duration, and dose of insulin.
3. State recommendations for site rotation, storage of insulin, and disposal of syringes.
4. State sign, symptoms, and treatment of hypoglycemia.
5. State intent to wear diabetes identification.
6. Describe self-care measures during illness.

Collaborative Problems

Potential Complication: Diabetic Ketoacidosis (DKA)

Potential Complication: Hypoglycemia

Potential Complication: Infections

Potential Complication: Vascular Disease

Potential Complication: Neuropathy

Potential Complication: Hyperglycemic Hyperosmolar State

Potential Complication: Retinopathy

Potential Complication: Nephropathy

Nursing Goal

The nurse will monitor for early signs and symptoms of (a) diabetic ketoacidosis, (b) hyperglycemic hyperosmolar state, (c) hypoglycemia, (d) infections, (e) vascular, (f) neurological, (g) retinal, and (h) renal complications, and collaboratively intervene to stabilize the client.

Indicators

- pH 7.35–7.45 (a, b)
- Fasting blood glucose 70–110 mg/dL (a, b, c)
- No ketones in urine (a, b)
- Serum sodium 1.35–1.45 mEq/L (a, b, h)
- Serum phosphates, 1.8–2.6 m Osm/kg (a, b, h)
- Serum osmolality, 280–295 m Osm/kg (a, b, h)
- BP <130/80 beats/min (e)
- Clear, oriented (a, b, e, f)
- Pulse 60–100 beats/min (e)
- Respiration 16–20 breaths/min (a, b, e)
- Capillary refill <3 seconds (e)
- Peripheral pulse, equal, full (e)
- Warm, dry skin (a, b, e)
- No change of vision (f, g)
- Deep tendon reflexes intact (f)
- Bowel sounds, present (f)
- White blood cells 300–10,800 mm (d)
- Urine, protein-negative (h)
- Creatinine 0.7–1.4 mg/dL (h)
- Blood urea nitrogen 5–25mg/dL (h)

Interventions	Rationales

1. Monitor for signs and symptoms of diabetic ketoacidosis (DKA):
  a. Recent illness/infection
  b. Blood glucose >300 mg/dL
  c. Moderate/large ketones
  d. Anorexia, nausea, vomiting, abdominal pain
  e. Kussmaul's respirations (deep, nonlabored)
  f. pH <7.35
  g. Decreased sodium, potassium, phosphates
  h. Dehydration
	1. When insulin is not available, blood glucose (BG) levels rise and the body metabolizes fat for energy-producing ketone bodies. Excessive ketone bodies cause headaches, nausea, vomiting, and abdominal pain. Increased respiratory rate and depth helps CO_2 excretion and reduces acidosis. Glucose inhibits water reabsorption in the renal glomerulus, leading to osmotic diuresis with loss of water, sodium, potassium, and phosphates. DKA occurs in Type 1 diabetes.

2. Explore with the client and significant others the actual or perceived effects of diabetes on:
  a. Finances
  b. Occupation (sick time)
  c. Lifestyle
  d. Energy level
  e. Relationships
	2. Common frustrations associated with diabetes stem from problems involving the disease itself, the treatment regimen, and the health care system. Recognizing that these problems are common indicates a need to use anticipatory guidance to prevent the associated frustrations.

3. Monitor for signs and symptoms of hyperglycemic hyperosmolar state coma:
  a. Blood glucose 600 to 2000 mg/dL
  b. Severe dehydration
  c. Serum osmolality >350 mOsm/kg
  d. Hypotension
  e. Altered sensorium
	3. Hyperglycemic hyperosmolar state coma is a state of marked dehydration and excessive hyperglycemia and occurs in Type 2 diabetes. Ketones are not present. Glucose inhibits water reabsorption in the renal glomerulus, leading to osmotic diuresis with loss of water, sodium, potassium, and phosphates. Cerebral impairment is due to intracellular dehydration.

4. Monitor cardiac status:
  a. Vital signs
  b. Skin color
  c. Capillary refill
  d. Peripheral pulses
  e. Serum potassium
	4. Severe dehydration may cause reduced cardiac output and compensatory vasoconstriction. Cardiac dysrhythmias may result from potassium imbalances.

5. Monitor for signs and symptoms of hypoglycemia:
  a. Blood glucose <70 mg/dL
  b. Pale, moist, cool skin
  c. Tachycardia, diaphoresis
  d. Jitteriness, irritability
  e. Incoordination
  f. Drowsiness
  g. Hypoglycemia unawareness
	5. Hypoglycemia may be caused by too much insulin, too little food, or too much physical activity. When blood glucose falls rapidly, the sympathetic system is stimulated to produce adrenaline, which causes diaphoresis, cool skin, tachycardia, and jitteriness (ADA, 2006). Hypoglycemia unawareness is a defect in the body's defense system that impairs the ability to feel the warning symptoms usually associated with hypoglycemia. The client may rapidly progress from alertness to unconsciousness.

6. Monitor for signs and symptoms of infection:
  a. Upper respiratory tract infection
  b. Urinary tract infection
  c. External otitis
  d. Red, painful, or warm skin
  e. Furunculosis
  f. Carbuncles
	6. Increased glucose in epidermis and urine promotes bacterial growth. The early diagnosis and treatment of infection in a client with diabetes is necessary, because infection is a leading cause of metabolic abnormalities.

7. Assess for risk factors and monitor for signs and symptoms of macrovascular complications:
  a. Family history of heart disease
  b. Male: over age 40
	7. Diabetes is associated with severe degenerative vascular changes. Lesions of the blood vessels strike at an earlier age and tend to produce more severe pathologic changes. Early atherosclerotic changes are probably caused by high

(continued on page 156)

Interventions	Rationales
c. Cigarette smoker d. Hypertension e. Hyperlipidemia f. Obesity g. Uncontrolled diabetes	blood glucose and lipid levels characteristic of persistent hyperglycemia. Atherosclerosis leads to premature coronary artery disease.
8. Monitor for signs and symptoms of retinopathy: a. Blurred vision b. Black spots c. "Cobwebs" d. Sudden loss of vision	8. Retinopathy does not cause visual symptoms until a fairly advanced stage, usually when macular edema or proliferative retinopathy has occurred. The incidence and severity of retinopathy are thought to be related to the duration and the degree of control of blood glucose (ADA, 2006).
9. Teach the client to have an annual ophthalmologic examination by an experienced ophthalmologist.	9. Early detection of retinopathy can successfully be treated with laser therapy.
10. Monitor for signs and symptoms of peripheral neuropathy: a. Uncontrolled diabetes b. Diagnosis of diabetes >10 years c. Pain d. Decreased sensation e. Decreased deep tendon response (Achilles and patella) f. Decreased vibratory sense g. Charcot's foot ulcer h. Decreased proprioception i. Paresthesia 11. Monitor for signs and symptoms of automatic neuropathy: a. Uncontrolled diabetes b. Diagnosis of diabetes >10 years c. Orthostatic hypotension d. Impotence e. Abnormal sweating f. Bladder paralysis g. Nocturnal diarrhea h. Gastroparesis	10,11. Among the most common and perplexing complications of diabetes, neuropathy is one of the earliest complications and may even be present on diagnosis. Sensory symptoms usually predominate and include numbness, tingling, pain, or loss of sensation. Current treatments include improved control of blood glucose and use of antidepressant drugs as well as aldose reductase inhibitors (ADA, 2006).
12. Monitor for signs and symptoms of nephropathy: a. Uncontrolled diabetes b. Diabetes ≥10 years c. Hypertension d. Proteinuria, bacteriuria, casts e. Elevated white blood cell (WBC) f. Abnormal BUN and creatinine	12. In nephropathy, the capillary basement membrane thickens, due to chronic filtering of high glucose. The membrane becomes more permeable, causing increased loss of blood proteins in urine. Increased filtration requirements increase the pressure in renal blood vessels, contributing to sclerosis.
13. Monitor for proteinuria: a. Consult with the physician to order a 24-hour urine test.	13. Clinical manifestations of nephropathy occur late in the disease. Proteinuria is the first sign of the disorder. A 24-hour urine test is more sensitive than a urinalysis to the presence of microalbumin. Alert the physician of decreased kidney function. When decreased kidney function is identified early, more aggressive therapy may be initiated.
14. Instruct the client on the importance of controlling blood pressure.	14. Blood pressure control is the most important therapy to prevent or ameliorate renal damage (ADA, 2006).

(continued on page 157)

Interventions	Rationales
15. Teach the client about the risk factors that may precipitate renal damage: a. Uncontrolled blood glucose b. Hypertension c. Neurogenic bladder d. Urethral instrumentation e. Urinary tract infection f. Nephrotoxic drugs	15. Making the client aware of risk factors may help to reduce renal impairment.

 ### Related Physician-Prescribed Interventions

Medications
Oral: Sulfonylureas, biguanides, thiazolidinediones, alpha-glucosidase inhibitors, meglitinide combination agents, insulin powder
Injectables:
 Insulin: Regular, intermediate, long-acting, combination (NPH & regular), insulin pump, exenatide (Byetta), pramlintide (Symlin)
 Other: Angiotensin-converting enzyme inhibitors (ACE inhibitors) Angiotensin II receptor blocker (ARB)
Intravenous Therapy. For hyperglycemic or hypoglycemic emergencies
Laboratory Studies. Blood glucose (BG), serum osmolality, 24-hour urine for protein, albumin & creatinine, creatinine clearance, glomerular filtration rate (GFR), electrolytes, oral glucose tolerance test (OGTT), glycosylated hemoglobin Hgb A_{Ic}, fructosamine (use to monitor only persons with anemia and diabetes mellitus)
Diagnostic Studies. Fasting blood glucose, glucose tolerance test.
Therapies. Self-monitoring blood glucose (SMBG), ADA meal plan, exercise

Documentation

Flow records
 Vital signs
 Blood glucose Hgb A_{Ic}
 Glycosylated hemoglobin lipids
 BUN/creatinine
Date last eye exam
Date last 24-hr urine test
Progress notes
 Client complications
 Abnormal labs
 Episodes hypoglycemia
 Changes in medications

Nursing Diagnoses

High Risk for Ineffective Therapeutic Regimen Management Related to Insufficient Knowledge of Diabetes, Monitoring of BG, Medications, Meal Planning, Treatment of Hypoglycemia, Weight Control, Sick Day Management, Exercise Routine, Foot Care, Risks of Complications

 NOC Compliance Behavior, Knowledge: Treatment Regimen, Participation in Health Care Decisions, Treatment Behavior: Illness or Injury

Goals

The goals for this diagnosis represent those associated with discharge planning. Refer to the discharge criteria.

NIC Anticipatory Guidance, Risk Identification, Learning Facilitation, Health Education, Teaching: Procedure/Treatment, Health System Guidance

Interventions	Rationales
1. Instruct the client and family on the components of diabetes treatment—meal planning, exercise, and medications—with the goal not to follow a diet, but to manage blood glucose, blood pressure and lipids (ACP Diabetes Care Guide, 2007).	1. Diabetes education prepares the client and family for effective self-management.
2. Explore with the client and family their experiences with diabetes mellitus and their perceptions of the effects of diabetes on finances, occupation, life style, energy levels, and relationships. Discuss also their perception of controlling blood glucose.	2. Common frustrations associated with diabetes stem from problems involving the disease itself, the treatment regimens, and the health care system. Sharing their perceptions can help with anticipatory guidance to reduce frustrations (Funnell & Kruger, 2004).
3. For clients already diagnosed with diabetes (not a new diagnosis) ask (ACP Diabetes Care Guide, 2007): a. What is the hardest for you to do in caring for your diabetes right now? b. What are you most concerned about? c. What would you like to do or change to improve your health? d. What can you do this week to [specify]? e. How can I help you? f. Do you have difficulty paying for your medications or supplies?	3,4. An effective strategy for behavior change is helping clients to establish self-management goals based on their needs, priorities, and values (ACP Diabetes Care Guide, 2007).
4. Instruct the client on specific strategies to reduce unhealthy behaviors (e. g., obesity, smoking, and sedentary life style).	
5. Explain to the client the risk of complications of diabetes: a. Chronic: • Coronary artery disease • Peripheral vascular disease • Retinopathy • Neuropathy • Nephropathy b. Acute: • Hypoglycemia • Diabetic Ketoacidosis • Hyperglycemia	5. When teaching the risks of complications, stress the importance of regular checkups with a health care provider, including ophthalmologic and podiatric specialists.
6. Teach the client the signs and symptoms of hyperglycemia: a. Blood glucose >200 mg/dL b. Polyuria c. Polydipsia d. Polyphagia e. Fatigue f. Blurred vision g. Weight loss	6. Elevated BG causes dehydration from osmotic diuresis. Potassium is elevated because of hemoconcentration. Because carbohydrates are not metabolized, the client loses weight (Porth, 2005).
7. Teach the client the causes of hyperglycemia: a. Increased food intake b. Decreased insulin c. Decreased exercise d. Infection/illness e. Dehydration	7. Increased food intake requires increased insulin or exercise; otherwise hyperglycemia will ensue. Infections, illnesses, or both increase insulin requirements.

(continued on page 159)

Interventions	Rationales
8. Discuss BG monitoring (Rizvi & Sanders, 2006):	8. BG monitoring assists clients to control diabetes by regulating food, exercise, and medications, and has become an essential component of diabetes management. BG monitoring has allowed flexible mealtimes, made strenuous exercise safe, and made successful pregnancy outcomes more likely.
a. Recommend a meter for BG monitoring based on the client's motivation, physical ability, and financial resources.	a. BG meters vary in ease of use, maintenance, and optional features. Helping the client to choose a monitor that best fits her or his needs is an important role for the educator.
b. Assist the client to obtain a third-party reimbursement for BG monitoring.	b. Comparative shopping and third-party reimbursement may reduce the expense of BG monitoring. Medicare will pay for BG supplies for anyone who has diabetes (ADA, 1997).
c. Discuss with the client his or her specific BG goal, the frequency of BG monitoring, and the value of recording the results.	c. BG records help the client and health care provider evaluate patterns of food intake, insulin administration, and exercise.
d. Teach the client the need for increased BG monitoring when meals are delayed, before exercise, and when sick.	d. These situations may change dietary or insulin requirements.
9. Assist the client in identifying the brand, type, dosage, action, and side effects of prescribed medications for controlling diabetes.	9. A client needs to know the dose, action, and side effects to make appropriate decisions for adjusting food intake and exercise.
10. Advise the client about prescription drugs and over-the-counter remedies, such as cough syrups and throat lozenges that affect BG levels.	10. Oral agents, insulin, glucagon, aspirin, and beta-adrenergic blockers decrease blood glucose; whereas corticosteroids, birth control pills, diuretics, and cold remedies containing decongestants increase BG.
11. Teach the client insulin administration and storage, including: a. Measuring an accurate dose b. Mixing insulin c. Injecting insulin d. Rotating injection sites e. Reusing syringes f. Injecting insulin through clothing	11. Return demonstration allows the nurse to evaluate the client's ability to administer insulin unassisted. Studies have found no evidence of infection when clients reuse syringes. Decreased cost has been the single most important motivation for clients to consider reusing syringes. Clients have been injecting insulin through clothing for more than 50 years without medical advice. A 1997 study found this technique to be safe and convenient. Using the same area repetitively may cause hypertrophy. Insulin is absorbed at different rates in the arms, abdomen, and thighs. It is recommended that rotation occur within the same anatomic area. For example, inject morning insulin into the abdomen, and evening insulin into the thighs (ADA, 2006).
12. Refer the client and family to a home health care nursing agency and to a nutritionist.	12. Continued monitoring and teaching at home will be needed after discharge.
13. Discuss strategies to improve nutrition even before the client sees a nutritionist: a. Provide a list of food sources of carbohydrates (CHO), protein, and vegetables that are low in fat. b. Teach the client to lower fat intake by: • trimming fat off meat • choosing whole grain pasta, rice, grains • avoiding fried foods • limiting salad dressings, selecting low fat	13. Balanced nutrition helps to maintain normal blood glucose level. The ADA recommends an individualized meal plan based on client assessment. The exchange list, food pyramid, and gram counting methods are all acceptable. Low fat foods, water as a beverage, and portion controls of CHO and protein can reduce weight and lower BG.

(continued on page 160)

Interventions	Rationales
c. Show the client and family a paper plate that is divided into quarter sections: • Fill ½ of plate with nonstarchy vegetables (not corn). • Fill ¼ with protein (meat, beans, fish, eggs). • Fill ¼ with carbohydrates (rice, potatoes, pasta, bread). d. Advise the client to: • Drink water. Limit diet soda, coffee, and tea. Avoid all sugar drinks (juice, soda, power drinks) • Eat breakfast every day (high fiber cereal, low fat milk) • Do not skip meals • Eat slowly • Avoid seconds • Order regular-size not oversized portions	
14. Encourage the client to access self-management information at American Diabetes Association (www.diabetes.org), National Diabetes Education Program (www.ndep.nih.gov/diabetes), American Dietetic Association (www.eatright.org)	14. The journals provide up-to-date information on research, new products, recipes, meal plans, and exercise.
15. Teach the signs and symptoms of hypoglycemia to the client and family. a. Mild hypoglycemia: • Sudden plunges • Tingling in hands, lips, and tongue • Cold, clammy, and pale skin. • Tachycardia/palpitations b. Moderate hypoglycemia (<50 mg/dL) • Uncooperative • Irritable • Often requires assistance c. Severe (<40 mg/dL) hypoglycemia (central nervous system): • Incoherent speech • Lack of motor coordination • Mental confusion • Seizure or coma/convulsions	15. Early detection of hypoglycemia enables prompt intervention and may prevent serious complications (ADA 1997). Insulin reaction, insulin shock, and hypoglycemia are all synonymous with low blood glucose (<70 mg/dL). Hypoglycemia may result from too much insulin, too little food, or too vigorous activity. Low BG may occur just before meal times, during or after exercise, and/or when insulin is at its peak action.
16. Teach the client to prevent hypoglycemia: a. Routine BG monitoring b. Scheduled meal plan c. BG monitoring before exercise or strenuous activity d. Guidelines for decreasing insulin or increasing food before exercise e. Awareness of changes in daily routines that may precipitate hypoglycemia f. Need to carry some form of glucose for emergencies g. Need to plan food intake carefully when drinking alcohol (drink one to two drinks only) h. Need to wear diabetes identification	16. Regular BG monitoring may help to minimize fluctuations in BG levels.
17. Teach the client self-management of hypoglycemia (<70 mg/dL): a. Take 15 grams of carbohydrates (3–4 oz. of juice, 4 oz. regular soda, 3 tsp. jelly, 8 oz milk, 3–5 glucose tablets) b. Wait 15 minutes, test BG again. Take another 15 grams of carbohydrates if BG is still <70 mg/dL.	17. a,b. Quick-acting carbohydrates (CHO) are needed to increase BG quickly. Slowly digested CHO helps to maintain BG levels if the client is 2 hours from the next meal.

(continued on page 161)

Interventions	Rationales
c. Do not overtreat hypoglycemia with excessive carbohydrates.	c. Commercial products may be more appropriate if the client tends to overeat during decreased BG episodes. Glucose gels or liquids are treatments of choice for a semiconscious person.
d. If hypoglycemia is severe or the client cannot swallow, administer 1 mg of glucagon subcutaneously (or IV). If the client does not respond within 15 minutes, seek emergency assistance.	d. Commercial glucagon is an injectable treatment for severe hypoglycemia. It is available by prescription and recommended for clients who may be confused or unconscious, and are unable to take food or drink by mouth. The stability of glucagon is short; therefore, it must be mixed just before use. Because glucagon must be administered by another person, the client's family or friends must be taught how to prepare and administer it in case of an emergency (ADA, 1996).

18. If hypoglycemia occurs at night or following significant exercise after BG level >69 mg/dL is established:
a. Have the client eat 1/2 bread and 1/2 meat exchange to avoid repeated episodes.
b. Teach the client examples of appropriate treatment for hypoglycemia:
  • *Fruit exchange* (15 g CHO):
    ½ cup fruit juice
    ½ cup regular (not diet) soda
    ½ cup apple sauce
    6–7 Lifesavers
  • *Bread exchange* (15 g CHO)
    6 saltines
    1 slice bread
    ½ English muffin
  • *Meat exchange*
    1 oz cheese
    ¼ cup cottage cheese
b. 1 tbsp peanut butter
c. Discuss commercial products available for treating hypoglycemia:
  • Dextrosol tablets (Orange Medical)
  • Glucose tablets (B-D)
  • Monoject gel (Sherwood)
  • Glutose liquid (Paddock)
  • Glucagon injection (Eli Lilly)
	18. Intensive monitoring and intravenous access is needed for successful management.

19. Teach the client the importance of achieving and maintaining normal weight. (Refer to the Obesity care plan for specific strategies.)	19. An obese client has fewer available insulin receptors. Weight loss restores the number of insulin receptors, making insulin more effective. Weight loss may also reduce or eliminate the need for oral agents.

20. Explain Sick Day Treatment:
a. Never fail to take diabetic medicine
b. Monitor blood glucose every 3–4 hours. Test urine for ketones when two BG levels are >250 mg/dL
c. Drink 6–8 ounces of water each hour
 	
d. Call health care provider or seek emergency room care if:
  • vomiting or diarrhea persists for more than 6 hours
  • ketone values are moderate or large
  • blood glucose levels are low (<70 mg/dL)
  • you do not know what to do
	20.
	a,b. Anticipating the effects of illness on the BG level may alert the client to take precautions. Extra fluids help to prevent dehydration.
	c. Immediate interventions are required to prevent dehydration and severe hypoglycemia.
	d. Early detection of ketones in urine can enable prompt intervention to prevent ketoacidosis. Clients with type I diabetes are susceptible to ketosis.

(continued on page 162)

Interventions	Rationales

21. Teach the client to take insulin and maintain carbohydrate (CHO) intake when ill by substituting liquids or easily digested solids for regular food. Assist the client to determine the total amount (in grams) of CHO needed in 24 hours. Instruct the client to *always* consume CHO, even when ill.
 	
Examples of CHO for sick days:
a. *Bread exchange* = 15 g CHO
  1 slice bread or toast
  ½ English muffin
  ½ bagel (2 oz)
  ½ cup cooked cereal
  6 saltines
  6 pretzels
  20 oyster crackers
b. *Fruit exchange* = 15 g CHO
  1 cup Gatorade
  ½ twin bar popsicle
  ½ cup orange juice
  ½ cup apple cider
  ½ cup unsweetened applesauce
  ½ cup ginger ale or cola (not diet)
c. CHO content of other foods
  ½ cup regular Jello = 24 g
  2 level tsp. sugar = 8 g
	21. Illness often causes loss of appetite. Liquids or semisoft foods may be substituted for the client's normal diet. A client on insulin therapy needs to maintain a consistent CHO intake that will supply glucose. When there is a lack of CHO, fats are used for energy. Ketones form from the metabolism of fat.

22. Explain the effects of exercise on glucose metabolism:
a. Explain the benefits of regular exercise:
  • Improved fitness
  • Psychological benefits (e.g., enhanced ability to relax, increased self-confidence, and improved self-image)
  • Reduction of body fat
  • Weight control
b. Explain that the goal is to engage in a total of 30 minutes of moderate-intensity physical activity every day. For example, walk 10,000 steps in a day (usual is 4000–6000 steps). Wear a pedometer to monitor and motivate. Refer also to www.walkinginfo.org.
c. Instruct the client to seek the advice of a health care provider before beginning an exercise program.
d. Teach the client to avoid injecting insulin into a body part that is about to be exercised.
e. Encourage the client to exercise with others or where other informed persons are nearby, and to always wear diabetes identification.
f. Explain how to reduce serious hypoglycemic episodes related to exercise:
  • Monitor BG before and after exercise.
  • Exercise when BG level tends to be higher, such as shortly after a meal.
  • Carry a source of sugar for emergency.
  • Identify a relative or friend who is willing and able to inject glucagon, if necessary.
  • Have glucagon available whenever strenuously exercising.
	22.
	a. Emphasizing the benefits of exercise may help the client to succeed with the prescribed exercise regimen (ADA, 2006).
	
	b. Exercise is contraindicated when BG level exceeds 300 mg/dL, because it causes a rise in BG and an increase in ketone production, as hepatic production of glucose becomes disproportionately greater than the body's use of insulin.
	c. Exercise may be contraindicated with certain complications (e.g., severe nephropathy, proliferative retinopathy).
	d. Insulin absorption increases in a body part that is exercised, which alters the insulin's absorption (ADA, 1996).
	e. Exercising with others ensures that assistance is available should hypoglycemia occur.
	
	f. Proper timing of exercise, monitoring BG, and adjusting food or insulin decreases the risk of exercise-induced hypoglycemia. In the event of a severe reaction, a semiconscious or unconscious client may require glucagon (ADA, 1996).

(continued on page 163)

Interventions	Rationales

23. Explain the importance of foot care and risks to the feet.
  a. Teach the importance of daily foot inspection.
  b. Teach the client to prevent foot problems:
    • Maintain normal BG and cholesterol levels.
    • Remove shoes and socks at every office visit.
    • Contact your health care provider at the first sign of a foot problem.
    • Trim toenails straight across; seek professional care regularly for corns, calluses, or ingrown/thickened toenails.
    • Make foot inspection part of the daily routine.
    • Avoid exposing the feet to temperature extremes.
    • Wear warm, natural-fiber socks and well-made, properly fitting shoes.
    • Nonsmoking status is essential.
	23. Foot lesions result from peripheral neuropathy, vascular disease, and superimposed infection. Feet that are deformed, insensitive, and ischemic are prime targets for lesions and susceptible to trauma.

24. Teach the client and family to contact a health care provider when any of these occur:
  a. Unexplained fluctuations in BG
  b. Unexplained urinary ketones
  c. A foot injury that does not show signs of healing in 24 hours
  d. Changes in vision
  e. Vomiting/diarrhea for more than 24 hours
  f. Signs of infection
	24. Diabetes makes the feet more prone to injury from decreased circulation. Daily inspections are vital to detect problems early. Injury can be reduced with proper shoes; proper nail trimming; attention to calluses, corns, and thickened nails; and avoiding extreme temperatures. Removing shoes and socks with each visit to a health care provider will remind the provider to examine the feet. Tobacco use will increase vasoconstriction and decrease circulation to the feet.

25. Provide informational materials and/or referrals that may assist the client to reach goals:
  a. Comprehensive Outpatient Diabetes
  b. Support groups
  c. *Diabetes Forecast, Diabetes Self-Management*, and *Clinical Diabetes*
  d. American Diabetes Association (www.diabetes.org/for)
  e. Other online sites, books, and/or DVDs on diabetes
  f. American Association of Diabetes Educators (AADE)
	25. A client who feels well-supported can cope more effectively. A chronically ill person with multiple stressors needs to identify an effective support system. Knowing a friend or neighbor with diabetes, participating in a walk-a-thon for the ADA, and reading about people successfully coping with diabetes are some helpful examples.

Documentation

Discharge summary record
    Client teaching
    Status of outcome achievement
    Referrals

Hepatitis (Viral)

Hepatitis is an inflammation of the liver caused by one of five different viral agents (Table 1). The effects of hepatitis range from mild and curable to chronic and fatal.

TABLE 1   Types of Viral Hepatitis

	Type A	Type B	Type C	Type D
Method of Transmission	Fecal–oral 98% Transfusion <2%	Parenteral Sexual Perinatal	Parenteral (IV drugs) 70% Sexual 6% Unknown 25%–30%	Primary Parenteral Sexually (rare) Perinatal
Severity, Chronicity	Never chronic, but can relapse	90% Recover 5%–10% Chronic	Subclinical infection; Can take 10–30 years to develop chronic hepatitis	
Incubation	2–6 weeks	4 weeks to 6 months	15–150 days	4–6 weeks
Complications	Fulminant hepatitis <1%	Fulminant hepatitis <1% Hepatocellular carcinoma	Cirrhosis 15%–20% Hepatocellular carcinoma 10%–20% Chronic hepatitis 75%	
Prevention	Preexposure HAURIX Postexposure immunoglobulin	Postexposure HBIG+ Recombivax Preexposure Recombivax	None	Vaccine against B will protect against D

■■■■■■ DIAGNOSTIC CLUSTER

Collaborative Problems	Refer to
△ PC: Fulminant Hepatic Failure	
△ PC: Portal Systemic Encephalopathy	Cirrhosis
△ PC: Hypokalemia	Cirrhosis
△ PC: Hemorrhage	Cirrhosis
△ PC: Drug Toxicity	Cirrhosis
△ PC: Renal Insufficiency	Renal Calculi

Nursing Diagnoses	Refer to
▲ High Risk for Infection Transmission related to contagious nature of viral agents	
▲ Imbalanced Nutrition: Less Than Body Requirements related to anorexia, epigastric distress, and nausea	Cirrhosis
△ High Risk for Ineffective Therapeutic Regimen Management related to lack of knowledge of condition, rest requirements, precautions to prevent transmission, nutritional requirements, and activity restrictions.	
△ Impaired Comfort related to pruritus secondary to accumulation of bilirubin pigment and bile salts	Cirrhosis
△ Pain related to swelling of inflamed liver	Pancreatitis

▲ This diagnosis was reported to be monitored for or managed frequently (75%–100%).
△ This diagnosis was reported to be monitored for or managed often (50%–74%).

Discharge Criteria

Before discharge, the client or family will

1. Describe the modes of disease transmission.
2. State signs and symptoms that they must report to a health care professional.

Collaborative Problems

Potential Complication: Fulminant Hepatic Failure

Nursing Goal

The nurse will detect early signs/symptoms of fulminant hepatic failure and collaboratively intervene to stabilize the client.

Indicators

- Blood glucose <140 mg/dL two hours after eating
- Prothrombin time (PT) 11–12.5 seconds
- Partial prothrombin time (PTT) 60–70 seconds
- Aspartate aminotransferase (AST)
  - Male 7–21 u/L
  - Female 6–18 u/L
- Alanine aminotransferase (ALT) 5–35 u/L
- Alkaline phosphatase 30–150 u/L
- Blood urea nitrogen (BUN) 5–25 mg/dL
- Serum electrolytes (refer to laboratory values in institution)
- Prealbumin 20–50 mg/dL
- Alert, oriented
- Pulse 60–100 beats/min
- BP >90/60, <140/90 mmHg
- Temperature 98–99.5°F
- Respiration 16–20 breaths/min
- EEG normal

Interventions	Rationales

1. Monitor for fulminant hepatic failure.
  a. Coagulation defects
  b. Renal failure
  c. Electrolyte imbalance
  d. Infection
  e. Hypoglycemia
  f. Encephalopathy
  g. Cerebral edema
	1. Fulminant hepatic failure is the sudden onset of severely impaired liver function. Older adults with hepatitis are at serious risk for this problem.

2. Refer to index of collaborative problems for specific interventions for each physiologic complication above.	

 Related Physician-Prescribed Interventions

Medications. Hepatitis C antivirals (acyclovir, ribavirin); antiemetics; antidiarrheals; antacids; interferon alpha, peginterferon (Hep-C); vitamins

Intravenous Therapy. Total parenteral therapy, protein hydrolysates

Laboratory Studies. Bilirubin; alkaline phosphatase; prothrombin time; serum albumin; hepatitis C viral load, hepatitis C genotype; hepatitis panels; serum alanine aminotransferase (ALT)

Diagnostic Studies. Liver scan, aspartate aminotransferase (AST), liver biopsy

Therapies. Dietary restrictions depending on fat and protein tolerance, bed rest

Documentation

Flow records
  Intake and output
Progress notes
  Evaluation of signs and symptoms

Nursing Diagnoses

High Risk for Infection Transmission Related to Contagious Nature of Viral Agents

(This diagnosis is not currently on the NANDA list but has been included for clarity or usefulness.)

NOC Infection Status, Risk Control, Risk Detection

Goal

The client will report precautions needed to prevent transmission.

Indicators

- Remain in isolation until noninfectious.
- Demonstrate meticulous hand-washing during hospitalization.

NIC Teaching: Disease Process, Infection Protection

Interventions	Rationales
1. Use appropriate universal body substance precautions for all body fluids: a. Wash hands before and after all client or specimen contact. b. Handle blood as potentially infectious. c. Wear gloves for potential contact with blood and body fluids. d. Place used syringes immediately in a nearby impermeable container; do not recap or manipulate the needle in anyway. e. Use protective eye wear if splatter with blood or body fluids is possible (e.g., bronchoscopy, oral surgery). f. Wear gowns when splash with blood or body fluids is anticipated. g. Handle all linen soiled with blood or body secretions as potentially infectious. h. Process all laboratory specimens as potentially infectious.	1. Refer to Table 1 for specific modes of transmission.
2. Use appropriate techniques for disposal of infectious waste, linen, and body fluids, and for cleaning contaminated equipment and surfaces.	2. These techniques help to protect others from contact with infectious materials and prevent disease transmission.
3. Refer the infection control practitioner for follow-up with the appropriate Health Department.	3. This referral is necessary to identify the source of exposure and other possibly infected persons.
4. Explain the importance of frequent hand-washing to the client, family, other visitors, and health care personnel.	4. Hand-washing removes organisms and breaks the chain of infection transmission.

Documentation

Flow records
Isolation precautions required
Discharge summary record
Client teaching

High Risk for Ineffective Therapeutic Regimen Management Related to Lack of Knowledge of Condition, Rest Requirements, Precautions to Prevent Transmission, Nutritional Requirements, and Contraindications

NOC Compliance Behavior, Knowledge: Treatment Regimen, Participation in Health Care Decisions, Treatment Behavior: Illness or Injury

Goals

The goals for this diagnosis represent those associated with discharge planning. Refer to the discharge criteria.

NIC Health Education, Health System Guidance, Learning Facilitation, Learning Readiness Enhancement, Risk Identification, Self-Modification Assistance

Interventions	Rationales
1. Explain the mode of infection transmission to the client and family. Refer to Table 1.	1. Understanding how infection can be transmitted is the first step in prevention.
2. If appropriate, explain to contacts such as family and peers that they should receive hepatitis B or A vaccines or immune globulin.	2. For their protection, family and associates should receive active or passive immunization for hepatitis B.
3. Explain the need to rest and to avoid strenuous activity.	3. As the liver repairs itself, excessive physical activity depletes the body of the energy needed for healing. Adequate rest prevents relapse. It may take 3 to 6 months for energy levels to return to normal.
4. Explain the need for a diet high in protein and calories. (Refer to the nursing diagnosis Imbalanced Nutrition in the Cirrhosis care plan.)	4. Protein and caloric requirements increase during periods of tissue healing.
5. Explain the hazards of certain medications: oral contraceptives, narcotics, sedatives, tranquilizers, and acetaminophen.	5. Certain drugs are hepatotoxic. Moreover, in hepatitis, impaired liver function slows drug metabolism; this causes drug levels to accumulate in the body.
6. Teach the client and family to watch for and report signs and symptoms of complications: a. Unusual bleeding (e.g., gums, stools) b. Hypokalemia (manifested by muscle cramps, nausea, vomiting) c. Confusion, altered speech patterns d. Increasing severity of symptoms e. Rapid weight loss or gain	6. Early recognition and reporting enable prompt intervention to prevent serious complications. a. Bleeding indicates decreased prothrombin time and clotting factors. b. Overproduction of aldosterone causes sodium and water retention and potassium excretion. c. Neurologic impairment results from cerebral hypoxia owing to high serum ammonia levels caused by the liver's impaired ability to convert ammonia to urea (Porth, 2007). d. Worsening symptoms indicate progressive liver damage. e. Rapid weight loss points to negative nitrogen balance; rapid weight gain points to fluid retention.

(continued on page 168)

Interventions	Rationales
7. Explain the importance of avoiding alcohol.	7. Alcohol increases hepatic irritation and may interfere with recovery. With Hepatitis C, alcohol leads to rapid progression of cirrhosis.
8. Stress the importance of follow-up care and laboratory studies.	8. Follow-up care enables evaluation of liver function and detection of relapse or recurrence. New therapies are available for severe liver disease.

Documentation

Discharge summary record
  Client teaching
  Outcome achievement
  Referrals when indicated

Hypothyroidism

In hypothyroidism, thyroid gland dysfunction results in a deficiency of thyroid hormones thyroxine (T_4) and triiodothyronine (T_3). These hormones are responsible for maintaining body metabolism. Factors that contribute to hypothyroidism are hypothalamic dysfunction, thyroid-releasing hormone or thyroid-stimulating hormone deficiency, iatrogenic (e.g., surgery) response, iodide medications (e.g., lithium), pituitary disorders, thyroid deficiencies or destruction (Porth, 2007).

 Time Frame
Initial diagnosis, secondary diagnosis

▪▪▪▪▪▪ DIAGNOSTIC CLUSTER*

Collaborative Problems

PC: Metabolic
PC: Myxedema Coma
PC: Atherosclerotic Heart Disease
PC: Hematologic
PC: Acute Organic Psychosis

Nursing Diagnoses	Refer to
Impaired Comfort related to cold intolerance secondary to decreased metabolic rate	
High Risk for Ineffective Therapeutic Regimen Management related to insufficient knowledge of condition, treatment regimen, signs and symptoms of complications, dietary management, pharmacological therapy, and activity restrictions.	

(continued on page 169)

Nursing Diagnoses	Refer to
Imbalanced Nutrition: Less Than Body Requirements related to intake greater than metabolic needs secondary to slowed metabolic rate	Corticosteroid Therapy
Constipation related to decreased peristaltic action secondary to decreased metabolic rate and decreased physical activity	General Surgery

* This medical condition was not included in the validation study.

Discharge Criteria

Before discharge, the client or family will

1. Describe dietary restrictions.
2. Relate the importance of adhering to the medication schedule.
3. Describe risk factors.
4. Relate signs and symptoms that must be reported to a health care professional.
5. Identify community resources available for assistance.

Collaborative Problems

Potential Complication: Metabolic

Potential Complication: Myxedema Coma

Potential Complication: Atherosclerotic Heart Disease

Potential Complication: Hematologic

Potential Complication: Acute Organic Psychosis

Nursing Goal

The nurse will detect early signs and symptoms of (a) metabolic dysfunction, (b) atherosclerotic heart disease, (c) hematologic dysfunction, and (d) acute psychosis, and collaboratively intervene to stabilize the client.

Indicators

- Temperature 98–99.5°F (a)
- Heart rhythm regular (a, b, c)
- Heart rate 60–100 beats/min (a, b, c)
- BP >90/60, <140/90 mmHg
- Respiration 16–20 breaths/min (a, c)
- Intact peripheral sensation (a)
- Alert, oriented, and calm (a, b, c, d)
- Intact memory (b, d)
- Clear speech (b, d)
- Intact muscle strength (b, d)
- Regular menses (a)
- Regular bowel movements (a)
- No jaundice (a)
- Urine, stool, emesis—negative for blood (c)
- No signs of bleeding, bruises (c)
- Thyroid-stimulating hormone 2–10 U/mL (a)
- Triiodothyronine (T_3) 0.2–0.6 µg/dL (a)
- Thyroxine (T_4) 5–12 µg/dL (a)
- Fasting Serum glucose 70–100 mg/dL (a)

Interventions	Rationales
1. Monitor metabolic function:	1. Deficiencies in circulating hormones reduce metabolism, thus affecting all body systems. Severity of signs and symptoms depends on the duration and degree of thyroid hormone deficiency (Porth, 2005).
a. Cardiac: • Decreased cardiac output • Low blood pressure or decreased pulse rate and pressure • Decreased or normal heart rate	a. Cardiac tissue changes, decreased stroke volume, and heart rate reduce cardiac output. Impaired peripheral circulation accounts for changes in cardiac performance.
b. Respiratory	b. Hypoventilation occurs partly because of mucopolysaccharide deposits in respiratory system, with subsequent decreased vital capacity. Hypercarbia also further decreases respiratory rate.
c. Neurologic: • Paresthesias of fingers and toes • Changes in affect, mentation, short-term memory, delusions • Slowed, slurred speech • Seizures	c. Hyponatremia may be responsible for some neurologic symptoms. Paresthesias result from direct metabolic changes on nerves and interstitial edema of surrounding tissues. Changes in affect, mentation, short-term memory, and delusions are caused by cerebral edema resulting from changes in adrenal gland affecting water retention, and by cerebral hypoxia resulting from decreased cerebral blood flow. Speech problems result from edema in the cerebellar region of the brain. Seizures may occur in up to 25% of people with long-standing hypothyroidism.
d. Musculoskeletal: • Muscle weakness • Pathologic fractures	d. Mucoprotein edema separating muscle fibers causes muscle weakness and stiffness. Pathologic fractures result from impaired calcium transport and use caused by decreased calcitonin levels (produced by the thyroid gland).
e. Gastrointestinal: • Constipation • Impaired digestion	e. GI tract motility is decreased because of mucoproteins in the interstitial spaces. Poor food digestion occurs throughout the GI tract because of mucosal atrophy and decreased production of hydrochloric acid.
f. Hormonal: • Hypoglycemia • Increased thyroid-stimulating hormone (TSH) • Decreased T_3 or T_4 • Menorrhagia or amenorrhea, decreased libido	f. Hypoglycemia results from changes in the adrenal cortex. Increased TSH usually confirms the diagnosis of primary hypothyroidism, which accounts for approximately 90% of cases of hypothyroidism. TSH levels tend to increase with age. Levothyroxine (T_4) and triiodothyronine (T_3) are produced and distributed by the thyroid gland; T_4 is responsible for maintaining a steady metabolic rate. Altered levels of sexual hormones in early hypothyroidism result in prolonged heavy menstrual periods and changes in libido. Prolonged hypothyroidism leads to amenorrhea, anovulation, and infertility, resulting from effects of myxedema on luteinizing hormone.
g. Integumentary: • Thickened, dry skin • Yellowish skin color in absence of jaundiced sclera • Thin, brittle nails, with transverse grooves • Coarse, dry hair with beginning hair loss (e.g., medial third of eyebrows)	g. Hyperkeratosis, an overgrowth of the horny layer of the epidermis, occurs with subsequent decrease in activity of sweat glands and resulting skin dryness. Monopolysaccharide accumulation in subcutaneous tissue results in thickened skin. Low-density lipoprotein, the primary plasma carrier of carotene, increases with low levels of thyroid hormones, resulting in yellowed skin. Dry skin, hair loss, and nail changes result in altered cell replication resulting from decreased thyroid hormones.
2. Monitor for myxedema coma: • Comatose • Hypothermia • Bradycardia • Hypoventilation • Hypotension • Hyponatremia • Hypoglycemia	2. Myxedema coma, although rare, may result from untreated progressive myxedema. It occurs more frequently in older women. Many of the cases occur when the individual with long-standing hypothyroidism is hospitalized for another condition. It carries a 50% mortality rate. Precipitating events for myxedema coma include infections, surgery, trauma, hypothermia, and effects of various drugs such as sedatives or hypnotics.

(continued on page 171)

Interventions	Rationales

3. Monitor a myxedematous client for signs and symptoms of myocardial ischemia and infarction after initiating thyroid hormone replacement:
  a. Abnormal rate or rhythm
  b. Palpitations
  c. Syncope
  d. Cardiac emergencies (e.g., arrest or ventricular fibrillation)
	3. As oxygen requirements increase with increased metabolism, angina may result if the client has atherosclerosis or coronary artery disease caused by reduced lipid metabolism with monopolysaccharide deposits in the myocardium (Porth, 2005).

4. Monitor for signs and symptoms of atherosclerotic heart disease:
  a. Elevated blood pressure
  b. Vertigo
  c. Chest pain
	4. Atherosclerosis can occur rapidly in a client with hypothyroidism, because the protein-bound iodine and T_4 levels are low and blood cholesterol levels are high. Sometimes a decrease in atherosclerosis occurs after thyroid hormone replacement is initiated. However, excessive doses of thyroid hormone replacement initially may result in vascular occlusion due to atherosclerosis.

5. Monitor for signs and symptoms of acute organic psychosis:
  a. Agitation
  b. Acute anxiety
  c. Paranoia
  d. Delusions
  e. Hallucinations
	5. Often a client with severe behavioral symptoms has an underlying psychiatric disorder that may not improve and actually may be exacerbated by thyroid hormone therapy.

6. Monitor for signs and symptoms of anemia:
  a. Fatigue
  b. Hypoxia
  c. Easy bruising
  d. Confusion
	6. Normochromic, normocytic anemia results from a decrease in erythrocyte mass as a compensatory response to decreased oxygen demand.

7. Monitor for signs of abnormal bleeding:
  a. Petechiae
  b. Bleeding gums
  c. Ecchymotic areas
  d. Blood in urine, stool, or emesis
	7. Thyroid hormone deficiencies cause increased capillary fragility, prolonged clotting time, and decreased platelet adhesiveness.

8. Avoid administering sedatives and narcotics, or reduce dosage to one-half or one-third the regular dose.	8. Slowed breakdown of these medications prolongs high circulating levels, resulting in heightened response and possibly respiratory depression.

 ### Related Physician-Prescribed Interventions

Medications. Levothyroxine, liothyronine
Intravenous Therapy. Not indicated
Laboratory Studies. Serum T_4, T_3; serum cholesterol; serum sodium; resin T_3 uptake; alkaline phosphate; thyroid-stimulating hormone assay (TSH); triglyceride levels
Diagnostic Studies. Radioactive iodine uptake, electrocardiogram, thyroid scan, MRI–head
Therapies. Weight loss diet

Documentation

Flow records
   Vital signs
   Intake and output
   Rhythm strips
Progress notes
   Unusual events

Nursing Diagnoses

Impaired Comfort Related to Cold Intolerance Secondary to Decreased Metabolic Rate (This diagnosis is currently not on the NANDA list and has been added for clarity and usefulness.)

NOC Symptom Control

Goals

1. The client will report episodes of cold intolerance.
2. The client will report improved tolerance to cold after body heat retention measures are employed.

NIC Pruritus Management, Fever Treatment, Environmental Management: Comfort

Interventions	Rationales

1. Monitor for signs of hypothermia:
  a. Rectal temperature <96°F
  b. Decreased pulse and respiration rate
  c. Cool skin
  d. Blanching, redness, or pallor
  e. Shivering
	1. Decreased circulating thyroid hormones reduce the metabolic rate; the resulting vasoconstriction increases the risk of hypothermia.

2. Explain measures to prevent chilling:
  a. Increase temperature in the living environment.
  b. Eliminate drafts.
  c. Use several blankets at night.
  d. Protect from cold exposure (e.g., wear several layers of clothing and wool hats, socks, and gloves.)
	2. Chilling increases the metabolic rate and puts increased stress on the heart.

3. Explain the need for rewarming *gradually* after exposure to cold, and for avoiding application of external heat to rewarm rapidly.	3. Vascular collapse can result from a rapid increase in metabolic rate by heating and the subsequent strain on the heart from the increased myocardial oxygen requirements.
4. Encourage the client to avoid smoking cigarettes.	4. Smoking further increases the vasoconstriction caused by a decreased metabolic rate, increasing susceptibility to cold in the body's peripheral areas.

Documentation

Flow records
  Vital signs including rectal temperature
Discharge summary record
  Client teaching
  Outcome achievements

High Risk for Ineffective Therapeutic Regimen Management Related to Insufficient Knowledge of Condition, Treatment Regimen, Signs and Symptoms of Complications, Dietary Management, Pharmacological Therapy, and Contraindications

NOC Compliance Behavior, Knowledge: Treatment Regimen, Participation in Health Care Decisions, Treatment Behavior: Illness or Injury

Goal

The goals for this diagnosis represent those associated with discharge planning. Refer to the discharge criteria.

NIC   Health Education, Health System Guidance, Learning
Facilitation, Learning Readiness Enhancement,
Risk Identification, Self-Modification Assistance

Interventions	Rationales
1. Explain the pathophysiology of hypothyroidism by using teaching aids (e.g., pictures, slide-tapes, models) appropriate to the client's or family's educational level.	1. Presenting relevant and useful information in an easily understandable format greatly decreases learning frustration and may help to increase compliance.
2. Explain risk factors that can be eliminated or modified: a. Exposure to cold b. Tobacco use c. Regular alcohol intake d. High-fat diet e. Stressors (e.g., emotional stress, infections)	2. The client's understanding that certain risk factors can be controlled may help to improve compliance with the therapeutic regimen. a–c. Exposure to cold as well as tobacco and alcohol use increase vasoconstriction. a–d. Decreased thyroid hormone levels increase blood lipids. a–e. Stress raises the metabolic rate in hypothyroidism.
3. Instruct the client and family to observe for and report signs and symptoms of disease complications: a. Progression of disease signs and symptoms b. Behavioral changes (e.g., agitation, confusion, delusions, paranoia, hallucinations) c. Angina d. Extreme fatigue e. Seizure activity f. Edema in the feet and ankles	3. Early detection and reporting complications enable prompt treatment.
4. Reinforce explanations for therapeutic diet. Consult a dietitian when indicated. a. Maintain a low-calorie diet. b. Have small portions of nutritious foods. c. Avoid excessive fluid intake. d. Eat foods rich in fiber. e. Avoid soybeans, white turnips, cabbage, and peanuts.	4. Understanding the reasons for the therapeutic diet may encourage the client to comply. a. A low-calorie diet compensates for a decreased metabolic rate. b. Small portions compensate for impaired digestion secondary to decreased production of hydrochloric acid. c. Limited fluid intake may help to reduce fluid retention secondary to increased capillary permeability. d. Increased fiber intake can help to increase gastrointestinal motility. e. These foods interfere with thyroid hormone production.
5. Explain why precautions are required when taking certain medications: a. Antihyperlipidemics, phenothiazines, sedatives, narcotics, anesthetics: Chemical reactions are slowed, causing delayed breakdown of medications and prolonged high circulating levels; this results in increased somnolence. b. Insulin: Thyroid hormones may increase blood glucose levels. c. Digitalis, indomethacin, anticoagulants: Delayed metabolism can potentiate their effects. d. Phenytoin (Dilantin), lovastatin (Mevacor), and carbamazepine (Tegretol) lower circulating T_4 levels by increasing rate of clearance. e. Lithium inhibits secretion of thyroid hormones from the thyroid gland.	5. Understanding that the delayed metabolism of medications can cause sustained elevated levels may encourage the client to adhere to the dosage schedule.

(continued on page 174)

Interventions	Rationales
6. Explain that the side effects of thyroid hormone therapy can produce signs and symptoms similar to those of hyperthyroidism: a. Tachycardia b. Increased respiratory rate c. Restlessness or irritability d. Heat intolerance e. Increased perspiration f. Diarrhea g. Osteopenia or reduction in bone density	6. Excessive dosage can cause hyperthyroidism and a too-rapid metabolic rate. These signs and symptoms tend to be less exaggerated in an elderly client than in a younger one. Studies have shown a 9%–13% decrease in bone density with use of thyroxine for more than 5 years (Franklyn & Sheppard, 1990).
7. Teach the client to observe for symptoms of a too-rapid change in metabolic rate: a. Headaches b. Palpitations c. Angina	7. The client must begin the medication regimen slowly so as to not significantly increase cardiac workload that would cause dysrhythmias and angina.
8. Explain the importance of continuing daily medication and periodic laboratory testing throughout the rest of the client's life. Explain the following: a. The client should take thyroid hormone at the same time each day. b. T_3 and T_4 testing should be done periodically to check thyroid hormone blood levels. c. The brand of thyroid replacement therapy should not be changed.	8. a,b. Fluctuations in drug blood levels produce signs and symptoms of hypothyroidism. c. Different brands of the drug are *not* bioequivalent.
9. Reinforce the need for follow-up care; note that it may take several months to achieve control.	9. Follow-up enables evaluation for signs of hypothyroidism or hyperthyroidism and laboratory tests to determine if medication adjustments are needed.

Documentation

Discharge summary record
    Discharge instructions
    Follow-up instructions
    Status at discharge
    Achievement of goals (family or individual)

Obesity

More than 97 million Americans are overweight or obese. Overweight is defined as having a body mass index (BMI) of 25–29.9 kg/m². BMI describes a person's weight relative to their height. It is significantly correlated with total body fat content. A BMI above 30 kg/m² defines obesity (Blackwell, Miller, & Chun, 2002), which is a complex problem involving social, psychological, and metabolic issues. Obesity is most commonly caused by overeating and insufficient exercise. Behavioral characteristics common to obese persons include the following:

- Response to external cues rather than internal cues as to when to eat or stop eating
- Eating in response to feelings of depression, elation, loneliness, sadness, or boredom
- Excessive eating in a short time span, followed by feelings of remorse
- Inactivity or underactivity (Dudek, 2006)

■■■■■■ **DIAGNOSTIC CLUSTER***

Nursing Diagnoses

Ineffective Health Maintenance related to imbalance between caloric intake and energy expenditure

Ineffective Coping related to increased food consumption secondary to response to external stressors

* This medical condition was not included in the validation study.

Discharge Criteria

Before discharge, the client or family will:

1. Relate caloric, nutritional, and exercise requirements.
2. State the condition of home behavioral management of food consumption and energy expenditure.
3. Relate community resources or professionals to contact after discharge.

Nursing Diagnoses

Ineffective Health Maintenance Related to Imbalance Between Caloric Intake and Energy Expenditure

NOC Health Promoting Behavior, Health Seeking Behavior, Knowledge: Health Promotion, Knowledge: Health Resources, Participation in Health Care Decisions, Risk Detection, Treatment Behavior: Illness

Goals

The client will commit to a weight loss program:

1. Identify present eating and exercise patterns.
2. Describe the relationship between metabolism, intake, and exercise.
3. Relate a plan to lose weight.

NIC Health Education, Self-Responsibility Facilitation, Health Screening, Risk Identification, Family Involvement Promotion

Interventions	Rationales
1. Increase the client's awareness of how body weight is affected by the balance between food intake and activity. Explain that successful weight reduction and maintenance hinge on achieving a balance between reduced caloric intake and increased caloric expenditure through regular exercise. To determine the number of calories the client should consume daily to reach and maintain his or her ideal weight, multiply the female client's ideal weight in pounds by 11, or the male client's by 12. One pound of fat roughly equals 3500 calories. Thus, to lose 2 pounds per week, the client must cut 7000 calories from her or his current weekly intake. Exercise caloric expenditure charts may be used to determine the calories burned during various activities.	1. Weight loss goals may be achieved through a combination of reduced caloric intake and increased caloric expenditure through exercise. Any increase in physical activity increases energy output and caloric deficits in a person following a reduced-calorie dietary regimen.

(continued on page 176)

Interventions	Rationales

2. Help the client to develop a safe, realistic weight-loss program that considers these factors:
  a. Amount of loss desired
  b. Duration of program
  c. Cost
  d. Nutritional soundness
  e. Compatibility with life style
	2. Realistic goals increase the likelihood of success. Successes give the client an incentive to continue the program.

3. Help the client to identify environmental factors that contribute to poor eating patterns by discussing the following (Dudek, 2006):
  a. Friends, family, coworkers: What are their habits? Would they be supportive?
  b. What types of food are found in the home? At parties? At work? In the lunch room?
  c. In what type of leisure or recreational activities does the client engage? Is the client sedentary?
  d. What route(s) does the client take to and from work? Does the client pass by fast food restaurants?
  e. Who does the housework? The gardening and yard work? Errands?
  f. How much television does the client watch?
  g. Has the client responded to any advertisements for rapid weight loss programs or devices?
	3. Helping the client to identify such external factors may increase his or her internal motivation to overcome them (Dudek, 2006).

4. Instruct the client to keep a diary for 1 week that includes these things:
  a. Food intake and exercise
  b. Location and times of meals
  c. Emotions during mealtimes
  d. Person(s) with whom the client ate
  e. Any skipped meals
  f. Snacks
	4. Such a diary helps the client to become aware of food intake patterns.

5. Discuss the hazards of the following activities:
  a. Eating while doing another activity, such as watching TV or reading
  b. Eating while standing; this can give the illusion of not eating a meal
  c. Eating out of boredom, stress, or another psychological reason
  d. Eating because everyone else is eating
	5. Certain situations may be identified as cues that trigger inappropriate eating.

6. Teach the client the basics of balanced nutritional intake, including supportive measures:
  a. Choose a diet plan that encourages high intake of complex carbohydrates and limited fat intake. Recommended U.S. dietary goals are 30% of total calories from fat, 12% from protein, 48% from complex carbohydrates, and 10% from simple carbohydrates.
  b. Be aware that the method of food preparation also affects total calorie and fat content. For example, a fried-chicken steak is a protein with a high fat content owing to its method of preparation (frying).
  c. Try to obtain as many calories as possible from fruits and vegetables instead of from meat and dairy products.
  d. Eat more chicken and fish, which contain less fat and total calories per ounce than red meat.
	6. Successful weight loss and long-term maintenance can be achieved through a diet low in fat and high in complex carbohydrates (Dudek, 2006).

(continued on page 177)

Interventions	Rationales
e. Limit high-fat salad dressings, especially those that contain mayonnaise (216–308 calories per 2-oz serving). f. Avoid fast foods that have a high-fat and total calorie content. g. When dining in a restaurant, make special requests (e.g., serve salad dressing on the side; omit sauce from entree). h. Plan meals in advance. i. If attending a party or dining out, plan your eating ahead of time and stick to the plan. j. When food shopping, prepare a shopping list and adhere to it. k. Involve the family in meal planning for better nutrition. l. Buy the highest quality ground beef to limit fat content. (Ground round has about 10% fat; regular hamburger, 25% fat.) m. Choose a wide variety of appropriate foods to reduce feelings of deprivation. n. Avoid eating at family-style buffets that increase the chance of overeating. o. Drink 8 to 10 glasses (8 oz) of water daily to help excrete the by-products of weight loss. p. Measure foods and count calories; keep records. q. Read food labels and note ingredients, composition, and total calories per serving. Choose low-fat or no-fat products when possible. Be aware that many prepared foods have hidden ingredients, such as salt and saturated fats, and that some so-called "natural" foods, such as granola, are high in fat and sugar. r. Eat slowly and chew food thoroughly. s. Experiment with spices, fat substitutes, and low-calorie recipes. t. Chew gum while preparing meals to deter eating while cooking.	
7. Discuss the benefits of exercise: a. Reduces caloric absorption b. Acts as an appetite suppressant c. Increases metabolic rate and caloric expenditure d. Preserves lean muscle mass e. Increases oxygen uptake f. Improves self-esteem and decreases depression, anxiety, and stress g. Aids restful sleep h. Improves body posture i. Provides fun, recreation, and diversion j. Increases resistance to degenerative diseases of middle and later years (e.g., cardiovascular disorders)	7. A significant amount of lean muscle mass (up to 30%) can be lost on a calorie-restricted diet. Exercise, on the other hand, minimizes this loss. Exercise also contributes to an overall feeling of well-being, which can positively influence self-esteem during dieting.
8. Help the client to develop a safe, realistic exercise program by considering the following factors: a. Motivation, personality, and life style b. Preferences (e.g., outdoors, classes, individual) c. Time availability d. Occupation: sedentary or active e. Safety (e.g., sports injuries, environmental hazards, risk of crime) f. Cost of club membership or equipment g. Age, physical size, and physical condition	8,9. The client is more likely to comply with a regular exercise program that is convenient and enjoyable. A gradually progressing exercise program minimizes discomfort and injury and encourages compliance.

(continued on page 178)

Interventions	Rationales
9. Discuss beginning an exercise program. If indicated, instruct the client to consult with a physician before starting. Advise the client as follows: a. Start slow and easy. b. Choose activities that exercise many parts of the body. c. Choose activities that are vigorous enough to cause "healthful fatigue." d. Read, consult with experts, and talk with friends and coworkers who exercise. e. Develop a regular exercise program and chart progress. f. Add supplemental activities (e.g., park far away and walk; work on garden; walk up stairs; spend weekends at leisure activities that require walking, such as festivals or art fairs). g. Eliminate time- and energy-saving devices when practicable. h. Work up to ½ to 1 hour of exercise per day at least 4 days per week. i. To maintain optimum conditioning, avoid lapses of more than 2 days between exercise sessions.	
10. Teach the client about the risks of obesity: a. Metabolic abnormalities b. Arteriosclerosis c. Hypertension d. Left ventricular hypertrophy e. Diabetes mellitus f. Gallbladder disease g. Increased risk of complications from surgery h. Respiratory disease i. Increased risk of cancer (e.g., breast, colon) j. Increased risk of accident and injury	10. The client must understand that obesity is a multiple-system health hazard. A diet high in fat and simple cholesterol contributes to atherosclerosis, diabetes, gallbladder disease, breast cancer, and colon cancer. A sedentary life style decreases muscle tone and strength; compromised mobility and balance increases the risk of falls and injury. Fatty tissue is less vascular and more susceptible to infection. Increased peripheral resistance causes increased cardiac workload, which raises blood pressure. Excessive abdominal fatty tissue compromises diaphragmatic movement, which can lead to hypoventilation.
11. Discuss the value of weekly goals versus the larger weight loss goal (e.g., will walk 20 minutes 3–5 days weekly).	11. Weekly goals enable achievement and foster compliance. Unsatisfactory habits can be targeted (e.g., the client doubles eating time by actively slowing consumption) and healthy habits can be promoted (e.g., the client eats plain popcorn as an evening snack). Because weight loss may vary from week to week, a primary focus on pounds lost may be discouraging.

Documentation

Progress notes
   Client teaching
Planning:
   Weight loss goal
   Exercise (type, frequency)
   Weekly goals

Ineffective Coping Related to Increased Food Consumption Secondary to Response to External Stressors

NOC Coping, Self-Esteem, Social Interaction Skills

Goal

The client will identify alternative responses to stressors besides eating.

Indicators

- Identify stressors contributing to overeating.
- Verbalize strengths.

 Coping Enhancement, Counseling, Emotional Support, Active Listening, Assertiveness Training, Behavior Modification

Interventions	Rationales

1. Assist the client to do the following:
  a. Alter ways of thinking (e.g., think of "cheating" as "off-target behavior"; "eating" as "energy intake"; "exercise" as "energy consumption").
  b. Reduce fears of loss of control (e.g., learn to take a taste without fear of a binge).
  c. Take risks and reward successes.
  d. Identify potential problem areas and have a definite plan for getting back "on target."
  e. Understand that weight management simply involves balancing energy intake and energy expenditure.
  f. Observe role models and understand that persons who maintain their weight are not "just lucky."
  g. Examine personal meanings for eating and food other than as a way to meet physiologic needs and sustain life.
	1. Our society places a high value on thinness and typically labels obese persons as undesirable and undisciplined. The measures listed here attempt to alter the client's attitude toward obesity, weight reduction, and exercise.

2. Encourage and assist the client to do the following:
  a. Contract reduction and exercise programs with realistic goals.
  b. Keep intake and exercise records.
  c. Post an admired photograph on the refrigerator.
  d. Increase knowledge about weight loss and exercise by talking with health-conscious friends, relatives, and associates.
  e. Make new friends who are health-conscious and active.
  f. Get a friend to join the program or to serve as a support person.
  g. Reward self for progress.
  h. Keep in mind that self-image and behavior are learned and can be unlearned.
  i. Build a support system of people who value growth and appreciate her or him as an individual.
  j. Be aware of rationalization (e.g., "lack of time" may actually be poor prioritization).
  k. Keep a list of positive outcomes.
	2. Significant weight loss takes many months. These activities help to increase the client's interest and maintain motivation throughout the long program.

3. If possible, involve the client's family in the weight-reduction program. Determine if support is present.	3. Family support is important. If support is not present, open discussions are needed to elicit family support.
4. Instruct the client to limit body measurements and weighing to once per week.	4. Fluctuations in body weight are common, especially in females, owing to water retention. Daily weights are misleading and often disheartening; body measurements provide a better indicator of losses. Moreover, consistent exercising results in lean muscle mass gain. Because muscle weighs more than fat, this may be reflected as weight gain on the scale.
5. Encourage the client to avoid persons who may sabotage weight loss attempts, if possible.	5. Certain persons and relationships may be threatened by the client's weight loss.

(continued on page 180)

Interventions	Rationales

6. Teach the client to do the following:
  a. Distinguish between an urge and actual hunger.
  b. Use distraction, relaxation, and guided imagery.
  c. Make a list of external cues or situations that lead to off-target behavior.
  d. List constructive actions to substitute for off-target behavior (e.g., take a walk).
  e. Post the list of alternative behaviors on the refrigerator.
  f. Adhere to the list and reward self when appropriate.
  g. Every 1 or 2 weeks, reevaluate whether the plan is realistic.
	6. Identification and reduction of inappropriate or destructive responses to stressors can be the critical factors for successful weight loss and maintenance.

Documentation

Progress Notes
Interactions

Pancreatitis

Pancreatitis is an inflammatory response and potential necrosis of pancreatic endocrine and exocrine cells resulting from activation of pancreatic enzymes. The most common causes are alcohol abuse and biliary tract obstruction related to gallstones (Munoz & Katerndahl, 2000). Mechanical causes are those that obstruct or damage the pancreatic duct system, such as cancer, cholelithiasis, abdominal trauma, radiation therapy, parasitic diseases, and duodenal disease. Metabolic causes are those that alter the secretory processes of the acinar cells, such as alcoholism, certain medications, genetic disorders, and diabetic ketoacidosis.

Miscellaneous etiologic factors include infections, ischemic injury, embolism, and hypovolemia. The substrates released cause local inflammation and pathology in and around the pancreas, and trigger systemic complications. The mortality rate for acute pancreatitis is 2%–9%, and rises to 20%–50% if hemorrhage is present (Munoz & Katerndahl, 2000).

 Time Frame
Initial diagnosis
Recurrent acute episode

■■■■■■ DIAGNOSTIC CLUSTER

Collaborative Problems

▲ PC: Hyperglycemia
▲ PC: Hypovolemia/Shock
▲ PC: Hypercalcemia
▲ PC: Delirium Tremens (refer to Alcohol Withdrawal care plan)
✳ PC: Acute Respiratory Distress Syndrome
✳ PC: Sepsis
✳ PC: Hematologic
✳ PC: Acute Renal Failure

(continued on page 181)

Nursing Diagnoses

▲ Acute Pain related to nasogastric suction, distention of pancreatic capsule, and local peritonitis

▲ Imbalanced Nutrition: Less Than Body Requirements related to vomiting, anorexia, impaired digestion secondary to decreased pancreatic enzymes

▲ Ineffective Denial related to acknowledgment of alcohol abuse or dependency

▲ High Risk for Ineffective Therapeutic Regimen Management related to lack of knowledge of disease process, treatments, contraindications, dietary management, and follow-up care

▲ This diagnosis was reported to be monitored for or managed frequently (75%–100%).
✳ This diagnosis was not included in the validation study.

Discharge Criteria

The client or family will:

1. Explain the causes of the symptoms.
2. Describe signs and symptoms that must be reported to a health care professional.
3. Relate the importance of adhering to dietary restrictions and avoiding alcohol.
4. If alcohol abuse is present, admit to the problem.
5. Relate community resources available for alcoholism.

Collaborative Problems

Potential Complication: Hyperglycemia

Potential Complication: Hypovolemia/Shock

Potential Complication: Hypercalcemia

Potential Complication: Acute Respiratory Distress Syndrome

Potential Complication: Sepsis

Potential Complication: Hematologic

Potential Complication: Acute Renal Failure

Nursing Goals

The nurse will detect early signs and symptoms of (a) cardiovascular complications, (b) respiratory complications, (c) metabolic complications, (d) alcohol withdrawal, (e) sepsis, (f) renal insufficiency, and (g) hematologic complications, and collaboratively intervene to stabilize the client.

Indicators

- Cardiac: rhythm regular, rate 60–100 beats/min (a)
- BP >90/60, <140/90 mmHg (a, b)
- Respiratory rate 16–20 breaths/min (a, b)
- Urinary output >5 mL/kg/h
- Capillary refill <3 seconds (a)
- Calm, alert (a, b)
- Dry skin (a, b)
- No nausea or vomiting (c, e)
- Temperature 98–99.5°F (c, e)
- White blood cells 4300–10,800 mm^3 56–190 IV/L (c, e)
- Serum amylase alkaline phosphatase 30–85 mU/mL (e)

- Fasting serum glucose 70–115 mg/dL (c)
- Aspartate aminotransferase (AST) (c)
  - Male: 7–21 u/L
  - Female: 6–18 u/L
- Alanine aminotransferase 5–35 U/L (c)
- Lactate dehydrogenase (LDH) 100–225 U/L (c)
- Hematocrit (g)
  - Male: 42%–52%
  - Female: 37%–47%
- Serum calcium 8.5–10.5 mg/dL (f)
- Oxygen saturation (pulse oximeter) >96% (a, b)
- pH 7.35–7.45 (a, b, c)
- Stool occult blood negative (g)
- Urine specific gravity 1.005–1.030 (f)
- Blood urea nitrogen (BUN) 10–20 mg/dL (e)
- Serum potassium 3.8–5 mEq/L (e)

Interventions	Rationales
1. Monitor for signs and symptoms of hypovolemia and shock: a. Increasing pulse rate, normal or slightly decreased blood pressure b. Urine output <30 mL/h c. Restlessness, agitation, change in mentation d. Increasing respiratory rate e. Diminished peripheral pulses f. Cool, pale, or cyanotic skin g. Thirst	1. The release of vasoactive compounds during autodigestion of the pancreas results in increased capillary permeability, causing a plasma shift from the circulatory system to the peritoneal cavity. Hypovolemic shock can result. The compensatory response to decreased circulatory volume is to increase blood oxygen by increasing heart and respiratory rates and to decrease circulation to the extremities, causing decreased pulse and cool skin. Diminished oxygen to the brain causes changes in mentation.
2. Monitor cardiovascular response and fluid volume carefully: • Blood pressure • Peripheral pulses • Capillary refill • Intake • Output	2. The degree of inflammation will influence the amount of fluid sequestered and the resulting hypovolemia.
3. Monitor for respiratory complications: a. Hypoxemia b. Atelectasis c. Pleural effusion	3. Sixty percent of deaths in acute pancreatitis occur in the first 7 days from respiratory complications. The cause is believed to be enzyme-induced inflammation of the diaphragm or pulmonary microvasculature (Munoz & Katerndahl, 2000).
4. Monitor for sepsis: a. Persistent abdominal pain or tenderness b. Prolonged fever c. Abdominal distention d. Palpable abdominal mass e. Vomiting, nausea f. Increased WBC count, increased C-reactive protein g. Persistent elevation of serum amylase h. Hyperbilirubinemia i. Elevated alkaline phosphatase j. Positive culture and Gram stain k. Jaundice	4. Septic complications from pancreatic abscess, infected pancreatic necrosis, and an infected pseudocyst have a high mortality rate (Munoz & Katerndahl, 2000). Twenty to thirty percent of people with acute pancreatitis will develop complications of necrosis.

(continued on page 183)

Interventions	Rationales

5. Monitor for signs and symptoms of hypocalcemia:
  a. Change in mental status
  b. Cardiac dysrhythmias
  c. Numbness, tingling of fingers, toes
  d. Muscle cramps
  e. Seizures
  f. Positive Chvostek sign (spasm of face after tapping)
  g. Positive Trousseau sign (contracture of fingers and hands after BP cuff is inflated above systolic BP for 3 minutes)
	5. Several causes of hypocalcemia have been proposed. Calcium may bind with free fats that are excreted owing to the lack of lipase and phospholipase needed for digestion. Low serum calcium levels produce increased neural excitability, resulting in muscle spasms (cardiac, facial, extremities) and central nervous system irritability (seizures). Hypomagnesemia may also cause hypocalcemia because it inhibits parathyroid hormone secretion (Bullock & Henze, 2000).

6. Monitor glucose levels in blood and urine.	6. Injury to pancreatic beta cells decreases insulin production; injury to pancreatic alpha cells increases glucagon production.

7. Monitor for signs and symptoms of hyperglycemia:
  a. Early signs:
    • Polyuria
    • Polydipsia
  b. Later manifestations (ketoacidosis):
    • Polyphagia
    • Fruity breath odor
    • Weakness
    • Warm, flushed, dry skin
    • Hypotension
    • Blood glucose >300 mg/dL
	7. Without insulin, cells cannot use glucose. Protein and fats are then metabolized, producing ketones. Ketoacidosis results, with the lungs and kidneys attempting to return the pH to normal. Increased urine excretion causes loss of water, sodium, potassium, magnesium, calcium, and phosphate. Respiration increases to reduce CO_2 levels.

8. Evaluate whether or not the client abuses alcohol.	8. Alcoholism contributes to pancreatitis by lowering gastric pH, which triggers release of pancreatic enzymes. Alcohol also triggers excess production of hydrochloric acid, which causes spasms and partial obstruction of the ampulla of Vater. Alcohol also directly irritates the pancreas, causing protein precipitates that obstruct the acinar ductules.

9. Monitor for signs and symptoms of alcohol withdrawal:
  a. Tremors
  b. Diaphoresis
  c. Anorexia, nausea, vomiting
  d. Increased heart rate and respiratory rate
  e. Agitation
  f. Hallucinations (visual or auditory)
  g. Delirium tremens (grand mal seizures, disorientation to time and place, panic level anxiety, visual hallucinations)
	9. Because chronic alcohol abuse can cause pancreatitis, the nurse must be alert for the signs even when the client denies alcoholism. Signs of alcohol withdrawal begin 24 hours after the last drink and can continue for 1 to 2 weeks. Refer to Alcohol Withdrawal care plan.

10. Consult with a physician for sedation in appropriate dosage to control symptoms.	10. Alcohol withdrawal often requires large doses of sedatives to prevent seizures.

11. Identify high-risk clients:
  a. At diagnosis:
    • Age >55 years
    • WBC count >16,000/mm³
    • Blood glucose >200 mg/dL
    • Serum lactate dehydrogenase >350 IU/L
    • Serum glutamic oxaloacetic transaminase >250 IU/L
    • Aspartate aminotransferase
	11. Ranson's prognostic signs have a 96% accuracy rate. People with fewer than three signs have a 1% mortality rate; three to four signs, 16% rate; five to six signs, 40% rate; and more than six signs, 100% rate (Munoz & Katerndahl, 2000).

(continued on page 184)

Interventions	Rationales
b. During initial 48 hours: • Hematocrit decrease >10 percentage points • Serum calcium level <8 mg/dL • Arterial PO_2 <60 mmHg • BUN rise >5 mg/dL • Base deficit >4 mEq/L • Estimated fluid sequestration >6000 mL	
12. Monitor for hematologic complications: a. Thrombosis b. Disseminated intravascular coagulation	12. Elevated levels of fibrinogen and factor VIII contribute to a hypercoagulable state (Munoz & Katerndahl, 2000).
13. Monitor: a. Coagulation profiles b. Hemoglobin and hematocrit c. Stool, urine, and GI drainage for occult blood d. For ecchymosis (blackened bruises)	13. Early detection of signs of bleeding or disseminated intravascular coagulation (DIC) can reduce morbidity.
14. Refer to collaborative problem index under thrombosis and disseminated intravascular coagulation for specific monitoring criteria.	
15. Monitor for renal insufficiency: a. Oliguria b. Elevated urinary sodium c. Elevated specific gravity d. Elevated BUN	15. Hypovolemia and hypotension activate the renin-angiotensin system; this results in increased renal vasculature resistance, which decreases renal plasma flow and glomerular filtration rate (Bullock & Henze, 2000).
16. Monitor for hypokalemia: a. Muscle weakness b. Polyuria c. Hypotension d. Electrocardiogram changes	16. Pancreatic enzymes are high in potassium; losses into the peritoneal cavity may result in a potassium deficiency.
17. Monitor for: a. Hiccups b. Cardiac rate, rhythms, and pattern c. Temperature	17. a. Hiccups may be related to phrenic nerve irritation resulting from subdiaphragmatic collection of purulent debris. b. Electrolyte imbalance can cause cardiac dysrhythmias. c. Fever in pancreatitis may indicate cholangitis, cholecystitis, peritonitis, intra-abdominal abscesses, or fistula.
18. Maintain strict nothing-by-mouth (NPO) status. Explain to the client that even ice chips are not allowed.	18. NPO reduces or ceases secretion of pancreatic enzymes, which reduces the inflammatory process.
19. Explain the use of nasogastric tube and suctioning.	19. Nasogastric suctioning is used to remove gastric juices, which, if present, will stimulate the release of secretions in the duodenum. These secretions, in turn, stimulate the pancreas to secrete enzymes.
20. If total parenteral nutrition (TPN) is used, refer to TPN care plan.	20. Oral intake should not be resumed until abdominal pain subsides and serum amylase levels are normal.

Related Physician-Prescribed Interventions

Medications. Antibiotic therapy, replacement pancreatic enzymes, vitamins, analgesics, insulin, antacids, anticholinergics, tranquilizers/sedatives, histamine H_2 receptor blockers, glucagon, somatostatin, calcitonin
Intravenous Therapy. Fluid/electrolyte replacement, TPN
Laboratory Studies. Fresh frozen plasma; CBC with differential; partial thromboplastin time (PTT); serum amylase; prothrombin time (PT); serum, trypsin/elastase C-reactive protein; creatine protein transaminase; coagulation studies; urine amylase; serum magnesium; serum lipase and bilirubin; serum ionized calcium; serum albumin, protein; serum isoamylase P_4; serum glucose; WBC; serum calcium and potassium; liver enzymes; triglycerides; arterial blood gases; LDH; AST
Diagnostic Studies. Computed tomographic (CT) scan, ultrasonography, endoscopy, endoscopic retrograde cholangiopancreatography, upper GI series
Therapies. NPO; peritoneal lavage; nasogastric suction; low-fat, high-protein, and moderate CHO diet

Documentation

Flow records
   Vital signs
   Intake and output
Progress notes
   Behavior, orientation
   Changes in physiologic status
   Actions taken
Response

Acute Pain Related to Nasogastric Suction, Distention of Pancreatic Capsule, and Local Peritonitis

 Comfort Level, Pain Control

Goal

The client will relate satisfactory relief after pain-relief interventions.

Indicators

- Relate factors that increase pain.
- Relate effective interventions.
- Rate pain level lower after measures.

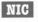 Pain Management, Medication Management, Emotional Support, Teaching: Individual, Heat/Cold Application, Simple Massage

Interventions	Rationales
1. Collaborate with client to determine what methods could be used to reduce the pain's intensity.	1. Pain related to pancreatitis produces extreme discomfort in addition to increasing metabolic activity, with a corresponding increase in pancreatic secretory activity.
2. Relate to the client your acceptance of his or her response to pain: a. Acknowledge the pain. b. Listen attentively to descriptions of the pain. c. Convey that you are assessing the pain because you want to understand it better. d. Ask the client to rate the pain (0–10) at its highest, and to rate the pain level that is satisfactory after relief measures.	2. A client who must try to convince health care providers that he or she is in pain becomes anxious, which intensifies the pain. Subjective assessment of pain can be quantified with a 0–10 scale.

(continued on page 186)

Interventions	Rationales
3. Provide accurate information and correct any misconceptions the client may have: a. Explain the cause of the pain. b. Relate how long the pain should last, if known.	3. Movement of inflammatory exudates and enzymes into the retroperitoneum produces a chemical burn to tissue, resulting in the pain of pancreatitis. The pain is severe and knife-like, twisting, or band-like. A client who is prepared for a painful experience through an explanation of the actual sensations tends to experience less stress than a client who receives vague or no explanation.
4. Provide nasogastric tube care, if indicated: a. Explain that the tube is used to reduce gastric contents, which reduces pancreatic secretions. b. Apply a water-soluble lubricant around the nares to prevent irritation. c. Monitor the nares for pressure points and signs of necrosis. Retape or reposition the tube when it gets detached or soiled. d. Provide frequent oral care with gargling; avoid alcohol-based mouthwashes that dry mucosa.	4. These interventions can reduce some discomfort associated with nasogastric tube use.
5. Explain the need for bed rest.	5. Rest decreases metabolism, reduces gastric secretions, and allows available energy to be used for healing.
6. Position the client sitting upright in bed with knees and spine flexed.	6. This position relieves tension on the abdominal muscles.
7. When the client is NPO, avoid all exposure to food (e.g., sight and smell).	7. The sight and smell of food can cause pancreatic stimulation.
8. Discuss with the physician the use of analgesics such as meperidine, barbiturates, and fentanyl. Avoid the PRN approach and morphine.	8. These analgesics do not cause spasm of the sphincter of Oddi (Munoz & Katerndahl, 2000). A regular time schedule maintains a steady drug blood level.
9. Explain the need for the following: a. To reduce pancreatic activity, advance diet slowly and avoid large meals. b. Take antacids to neutralize gastric acid. c. Restrict dietary fats (e.g., fried foods, ice cream, whole milk, nuts, gravies, meat fat, bacon) that require pancreatic enzymes for digestion.	9. Decreasing pancreatic enzyme release through modifications in eating habits may reduce the pain of pancreatitis.

Documentation

Medication administration record
    Type, route, and dosage of all medications
Progress notes
    Status of pain
    Degree of relief from pain-relief measures

Imbalanced Nutrition: Less Than Body Requirements Related to Vomiting, Anorexia, Impaired Digestion Secondary to Decreased Pancreatic Enzymes

NOC Nutritional Status, Teaching: Nutrition

Goal

The client will ingest daily nutritional requirements in accordance with activity level and metabolic needs.

Indicators

- Describe reasons for dietary restrictions.
- Weigh within norm for height and age.

NIC Nutrition Management, Nutritional Monitoring

Interventions	Rationales
1. Promote foods that stimulate eating and increase calorie consumption.	1. Nausea and fear of pain associated with eating negatively influence appetite.
2. Maintain good oral hygiene before and after meals.	2. This decreases microorganisms that can cause foul taste and odor that inhibit appetite.
3. Offer small, frequent feedings.	3. Small, frequent feedings can reduce malabsorption and distention by decreasing protein metabolized at one time.
4. Determine what time of the day the client's appetite is greatest and plan the most nutritious meal for this time.	4. This can help to ensure intake of nutrients needed for cell growth and repair.
5. Explain the need for a high-carbohydrate, low-protein, low-fat diet.	5. A diet low in protein and fat reduces secretion of secretin and cholecystokinin, thus decreasing autodigestion and destruction of pancreatic cells (Dudek, 2006).
6. Explain the need to avoid alcohol, caffeine, and gas-forming and spicy foods.	6. Alcohol produces hypersecretion of protein in pancreatic secretions that causes protein plugs and obstructs pancreatic ducts. Caffeine and spicy foods increase gastric and pancreatic secretions. Gas-forming foods increase gastric distention (Dudek, 2006).

Documentation

Flow records
  Intake (amount, type, time)
  Weight
  Output (urine, stool, vomitus)

Ineffective Denial Related to Acknowledgment of Alcohol Abuse or Dependency

NOC Anxiety Level, Coping, Social Support, Substance Addiction Consequences, Knowledge: Substance Abuse Control, Knowledge: Disease Process

NIC Coping Enhancement, Anxiety Reduction, Counseling, Mutual Goal Setting, Substance Abuse Treatment, Support System Enhancement, Support Group

Goal

The client will acknowledge an alcohol/drug abuse problem.

Indicators

- Explain the psychologic and physiologic effects of alcohol or drug use.
- Abstain from alcohol/drug use.

Interventions	Rationales
1. Approach client nonjudgmentally. Some causes of pancreatitis are not alcohol-related. Be aware of your own feelings regarding alcoholism.	1. The client probably has been reprimanded by many and is distrustful. The nurse's personal experiences with alcohol may increase or decrease empathy for the client.
2. Help the client to understand that alcoholism is an illness, not a moral problem.	2. Historically alcoholics have been viewed as immoral and degenerate. Acknowledgment of alcoholism as a disease can increase the client's sense of trust.
3. Assist the client to examine how drinking has affected relationships, work, and so on. Ask how he or she feels when not drinking.	3. During acute pancreatitis, the client may be more likely to acknowledge his or her drinking problem.
4. Encourage significant others to discuss with the client how alcohol has affected their lives.	4. Confrontation with family and peers may help to break down the client's denial.
5. Focus on how the client can avoid alcohol and recover, not on reasons for drinking.	5. The client may try to focus on the reasons for using alcohol in an attempt to minimize the problem's significance.
6. Explain that inpatient treatment programs or self-help groups are critical for assistance in recovering. Specific treatment programs include lectures, psychotherapy, peer assistance, recreational therapy, and support groups.	6. Participation in a structured treatment program greatly increases the chance of successful recovery from alcoholism.
7. If sanctioned, schedule interactions with recovering alcoholics.	7. Recovering alcoholics provide honest, direct confrontation with the realities of alcoholism.
8. If sanctioned, schedule a visit with an expert from a detoxification program for ongoing treatment.	8. Affording the client direct contact with an expert who can help can promote a sense of hope.
9. Refer the family to Al-Anon and Al-Ateen as appropriate.	9. The client's family needs assistance to identify enabling behavior and strategies for dealing with a recovering or existing alcoholic (Smith-DiJulio, 2006).
10. Refer to care plan on Alcohol Withdrawal.	

Documentation

Progress notes
   Dialogues
Discharge summary record
Client teaching
   Outcome achievement
   Referrals

High Risk for Ineffective Therapeutic Regimen Management Related to Lack of Knowledge of Disease Process, Treatments, Contraindications, Dietary Management, and Follow-up Care

NOC Compliance Behavior, Knowledge: Treatment Regimen, Participation in Health Care Decisions, Treatment Behavior: Illness or Injury

Goals

The goals for this diagnosis represent those associated with discharge planning. Refer to the discharge criteria.

NIC   Health Education, Health System Guidance, Learning Facilitation, Learning Readiness Enhancement, Risk Identification, Self-Modification Assistance

Interventions	Rationales
1. Explain the causes of acute and chronic pancreatitis.	1. Inaccurate perceptions of health status usually involve misunderstanding the nature and seriousness of the illness, susceptibility to complications, and need for restrictions to control illness.
2. Teach the client to report these symptoms: a. Steatorrhea b. Severe back or epigastric pain c. Persistent gastritis, nausea, or vomiting d. Weight loss e. Elevated temperature	2. These symptoms can indicate worsening of inflammation and increased malabsorption. An elevated temperature could indicate infection or abscess formation.
3. Explain the relationship of hyperglycemia to pancreatitis; teach the client to observe for and report signs and symptoms.	3. Early detection and reporting enables prompt intervention to prevent serious complications.

Documentation

Discharge summary record
    Client teaching
    Outcome achievement
    Referrals, when indicated

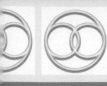

GASTROINTESTINAL DISORDERS

Gastroenterocolitis/Enterocolitis

An infectious agent (bacterial or viral) can cause inflammation of the stomach and intestines (gastroenterocolitis) or both the small and large colons (enterocolitis). Enterocolitis causes cramps and diarrhea, whereas gastroenterocolitis produces nausea, vomiting, diarrhea, and cramps. Hospitalization is indicated with severe fluid and electrolyte imbalances or for high-risk clients (older adults, clients with diabetes, clients with compromised immune systems) (Cheskin & Lacy, 2003).

 Time Frame
Acone episode

■■■■■■ **DIAGNOSTIC CLUSTER***

Collaborative Problems

PC: Fluid/Electrolyte Imbalance

Nursing Diagnoses

High Risk for Deficient Fluid Volume related to losses secondary to vomiting and diarrhea

Acute Pain related to abdominal cramping, diarrhea, and vomiting secondary to vascular dilatation and hyperperistalsis

High Risk for Ineffective Therapeutic Regimen Management related to lack of knowledge of condition, dietary restrictions, and signs and symptoms of complications

*This medical condition was not included in the validation study.

Discharge Criteria

Before discharge, the client or family will

1. Describe the causes of gastroenteritis and its transmission.
2. Identify dietary restrictions that promote comfort and healing.
3. State signs and symptoms of dehydration.
4. State signs and symptoms that must be reported to a health care professional.

Collaborative Problems

Potential Complication: Fluid/Electrolyte Imbalance

Nursing Goals

The nurse will detect early signs and symptoms of (a) dehydration and (b) electrolyte imbalances and collaboratively intervene to stabilize client.

Indicators

- Urine output >5 mL/kg/h (a, b)
- Urine specific gravity 1.005–1.030 (a)
- Moist skin/mucous membranes (a)
- Serum sodium 135–145 mEq/L (b)
- Serum potassium 3.8–5 mEq/L (b)
- Serum chloride 95–105 mEq/L (b)

Interventions	Rationales

1. Monitor for signs and symptoms of dehydration:
  a. Dry skin and mucous membrane
  b. Elevated urine specific gravity
  c. Thirst
	1. Rapid propulsion of feces through the intestines decreases water absorption. Low circulatory volume causes dry mucous membranes and thirst. Concentrated urine has an elevated specific gravity.

2. Carefully monitor intake and output.	2. Intake and output records help to detect early signs of fluid imbalance.

3. Monitor for electrolyte imbalances:
  a. Sodium
  b. Chloride
  c. Potassium
	3. Rapid propulsion of feces through the intestines decreases electrolyte absorption. Vomiting also causes electrolyte loss.

 Related Physician-Prescribed Interventions

Medications. Antidiarrheals, antiemetics, antibiotics (if bacterial)
Intravenous Therapy. Fluid/electrolyte replacement
Laboratory Studies. CBC with differential; stool examination/cultures for amoeba, bacteria, parasites, leukocytes; electrolytes
Diagnostic Studies. Endoscopy (if severe)
Therapies. Diet, as tolerated (e.g., clear fluids, full fluids, bland, soft); oral electrolyte preparations

Documentation

Flow records
  Intake and output
  Stools (amount, consistency)

Nursing Diagnoses

High Risk for Deficient Fluid Volume Related to Losses Secondary to Vomiting and Diarrhea

(If client is NPO, this is then a collaborative problem: refer to index: PC: Hypovolemia.)

NOC Electrolyte & Acid/Base Balance, Fluid Balance, Hydration

Goal

The client will have a urine specific gravity between 1.005 and 1.030.

Indicators

- Intake is 1.5 mL of fluids every 24 hours.
- Urinate at least every 2 hours.

NIC Fluid/Electrolyte Management, Fluid Monitoring

Interventions	Rationales

1. Monitor for early signs and symptoms of fluid volume deficit:
  a. Dry mucous membranes (lips, gums)
  b. Amber urine
  c. Specific gravity >1.025
	1. Decreased circulating volume causes drying of tissues and concentrated urine. Early detection enables prompt fluid replacement therapy to correct deficits.

(continued on page 192)

Interventions	Rationales
2. Monitor parenteral fluid infusion and administer parenteral antiemetic medications as ordered.	2. Antiemetics prevent vomiting by inhibiting stimuli to the vomiting center.

3. Provide fluids often and in small amounts so that the urge to urinate occurs every 2 hours:
  a. Broths
  b. Noncarbonated soft drinks
  c. Electrolyte-supplemented drinks
  d. Apple juice
 	
4. Instruct to
  a. Avoid products (drinks, gum) with sorbitol.
  b. Put a small amount (1/4 teaspoon) of sugar in carbonated beverages.
	3,4. Carbonated beverages replace sodium and potassium lost in diarrhea and vomiting.
	  a. Sorbitol can cause or aggravate diarrhea.
	  b. Sugar will disperse bubbles to reduce gastric distention.

5. Monitor intake and output, making sure that intake compensates for output.	5. Output may exceed intake that already may be inadequate to compensate for insensible losses. Dehydration may decrease glomerular filtration rate, making output inadequate to clear wastes properly and leading to elevated BUN and electrolyte levels.
6. Weigh the client daily.	6. Accurate daily weights can detect fluid loss.

Documentation

Flow records
  Vital signs
  Intake and output
  Daily weights
  Medications
  Vomiting episodes

Acute Pain Related to Abdominal Cramping, Diarrhea, and Vomiting Secondary to Vascular Dilatation and Hyperperistalsis

NOC Comfort Level, Pain Control

Goal

The client will report less painful symptoms.

Indicators

• Report reduced abdominal cramping.
• List foods and fluids to avoid.

NIC Pain Management, Medication Management, Emotional Support, Teaching: Individual, Heat/Cold Application, Simple Massage

Interventions	Rationales
1. Encourage the client to rest in the supine position with a warm heating pad on the abdomen.	1. These measures promote GI muscular relaxation and reduce cramping.

(continued on page 193)

Interventions	Rationales
2. Encourage frequent intake of small amounts of cool clear liquids (e.g., dilute tea, flat ginger ale, Jell-O, water): 30 to 60 mL every ½ to 1 hour.	2. Small amounts of fluids do not distend the gastric area, and thus do not aggravate the symptoms.
3. Eliminate unpleasant sights and odors from the client's environment.	3. Unpleasant sights or odors can stimulate the vomiting center.
4. Instruct the client to avoid these items: a. Hot or cold liquids b. Foods containing fat or fiber (e.g., milk, fruits) c. Caffeine	4. Cold liquids can induce cramping; hot liquids can stimulate peristalsis. Fats also increase peristalsis, and caffeine increases intestinal motility.
5. Protect the perianal area from irritation.	5. Frequent stools of increased acidity can irritate perianal skin.

Documentation

Flow records
   Intake and output
   Tolerance of intake
   Stools (frequency, characteristics, consistency)
   Bowel sounds

High Risk for Ineffective Therapeutic Regimen Management Related to Lack of Knowledge of Condition, Dietary Restrictions, and Signs and Symptoms of Complications

NOC Compliance Behavior, Knowledge: Treatment Regimen, Participation in Health Care Decisions, Treatment Behavior: Illness or Injury

Goal

The goals for this diagnosis represent those associated with discharge planning. Refer to the discharge criteria.

NIC Health Education, Health System Guidance, Learning Facilitation, Learning Readiness Enhancement, Risk Identification, Self-Modification Assistance

Interventions	Rationales
1. Discuss the disease process in understandable terms; explain the following: a. Causative agents b. Reason for enteric precautions c. Preventive measures d. Importance of scrupulous hand-washing	1. The client's understanding may increase compliance with dietary restrictions and hygiene practices.
2. Explain dietary restrictions: a. High-fiber foods (e.g., bran, fresh fruit) b. High-fat foods (e.g., whole milk, fried foods) c. Very hot or cold fluids d. Caffeine e. High carbohydrate foods	2. These foods can stimulate or irritate the intestinal tract.

(continued on page 194)

Interventions	Rationales

3. Instruct on dietary options:
  a. Rice
  b. Toast, crackers
  c. Bananas
  d. Tea
  e. Apple juice/sauce
	3. Foods with complex carbohydrates facilitate fluid absorption into the intestinal mucosa (Cheskin & Lacy, 2003).

4. Teach the client and family to report these symptoms:
  a. Inability to retain fluids
  b. Dark amber urine persisting for more than 12 hours
  c. Bloody stools
	4. Early detection and reporting of the signs of dehydration enable prompt interventions to prevent serious fluid or electrolyte imbalances.

5. Explain the benefits of rest and encourage adequate rest.	5. Inactivity reduces peristalsis and allows the GI tract to rest.

6. Explain preventive measures:
  a. Proper food storage/refrigeration
  b. Proper cleaning of kitchen utensils especially wooden cutting boards
  c. Hand-washing before and after handling food
	6. The most common cause of gastroenteritis is ingestion of bacteria-contaminated food.

7. Instruct to wash hands and:
  a. Sanitize surface areas with disinfectants that contain high proportion of alcohol.
  b. Suspend eating utensils and thermometers in alcohol solution, or use dishwasher for eating utensils and dishes.
  c. Do not permit sharing of objects used by ill person (toys, games).
	7. The spread of bacteria and viruses can be controlled by disinfecting surface areas (bathrooms) and eating utensils. Disinfectants with low proportions of alcohol are ineffective against some bacteria and viruses.

8. If stool culture is needed, instruct to refrigerate stool in container until transported to lab. Advise only to send watery stool for culture.	8. Most bacteria that cause diarrhea die quickly at room temperature.
9. Explain the risks of ill persons working in food service, institutions, elementary school, and day care.	9. The risk for transmission is high, especially in such groups as children and the elderly.

Documentation

Discharge summary record
  Discharge instructions
  Progress toward goal attainment
  Status at discharge

Inflammatory Bowel Disease

Inflammatory bowel disease (IBD) is a generic term comprising both Crohn disease and ulcerative colitis. Both are inflammatory conditions of the GI tract and have similar clinical presentations. Crohn disease has transmural lesions that can involve the entire intestinal tract. Ulcerative colitis consists of mucosal inflammation limited to the colon involving the rectal mucosa 95% of the time (Arcangelo & Peterson, 2005; Cheskin & Lacy, 2003). Crohn disease can involve the entire intestinal tract from the mouth to the anus, with discontinuous focal ulceration, fistula formation, and perianal involvement. Small bowel or upper GI involvement, fistulas, fissures, and abscesses are absent. The causes of IBD are not known.

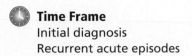
Time Frame
Initial diagnosis
Recurrent acute episodes

██ ▄▄██ **DIAGNOSTIC CLUSTER**

Collaborative Problems

▲ PC: Fluid/Electrolyte Imbalances
▲ PC: Intestinal Obstruction
▲ PC: GI Bleeding
▲ PC: Anemia
△ PC: Fistula/Fissure/Abscess
△ PC: Renal Calculi
▲ PC: Growth Retardation

Nursing Diagnoses

▲ Chronic Pain related to intestinal inflammatory process

▲ Imbalanced Nutrition: Less Than Body Requirements related to dietary restrictions, nausea, diarrhea, and abdominal cramping associated with eating or painful ulcers of the oral mucous membrane

▲ Diarrhea related to intestinal inflammatory process

△ High Risk for Ineffective Coping related to chronicity of condition and lack of definitive treatment

△ High Risk for Ineffective Therapeutic Regimen Management related to lack of knowledge of condition, diagnostic tests, prognosis, treatment, and signs and symptoms of complications

Related Care Plan

Corticosteroid Therapy

▲ This diagnosis was reported to be monitored for or managed frequently (75%–100%).
△ This diagnosis was reported to be monitored for or managed often (50%–74%).

Discharge Criteria

Before discharge, the client or family will

1. Discuss management of activities of daily living.
2. State signs and symptoms that must be reported to a health care professional.
3. Verbalize an intent to share feelings and concerns related to IBD with significant others.
4. Identify available community resources or self-help groups.

Collaborative Problems

Potential Complication: Fluid/Electrolyte Imbalances

Potential Complication: Intestinal Obstruction

Potential Complication: GI Bleeding

Potential Complication: Anemia

Potential Complication: Fistula/Fissure/Abscess

Potential Complication: Renal Calculi
Potential Complication: Growth Retardation

Nursing Goal

The nurse will detect early signs/symptoms of (a) fluid/electrolyte imbalances, (b) intestinal obstruction, (c) abscess, (d) GI bleeding, (e) anemia, and (f) renal calculi.

Indicators

- Temperature 98–99.5°F (c, f)
- Respiratory rate 16–20 breaths/min (a, d)
- Normal breath sounds, no adventitious sounds (a, d)
- Normal relaxed, quiet, even breathing (a, d)
- Peripheral pulses full, bounding (a)
- Pulse 60–100 beats/min (a)
- Blood pressure >90/60, <140/90 mmHg
- Serum pH 7.35–7.45
- Warm, dry skin (a)
- Pinkish, ruddy brownish, or olive skin tones
- Calm, oriented (d)
- No nausea or vomiting (b)
- Urine output >5 ml/kg/h (a, f)
- Urine specific gravity 1.005–1.030 (a, f)
- Blood urea nitrogen 5–25 mg/dL (f)
- Serum prealbumin 20–50 mg/dL (f)
- Red blood cells (e)
  Male 4.6–5.9 million/mm^3
  Female 4.2–5.4 million/mm^3
- White blood count 4,300–10,800 mm^3 (c)
- Serum potassium 3.5–5.0 mEq/L (a)
- Creatinine clearance (a)
  Male 95–135 mL/mm
  Female 85–125 mL/mm
- Serum sodium 135–145 mEq/L (a)
- Capillary refill <3 seconds
- Bowel sounds present in all quadrants (b)
- Stool occult blood negative
- Usual weight (a)
- No abdominal pain (b)
- B$_{12}$ 130–785 pg/mL (e)
- Folate 2.5–20 ng/mL (e)
- Hemoglobin (d, e)
  Males 13.18 gm/dL
  Females 12.16 gm/dL
- No abdominal pain (c)
- No rectal pain or discharge (c)

Interventions	Rationales

1. Monitor laboratory values for electrolyte imbalances:
    a. Potassium
    b. Sodium
    c. Calcium
    d. Phosphorus
    e. Magnesium
    f. Zinc
	1. Chronic diarrhea and inadequate oral intake can deplete electrolytes. Small intestine inflammation impairs absorption of fluid and electrolytes (Bullock & Henze, 2000).

(continued on page 197)

Interventions	Rationales

2. Monitor for signs and symptoms of dehydration:
   a. Tachycardia
   b. Dry skin/mucous membrane
   c. Elevated urine specific gravity
   d. Thirst
	2. When circulating volume decreases, heart rate increases in an attempt to supply tissues with oxygen. Low circulatory volume causes dry mucous membranes and thirst. Concentrated urine has an elevated specific gravity.

3. Monitor intake and output.	3. Intake and output monitoring provides early detection of fluid imbalance.
4. Collect 24-hour urine samples weekly for evaluation of electrolytes, calcium, phosphates, urea, and nitrogen.	4. This enables evaluation of electrolyte status and renal function.

5. Monitor for signs and symptoms of intestinal obstruction:
   a. Wavelike abdominal pain
   b. Vomiting (gastric juices, bile, progressing to fecal material)
   c. Abdominal distention
   d. Change in bowel sounds (initially hyperactive, progressing to none)
	5. Inflammation and edema cause the obstruction. Intestinal contents are then propelled toward the mouth instead of the rectum.

6. If you suspect intestinal obstruction, withhold all food and fluids and notify the physician.	6. Avoidance of foods and fluids prevents further distention and prepares the GI tract for surgery.

7. Monitor for signs and symptoms of fistula, fissures, or abscesses:
   a. Purulent drainage
   b. Fecal drainage from vagina
   c. Increased abdominal pain
   d. Burning rectal pain following defecation
   e. Perianal induration, swelling, redness, and cyanotic tags
   f. Signs of sepsis (e.g., fever, increased WBC count)
	7. The inflammation and ulceration of Crohn disease can penetrate the intestinal wall and form an abscess or fistula to other parts of the intestine or skin. Abscesses and fistulas may cause cramping, pain, and fever, and may interfere with digestion. Sepsis may arise from seeding of the bloodstream from fistula tracts or abscess cavities (Bullock & Henze, 2000).

8. Monitor for signs and symptoms of GI bleeding:
   a. Decreased hemoglobin and hematocrit
   b. Fatigue
   c. Irritability
   d. Pallor
   e. Tachycardia
   f. Dyspnea
   g. Anorexia
	8. Chronic inflammation can cause erosion of vessels and bleeding.

9. Monitor for signs of anemia:
   a. Decreased hemoglobin
   b. Decreased red blood cells
   c. B_{12} deficiency
   d. Folate deficiency
	9. Anemia may result from GI bleeding, bone marrow depression (associated with chronic inflammatory diseases), and inadequate intake or impaired absorption of vitamin B_{12}, folic acid, and iron. Sulfasalazine therapy can cause hemolysis, which contributes to anemia (Bullock & Henze, 2000).

10. Monitor for signs and symptoms of urolithiasis (refer to the Renal Calculi [Urolithiasis] care plan if they occur):
   a. Flank pain
   b. Fever, chills
	10. Severe diarrhea can lead to a decreased volume of concentrated urine. This, combined with intestinal bicarbonate loss and lowered pH, leads to the development of urate stones. With ileal resection or severe IBD, the calcium normally available to bind with oxalate binds instead with fatty acids, freeing dietary oxalate for absorption. Decreased urine volume enhances the precipitation of calcium oxalate in the kidney, predisposing to stone formation (Bullock & Henze, 2000).

(continued on page 198)

Interventions	Rationales
11. Monitor an adolescent client for signs of growth retardation: a. Delayed bone growth b. Weight loss c. Delayed development of secondary sex characteristics	11. Possible causes include decreased nutritional intake, loss of protein and nutrients by rapid passage through the GI tract, increased metabolic requirements secondary to bowel inflammation, and corticosteroid therapy (Cheskin & Lacy, 2003).

❱ Related Physician-Prescribed Interventions

Medications. Aminosalicylates, immunosuppressants, antibiotics, corticosteroids, IgG (infliximab) (oral, enemas), vitamins/minerals, erythropoietin, tumor necrosis factor inhibitors, opioids, $5HT_4$ receptor antagonist

Intravenous Therapy. Fluid/electrolyte replacement, 5-aminosalicylic acid

Laboratory Studies. Stool specimens (bacteria), ova, parasites; CBC; serum protein electrophoresis; serum electrolytes; sedimentation rate; blood urea nitrogen; alkaline phosphatase; creatinine; prothrombin time

Diagnostic Studies. Endoscopy, biopsy (rectal), GI x-ray film, D-xylose test, colonoscopy, barium enema, abdominal MRI, abdominal CT scan

Therapies. Low-residue, high-protein diet; surgery; total parenteral nutrition

Documentation

Flow records
  Abnormal laboratory values
  Vital signs
  Intake and output
  Bowel sounds
  Diarrhea episodes
  Vomiting episodes
  Drainage (wound, rectal, vaginal)
  Urine specific gravity

Nursing Diagnoses

Chronic Pain Related to Inflammatory Intestinal Process

NOC Comfort Level, Pain: Disruptive Effects, Pain Control, Depression Control

Goal

The client will relate improvement of pain and an increase in ability to perform activities of daily living (ADLs).

Indicators

- Relate that others acknowledge and validate the pain.
- Practice noninvasive pain relief measures to manage pain.

NIC Pain Management, Medication Management, Exercise Promotion, Mood Management, Coping Enhancement

Interventions	Rationales
1. Acknowledge the reality of the client's pain.	1. Acknowledging and validating a client's pain may help reduce his or her anxiety, which can decrease pain.
2. Have the client rate pain intensity on a scale of 1 to 10 (1 = no pain; 10 = greatest pain possible), and level of pain tolerance (1 = can tolerate; 10 = cannot tolerate at all).	2. Such a rating scale provides a good method of evaluating the subjective experience of pain.
3. Determine the relationship between eating and drinking and abdominal pain.	3. The client may link eating or drinking to the onset of abdominal pain and may limit intake to avoid pain.
4. Determine the relationship between passage of stool or flatus and pain relief.	4. Pain not relieved by passage of feces or flatus may be a sign of intestinal obstruction or peritonitis.
5. Determine the effects of chronic pain on the client's life style.	5. Chronic pain can cause withdrawal, depression, anger, and dependency.
6. Determine if pain occurs during the night.	6. Abdominal cramps or a feeling of urgency to defecate may awaken the client at night. This usually occurs less often in Crohn disease than in ulcerative colitis.
7. Provide for pain relief: a. Assist with position changes. b. Apply a warm heating pad to the abdomen, *except* during an acute flareup of IBD. c. Encourage relaxation exercises. d. Encourage diversional activities, such as family visits, telephone calls, and involvement in self-care.	7. a. Repositioning may help to move air through the bowel and relieve cramps. b. Warmth relaxes abdominal muscles. c. Relaxation may enhance the therapeutic effects of pain medication. d. Diversion may help to distract the client from pain.
8. Evaluate the effectiveness of the pain management plan.	8. Frequent evaluation of pain relief enables regimen adjustment for maximum effectiveness. Failure to manage chronic pain may lead to depression.

Documentation

Medication administration record
   Type, dosage, and route of all medications
Progress notes
   Pain descriptions
   Unsatisfactory relief from pain relief measures

Imbalanced Nutrition: Less Than Body Requirements Related to Dietary Restrictions, Nausea, Diarrhea, and Abdominal Cramping Associated with Eating or Painful Ulcers of the Oral Mucous Membrane

NOC Nutritional Status, Teaching: Nutrition

Goal

The client will have positive nitrogen balance as evidenced by weight gain of 2–3 lb/wk.

Indicators

• Verbalize understanding of nutritional requirements.
• List foods to avoid.

NIC Nutrition Management, Nutritional Monitoring

Interventions	Rationales

1. Administer total parenteral nutrition (TPN) therapy, as ordered, and intervene as follows:
  a. Teach long-term venous access catheter care. (Refer to the Long-Term Venous Access Devices care plan for more information.)
 	
  b. Maintain nothing-by-mouth (NPO) status.
 	
  c. Provide psychosocial support and reassurance during bowel rest and TPN.
  d. Assist the client to ambulate with an intravenous pole.
	1. On TPN therapy:
	  a. TPN is the treatment of choice when weight loss, nutritional depletion, and symptoms of IBD are severe. In TPN, the client requires 45 to 50 kcal and about 2 g of protein/kg of body weight/day to remain in positive nitrogen balance. This allows weight gain of about 8 oz/day. Clients with ulcerative colitis do not benefit from TPN therapy as greatly as do those with Crohn disease.
	  b. NPO status decreases the mechanical, physical, and chemical activities of the bowel.
	  c. Prolonged NPO status is disturbing both socially and psychologically.
	  d. Ambulation enhances the client's sense of well-being and helps to maintain or improve physical conditioning.

2. Wean the client from TPN feedings when ordered (Dudek, 2006):
  a. Use a relaxed, confident, consistent approach to TPN catheter care.
  b. Provide emotional support during the weaning process.
 	
  c. Reassure the client that weight loss during the first week off TPN is due to fluid loss.
  d. Help client to set realistic expectations for gaining weight after discontinuation of TPN.
 	
  e. Encourage use of high-protein drinks with meals.
 	
  f. Arrange for a dietitian to spend time with the client.
	2. Weaning from TPN:
	
	  a,b. A client receiving TPN typically views the TPN catheter as his or her "lifeline." He or she may feel protective of it and question the expertise of the professional staff caring for it.
	  a,c. The client generally loses 4 to 5 lb of fluid during the first week off TPN.
	  a,d. The client may expect to gain weight on oral feeding at the same rate as when on TPN; however, this is not a realistic expectation.
	  a,e. Dietary supplements may be needed to meet nutritional requirements.
	  a,f. Consultation may be needed to plan an adequate dietary regimen.

3. Assist the client in resuming oral food intake:
 	
  a. Encourage liquids with caloric value rather than coffee, tea, water, or diet soda.
  b. Assess the client's acceptance of and response to oral fluid intake.
  c. Start formula feedings in dilute form and progress to full strength, as tolerated.
 	
  d. Offer a variety of flavors of elemental feedings and keep them chilled.
 	
  e. Assist with progression to soft, bland, and low-residue solids and encourage small frequent feedings high in calories, protein, vitamins, and carbohydrates.
  f. Teach the client to avoid raw fruits, vegetables, condiments, whole-grain cereals, gas-forming and fried foods, alcohol, and iced drinks.
  g. As ordered, supplement the client's diet with folic acid, ascorbic acid, iron, calcium, copper, zinc, vitamin D, and vitamin B_{12}.
	3. The client may need encouragement to resume oral intake, because he or she may resist for fear of pain.
	  a. Calorie-rich liquids can help to prevent malnutrition.
	
	  b. The ability to absorb nutrients must be evaluated daily.
	
	  c. If the client cannot tolerate a regular diet, elemental feedings may be ordered. They are better tolerated because they are residue-free, low in fat, nutritionally balanced, and digested mainly in the upper jejunum. They do not stimulate pancreatic, biliary, and intestinal secretions as does regular food.
	  d. Elemental diets have an unpleasant odor and taste because of the presence of amino acids. Adding flavor and keeping them chilled increase their palatability.
	  e. Gradual introduction of solid foods is needed to reduce pain and increase tolerance.
	
	  f. These foods and liquids can irritate the GI tract.
	
	  g. Nutrient deficiencies result from decreased oral intake, malabsorption, or both.

Documentation

Flow records
    Acceptance of food
    Tolerance of food
    Type and amount of food taken orally
    Daily weight
Progress notes
    Energy level

Diarrhea Related to Intestinal Inflammatory Process

NOC Bowel Elimination, Electrolyte & Acid/Base Balance, Fluid Balance, Hydration, Symptom Control

Goal

The client will report less diarrhea.

Indicators

* Describe factors that cause diarrhea.
* Explain the rationales for interventions.
* Have fewer episodes of diarrhea.
* Verbalize signs and symptoms of dehydration and electrolyte imbalances.

NIC Bowel Management, Diarrhea Management, Fluid/Electrolyte Management, Nutrition Management, Enteral Tube Feeding

Interventions	Rationales

1. Assess for the following:
  a. Decreased number of stools
  b. Increased consistency of stools
  c. Decreased urgency to expel stool
	1. Stool assessment helps to evaluate the effectiveness of antidiarrheal agents and dietary restrictions.

2. Maintain an odor-free client environment:
  a. Empty the bedpan or commode immediately.
  b. Change soiled linens.
  c. Provide a room deodorizer.
	2. Fecal odor can cause embarrassment and self-consciousness and can increase the stress of living with IBD.

3. Provide good perianal care.	3. Perianal irritation from frequent liquid stool should be prevented.
4. Decrease physical activity during acute episodes of diarrhea.	4. Decreased physical activity decreases bowel peristalsis.
5. Determine the relationship between diarrheal episodes and ingestion of specific foods	5. Identification of irritating foods can reduce diarrheal episodes.

6. Observe for signs and symptoms of electrolyte imbalance:
  a. Decreased serum potassium
 	
  b. Decreased serum sodium
	6. Electrolyte imbalance:
	  a. In osmotic diarrhea, impaired fluid absorption by the intestines is caused by ingested solutes that cannot be digested or by a decrease in intestinal absorption. Water and electrolytes are drawn into the intestine in greater quantities than can be absorbed, and the diarrheal fluid is high in potassium (Bullock & Henze, 2000).
	  b. Secretory diarrhea occurs when the gut wall is inflamed or engorged or when it is stimulated by bile salts. The resulting diarrheal stool is high in sodium.

(continued on page 202)

Interventions	Rationales
7. Replace fluid and electrolytes with oral fluid containing appropriate electrolytes: a. Gatorade, a commercial preparation of glucose-electrolyte solution b. Apple juice, which is high in potassium but low in sodium c. Colas, root beer, and ginger ale that contain sodium but negligible potassium.	7. The type of fluid replacement depends on the electrolyte(s) needed.

Documentation

Flow records
    Intake and output
    Number of stools
    Consistency of stools
Medication administration record
    Frequency of as-needed antidiarrheal medication

High Risk for Ineffective Coping Related to Chronicity of Condition and Lack of Definitive Treatment

NOC Coping, Self-Esteem, Social Interaction Skills

Goal

The client will make appropriate decisions to cope with condition.

Indicators

- Verbalize factors that contribute to anxiety and stress.
- Verbalize methods to improve the ability to cope with the chronic condition.

NIC Coping Enhancement, Counseling, Emotional Support, Active Listening, Assertiveness Training, Behavior Modification

Interventions	Rationales
1. Clear up misconceptions about IBD. Stress that psychologic symptoms are a reaction to, not the cause of, IBD.	1. Correcting misconceptions may help to reduce the guilt associated with this belief.
2. Identify and minimize factors that contribute to anxiety: a. Explain all diagnostic tests and support the client during each procedure. b. Do not label the client as "demanding" or a "big baby."	2. Understanding procedures can reduce anxiety. Labels lead to overt or subtle rejection by others and further exaggerate the client's feelings of helplessness and isolation.
3. Allow the client to have some control over care. Demonstrate acceptance and concern when caring for the client.	3. A client with IBD typically feels as if he or she has lost control over other aspects of life.
4. Set appropriate limits if the client demands constant attention. Explain that frequent checks will be made at specified intervals to ensure that needs are met.	4. Demanding behavior is a sign of fear and dependency. If the client feels sure that the caregiver will return, he or she will feel more secure and be less demanding of time.
5. Set aside 15 to 30 minutes a day to allow the client time to verbalize fears and frustrations.	5. The nurse can use this time to help the client develop new, more effective coping strategies.
6. Reinforce effective coping strategies.	6. Reinforcement may promote continued use of effective coping strategies.

(continued on page 203)

Interventions	Rationales
7. Involve family members or significant others in care, if possible.	7. Family members and others play a very important role in supporting clients and helping them to cope with and accept their disease.
8. Refer the client and family to the National Foundation for Ileitis and Colitis. (Each state has a chapter that offers self-help support groups for clients and families, and annual conferences on coping with inflammatory bowel disease.)	8. Discussing IBD with others with the same problem can reduce feelings of isolation and anxiety. Sharing experiences in a group led by professionals gives the client the benefit of others' experiences with IBD and the interpretation of those experiences by health care professionals.
9. Refer to the nursing diagnosis Ineffective Individual Coping in the Ostomy care plan for role-playing strategies to increase coping abilities.	

Documentation

Progress notes
    Participation in self-care
    Emotional status
    Interactions with staff and significant others

High Risk for Ineffective Therapeutic Regimen Management Related to Lack of Knowledge of Condition, Diagnostic Tests, Prognosis, Treatment, and Signs and Symptoms of Complications

NOC Compliance Behavior, Knowledge: Treatment Regimen, Participation in Health Care Decisions, Treatment Behavior: Illness or Injury

Goal

The goals for this diagnosis represent those associated with discharge planning. Refer to the discharge criteria.

NIC Health Education, Health System Guidance, Learning Facilitation, Learning Readiness Enhancement, Risk Identification, Self-Modification Assistance

Interventions	Rationales
1. Explain the diagnostic tests:	1. Explanations of what to expect can reduce the client's anxiety associated with the unknown.
a. Colonoscopy is done to explore the large intestine with a long, flexible tube. A clear liquid diet is maintained for 24 to 48 hours before the procedure, and a cleansing enema may be given before the examination. Medication is given to promote relaxation and aid insertion of the lubricated tube into the anus. The procedure takes about one hour. The client may feel pressure and cramping; breathing slowly and deeply may help relieve discomfort.	a. Colonoscopy may be used to diagnose the medical problem. Polyps can be removed and tissue collected for further study. The procedure may reduce the need for surgery.
b. GI x-ray films: The role of the barium enema is to determine the extent of the disease early in its progression. It also helps the endoscopist determine the configuration of the colon and indicates suspicious areas that should be observed directly by endoscopy.	b. Contrast studies of the colon using barium have been used historically as a surveillance technique. The repetition of barium enema every 6 to 12 months raises the question of the effect of long-term radiation on intestinal mucosa that is already at risk.

(continued on page 204)

Interventions	Rationales
c. Biopsy to differentiate ulcerative colitis and Crohn disease and to detect dysplasia.	c. If dysplasia is found in multiple areas of the colon, the client is in a high-risk group for developing carcinoma of the colon.
d. Blood tests: • CBC • Serum electrolytes • BUN • Creatinine • Serum protein electrophoresis • Sedimentation rate • Alkaline phosphatase	d. Bone marrow depression of blood cells may be present with fulminating types of colitis. The white blood count may be elevated and the sedimentation rate increased. Electrolyte imbalance is common with severe acute IBD. A decreased serum albumin and negative nitrogen balance may result from decreased protein intake and increased metabolic needs. Anemia may be caused by iron deficiency or by chronic inflammation.
2. Explain the familial aspects of IBD. Although the cause of IBD is unknown, 15%–35% of clients with IBD have a relative with the disorder; thus, it is considered a familial disorder. 3. Explain the possible etiology of IBD; theories center on the body's immune system and include the following: a. Hypersensitivity reaction in the gut b. Autoimmune antibody–mediated damage to the epithelial cells c. Tissue deposition of antigen–antibody complexes d. Lymphocyte-mediated cytotoxicity e. Impaired cellular immune mechanisms Emotional and psychological factors have not been identified or implicated in the etiology of IBD. However, stress seems to provoke hyperreactivity of the colon in susceptible persons.	2,3. A client with IBD may have been led to believe that anxiety or psychological problems caused the disorder. Dispelling this belief can help the client to accept the disorder and encourage compliance with treatment.
4. Discuss the prognosis of IBD. IBD typically is a chronic illness with remissions and relapses. In Crohn disease, the client is much more likely to develop fistulas and abscesses. In ulcerative colitis, the client is more likely to develop toxic megacolon and carcinoma of the colon. In ulcerative colitis, total colectomy and ileostomy is considered a cure because ulcerative colitis involves only the colon. Crohn disease can affect any portion of the intestinal tract and tends to recur in the proximal bowel even after colectomy.	4. A client can usually deal with a frank and realistic discussion of the prognosis better than with a lack of information about the prognosis.
5. Discuss the treatment of IBD: a. Medical • Medications • Diet (Refer to the nursing diagnosis Altered Nutrition: Less Than Body Requirements in this care plan.) • TPN and bowel rest (Refer to the nursing diagnosis Altered Nutrition: Less Than Body Requirements in this care plan.) b. Surgical (ulcerative colitis) • Bowel resection A. Total colectomy and ileostomy (Refer to the Ileostomy care plan.) B. Partial colectomy and colostomy (Refer to the Colostomy care plan.) • Incision, drainage, or resection of perianal fistulas and abscesses	5. Treatment of IBD is symptomatic. b. Surgical treatment is indicated only when medical treatment fails and the client becomes disabled. Surgery for Crohn disease is not curative, because of recurrence in remaining intestines.
6. Explain the potential complications of IBD. (Refer to the Collaborative Problems in this care plan for specific signs and symptoms):	6. The client's understanding of IBD complications can help to ensure early detection and enable prompt treatment.

(continued on page 205)

Interventions	Rationales
a. Fissures, fistulas, and perianal abscesses	
b. Anemia	b. Anemia may result from either malabsorption of iron (vitamin B_{12}) or folate deficiency.
c. Toxic megacolon marked by a sharp increase in number of stools and flatus, bloody diarrhea, increasing abdominal pain and distention, and hypoactive or absent bowel sounds	
d. Intestinal obstruction or perforation	
e. Erythema nodosum or pyoderma gangrenosum: A condition exhibiting red, raised, and tender nodules, erythema nodosum occurs in 5%–15% of clients with IBD.	
f. Arthritis, migratory polyarthritis, or ankylosing spondylitis	f. The National Cooperative Crohn's Disease Study reported that 14% of clients studied had arthritis or arthralgia at the time of diagnosis.
g. Ocular lesions	g. Conjunctivitis, iritis, uveitis, or episcleritis occurs in 3%–10% of clients with IBD.
h. Nephrolithiasis	h. Severe diarrhea can lead to decreased volume of concentrated urine. This, combined with intestinal bicarbonate loss and decreased pH, leads to the development of urate stones. With ileal resection or extensive IBD, the calcium normally available to bind with oxalate instead binds with fatty acids, freeing dietary oxalate for absorption. Decreased urine volume leads to increased precipitation of calcium oxalate in the kidneys.
i. Cholelithiasis	i. Gallstones occur in 30%–35% of clients with Crohn disease of the terminal ileum. The ileal dysfunction causes bile acid malabsorption and a decrease in the concentration of bile salts. The decrease in bile salt to cholesterol ratio predisposes the client to the precipitation of cholesterol stones.
j. Colon cancer	j. The incidence of colon cancer is 10–20 times greater in clients with ulcerative colitis than in the general population. The etiology of cancer in IBD is unknown. Close surveillance is needed because cancer may mimic the signs and symptoms of IBD.
k. Growth retardation	k. Growth is impaired in 30%–50% of young clients with IBD occurring before puberty. Possible causes include decreased nutritional intake, loss of protein and nutrients by rapid passage through the GI tract, increased metabolic requirements secondary to inflammatory bowel, and corticosteroid therapy.
7. Teach the importance of maintaining optimal hydration.	7. Optimal hydration prevents dehydration and reduces the risk of renal calculi formation.
8. Avoid oral contraceptives and tobacco use.	8. These two agents have been found to exacerbate Crohn disease but not ulcerative colitis (Arcangelo & Peterson, 2001).
9. Teach measures to preserve perianal skin integrity: a. Use soft toilet tissue. b. Cleanse area with mild soap after bowel movements. c. Apply a protective ointment (e.g., A&D, Desitin, Sween Cream).	9. These measures can help prevent skin erosion from diarrheal irritation.
10. Teach the client to report the following signs and symptoms: a. Increasing abdominal pain or distention b. Persistent vomiting c. Unusual rectal or vaginal drainage or rectal pain d. Change in vision	10. Early reporting enables prompt intervention to reduce the severity of complications. a. Increasing abdominal pain or distention may indicate obstruction or peritonitis. b. Persistent vomiting may point to obstruction. c. Unusual drainage or rectal pain may indicate abscesses or fistulas. d. Vision changes may indicate ocular lesions.

(continued on page 206)

Interventions	Rationales
e. Continued amber urine f. Flank pain or ache g. Heart palpitations	e. Amber urine indicates dehydration. f. Flank pain may indicate renal calculi. g. Palpitations may point to potassium imbalance.
11. Provide information on available community resources (e.g., self-help groups, counseling) and client education material on how to live with IBD.	11. Communicating with others with IBD may help the client to cope better with the disorder's effect on his or her lifestyle.

Documentation

Discharge summary record
Client teaching
Outcome achievement or status
Referrals, if indicated

Peptic Ulcer Disease

Peptic ulcer disease involves erosion in the mucosal wall of the stomach, pylorus, duodenum, or esophagus. The eroded areas are circumscribed and occur only in the areas of the gastrointestinal tract exposed to hydrochloric acid and pepsin. Duodenal ulcers are usually caused by hypersecretion of gastric acid. Peptic ulcers are primarily caused by *Helicobacter pylori* bacterium and long-term use of nonsteroidal anti-inflammatory drugs (NSAIDs). Other causes are cancer and hypersecretory disorders such as Zollinger-Ellison syndrome. With gastric ulcers, gastric acid secretion may be normal or even subnormal. Stress ulcers are usually found in the fundus of the stomach. A major physiologic stress causes an imbalance of aggressive factors that promote ulceration (e.g., acid, bile, urea) and defense factors that protect against ulceration: mucosal barrier, mucosal blood flow, mucus secretion, epithelial regeneration, and prostaglandins. The incidence of stress ulcers in critically ill clients is nearly 100%. *Helicobacter pylori* is an organism found in gastric epithelium. Eradication of *H. pylori* accelerates duodenal ulcer healing (Damianos & McGarrity, 1997; National Institutes of Health [NIH], 1994).

 Time Frame
Initial diagnosis
Recurrent acute episodes

■■■■■■ DIAGNOSTIC CLUSTER

Collaborative Problems

▲ PC: Hemorrhage
▲ PC: Stress Ulcer
△ PC: Pyloric Obstruction

Nursing Diagnoses

▲ Acute/Chronic Pain related to lesions secondary to increased gastric secretions

△ High Risk for Ineffective Therapeutic Regimen Management related to lack of knowledge of disease process, contraindications, signs and symptoms of complications, and treatment regimen

▲ This diagnosis was reported to be monitored for or managed frequently (75%–100%).
△ This diagnosis was reported to be monitored for or managed often (50%–74%).

Discharge Criteria

Before discharge, the client or family will

1. Identify the causes of disease symptoms.
2. Identify behaviors, substances, or foods that may alter gastric activity.
3. Identify necessary adjustments to prevent ulcer formation.
4. State signs and symptoms that must be reported to a health care professional.
5. Relate community resources that can provide assistance with life style modifications.

Collaborative Problems

Potential Complication: Hemorrhage
Potential Complication: Stress Ulcer
Potential Complication: Pyloric Obstruction

Nursing Goal

The nurse will detect early signs and symptoms of (a) hemorrhage, (b) stress ulcer, and (c) pyloric obstruction and collaboratively intervene to stabilize client.

Indicators

- Heart rate 60–100 beats/min (a)
- Cardiac rhythm regular (b)
- Respiratory rate 16–20 breaths/min (c)
- BP >90/60, <40/90 mmHg (d)
- Urinary output >5 mL/kg/h
- No abdominal pain (b, c)
- Alert, oriented, calm (a, b, c)
- Dry, warm skin
- Capillary refill <3 seconds (a, b, c)
- Gastric pH 3.5–5.0 (b)
- Gastric aspirates negative for occult blood (b)

Interventions	Rationales

1. Identify clients at high risk for stress ulcers
  a. Shock, hypotension
  b. Prolonged mechanical ventilation
  c. Multiple trauma
  d. Major surgery (>3 hours)
  e. Sepsis
  f. Head injury
  g. Acute renal, hepatic failure
  h. Respiratory insufficiency
  i. Cardiovascular disease
  j. Severe vascular disease
  k. Burns (>35% of body)
	1. Decreased blood supply to mucosa limits the production of bicarbonate, which results in an inability to control hydrogen ions. These ions damage mucosal cells and capillaries, which leads to the formation of mucosal lesions. Ischemia with a hypersecretion of gastric acid and pepsinogen also interferes with blood flow to the mucosa. Normally, this limited diffusion and bicarbonate neutralization maintain a slightly acid mucosa. Epithelial cells of the stomach are sensitive to even slight decreases in blood supply, which results in necrosis (Porth, 2007).

2. Monitor for occult blood in gastric aspirates and bowel movements.	2. Frequent and careful assessment can help diagnose bleeding before the client's status is severely compromised.

3. Monitor gastric pH every 2 to 4 hours.
 	
  a. Use pH paper with a range from 0 to 7.5.
  b. Use good light to interpret the color on the pH paper.
	3. Maintenance of gastric pH below 5 has decreased bleeding complications by 89% (Eisenberg, 1990).
	a,b. The user error in pH testing is considerable.

(continued on page 208)

Interventions	Rationales
c. Position client on left side, lying down.	c. The left-side-down position allows the tip of the naso-gastric or gastrostomy tube to move into the greater curvature of the stomach and usually below the level of gastric fluid.
d. Use two syringes (>30 mL) to obtain the aspirate. Aspirate a gastric sample and discard. Use aspirate in second syringe for testing.	d. The first aspirate will clear the tube of antacids and other substances that can alter the pH of the sample.
4. Evaluate for other factors that will affect the pH readings. a. Medications (e.g., cimetidine) b. Tube feeding c. Irrigations	4. False positives and negatives can result when aspirate contains certain substances.
5. Consult with the physician for the specific prescription for titration ranges of pH and antacid administration.	5. Most investigators recommend a pH range of 3.5–5.0 volume increases blood oxygen by increasing heart and respiratory rates and decreases circulation to extremities; this is marked by changes such as decreased pulse and cool skin. Diminished oxygen to the brain causes changes in mentation.
6. Monitor for signs and symptoms of hemorrhage and report promptly: a. Hematemesis b. Dizziness c. Generalized weakness d. Melena e. Increasing pulse rate with normal or slightly decreased blood pressure f. Urine output <30 mL/h g. Restlessness, agitation, change in mentation h. Increasing respiratory rate i. Diminished peripheral pulses j. Cool, pale, or cyanotic skin k. Thirst	6. Hemorrhage is the most common complication of peptic ulcer disease and occurs in 15%–20% of clients. Signs and symptoms of hemorrhage may be insidious and present gradually, or may have a sudden onset.
7. If saline lavage is ordered, use tepid saline.	7. Ice saline lavages have been shown to damage stomach mucosa and promote bleeding.

 ### Related Physician-Prescribed Interventions

Medications. Bismuth subsalicylate, sedatives, tetracycline, misoprostol, histamine-2 (H$_2$) receptor antagonists, anticholinergics, antacids, sucralfate, triple therapy for *H. pylori* (clarithromycin, metronidazole, amoxicillin), proton pump inhibitors, prostaglandins

Intravenous Therapy. Variable, depending on severity of illness

Laboratory Studies. Serum gastrin, guaiac testing, CBC, stool antigen test, electrolytes, immunoglobin A anti-h (detects *H. pylori* antibodies)

Diagnostic Studies. Fasting gastric levels, barium study, endoscopy with biopsy, arteriography, C urea breath test

Therapies. NPO or diet as tolerated, nasogastric intubation/gastrostomy

Documentation

Flow records
    Vital signs
    Intake and output
    Weight
    Gastric pH

Stool characteristics
Bowel sounds
Progress notes
Unusual events

Acute/Chronic Pain Related to Lesions Secondary to Increased Gastric Secretions

NOC Comfort Level, Pain Control

Goal

The client will report improvement of pain and an increase in daily activities.

Indicators

- Report symptoms of discomfort promptly.
- Verbalize increased comfort in response to treatment plan.
- Identify changes in life style to reduce recurrence.

NIC Pain Management, Medication Management, Emotional Support, Teaching: Individual, Heat/Cold Application, Simple Massage

Interventions	Rationales
1. Explain the relationship between hydrochloric acid secretion and onset of pain.	1. Hydrochloric acid (HCl) presumably is an important variable in the appearance of peptic ulcer disease. Because of this relationship, control of HCl secretion is considered an essential aim of treatment (Porth, 2006).
2. Explain the risks of nonsteroidal anti-inflammatory drugs (NSAIDs) (e.g., Motrin, Aleve, Relafen).	2. NSAIDs cause superficial irritation of the gastric mucosa and inhibit the production of prostaglandins that protect gastric mucosa (Arcangelo & Peterson, 2007).
3. Administer antacids, anticholinergics, sucralfate, and H_2 blockers, as directed.	3. HCl secretion can be regulated by neutralizing it with various drug therapies.
4. Encourage activities that promote rest and relaxation.	4. Relaxation of muscles decreases peristalsis and decreases gastric pain.
5. Help the client to identify irritating substances (e.g., fried foods, spicy foods, coffee).	5. Avoidance of irritating substances can help to prevent the pain response.
6. Teach diversional techniques for stress reduction and pain relief.	6. The relationship between stress and peptic ulcer disease is based on the higher incidence of peptic ulcers in those with chronic anxiety.
7. Advise the client to eat regularly and to avoid bedtime snacks.	7. Contrary to popular belief, certain dietary restrictions do not reduce hyperacidity. Individual intolerances first must be identified and used as a basis for restrictions. Avoidance of eating prior to bedtime may reduce nocturnal acid levels by eliminating the postprandial stimulus to acid secretion. During the day, regular amounts of food particles in the stomach help to neutralize the acidity of gastric secretions.
8. Encourage the client to avoid smoking and alcohol use.	8. Smoking decreases pancreatic secretion of bicarbonate; this increases duodenal acidity. Tobacco delays the healing of gastric duodenal ulcers and increases their frequency (Katz, 2003).

(continued on page 210)

Interventions	Rationales
9. Encourage the client to reduce intake of caffeine-containing and alcoholic beverages, if indicated.	9. Gastric acid secretion may be stimulated by caffeine ingestion. Alcohol can cause gastritis.
10. Teach the client the importance of continuing treatment even in the absence of pain	10. Dietary restrictions and medications must be continued for the prescribed duration. Pain may be relieved long before healing is complete.

Documentation

Progress record
    Complaints of pain
    Response to treatment plan

High Risk for Ineffective Management of Therapeutic Regimen Related to Lack of Knowledge of Disease Process, Contraindications, Signs and Symptoms of Complications, and Treatment Regimen

NOC Compliance Behavior, Knowledge: Treatment Regimen, Participation in Health Care Decisions, Treatment Behavior: Illness

Goals

The goals for this diagnosis represent those associated with discharge planning. Refer to discharge criteria.

NIC Health Education, Health System Guidance, Learning Facilitation, Learning Readiness Enhancement, Risk Identification, Self-Modification Assistance

Interventions	Rationales
1. Explain the pathophysiology of peptic ulcer disease, using terminology and media appropriate to the client's and family's levels of understanding.	1. Understanding helps to reinforce the need to comply with restrictions and may improve compliance.

2. To reduce the risk of recurrence, explain behaviors that can be modified or eliminated:
  a. Tobacco use
  b. Excessive alcohol intake
  c. Intake of caffeine-containing beverages and foods
  d. Large quantities of dairy products
	2. Alcohol on an empty stomach causes gastritis. Smoking decreases pancreatic secretion of bicarbonate; this increases duodenal acidity. Excessive calcium and protein cause more gastric acid production (Katz, 2003).

3. If the client is being discharged on antacid therapy, teach the following (Arcangelo & Peterson, 2007):
  a. Chew tablets well and follow with a glass of water to enhance absorption.
  b. Lie down for ½ hour after meals to delay gastric emptying.
  c. Take antacids 1 hour after meals to counteract the gastric acid stimulated by eating.
  d. Avoid antacids high in sodium (e.g., Gelusil, Amphojel, Mylanta II); excessive sodium intake contributes to fluid retention and elevated blood pressure.
	3. Proper self-administration of antacids can enhance their efficacy and minimize side effects.

(continued on page 211)

Interventions	Rationales

4. If the client is being discharged on therapy for *H. pylori*, explain
  • The relationship of H. pylori and gastric ulcers, including its occurrence and reoccurrence
  • The need to be on therapy for 14 days
  • The need to take all three types of medication.
	4. Triple therapy for 2 weeks eradicates *H. pylori* at a 90% rate. Eradication of *H. pylori* promotes healing of the ulcer and prevents reoccurrence for at least 7 years. *H. pylori* is also present in 90% of persons with cancer of the stomach.

5. Discuss the importance of continued treatment, even in the absence of overt symptoms.	5. Continued therapy is necessary to prevent recurrence or development of another ulcer.

6. Instruct the client and family to watch for and report these symptoms:
  a. Red or black stools
  b. Bloody or brown vomitus
  c. Persistent epigastric pain
  d. Sudden, severe abdominal pain
  e. Constipation (not resolved)
  f. Unexplained temperature elevation
  g. Persistent nausea or vomiting
  h. Unexplained weight loss
	6. These signs and symptoms may point to complications such as peritonitis, perforation, or GI bleeding. Early detection enables prompt intervention.

7. Explain the risks of aspirin and nonsteroidal anti-inflammatory drugs (NSAIDs).	7. Aspirin disrupts the gastric mucosa and causes ulcer formation. Enteric-coated and buffered aspirin are also ulcerogenic. NSAIDs can also cause ulcers, especially in persons older than 60 years (Katz, 2003).
8. Refer to community resources, if indicated (e.g., smoking cessation program, stress management class).	8. The client may need assistance with life style changes after discharge.

Documentation

Discharge summary record
  Client teaching
  Status of goal achievements
  Referrals
For a Care map on peptic ulcer disease, visit http://thePoint.lww.com

Acute Kidney Failure

Acute kidney failure (AKF) is a syndrome characterized by an abrupt deterioration of renal function, resulting in the accumulation of metabolic wastes, fluids, and electrolytes, and usually accompanied by a marked decline in urinary output. ARF is one of the few types of total organ failure that may be reversible if the underlying cause is corrected (Baird, Keen, & Swearingen, 2005; Shigehiko et al., 2005). Although ARF has many causes, ischemia and toxicity are the most common. Depending on where the problem originates, ischemia and toxicity also determine if ARF is prerenal, intrarenal, or postrenal (Wagner, Johnson, & Kidd, 2006).

Prerenal ARF occurs when decreased blood flow to the kidneys causes ischemia of the nephrons. Blood loss, severe dehydration, septicemia, and cardiogenic shock are common underlying causes of prerenal ARF. *Intrarenal ARF* is associated with damage to the renal parenchyma. Prerenal ARF can trigger the problem, but a major cause of intrarenal ARF and ARF in general is acute tubular necrosis (damage to the renal tubules caused by ischemia or toxins). *Postrenal ARF* occurs as a result of conditions that block urine flow, causing it to back up into the kidneys. Prostatic hypertrophy, urethral obstruction (usually bilateral), and bladder outlet obstruction are common causes of postrenal ARF (Eachempati, Wang, Hydo, Shou, & Barie, 2007; Kohtz & Thompson, 2007).

 Time Frame
Initial diagnosis (post intensive care)
Recurrent acute episodes

▰▰▰▰▰ DIAGNOSTIC CLUSTER

Collaborative Problems

▲ PC: Fluid Overload
▲ PC: Metabolic Acidosis
▲ PC: Electrolyte Imbalances
✳ PC: Acute Albuminemia
  PC: Hypertension
  PC: Pulmonary Edema
  PC: Arrhythmias
  PC: Gastrointestinal Bleeding

Nursing Diagnoses	Refer to
▲ High Risk for Infection related to invasive procedure	
△ Imbalanced Nutrition: Less Than Body Requirements related to anorexia, nausea, vomiting, loss of taste, loss of smell, stomatitis, and unpalatable diet	Chronic Kidney Disease
✳ High Risk for Injury related to stress, retention of metabolic wastes and end products, altered capillary permeability, and platelet dysfunction	Chronic Kidney Disease

(continued on page 213)

Related Care Plans

Hemodialysis or Peritoneal Dialysis
Chronic Kidney Disease

▲ This diagnosis was reported to be monitored for or managed frequently (75%–100%).
△ This diagnosis was reported to be monitored for or managed often (50%–74%).
✳ This diagnosis was not included in the validation study.

Discharge Criteria

Before discharge, the client or family will

1. Relate the intent to comply with agreed-on restrictions and follow-up.
2. State signs and symptoms that must be reported to a health care professional.
3. Identify how to reduce the risk of infection.

Collaborative Problems

Potential Complication: Fluid Overload

Potential Complication: Metabolic Acidosis

Potential Complication: Electrolyte Imbalances

Potential Complication: Hypertension

Potential Complication: Pulmonary Edema

Potential Complication: Arrhythmias

Potential Complication: Decreased level of consciousness (to coma)

Potential Complication: Gastrointestinal Bleeding

Nursing Goal

The nurse will detect early signs and symptoms of (a) fluid overload, (b) metabolic acidosis, (c) electrolyte imbalances, (d) hypertension, (e) pulmonary edema, (f) arrhythmias, (g) decreased level of consciousness, (h) gastrointestinal bleeding, and will intervene collaboratively to stabilize the client.

Indicators

- Alert, calm, oriented (a, c, g)
- BP >90/160, <140/90 mmHg (a, d, e)
- Respiration relaxed and rhythmic (a, e)
- Pulse 60–100 beats/min (a, e, f, g)
- Respiration 16–20 breaths/min (a, e, f, g)
- EKG normal sinus rhythm (b, c, f)
- Flat neck veins (a)
- No edema (pedal, sacral, periorbital) (a)
- No seizure activity (b, c, g)
- No complaints of numbness/tingling in fingers or toes (b, c)
- No muscle cramps (b, c)
- Intact strength (b, c)
- Skin warm, dry, usual color (a, e, f, g, h)
- Serum albumin 3.5–5 g/dL (b, c)
- Serum prealbumin 1–3 g/dL (b, c)
- Serum sodium 135–145 mEq/L (b, c)
- Serum potassium 3.8–5 mEq/L (b, c)
- Serum calcium 8.5–10.5 mg/dL (b, c)
- Serum phosphates 125–300 mg/dL (b, c)

- Blood urea nitrogen 10–20 mg/dL (b)
- Creatinine 0.2–0.8 mg/dL (b)
- Alkaline phosphate 30–150 IU/mL (b)
- Creatinine clearance 100–150 mL/min (a, b)
- Oxygen saturation (SaO$_2$) >94% (a, e, g)
- Carbon dioxide (PaCO$_2$) 35–45 mmHg (a)
- Urine output >5 mL/kg/h (a, h)
- Urine specific gravity 1.005–1.030 (a)
- Usual or desired weight (a)
- Bowel sounds all quadrants (c)
- Normal stool formation (h)
- No vomitus positive for hemoglobin (h)

Interventions	Rationales
1. Monitor for signs of fluid overload: a. Weight gain b. Increased blood pressure and pulse rate, neck vein distention c. Dependent edema (periorbital, pedal, pretibial, sacral) d. Adventitious breath sounds (e.g., wheezes, crackles) e. Urine specific gravity <1.010	1. The oliguric phase of acute kidney failure usually lasts from 5 to 15 days and often is associated with excess fluid volume. Functionally, the changes result in decreased glomerular filtration, tubular transport of substances, urine formation, and renal clearance (Burger, 2004).
2. Weigh client daily or more often, if indicated. Ensure accuracy by weighing at the same time every day on the same scale and with the client wearing the same amount of clothing.	2. Weighing the client daily can help to determine fluid balance and appropriate fluid intake.
3. Maintain strict intake and output records; determine net fluid balance and compare with daily weight loss or gain for correlation.	3. A 1-kg weight gain should correlate with excess intake of 1 L (1 L of fluid weighs 1 kg, or 2.2 lb).
4. Inform the client about fluid management goals.	4. The client's understanding can help gain his or her cooperation.
5. Adjust the client's fluid intake so it approximates fluid loss plus 300 to 500 mL/day. Consider all sensible and insensible losses when calculating replacement fluids.	5. Careful replacement can prevent fluid overload.
6. Distribute fluid intake fairly evenly throughout the entire day and night.	6. Toxins can accumulate with decreased fluid and cause nausea and sensorium changes. It may be necessary to match fluid intake with loss every 8 hours or even every hour if the client is critically imbalanced.
7. Encourage the client to express feelings and frustrations; give her or him positive feedback.	7. Fluid and diet restrictions can be extremely frustrating.
8. Consult with dietitian regarding fluid plan and overall diet.	8. Fluid content of nonliquid food, amount and type of liquids, liquid preferences, and sodium content are all important in fluid management.
9. Administer oral medications with meals whenever possible. If medications must be administered between meals, give with the smallest amount of fluid necessary.	9. This prevents the fluid allowance from being used up unnecessarily.
10. Avoid continuous IV fluid infusion whenever possible. Dilute all necessary IV drugs in the smallest amount of fluid safe for IV administration.	10. A small IV bag, Buretrol, or an infusion pump is preferred to avoid accidental infusion of a large volume of fluid.

(continued on page 215)

Interventions	Rationales
11. Monitor for signs and symptoms of metabolic acidosis: a. Rapid, shallow respiration b. Headache c. Nausea and vomiting d. Low plasma bicarbonate e. Low arterial blood pH (<7.35) f. Behavior changes, drowsiness, and lethargy	11. Acidosis results from the kidney's inability to excrete hydrogen ions, phosphates, sulfates, and ketone bodies. Bicarbonates are lost when the kidney reduces its reabsorption. Hyperkalemia, hyperphosphatemia, and decreased bicarbonate levels aggravate metabolic acidosis. Excessive ketone bodies cause headaches, nausea, vomiting, and abdominal pain. Increases in respiratory rate and depth enhance CO_2 excretion and reduce acidosis. Acidosis affects the central nervous system (CNS) and can increase neuromuscular irritability because of the cellular exchange of hydrogen and potassium (Bhardwaj, Mirski, & Ulatowski, 2004).
12. Limit fat and protein intake. Ensure caloric intake (consult dietitian for appropriate diet).	12. Fats and protein are not used as main energy sources, so acidic end products do not accumulate.
13. Assess for signs and symptoms of hypocalcemia, hypokalemia, and alkalosis as acidosis is corrected.	13. Rapid correction of acidosis may cause rapid excretion of calcium and potassium and rebound alkalosis.
14. Consult with physician to initiate bicarbonate/acetate dialysis if above measures do not correct metabolic acidosis. a. Bicarbonate dialysis for severe acidosis: Dialysate—$NaHCO_3 = 100$ mEq/L b. Bicarbonate dialysis for moderate acidosis: Dialysate—$NaHCO_3 = 60$ mEq/L	14. The acetate anion that the liver converts to bicarbonate is used in dialysate to combat metabolic acidosis. Use of bicarbonate dialysis is indicated for clients with liver impairment, lactic acidosis, or severe acid–base imbalance.
15. Monitor for signs and symptoms of hypernatremia with fluid overload: a. Thirst b. CNS effects ranging from agitation to convulsions c. Edema, weight gain d. Hypertension e. Tachycardia f. Dyspnea g. Rales	15. Hypernatremia results from excessive sodium intake or increased aldosterone output. Water is pulled from the cells, which causes cellular dehydration and produces CNS symptoms. Thirst is a compensatory response to dilute sodium (Baird, Keen, & Swearingen, 2005).
16. Maintain sodium restriction.	16. Hypernatremia must be corrected slowly to minimize CNS deterioration.
17. Monitor for signs and symptoms of hyponatremia: a. CNS effects ranging from lethargy to coma b. Weakness c. Abdominal pain d. Muscle twitching or convulsions e. Nausea, vomiting, and diarrhea	17. Hyponatremia results from sodium loss through vomiting, diarrhea, or diuretic therapy; excessive fluid intake; or insufficient dietary sodium. Cellular edema, caused by osmosis, produces cerebral edema, weakness, and muscle cramps.
18. Monitor for signs and symptoms of hyperkalemia: a. Weakness to paralysis b. Muscle irritability c. Paresthesias d. Nausea, abdominal cramping, or diarrhea e. Irregular pulse f. Electrocardiogram (ECG) changes: tall, tented T-waves, ST segment depression, prolonged PR interval (>0.2 second), first-degree heart block, bradycardia, broadening the ORS complex, eventual ventricular fibrillation, and cardiac standstill	18. Hyperkalemia results from the kidney's decreased ability to excrete potassium or from excess intake of potassium. Acidosis increases release of potassium from cells. Fluctuations in potassium affect neuromuscular transmission; this produces cardiac dysrhythmias, reduces action of GI smooth muscle, and impairs electrical conduction (Baird, Keen, & Swearingen, 2005).

(continued on page 216)

Interventions	Rationales

19. Intervene for hyperkalemia:
   a. Restrict potassium-rich foods and fluids. Do not allow salt substitute that contains potassium as the cation.
   b. Hemodialysis on a potassium-free bath removes K+ rapidly and efficiently from the plasma.
   c. Administer blood transfusions during hemodialysis to remove excess K+.
	19. High potassium levels necessitate a reduced potassium intake. Prolonged dwell time during dialysis increases potassium excretion.

20. Monitor for signs and symptoms of hypokalemia:
   a. Weakness or paralysis
   b. Decreased or no deep-tendon reflexes
   c. Hypoventilation
   d. Polyuria
   e. Hypotension
   f. Paralytic ileus
   g. ECG changes: U wave, flat T-wave, dysrhythmias, and prolonged Q-T interval
   h. Increased risk of digitalis toxicity
   i. Nausea, vomiting, and anorexia
	20. Hypokalemia results from losses associated with vomiting, diarrhea, or diuretic therapy or from insufficient potassium intake. Hypokalemia impairs neuromuscular transmission and reduces the efficiency of respiratory muscles. Kidneys are less sensitive to antidiuretic hormone (ADH) and thus excrete large quantities of dilute urine. Gastrointestinal smooth muscle action is also reduced. Abnormally low potassium levels also impair electrical conduction of the heart (Shigehiko et al., 2005).

21. Intervene for hypokalemia. Encourage increased intake of potassium-rich foods.	21. Increased dietary potassium intake helps to ensure potassium replacement.

22. Monitor for signs and symptoms of hypocalcemia:
   a. Altered mental status
   b. Numbness or tingling in fingers and toes
   c. Muscle cramps
   d. Seizures
   e. ECG changes: prolonged Q-T interval, prolonged ST segment, and dysrhythmias
	22. Hypocalcemia results from the kidneys' inability to metabolize vitamin D (needed for calcium absorption); retention of phosphorus causes a reciprocal drop in serum calcium level. Low serum calcium level produces increased neural excitability resulting in muscle spasms (cardiac, facial, extremities) and CNS irritability (seizures). It also causes cardiac muscle hyperactivity as evidenced by ECG changes (Baird, Keen, & Swearingen, 2005).

23. Intervene for hypocalcemia. Administer a high-calcium, low-phosphorus diet.	23. Elevated phosphate levels lower serum calcium level, necessitating dietary replacement.

24. Monitor for signs and symptoms of hypermagnesemia:
   a. Weakness
   b. Hypoventilation
   c. Hypotension
   d. Flushing
   e. Behavioral changes
	24. Hypermagnesemia results from the kidneys' decreased ability to excrete magnesium. Its effects include CNS depression, respiratory depression, and peripheral vasodilation (Baird, Keen, & Swearingen, 2005; Wagner, Johnson, & Kidd, 2006).

25. Monitor for signs and symptoms of hyperphosphatemia:
   a. Tetany
   b. Numbness or tingling in fingers and toes
	25. Hyperphosphatemia results from the kidneys' decreased ability to excrete phosphorus. Elevated phosphorus itself does not cause the symptoms, but contributes to tetany and other short-term neuromuscular symptoms (Baird, Keen, & Swearingen, 2005; Wagner, Johnson, & Kidd, 2006).

26. For a client with hyperphosphatemia, administer phosphorus-binding antacids, calcium supplements, or vitamin D, and restrict phosphorus-rich foods.	26. The client needs supplements to overcome vitamin D deficiency and to compensate for a calcium-poor diet. High phosphate decreases calcium, which increases parathyroid hormone (PTH). PTH is ineffective in removing phosphates (as a result of kidney failure), but causes calcium reabsorption from the bones and decreases tubular reabsorption of phosphate.

(continued on page 217)

Interventions	Rationales

27. Monitor for signs and symptoms of hypertension:
  a. Headache
  b. Fatigue
  c. Dizziness
  d. Blurred vision.
	27. Hypertension is a common manifestation of renal failure. It is caused by systemic and central fluid volume excess and increased renin production. In the presence of renal ischemia the renin-angiotensin system is triggered, which results in increased blood pressure and increased renal blood flow (Baird, Keen, & Swearingen, 2005).

28. Monitor for signs and symptoms of pulmonary edema:
  a. Pink frothy sputum
  b. Dyspnea
  c. Anxiety
  d. Excessive sweating and pale skin
	28. Pulmonary edema is usually a result of cardiac failure but can also be caused by renal failure due to fluid volume excess and electrolyte imbalance (Wagner, Johnson, & Kidd, 2006).

29. Monitor for signs and symptoms of decreased level of consciousness:
  a. Fatigue and lethargy
  b. Altered mental status
  c. Decreased range of movement
	29. A decrease in mental functioning is a direct result of an accumulation of nitrogenous waste products from impaired renal excretion and metabolic acidosis (Wagner, Johnson, & Kidd, 2006).

30. Monitor for signs and symptoms of gastrointestinal bleeding:
  a. Vomiting of blood
  b. Black tarry stool
  c. Tachycardia
  d. Hypotension
  e. Abdominal pain
	30. Increasing levels of uremic toxins are the primary contributors to gastrointestinal (GI) manifestations. As urea decomposes in the GI tract, it releases ammonia. Ammonia in the GI tract increases capillary fragility and GI mucosal irritation, small mucosal ulcerations may develop, causing GI bleeding (Wagner, Johnson, & Kidd, 2006).

Related Physician-Prescribed Interventions

Medications. Diuretics; antihypertensives; electrolyte inhibitors or replacements (e.g., calcium gluconate, aluminum hydroxide gels)

Intravenous Therapy. Fluid and electrolyte replacement

Laboratory Studies. Urine pH, osmolality, creatinine clearance, specific gravity, sodium, HCO_3, casts, protein, RBCs, hemoglobin, albumin, serum pH, prealbumin, blood urea nitrogen, creatinine

Diagnostic Studies. ECG; x-ray film (kidney-ureter-bladder [KUB]); retrograde pyelogram

Therapies. Dialysis, pulse oximetry, indwelling catheter, fluid restrictions

Documentation

Flow records
  Vital signs
  Respiratory assessment
  Weight
  Edema (sites, amount)
  Specific gravity
  Intake and output
  Complaints of nausea, vomiting, or muscle cramps
  Treatments
Progress notes
  Changes in behavior and sensorium
  ECG changes

Nursing Diagnoses

High Risk for Infection Related to Invasive Procedure

NOC Infection Status, Immune Status

Goal

The client will continue to be infection free.

Indicators

- Describe the reasons for increased susceptibility.
- Relate precautions to prevent infection.

NIC Infection Control, Health Education

Interventions	Rationales
1. Instruct the client about his or her increased susceptibility to infection and responsibility in prevention.	1. Infections are a leading cause of death in acute kidney failure; urinary tract infection is a major culprit. A client with acute kidney failure has altered immunity and nutritional status, disruptive biochemical status, poor healing potential, edema, and decreased activity—all of which predispose him or her to infection. Therefore, implementation of preventive measures is mandated (Baird, Keen, & Swearingen, 2005; Wagner, Johnson, & Kidd, 2006).

2. Use an indwelling bladder catheter only when necessary, for the shortest time possible, and with diligent care.
 	
3. Avoid other invasive procedures as much as possible:
  a. Repeated venous punctures
  b. IV lines
  c. Central venous lines
  d. Arterial catheters
	2,3. Avoiding catheters and invasive procedures helps to prevent introducing microorganisms into the body (Baird, Keen, & Swearingen, 2005; Wagner, Johnson, & Kidd, 2006).

4. Whenever possible, avoid placing the client with a roommate who has an indwelling catheter, urinary tract infection, or upper respiratory infection.	4. Selected isolation can decrease risk of cross-contamination and possible spread of infection.
5. Use aseptic technique with all invasive procedures and when caring for lines, catheters, dressing changes, suctioning, and dialysis accesses. Do not use venous access catheters for blood sampling.	5. Each disruption of invasive lines introduces microorganisms. Aseptic technique reduces the quantity of microorganisms introduced.

6. Assess for and report signs of infection at invasive sites:
  a. Redness
  b. Swelling
  c. Drainage
  d. Warmth
	6. Traumatized tissue predisposes to inflammation and infection. Uremic toxins decrease neutrophil phagocytosis and chemotaxis that increase susceptibility to infection (Baird, Keen, & Swearingen, 2005; Wagner, Johnson, & Kidd, 2006).

7. Never cannulate an inflamed area of an arteriovenous fistula.	7. Cannulation will increase the risk of introducing microorganisms.
8. Teach the client to avoid contacting people with any infection, especially an upper respiratory tract infection.	8. Selected isolation can help to protect client against contacting an infection.
9. Use written signs to alert visitors to wash hands before and after contact with the client.	9. Handwashing reduces risk of cross-contamination.

Documentation

Flow records
    Urine color and other characteristics
Progress notes
    Redness, swelling, drainage, or warmth at sites

Chronic Kidney Disease

Chronic renal failure (CRF) refers to the slow, progressive, and irreversible destruction of the kidneys over a period of months to years. CRF can result from a primary renal disorder (e.g., glomerulonephritis or polycystic kidney disease), or as a secondary disorder (e.g., as a complication of diabetes mellitus or hypertension). However, the most common causes of CRF are diabetes, hypertension, and glomerulonephritis, as well as congenital and hereditary factors.

There are five stages of CRF, as outlined in Table 1. CRF is a progression through an abnormally low and deteriorating glomerular filtration rate which is usually determined indirectly by the creatinine level in blood serum (Wagner, Johnson, & Kidd, 2006; Lewis et al., 2004; Porth, 2002). The kidney cannot maintain metabolic, fluid, and electrolyte balance; this results in uremia. As the condition progresses, dialysis or transplantation is considered.

Recent studies, which include observational analyses, are earnestly puzzled by the interrelationship of anemia and erythropoietin resistance in clients with chronic kidney disease. The sicker the client and the more prolonged his or her sickness, the longer anemia is present and the greater the cumulative erythropoietin dose that must be administered to achieve the target hemoglobin level. The observational studies have illustrated how higher hemoglobin levels correlate with lower hospitalization rates, fewer cardiovascular events, and better survival in dialysis clients. One such report demonstrated a lower mortality rate among hemodialysis clients who maintained hemoglobin levels between 12 and 13 g/dL (Coyne, 2007).

 Time Frame
Acute exacerbations

TABLE 1	Stages of Chronic Kidney Disease: A Clinical Action Plan		
Stage	Description	GFR (mL/min/1.73 m²)	Action*
1	Kidney damage with normal or increased GFR	>90	Diagnosis and treatment; treatment of comorbid conditions; slowed progression; CVD risk reduction
2	Kidney damage with mild, decreased GFR	60–89	Estimating progression
3	Moderate, decreased GFR	30–59	Evaluating and treating complications
4	Severe, decreased GFR	15–29	Preparation for kidney replacement therapy
5	Kidney failure	<15 (or dialysis)	Replacement (if uremia present)

Chronic kidney disease is defined as either kidney damage or GFR, 60 mL/min/1.73 m² for ≥ 3 months. Kidney damage is defined as pathologic abnormalities or markers of damage including abnormalities in blood or urine tests or imaging studies.

*Includes actions form preceding stages

■■■■■ DIAGNOSTIC CLUSTER

Collaborative Problems	Refer to
△ PC: Fluid Imbalance	
▲ PC: Anemia	
PC: Hyperparathyroidism	
PC: Pathological Fractures	
△ PC: Polyneuropathy	
△ PC: Hypoalbuminemia	
△ PC: Congestive Heart Failure	
△ PC: Metabolic Acidosis	
△ PC: Pleural Effusion	
PC: Pericarditis, Cardiac Tamponade	Acute Kidney Failure
▲ PC: Fluid/Electrolyte Imbalance	Acute Kidney Failure
▲ PC: Fluid Overload	Hemodialysis
✳ PC: Hypertension	
PC: Cardiac Arrest	Myocardial Infarction
PC: Peripheral Neuropathy	Diabetes Mellitus

Nursing Diagnoses	Refer to
△ Imbalanced Nutrition: Less Than Body Requirements related to anorexia, nausea, vomiting, and loss of taste or smell, stomatitis, and unpalatable diet	
Ineffective Sexuality Patterns related to decreased libido, erectile dysfunction, amenorrhea, or sterility	
△ Powerlessness related to feeling of loss of control and life style restrictions	
▲ High Risk for Ineffective Therapeutic Regimen Management related to insufficient knowledge of condition, dietary restrictions, daily recording, pharmacological therapy, and signs and symptoms of complications, and insufficient resources (e.g., financial, caregiver), follow-up visits, and community resources	
▲ High Risk for Infection related to invasive procedures	Acute Kidney Failure
△ Impaired Comfort related to calcium phosphate or urate crystals on skin	Cirrhosis

Related Care Plans

Hemodialysis
Acute Kidney Failure
Cirrhosis

▲ This diagnosis was reported to be monitored for or managed frequently (75%–100%).

△ This diagnosis was reported to be monitored for or managed often (50%–74%).

✳ This diagnosis was not included in the validation study.

Discharge Criteria

Before discharge, the client or family will

1. Describe dietary restrictions, medications, and treatment plan.
2. Maintain contact and follow-up with health care providers (including dialysis, if needed).
3. Keep complete daily records, as instructed.
4. Verbalize available community resources.
5. Relate the intent to comply with agreed-on restrictions and follow-up.
6. State the signs and symptoms that must be reported to a health care professional.
7. Relate the importance of an outlet for feelings and concerns.

Collaborative Problems

Potential Complication: Fluid Imbalance

Potential Complication: Anemia

Potential Complication: Hyperparathyroidism

Potential Complication: Pathological Fractures

Potential Complication: Polyneuropathy

Potential Complication: Hypoalbuminemia

Potential Complication: Congestive Heart Failure

Potential Complication: Metabolic Acidosis

Potential Complication: Pleural Effusion

Potential Complication: Pericarditis, Cardiac Tamponade

Potential Complication: Hypertension

Potential Complication: Cardiac Arrest

Potential Complication: Peripheral Neuropathy

Nursing Goal

The nurse will monitor for early signs and symptoms of (a) fluid imbalance, (b) anemia, (c) hyperparathyroidism, (d) pathological fractures, (e) polyneuropathy, (f) hypoalbuminemia, (g) congestive heart failure, (h) metabolic acidosis, (i) pleural effusion, and (j) pericarditis/cardiac tamponade, (k) Hypertension, (l) cardiac arrest, (m) peripheral neuropathy, and will intervene collaboratively to stabilize the client.

Indicators

- Alert, calm, oriented (a, g, l, m)
- Respiration 16–20 breaths/min (g, h, i, l)
- Respiration relaxed and rhythmic (g, h, i, l)
- Breath sounds present all lobes (g, i)
- Pulse 60–100 beats/min (a, g, h, l)
- EKG normal sinus rhythm (c, d, e, f, g, l)
- BP >90/60, <140/90 mmHg (g, h, j, k, l)
- Temperature 98.5–99°F (j)
- No seizure activity (c)
- Flat neck veins (g, j)
- Full range of motion (c, m)
- No complaints of numbness of toes/fingers (e, m)
- No complaints of palpitations (g, l)
- Sensation intact (e, m)
- Strength intact (c, e, m)
- No foot drop (e)

- Intact reflexes (e)
- No or minimal edema (a, f)
- Ideal or desired weight (a, f)
- Urine output >5 mL/kg/h (a, f)
- No substernal pain (a, i, l)
- Red blood cells 4,000,000–6,200,000 mm^3 (b)
- White blood cells 48,000–100,000 mm^3 (j)
- Hematocrit (b)
  - Male 42%–50%
  - Female 40%–48%
- Hemoglobin (b)
  - Male 13–18 g/dL
  - Female 12–16 g/dL
- Serum albumin 3.5–5 g/dL (f)
- Serum prealbumin 1–3 g/dL (f)
- Total cholesterol <200 mg/dL (f)
- Transferrin saturation 230–320 mg/dL (b)
- Serum ferritin (b)
  - Males 29–438 ng/mL
  - Females 9–219 ng/mL
- Serum potassium 3.8–5 mEq/L (b, l)
- Serum sodium 135–145 mEq/L (a, l)
- Serum calcium 8.5–10.5 mg/dL (c, l)
- Folic acid 2.5–20 ng/mL (b)
- Vitamin B$_{12}$ 13–785 pg/mL (b)
- Serum phosphate 125–300 mg/dL (c, d)
- Blood urea nitrogen 10–20 mg/dL (h, l)
- Creatinine 0.2–0.8 ng/mL (h, l)
- Negative DEXA scan (c, d)
- Alkaline phosphatase 30–150 m/UmL (c)
- Urine sodium 130–200 mEq/24h (a)
- Creatinine clearance 100–150 mL/min (f)
- Oxygen saturation (SaO$_2$) >94% (a, h, l)
- Carbon dioxide (PaCO$_2$) 35–45 mmHg (a, h)

Interventions	Rationales

1. Monitor for fluid imbalances:
  a. Weight changes
  b. BP changes
  c. Increased pulse
  d. Increased respirations
  e. Neck vein distention
  f. Dependent, peripheral edema
  g. Increased fluid intake
  h. Increased sodium intake
  i. Orthostatic hypotension (decreased fluid volume)
	1. Fluid imbalance, usually hypervolemia, results from failure of kidney to regulate extracellular fluids by decreased sodium and water elimination.

2. Consult with nephrology staff if fluid volume changes. 3. Refer to Dialysis care plans for specific fluid management strategies.	2,3. Adjustments to the dialysis treatment may be needed.
4. Frequently monitor vital signs, particularly blood pressure and pulse.	4. Circulating volume must be monitored with chronic kidney disease to prevent severe hypervolemia.

(continued on page 223)

Interventions	Rationales
5. Monitor hematocrit each treatment.	5. A decline is directly proportional to the frequency and volume of blood loss associated with phlebotomy-related blood drawing and blood loss during dialysis (Baird, Keen, & Swearingen, 2005; Wagner, Johnson, & Kidd, 2006).
6. Administer bulk-forming laxatives or stool softeners if client is constipated. Avoid magnesium-containing laxatives.	6. Certain laxatives elevate serum magnesium levels. Clients with kidney disease already have difficulty excreting usual intake of magnesium in foods.
7. Monitor for manifestations of anemia: a. Dyspnea b. Fatigue c. Tachycardia d. Palpitations e. Pallor of nail beds and mucous membranes f. Low hemoglobin and hematocrit g. Bruising	7. Causes of anemia in chronic kidney disease include these (Coyne, 2007; Baird, Keen, & Swearingen, 2005; Wagner, Johnson, & Kidd, 2006): a. Decreased RBC production resulting from decreased erythropoietin production b. Decreased RBC survival time owing to elevated uremic toxins c. Loss of blood through GI bleeding d. Blood loss during hemodialysis from membrane rupture, hemolysis, and residual dialyzer blood loss e. Dilution caused by volume overload f,g. Phlebotomy-related blood drawing
8. Avoid unnecessary collection of blood specimens. Coordinate blood draws with predialysis starting times.	8. Blood loss occurs with every blood collection.
9. Instruct the client to use a soft toothbrush and to avoid vigorous nose blowing, constipation, and contact sports.	9. Trauma should be avoided to reduce risk of bleeding and infection.
10. Demonstrate the pressure method to control bleeding, should it occur.	10. Direct, constant pressure prevents excess blood loss.
11. If the client is on epoetin alfa therapy (Coyne, 2007), a. Monitor: • Blood pressure (three times weekly) • Hematocrit and reticulocyte levels (every week) • Transferrin saturation serum ferritin values (monthly, then quarterly when on maintenance) • Serum potassium (twice a month) b. Monitor folic acid and vitamin B_{12}. c. Monitor aluminum levels.	11. Epoetin alfa is a synthetic erythropoietin administered three times weekly until the hematocrit reaches 33%–36% with the dose tapered as needed for maintenance (Coyne, 2007). a. • Epoetin alfa increases blood viscosity and can increase blood pressure and thrombus formation in vascular access sites. • Epoetin alfa needs sufficient iron to be effective. Stop IV iron therapy two weeks before testing. b. Epoetin alfa needs sufficient quantities of these elements to be effective. c. Excessive aluminum levels may interfere with erythropoiesis and epoetin alfa effectiveness.
12. If the client is on epoetin alfa and the hematocrit drops (Coyne, 2007; Kee, 2004), a. Evaluate iron status and if the client has been compliant in iron therapy. b. Evaluate aluminum levels. c. Advise the client to eliminate aluminum antacids. d. Evaluate for blood loss.	12. a. Compliant clients may need increased iron therapy or parenteral therapy. Noncompliant clients will be assessed for reasons (Coyne, 2007). b. If abnormal, report to physician or nurse practitioner. c. They may cause increased serum aluminum levels. d. Reasons for blood loss are GI, menses, dialysis procedure, blood testing, and surgical access declotting procedures.

(continued on page 224)

Interventions	Rationales
e. Assess for underlying causes: • Vitamin deficiencies • Osteitis fibrosa • Hematologic disease f. Assess for signs/symptoms of infection (Coyne, 2007; Wagner, Johnson, & Kidd, 2006). • Sudden loss of responsiveness to recombinant human erythropoietin-alfa (rHuEPO) • Febrile episode • Erythema, pain, tenderness, drainage at access site joint pain • Serum iron and transferrin saturation with normal or increased serum ferritin • Recent invasive procedure	e. Underlying causes of blood loss or anemia will need to be diagnosed and corrected. f. Release of iron from the reticuloendothelial system is impaired during localized or septicemic inflammation. This decreased ability to transfer stored iron leads to normal or increased serum ferritin with normal or decreased transferrin saturation and serum iron (Coyne, 2007; Wagner, Johnson, & Kidd, 2006).
13. Monitor for manifestations of hyperparathyroidism: a. The symptoms of hyperparathyroidism can be remembered by the rhyme *moans, groans, stones, bones, and psychiatric overtones* (Lewis et al., 2004). <u>Moans</u> = complaints of not feeling well <u>Groans</u> = abdominal pain, gastroesophageal reflux <u>Stones</u> = renal stones <u>Bones</u> = bone pain secondary to osteoporosis <u>Psychiatric overtones</u> = lethargy, fatigue, depression, and memory problems (Lewis et al., 2004). b. Low serum calcium level (<9 mg/100 mL) c. Elevated serum phosphate level (>4.5 mg/100 mL) d. Elevated alkaline phosphatase level (>90 IU/L) e. Limited mobility f. Itching g. Deposits of calcium in joints, arteries, arterioles, soft tissue, and other sites h. Demineralization of bones, causing osteoporosis (seen on x-ray film and bone scan)	13. Phosphate clearance ceases when the glomerular filtration rate (GFR) falls below 10%. Despite a high level of parathormone and as reabsorption of calcium and phosphate from bone takes place, the plasma phosphate level also rises. This additional phosphate cannot be disposed of through the renal route, preventing increased serum calcium concentration and stimulating increased parathyroid secretion. A secondary hyperparathyroidism develops, contributing to bone degeneration (Baird, Keen, & Swearingen, 2005; Wagner, Johnson, & Kidd, 2006).
14. Inspect the client's gait, range of motion of joints, and muscle strength. Palpate joints for enlargement, swelling, and tenderness.	14. Identification of mobility problems points to the need for a structured exercise program.
15. As indicated, develop a plan of weight-bearing exercise (e.g., walking). Avoid immobilization, if possible.	15. Exercise helps to maintain strength and mobility and decrease calcium reabsorption. Immobilization increases protein catabolism and bone demineralization.
16. Ask the client about signs and symptoms of hypocalcemia: a. Tetany b. Carpopedal spasms c. Seizures d. Confusion e. Numbness and tingling fingertips and toes	16. Kidney disease causes decreased absorption of calcium caused by the kidney's inability to metabolize vitamin D and by loss of calcium with phosphorus retention (Porth, 2002; Baird, Keen, & Swearingen, 2005; Wagner, Johnson, & Kidd, 2006).
17. Monitor ECG for prolonged Q-T interval, irritable dysrhythmias, and A-V conduction defects.	17. Calcium imbalances can cause cardiac muscle hyperactivity (Porth, 2002; Baird, Keen, & Swearingen, 2005; Wagner, Johnson, & Kidd, 2006).

(continued on page 225)

Interventions	Rationales
18. Monitor for manifestations of osteodystrophy osteoporosis: a. Evidence of bone degeneration on x-ray film b. Incidence of pathological fractures c. Elevated serum phosphate level d. Bone pain e. Limited mobility f. Swelling of surrounding tissues and skin	18. Osteodystrophy is a decrease in bone density from inadequate mineralization. Factors that contribute to bone changes are elevated phosphate levels, impaired renal activation of vitamin D, and hyperparathyroidism (Porth, 2005).
19. Request a dietary consultation regarding calcium intake.	19. A consultation is necessary to evaluate the need for increased calcium in the diet.
20. Review medication dosage and the importance of taking phosphate binders (Basaljel, Amphojel, etc.).	20. These medications reduce phosphate loss.
21. Increase calcium level in dialysate, if indicated.	21. Supplemental calcium may be required to maintain calcium balance.
22. Monitor for manifestations of polyneuropathy (peripheral neuropathy): a. Decreased sensation in feet b. Numbness and burning of feet c. Muscle cramps d. Restlessness of legs: creeping, crawling, prickling, and itching sensations e. Loss of muscle strength f. Foot drop g. Decreased vibratory perception h. Abnormal deep tendon reflexes	22. Peripheral neuropathy results from demyelination of large muscle fibers and axonal degeneration secondary to uremia and decreased glomerular filtration rate (GFR). Symptoms of peripheral neuropathy usually do not occur until GFR is below 1 mL/min. Other possible etiologies include pyridoxine deficiencies, especially during isoniazid (INH) or hydralazine use; biotin deficiencies; vitamin B_{12} deficiencies; and acid–base and electrolyte imbalances. Neuropathy usually is bilateral and distal, and occurs in lower extremities first.
23. Caution the client to check for skin pressure sores, and to eliminate hazards such as prolonged pressure, ill-fitting shoes, and thermal or friction burns.	23. Peripheral neuropathies can cause loss of sensation and temperature perception.
24. Provide for movement and mobility: range of motion exercises, as indicated.	24. Movement often relieves the pain from neuropathies.

25. Monitor for manifestations of decreased albumin levels:
a. Serum albumin <3.5 g/dL and proteinuria (<100–150 mg protein/24 hours)
b. Edema formation: pedal, facial, sacral
c. Hypovolemia, increased hematocrit/hemoglobin
d. Signs and symptoms of negative nitrogen balance:
  • Decreased serum cholesterol
  • Decreased caloric intake (<45 Kcal/kg)
  • Decreased protein intake (<0.75 g/kg)
  • Delayed wound healing
  • Muscle wasting
	25. When albumin is lost through urinary excretion or peritoneal dialysis, the liver responds by increasing production of plasma proteins. When the loss is great, however, the liver cannot compensate and hypoalbuminemia results. Edema formation results from decreased plasma proteins and consequent decreased plasma oncotic pressure that causes a fluid shift from the vascular to the interstitial compartment. Hypovolemia can result from fluid loss, which leads to hemoconcentration and a consequent increase in hemoglobin and hematocrit. If the volume loss becomes great, shock occurs (Porth, 2005; Baird, Keen, & Swearingen, 2005; Wagner, Johnson, & Kidd, 2006).
	
	  A negative nitrogen balance results from protein and caloric malnutrition, leading to an oxygen and nutrient deficit that causes cellular catabolism, cell breakdown, and nitrogen loss. Humoral defenses to infection are depressed owing to protein loss, and general protein reserves are depleted resulting in slowed healing.

(continued on page 226)

Interventions	Rationales
26. Administer IV salt-free albumin per physician's order; avoid diuretics.	26. Parenteral administration of albumin-containing solutions results only in a transient increase in serum albumin concentrations; however, it is helpful to circumvent life-threatening hypotension. Diuretics are contraindicated if the plasma volume is low and in low-output kidney disease.
27. Hold a dietary consultation for nutritional assessment and to provide for the following: a. Fluid restrictions (with massive edema) b. Low-sodium diet c. Adequate calorie and protein intake d. Low-protein diet with high biological protein (meats, poultry, cheese, milk)	27. With chronic kidney disease (on dialysis), protein usually is restricted to 0.75 to 1.25 g/kg, with emphasis on high biological value protein. High biological value proteins supply the essential amino acids necessary for cell growth and repair, but produce less urea nitrogen during metabolism. Calories should be generous (35 to 45 Kcal/kg) to allow use of the minerals in protein for tissue maintenance. Tissue catabolism can develop when protein intake is inadequate. Catabolism increases BUN levels, acidosis, and hyperkalemia. (*Note:* Because of the greater permeability of the peritoneal membrane, protein loss is larger in chronic peritoneal dialysis than in hemodialysis; therefore, more protein may be needed in the diet to offset hypoalbuminemia.) A low-sodium diet may be beneficial to prevent additional fluid retention. The client should not become totally edema-free, however, because of the dangers of hypovolemia and hypotension.
28. Evaluate daily: a. Weight b. Fluid intake and output records c. Circumference of the edematous part(s) d. Laboratory data: hematocrit, serum potassium, and plasma protein in specific serum albumin	28. As GFR decreases and the functioning nephron mass continues to diminish, the kidneys lose the ability to concentrate urine and to excrete sodium and water; this results in hypervolemia.
29. Monitor for signs and symptoms of congestive heart failure (CHF) and decreased cardiac output: a. Gradual increase in heart rate b. Increased shortness of breath c. Diminished breath sounds, rales d. Decreased systolic BP e. Presence of or increase in S_3 and/or S_4 f. Gallop g. Peripheral edema h. Distended neck veins	29. Diminished urinary output causes volume retention that can lead to cardiomegaly and CHF. This results in reduced ability of left ventricle to eject blood and consequent decreased cardiac output and increased pulmonary vascular congestion. This causes fluid to enter the pulmonary tissue, leading to respiratory distress, rales, productive cough, and cyanosis (Shlipak et al., 2005; Baird, Keen, & Swearingen, 2005).
30. Encourage adherence to strict fluid restrictions: 800 to 1000 mL/24 hours or 24-hour urine output plus 500 mL.	30. A client who presents with evidence of fluid overload requires fluid restriction based on urine output. In an anuric client, restriction generally is 800 mL/day, which accounts for insensible losses from metabolism, the GI tract, perspiration, and respiration (Castner & Douglas, 2005).
31. Reevaluate and reestablish the client's optimal "dry" weight—that weight at which a client is free of any signs or symptoms of overload and maintains a normal blood pressure.	31. A client with chronic kidney disease is prone to fluctuations in weight, necessitating frequent reevaluation for optimal fluid balance. Accepted inter-dialytic weight gain is 1 to 2 lb per 24 hours (Dinwiddie, Burrows-Hudson, & Peacock, 2006).

(continued on page 227)

Interventions	Rationales
32. Collaborate with physician or dietitian in planning an appropriate diet. Encourage adherence to a low-sodium diet (2–4 g/24 h).	32. Sodium restrictions should be adjusted based on urine sodium excretion and serial weights (Castner & Douglas, 2005).
33. Monitor for manifestations of pleural effusion: a. Variable dyspnea b. Pleuritic pain c. Diminished and delayed chest movement on involved side d. Bulging of intercostal spaces (in massive effusion) e. Decreased breath sounds over site of pleural effusion f. Decreased vocal and tactile fremitus g. Increased rate and depth of respirations	33. A pleural effusion is a collection of fluid, either transudates or exudates, in the pleural cavity. Transudates are seen in chronic kidney disease and result from a rise in pulmonary venous pressure secondary to fluid overload. This transudation also may occur owing to the hypoproteinemia often seen in chronic kidney disease.
34. Monitor for manifestations of pericarditis: a. Pericardial friction rub b. Elevated temperature c. Elevated white blood cell count d. Substernal or precordial pain increasing during inspiration	34. Pericarditis results from irritation by accumulated serum nitrogenous wastes.
35. Explain the causes of pain to the client.	35. The client may fear that chest pain is signaling a heart attack.
36. Monitor for signs and symptoms of cardiac tamponade: a. Rapid decrease in blood pressure b. Narrowed pulse pressure c. Muffled heart sounds d. Distended neck veins e. Decreased blood pressure during hemodialysis with intolerance to ultrafiltration f. Cardiac arrhythmias (Baird, Keen, & Swearingen, 2005).	36. Exaggerated signs and symptoms of effusion implicate worsening pericarditis, pericardial effusion, and slowly developing cardiac tamponade. It can develop at any time in a client with uremic pericarditis.
37. Discuss with the physician the need for changing to peritoneal dialysis until pericarditis resolves.	37. Heparin infusion exacerbates the bloody effusions of pericarditis and increases the risk of cardiac tamponade.

 Related Physician-Prescribed Interventions

Medications. Diuretics; electrolyte inhibitors or replacements (e.g., calcium gluconate, aluminum hydroxide gels); anti-hypertensives; epoetin alfa, iron; vitamins and minerals

Erythropoietin & Iron Replacement Therapy

Intravenous Therapy. Fluid or electrolyte replacement

Laboratory Studies. Urine (pH, osmolality, creatinine clearance, specific gravity, sodium HCO_3, casts, protein, RBC); serum osmolality; serum protein; hemoglobin; RBC count; blood urea nitrogen (BUN), creatinine; serum pH; electrolytes; transferrin saturation; serum glucose; ferritin, serum iron; albumin, prealbumin

Diagnostic Studies. ECG; renal arteriogram; ultrasound; x-ray films (kidney-ureter-bladder [KUB]); renal biopsy; retrograde pyelogram; x-ray film (feet, hands, spine)

Therapies. Hemodialysis, dietary restrictions dependent on laboratory findings, indwelling catheter, fluid restrictions

Documentation

Flow records
    Weight (actual, dry)
    Vital signs
    Laboratory values
    Intake and output

Evidence of bleeding (e.g., blood in stool, bruises)
Status of edema
Progress notes
Chest complaints

Nursing Diagnoses

Imbalanced Nutrition: Less than Body Requirements Related to Anorexia, Nausea and Vomiting, Loss of Taste or Smell, Stomatitis, and Unpalatable Diet

NOC Nutritional Status, Teaching: Nutrition

Goal

The client will relate the importance of adequate nutritional intake and complying with the prescribed dietary regimen.

Indicators

• Has no nutritional deficiencies
• Has minimal or no edema
• Maintains ideal or desired weight

NIC Nutrition Management, Nutritional Monitoring

Interventions	Rationales

1. Establish nutritional goals with the client/family and a plan of care to achieve them.
  a. Consult the dietitian for assistance with nutritional assessment, identifying nutritional goals, prescribing diet modifications, and providing nutritional instruction to client.
  b. Reinforce the dietary instructions and provide written materials for verbal orders.
	1.
	  a. A properly prescribed diet is essential in management of chronic kidney disease to prevent uremic toxicity, fluid and electrolyte imbalances, and catabolism.
	
	  b. Empathy and reinforcement of dietary instructions can increase compliance with diet restrictions (Lewis et al., 2004).

2. Discuss dietary options rather than restrictions.	2. Clients and families will become discouraged if the diet is too restrictive and unpalatable (Lewis et al., 2004).
3. Encourage the client to verbalize his or her feelings and frustrations about diet modifications.	3. The client should be given as much control as possible over his or her diet—for example, have the client make a list of food and fluid preferences and dislikes and try to incorporate these into the prescribed diet (Lewis et al., 2004).
4. Provide for and encourage good oral hygiene before and after meals.	4. Proper oral hygiene reduces microorganisms and helps prevent stomatitis.
5. Provide a pleasant environment during mealtimes and assist as indicated.	5. Appetite is stimulated in a relaxed, pleasant setting.
6. Administer vitamins and phosphate binders, as ordered.	6. Supplements control plasma phosphate levels and help to maintain nutritional status.

(continued on page 229)

Interventions	Rationales
7. Evaluate, with client and dietitian, the client's nutritional status and the diet's effectiveness.	7. Continued evaluation enables alteration of diet according to the client's specific nutritional needs.
8. Explain the need for the client to eat the maximum protein allowed on the diet.	8. Adequate protein is needed to prevent protein catabolism and muscle wasting (Lewis et al., 2004).
9. Discuss methods for reducing potassium intake, if indicated. a. Drain canned fruits. b. Eat cooked vegetables, pasta, and cereals. c. Soak fresh vegetables in water before cooking. Use fresh water to cook.	9. Clients with chronic kidney disease (not on dialysis) usually must restrict potassium intake to 38 to 46 mEq/day. Certain foods are lower in potassium. Soaking vegetables removes 50% of the potassium (Lewis et al., 2004).
10. Prepare for and administer total parenteral nutrition (TPN), as ordered. (Refer to the TPN care plan for more information.)	10. For a client who cannot maintain nutritional status through the GI route, TPN can provide amino acids necessary for healing, especially renal tissue, and for preventing a catabolic state.
11. Prepare for dialysis, as indicated, and monitor for potential complications. (Refer to the Hemodialysis and Peritoneal Dialysis care plans for more information.)	11. Dialysis is indicated for rising BUN that dietary management cannot control. It also may be necessary to remove excess fluid administered with TPN.
12. Work with the client to develop a plan to incorporate the diet prescription successfully into her or his daily life.	12. Collaboration provides opportunities for the client to exert control; this tends to increase compliance.

Documentation

Flow records
Nursing
    Daily weights
    Intake (specify food types and amounts)
    Output
    Mouth assessment
Discharge summary records
    Client teaching
    Referrals

Ineffective Sexuality Patterns Related to Decreased Libido, Erectile Dysfunction, Amenorrhea, or Sterility

 NOC Body Image, Self-Esteem, Role Performance, Sexual Identity: Acceptance

Goal

The client will discuss own feelings and partner's concerns regarding sexual functioning.

Indicators

• Relate the causes of decreased libido and impaired sexual functioning.
• Verbalize an intention to discuss concerns with partner.
• Verbalize an intention to seek professional help with concerns of decreased and or impaired sexual functioning.

NIC Behavior Management: Sexual, Counseling, Emotional Support, Active Listening, Teaching: Sexuality

Interventions	Rationales
1. Explore the client's patterns of sexual functioning; encourage him or her to share concerns. Assume that all clients have had some sexual experience and convey a willingness to discuss feelings and concerns.	1. Many clients are reluctant to discuss sexuality. The proper approach can encourage them to share feelings and concerns.
2. Explain the possible effects of chronic kidney disease on sexual functioning and sexuality.	2. Explaining that impaired sexual functioning has a physiologic basis and can induce feelings of inadequacy and decreased self-esteem; this actually may help improve sexual function.
3. Reaffirm the need for frank discussion between sexual partners.	3. Both partners probably have concerns about sexual activity. Repressing these feelings affects the relationship adversely.
4. Explain how the client and partner can use role-playing to discuss sexual concerns.	4. Role-playing helps a client and his or her partner to gain insight by placing themselves in the other's position and allows more spontaneous sharing of fears and concerns.
5. Reaffirm the need for closeness and expressions of caring through touching, massage, and other means.	5. Sexual pleasure and gratification is not limited to intercourse. Other expressions of caring may prove more meaningful.
6. Suggest that sexual activity need not always culminate in intercourse, but that the partner can reach orgasm through noncoital manual or oral stimulation.	6. Sexual gratification is an individual matter. It is not limited to intercourse, but includes closeness, touching, and giving pleasure to others.
7. Explain the function of a penile prosthesis: point out that both semirigid and inflatable penile prostheses have high rates of success.	7. Explaining penile prostheses can give the client hope for renewed sexual function.
8. Refer the client to a certified sex or mental health professional, if desired.	8. Certain sexual problems require continuing therapy and the advanced knowledge of specialists.

Documentation

Progress notes
  Dialogues
    Client teaching

Powerlessness Related to Progressive Disabling Nature of Illness

NOC Depression Control, Health Beliefs: Perceived Control, Participation in Health Care Decisions

Goal

The client will participate in decision-making for plan of care.

Indicators

- Identify personal strengths.
- Identify factors that she or he can control.

NIC Mood Management, Teaching: Individual, Decision-Making Support, Self-Responsibility Facilitation, Health System Guidance, Spiritual Support

Interventions	Rationales

1. Explore the condition's effects on the following:
  a. Occupation
  b. Leisure and recreational activities
  c. Role responsibilities
  d. Relationships
  e. Finances
	1. Illness can negatively affect the client's self-concept and ability to achieve goals. Specifically, in chronic kidney disease, fatigue can interfere with the client's abilities to work and play.

2. Determine the client's usual response to problems.	2. To plan effective interventions, the nurse must determine if the client usually seeks to change her or his own behaviors to control problems, or if she or he expects others or external factors to control problems.
3. Encourage the client to verbalize his or her concerns about potential changes in body image, life style, close relationships, role expectations, and life goals.	3. Clients with chronic kidney disease experience the formal loss of self. Former self-image changes negatively because of a restricted life style, social isolation, unmet expectations, and dependence on others (Lewis et al., 2004; Katz, 2006).
4. Help the client to identify personal strengths and assets.	4. Clients with chronic illness need assistance to not see themselves as helpless victims. People with a sense of hope, self-control, direction, purpose, and identity can better meet the challenges of their disease (Lewis et al., 2004).
5. Assist the client to identify energy patterns and to schedule activities around these patterns.	5. A review of the client's daily schedule can help the nurse and the client to plan activities that promote feelings of self-worth and dignity, and to schedule appropriate rest periods to prevent exhaustion.
6. Discuss the need to accept help from others and to delegate some tasks.	6. The client may need assistance to prevent exhaustion and hypoxia.
7. Help the client seek support from other sources (e.g., self-help groups, support groups).	7. The client may benefit from opportunities to share similar experiences and problem-solving strategies with others in the same situation.
8. Encourage the client to make decisions that might increase her or his ability to cope.	8. Self-concept can be enhanced when clients actively engage in decisions regarding health and life style.
9. Develop a plan of care with the client that reinforces positive coping mechanisms, uses personal strengths, and acknowledges limitations.	9. Research has shown that clients who adjust their aspiration levels to fit their new circumstances have a higher quality of life (Lewis et al., 2004).
10. Provide adequate information about the multiple facets of the illness and therapy options.	10. This will help to increase active participation in care.
11. Provide anticipatory guidance and counseling.	11. Therapy can address major stressors to be encountered.
12. Provide opportunities for the client to meet others who have had similar experiences.	12. Sharing experiences can help a client identify previously unknown options.

Documentation

Progress notes
  Interactions with the client

High Risk for Ineffective Therapeutic Regimen Management Related to Insufficient Knowledge of Condition, Dietary Restrictions, Daily Recording, Pharmacological Therapy, Signs/Symptoms of Complications, Follow-up Visits, and Community Resources

NOC Compliance Behavior, Knowledge: Treatment Regimen, Participation in Health Care Decisions, Treatment Behavior: Illness

Goals

The goals for this diagnosis represent those associated with discharge planning. Refer to the discharge criteria.

NIC Anticipatory Guidance, Learning Facilatation, Risk Identification, Health Education, Teaching: Procedure/Treatment, Health System Guidance

Interventions	Rationales
1. Develop and implement a teaching plan using techniques and tools appropriate to the client's understanding. Plan several teaching sessions.	1. Presenting relevant and useful information in an understandable format greatly reduces learning frustration and enhances teaching efforts. Some factors specific to a client with chronic kidney disease influence the teaching–learning process (Lewis et al., 2004): • Depressed mentation that necessitates repeating information • Short attention span that may limit teaching sessions to 10–15 minutes • Altered perceptions that necessitate frequent clarification and reassurance • Sensory alterations that cause a better response to ideas presented using varied audiovisual formats.

2. Implement teaching that includes but is not limited to renal function (Lewis et al., 2004).
  a. Normal function
  b. Altered function
   • Disease process
   • Causes
   • Physiologic and emotional responses to uremia
 Treatment modalities
  a. Conservative management
  b. Hemodialysis
   • Home staff-assisted, self-care, daily dialysis
   • In-center (staff-assisted, self-care)
  c. Peritoneal dialysis
   • Continuous ambulatory peritoneal dialysis (CAPD)
   • Continuous cycling peritoneal dialysis (CCPD)
   • Intermittent peritoneal dialysis (IPD)
  d. Transplantation:
   • Living related/unrelated donor
   • Cadaveric donor
   • Multiple organ transplantation
  e. No treatment
 Renal replacement therapies
  a. Definitions
  b. Process/procedures
  c. Vascular/peritoneal access
  d. Availability
  e. Benefits/risks
  f. Life style adaptation
  g. Nutritional considerations
  h. Mobility/activity/rehabilitation
  i. Financial considerations
	2. Amount and depth of teaching will depend on the client's present readiness to learn. Several sessions will be needed; include written materials to take home.

(continued on page 233)

Interventions	Rationales

Laboratory, x-rays, routine tests
a. Purpose of each
b. Expected ranges
c. Monitoring frequency
Nutrition
a. Incorporation of prescribed diet into life style
b. Shopping, preparation, dining out
c. Nutritional requirements
  • Energy
  • Protein
  • Sodium and water
  • Potassium
  • Vitamins
  • Calcium and phosphorus
Medication therapy
a. Identification/name
b. Purpose
c. Dosage
d. Route
e. Side effects
f. Instructions for missed dose
g. Drug interactions
h. Relationship to diet
i. Avoidance of over-the-counter medications
j. Use of complementary and/or alterative
   medicine/treatments
Psychosocial issues
a. Emotional aspects: coping, self-concept
b. Sexual function
c. Rehabilitation
d. Energy/activity level
e. Body image
Financial aspects
a. Medicare/Medicaid/other pay or sources
b. Disability
Client involvement
a. Client's rights
b. Client's responsibilities
c. Advanced directives
d. Long-term care program
e. Short-term care plan
f. Medical record
  • Access for client review
  • Confidentiality	

3. Encourage the client to verbalize anxiety, fears, and questions.	3. Recognizing the client's fear of failure to learn is vital to successful teaching.

4. Identify factors that may help to predict noncompliance:
  a. Lack of knowledge
  b. Noncompliance in the hospital
  c. Failure to perceive disease's seriousness or chronicity
  d. Belief that the condition will "go away" on its own
  e. Belief that the condition is hopeless
	4. Openly addressing barriers to compliance may help to minimize or eliminate these barriers.

5. Include significant others in teaching sessions. Encourage them to provide support without acting as "police."	5. Significant others must be aware of the treatment plan so they can support the client. "Policing" the client can disrupt positive relationships.

(continued on page 234)

Interventions	Rationales
6. Emphasize to the client that, ultimately, it is his or her choice and responsibility to comply with the therapeutic regimen.	6. The client must understand that he or she has control over choices and that his or her choices can improve or impair health.
7. If cost of medications is a financial burden for the client, consult with social services.	7. A referral for financial support can prevent discontinuation because of financial reasons.
8. Assist the client to identify her or his ideal or desired weight.	8. Establishing an achievable goal may help to improve compliance.
9. Teach the client to record weight and urinary output daily.	9. Daily weight and urine output measurements allow the client to monitor her or his own fluid status, and limit fluid intake accordingly.
10. Explain the signs and symptoms of electrolyte imbalances and the need to watch for and report them. (See Collaborative Problems in this entry for more information.)	10. Early detection of electrolyte imbalance enables prompt intervention to prevent serious complications.
11. Teach the client measures to reduce risk of urinary tract infection: a. Perform proper hygiene after toileting to prevent fecal contamination of urinary tract. b. To prevent urinary stasis, drink the maximum fluids allowed.	11. Repetitive infections can cause further renal damage.
12. Reinforce the need to comply with diet and fluid restrictions and follow-up care. Consult with the dietitian regarding fluid plan and overall diet.	12. Compliance reduces the risk of complications.
13. Teach the client who has fluid restrictions to relieve thirst by other means: a. Sucking on a lemon wedge, a piece of hard candy, a frozen juice pop, or an ice cube b. Spacing fluid allotment over 24 hours	13. Strategies to reduce thirst without significant fluid intake reduce risk of fluid overload.
14. Encourage the client to express feelings and frustrations; give positive feedback for adherence to fluid restrictions.	14. Fluid and diet restrictions can be extremely frustrating; positive feedback and reassurance can contribute to continued compliance.
15. Explain importance of Epoetin alfa therapy and iron supplements to achieve an Hct of 33%–36%.	15. When Hct is maintained between 33% and 36%, there are incremental improvements in survival, left ventricle hypertrophy, exercise capacity, cognitive function, sleep dysfunction, and overall quality of life (Coyne, 2007; Baird, Keen, & Swearingen, 2005).
16. Teach the client to take oral medications with meals whenever possible. If medications must be administered between meals, give with the smallest amount of fluid possible.	16. Planning can reduce unnecessary fluid intake and conserve fluid allowance.
17. Encourage the client to maintain his or her usual level of activity and continue activities of daily living to the extent possible.	17. Regular activity helps to maintain strength and endurance and promotes overall well-being.

(continued on page 235)

Interventions	Rationales
18. Teach the client and family to watch for and report the following: a. Weight gain or loss greater than 2 lb b. Shortness of breath c. Increasing fatigue or weakness d. Confusion, change in mentation e. Palpitations f. Excessive bruising; excessive menses; excessive bleeding from gums, nose, or cut; blood in urine, stool, or vomitus g. Increasing oral pain or oral lesions	18. Early reporting of complications enables prompt intervention (Lewis et al., 2004). a. Weight gain greater than 2 lb may indicate fluid retention; weight loss may point to insufficient intake. b. Shortness of breath may be an early sign of pulmonary edema. c. Increasing fatigue or weakness may indicate increasing uremia. d. Confusion or other changes in mentation may point to acidosis or fluid and electrolyte imbalances. e. Palpitations may indicate electrolyte imbalances (K, Ca). f. Excessive bruising, excessive menses, and abnormal bleeding may indicate reduced prothrombin, clotting factors III and VIII, and platelets. g. Oral pain or lesions can result as excessive salivary urea is converted to ammonia in the mouth, which is irritating to the oral mucosa.
19. Discuss with the client and family any anticipated disease-related stressors: a. Financial difficulties b. Reversal of role responsibilities c. Dependency	19. Discussing the nonphysiologic effects of chronic kidney disease in family dynamics can help the client and family to identify effective coping strategies (Lewis et al., 2004).
20. Provide information about or initiate referrals to community resources (e.g., American Kidney Association, counseling, self-help groups, peer counseling, Internet information sites, publications).	20. Assistance with home management and dealing with the potential destructive effects on the client and family may be needed.

Documentation

Discharge summary record
Client teaching
Outcome achievement or status
Referrals, if indicated

Cerebrovascular Accident (Stroke)

Cerebrovascular accident (CVA), or stroke, involves a sudden onset of neurological deficits because of insufficient blood supply to a part of the brain, leading to cellular damage and cellular death (Parker-Frizzell, 2005). In 80% of cases, insufficient blood supply is caused by ischemia, usually secondary to atherosclerosis, a localized thrombus, an embolism originating elsewhere in the body, or by systemic hypoperfusion. In 20% of cases, insufficient blood supply is caused by hemorrhage from a ruptured blood vessel (Caplan, 2007). Symptoms are dependent on infarct location (Santoni-Reddy, 2006).

Preventable and costly, stroke, or brain attack, is the third leading cause of death and the leading cause of long-term disability in the United States (American Stroke Association, 2007). A recent estimate from the American Heart Association is that at least 700,000 new or recurrent strokes occur each year (American Stroke Association, 2007; Pajeau, 2002; Rosamond et al., 2007; Sacco et al., 2006)

Preventing first and recurrent strokes requires prompt identification of vulnerable clients. Some risk factors can be modified (Pajeau, 2002; Rosamond et al., 2007; Sacco et al., 2006), including hypertension, cigarette smoking, unhealthy eating habits, sedentary life style, lipid imbalance, poor glycemic control, cocaine use, and alcohol abuse (Parker-Frizzell, 2005; Rosamond et al., 2007; Sacco et al., 2006). Nonmodifiable risk factors include age, gender, genetic predisposition, history of previous stroke, transient ischemic attacks (TIAs), other cardiac conditions (Pajeau, 2002; Rosamond et al., 2007; Sacco et al., 2006), pregnancy, menopause, and sickle cell disease (Rosamond et al., 2007).

The primary assessment should focus on identifying the cause/s of the neurologic symptoms. If stroke is considered, it must be determined whether it is ischemic or hemorrhagic. Initial goals should include ensuring medical stability, quickly reversing the conditions that contribute to client's problem, identifying the pathophysiologic basis for the client's neurologic symptoms, and screening for potential contraindications for thrombolysis in acute ischemic stroke (Oliveira-Filho & Koroshetz, 2007). Thrombolytics should be given within 180 minutes of symptom onset (Parker-Frizzell, 2005).

 Time Frame
Initial diagnosis
Recurrent episodes

■■■■■■ DIAGNOSTIC CLUSTER

Collaborative Problems

▲ PC: Increased Intracranial Pressure

✱ PC: Pneumonia, Atelectasis

▲ PC: Adult Respiratory Distress Syndrome

✱ PC: Seizures

✱ PC: Gastrointestinal (GI) Bleeding

✱ PC: Hypothalamic Syndromes

Nursing Diagnoses	Refer to
▲ Impaired Communication related to the effects of hemisphere (left or right) damage on language or speech.	
▲ High Risk for Injury related to visual field, motor, or perception deficits	

(continued on page 237)

Nursing Diagnoses	Refer to
▲ Impaired Physical Mobility related to decreased motor function of (specify) secondary to damage to upper motor neurons	
▲ Functional Incontinence related to inability and difficulty in reaching toilet secondary to decreased mobility or motivation	
▲ Impaired Swallowing related to muscle paralysis or paresis secondary to damage to upper motor neurons	
▲ Self-Care Deficit related to impaired physical mobility or confusion	Immobility or Unconsciousness
△ Unilateral Neglect related to (specify site) secondary to right hemispheric brain damage	
△ High Risk for Ineffective Therapeutic Regimen Management related to altered ability to maintain self at home secondary to sensory/motor/cognitive deficits and lack of knowledge of caregivers of home care, reality orientation, bowel/bladder program, skin care, signs and symptoms of complications, and community resources	
△ Total Incontinence related to loss of bladder tone, loss of sphincter control, or inability to perceive bladder cues	Neurogenic Bladder
△ High Risk for Disturbed Self-Concept related to effects of prolonged debilitating condition on achieving developmental tasks and life style	Multiple Sclerosis
✳ Disuse Syndrome	Immobility or Unconsciousness
Related Care Plan	
Immobility or Unconsciousness	

▲ This diagnosis was reported to be monitored for or managed frequently (75%–100%).
△ This diagnosis was reported to be monitored for or managed often (50%–74%).
✳ This diagnosis was not included in the validation study.

Discharge Criteria

Before discharge, the client or family will

1. Describe measures for reducing or eliminating selected risk factors.
2. Relate intent to discuss fears and concerns with family members after discharge.
3. Identify methods for management (e.g., of dysphagia, of incontinence).
4. Demonstrate or relate techniques to increase mobility.
5. State signs and symptoms that must be reported to a health care professional.
6. Relate community resources that can provide assistance with management at home.

Collaborative Problems

Potential Complication: Increased Intracranial Pressure (ICP)

Potential Complication: Pneumonia, Atelectasis

Potential Complication: Adult Respiratory Distress Syndrome
Potential Complication: Seizures
Potential Complication: GI Bleeding
Potential Complication: Hypothalamic Syndromes

Nursing Goal

The nurse will detect early signs/symptoms of (a) increased ICP, (b) hypoxia, (c) pneumonia, (d) seizures, (e) GI bleeding, and (f) hypothalamic dysfunction, and collaboratively intervene to stabilize the client.

Indicators

- Alert, oriented (a, b, c, d)
- Pulse 60–100 beats/min (a, b, c, e)
- BP >90/60, <140/90 mmHg (a, b, c, e)
- Respiration 16–20 breaths/min (a, b, c,)
- Pupils equal, reactive to light (a, d)
- Temperature 98–99.5°F (c, d)
- Breath sounds equal, no adventitious sounds (a, c)
- Oxygen saturation (pulse oximetry) (SaO_2) >95 (a, b, c)
- Stool negative for occult blood (e)
- Urine specific gravity 1.005–1.030 (a, b, e)
- Serum sodium 135–145 mEq/L (f)

Interventions	Rationales
1. Monitor for signs and symptoms of increased intracranial pressure (ICP).	1. Cerebral tissue is compromised by deficiencies of cerebral blood supply caused by hemorrhage, hematoma, cerebral edema, thrombus, or emboli. Monitoring ICP is an indicator of cerebral perfusion.
a. Assess the following (Sheth, 2007): • Best eye opening response: spontaneously to auditory stimuli or to painful stimuli, or no response • Best motor response: obeys verbal commands, localizes pain, flexion-withdrawal, flexion-decorticate, extension-decerebrate, or no response • Best verbal response: oriented to person, place, and time; confused conversation, inappropriate speech, incomprehensible sounds, or no response	a. The Glasgow Coma Scale evaluates the client's ability to integrate commands with conscious and involuntary movements. Cortical function can be assessed by evaluating eye opening and motor response. No response may indicate damage to the midbrain.
b. Assess for changes in vital signs: • Pulse changes: slowing rate to 60 or below or increasing rate to 100 or above • Respiratory irregularities: slowing of rate with lengthening periods of apnea • Rising blood pressure or widening pulse pressure	b. These vital sign changes may reflect increasing ICP. • Changes in pulse may indicate brainstem pressure by being slowed at first, then increasing to compensate for hypoxia. • Respiratory patterns vary with impairments at various sites. Cheyne-Stokes breathing (a gradual increase followed by a gradual decrease, then a period of apnea) points to damage in both cerebral hemispheres, midbrain, and upper pons. Ataxic breathing (irregular, with random sequence of deep and shallow breaths) indicates medullar dysfunction. • Blood pressure and pulse pressure changes are late signs indicating severe hypoxia.

(continued on page 239)

Interventions	Rationales
c. Assess pupillary responses: • Inspect the pupils with a flashlight to evaluate size, configuration, and reaction to light. Compare both eyes for similarities and differences. • Evaluate gaze to determine whether it is conjugate (paired, working together), or if eye movements are abnormal. • Evaluate eyes' ability to adduct and abduct. d. Note the presence of the following (Sheth, 2007): • Vomiting • Headache (constant, increasing in intensity, or aggravated by movement or straining) • Subtle changes (e.g., lethargy, restlessness, forced breathing, purposeless movements, and changes in mentation)	c. Pupillary changes indicate pressure on oculomotor or optic nerves. • Pupil reactions are regulated by the oculomotor nerve (cranial nerve III) in the brain stem. • Conjugate eye movements are regulated from parts of the cortex and brain stem. • Cranial nerve VI, or the abducent nerve, regulates abduction and adduction of the eyes. Cranial nerve IV, or the trochlear nerve, also regulates eye movement. d. • Vomiting results from pressure on the medulla that stimulates the brain's vomiting center. • Compression of neural tissue movement increases ICP and pain. • These changes may be early indicators of ICP changes.
2. Elevate the head of the bed 15–30 degrees unless contraindicated. Avoid changing position rapidly. Ischemic stroke clients should remain as flat as possible for the first 24 hours only (Oliveira-Filho & Koroshetz, 2007).	2. Slight head elevation can aid venous drainage to reduce cerebrovascular congestion. Flat positioning improves cerebral blood flow by 20% in ischemic stroke; recommended for the first 24–48 hours only to prevent complications related to immobility (Oliveira-Filho & Koroshetz, 2007).
3. Avoid the following: a. Carotid massage b. Neck flexion or rotation >45 degrees c. Digital anal stimulation d. Breath holding, straining e. Extreme flexion of hips and knees	3. These situations or maneuvers can increase ICP. a. Carotid massage slows heart rate and reduces systemic circulation; this is followed by a sudden increase in circulation. b. Neck flexion or extreme rotation disrupts cerebrospinal fluid and venous drainage from intracranial cavity. c–e. These activities initiate Valsalva maneuver, which impairs venous return by constricting the jugular veins and increases ICP.
4. Consult with the physician for stool softeners, if needed.	4. Stool softeners prevent constipation and straining that initiate Valsalva maneuver.
5. Maintain a quiet, calm, softly lit environment. Plan activities to minimize ICP.	5. These measures promote rest and decrease stimulation, helping to decrease ICP. Suctioning, position changes, and neck flexion in succession will markedly increase cranial pressure.
6. Monitor for signs and symptoms of pneumonia: a. Increased respiratory rate b. Fever, chills (sudden or insidious) c. Productive cough d. Diminished or absent breath sounds e. Pleuritic pain	6. Pneumonia is a common complication of many major illnesses. Swallowing, respiratory therapy, and deep breathing exercises help to decrease the risk of pneumonia (American Heart Association, 2007a; American Stroke Association, 2001). a. Increased respiratory rate is a compensatory mechanism for hypoxia. b. Bacteria can act as pyrogen by raising the hypothalamic thermostat through the production of endogenous pyrogen that may mediate through prostaglandins. Chills can occur when the temperature setpoint of the hypothalamus changes rapidly. c. Productive cough indicates increased mucus production in response to irritant (bacteria). d. Airflow through the tracheobronchial tree is affected or obstructed by the presence of fluid or mucus. e. Pleuritic pain results from the rubbing together of inflamed pleural surfaces during respiration.

(continued on page 240)

Interventions	Rationales
7. Monitor for signs and symptoms of atelectasis:	7. Inactivity can cause retained secretions, leading to obstruction or infection.
a. Pleuritic pain	a. Pleuritic pain results from the rubbing together of inflamed pleural surfaces during respiration.
b. Diminished or absent breath sounds c. Dull percussion sounds over area	b,c. Changes in breath and percussion sounds represent increased density of lung tissue secondary to fluid accumulation.
d. Tachycardia e. Increased respiratory rate	d,e. Tachycardia and tachypnea are compensatory mechanisms for hypoxia.
f. Elevated temperature	f. Bacteria can act as pyrogen by raising the hypothalamic thermostat through the production of endogenous pyrogen, which may mediate through prostaglandins. Hyperthermia worsens brain injury—for every 1°C increase in body temperature, the risk of poor outcome increases by 2.2%. Clients should be kept normothermic (Caplan, 2007; Oliveira-Filho & Koroshetz, 2007; Santoni-Reddy, 2006).
g. Marked dyspnea	g. Dyspnea indicates hypoxia.
h. Cyanosis	h. Cyanosis indicates vasoconstriction in response to hypoxia.
8. Monitor high-risk clients closely for changes in respiratory status. Report changes immediately.	8. CVA clients who have pneumonia, sepsis, ICP, or gastric aspirations are at high risk for adult respiratory distress syndrome (ARDS). Mortality rate for ARDS is 50%–60%.
9. Monitor for signs and symptoms of ARDS: a. Respiratory discomfort b. Noisy tachypnea c. Tachycardia d. Diffuse rales and rhonchi	9. Damaged type II cells release inflammatory mediators that increase alveolocapillary membrane permeability, causing pulmonary edema. Decreased surfactant production decreases alveolar compliance. Respiratory muscles must greatly increase inspiratory pressures to inflate lungs.
10. Monitor hydration status by evaluating the following: a. Oral intake b. Parenteral therapy (Santoni-Reddy, 2006) c. Intake and output d. Urine specific gravity	10. A balance must be maintained to ensure hydration to liquefy secretions to maintain euvolemia. Use isotonic solutions (e.g., 0.9% sodium chloride); nonisotonic solutions can worsen cerebral edema, increasing ICP (Santoni-Reddy, 2006). *Note:* hypervolemia may be desired to prevent/treat cerebral vasospasm. Significantly increased amounts of urine output may indicate diabetes insipidus.
11. Monitor the effectiveness of airway clearance by evaluating (Oliveira-Filho & Koroshetz, 2007): a. Effectiveness of cough effort b. Need for tracheobronchial suctioning	11. Lower cranial deficits can affect swallowing ability. The prevalence of aspiration post-CVA is reported to be 25%–30%. Endotracheal intubation may be necessary to protect the airway (Oliveira-Filho & Koroshetz, 2007).
12. Monitor for seizures.	12. Ischemic areas may serve as epileptogenic foci or metabolic disturbances can lower the seizure threshold (American Stroke Association, 2001).
13. Refer to the Seizure Disorders care plan, if indicated.	
14. Monitor stools for blood.	14. Hypersecretion of gastric juices occurs during periods of stress.
15. Monitor for: a. Low serum sodium b. Elevated urine sodium c. Elevated urine specific gravity	15. Damage to the hypothalamic region may result in increased secretion of antidiuretic hormone (ADH).

(continued on page 241)

Interventions	Rationales
16. Monitor for diabetes insipidus (Santoni-Reddy, 2006): 　a. Excess urine output 　b. Extreme thirst 　c. Elevated serum sodium 　d. Low specific gravity	16. Compression of posterior pituitary gland or its neuronal connections can cause a decrease of ADH.
17. Monitor body temperature.	17. Hypothalamic pituitary compression can compromise the temperature-regulating mechanism.
18. Monitor for inability to maintain a functional airway (Oliveira-Filho & Koroshetz, 2007) 　a. $SpO_2 < 94\%$ 　b. Labored or shallow respiration 　c. Periods of apnea 　d. Cyanosis	18. Increased ICP can lead to decreased respiratory drive. Hypoventilation increases serum carbon dioxide levels, leading to vasodilation, further increasing ICP. Endotracheal intubation may be necessary to support respiratory efforts (Caplan, 2007; Oliveira-Filho & Koroshetz, 2007). Maintain SpO_2 above 94% to prevent brain injury (Santoni-Reddy, 2006).
19. Monitor for hypertension (Oliveira-Filho & Koroshetz, 2007)	19. Hypertension may be a compensatory mechanism to increase cerebral perfusion. Treatment is not recommended in ischemic stroke, unless systolic BP >220 mmHg or diastolic BP >120 mmHg. In both ischemic and hemorrhagic stroke, sudden drops in blood pressure should be avoided (Oliveira-Filho & Koroshetz, 2007). BP in nonchronic hypertensive clients usually returns to normal within 2 weeks of stroke (Smith, Johnston, & Easton, 2005).
20. Monitor for cerebral vasospasm (Santoni-Reddy, 2006) 　a. Change in level of consciousness 　b. Seizures	20. Cerebral vasospasm occurs in intracranial hemorrhage, especially subarachnoid hemorrhage, and accounts for 40%–50% of associated mortality. Vasospasm occurs 4–14 days after initial bleed (Santoni-Reddy, 2006).
21. Monitor blood sugar (Parker-Frizzell, 2005)	21. Hyperglycemia is associated with poor outcomes; serum glucose levels should be kept <200 mg/dL (Parker-Frizzell, 2005; Smith et al., 2005). HbA_{1c} should be ≤7% (Sacco et al., 2006).

 ## Related Physician-Prescribed Interventions

Medications. Anticonvulsants, antihypertensives, stool softeners, peripheral vasodilators, corticosteroids, anticoagulants, antiplatelets (e.g., aspirin, ticlopidine, abciximab), analgesics, antipyretics, thrombolytics, anxiolytics, barbiturates, osmotic diuretics, H_2 blockers, calcium channel blockers, antiemetics.

Intravenous Therapy. Fluid/electrolyte replacements (isotonic fluids)

Laboratory Studies.

All clients: Complete blood count, urinalysis, chemistry profile, sedimentation rate, prothrombin time and INR (international normalized ratio), partial thromboplastin time, RPR (rapid plasma reagin) serology, single-photon tomography, cardiac enzymes and troponin, serum glucose, oxygen saturation (7).

Selected clients: Liver function tests, toxicology screen, blood alcohol level, pregnancy tests, arterial blood gas, type and crossmatch, antiphospholipid antibodies, Hemoglobin A_{1c}.

Diagnostic Studies. Computed tomography (CT) scan of head (noncontrast), lumbar puncture, cerebral angiography, magnetic resonance imaging (MRI), positron emission tomography (PET) scan, brain scan, Doppler ultrasonography, electroencephalography (EEG), electrocardiogram, transesophageal echocardiogram (TEE), transthoracic echocardiogram, intracranial pressure monitoring

Therapies. Swallowing studies, antiembolism stockings, speech therapy, physical therapy, occupational therapy, craniotomy, endarterectomy, ventriculostomy

Documentation

Flow records
    Neurologic assessment
    Vital signs
Complaints of vomiting or headache
Changes in status
Respiratory assessment

Nursing Diagnoses

Impaired Communication Related to the Effects of Hemisphere (Left or Right) Damage on Language or Speech

NOC Communication Ability

Goal

The client will report improved satisfaction with ability to communicate.

Indicators

- Demonstrate improved ability to express self and understand others.
- Report decreased frustration during communication efforts.

NIC Communication Enhancement: Speech Deficit, Active Listening, Socialization Enhancement

Interventions	Rationales
1. Differentiate between language disturbances (dysphagia/aphasia) and speech disturbances (dyspraxia/apraxia).	1. Language involves comprehension and transmission of ideas and feelings. Speech is the mechanics and articulations of verbal expression.
2. Collaborate with a speech therapist to evaluate the client and create a plan (American Heart Association, 2003).	2. A detailed assessment is required to diagnose a language dysfunction. Most clients have more than one type of dysfunction (National Institute of Neurological Disorders and Stroke, 2000).
3. Provide frequent, short, therapy and practice sessions. Try to incorporate topics of interest to the client.	3. These sessions are more beneficial than lengthy, infrequent ones (National Institute of Neurological Disorders and Stroke, 2000).
4. Provide an atmosphere of acceptance and privacy: a. Do not rush. b. Speak slowly and in a normal tone. c. Decrease external noise and distractions (American Heart Association, 2003). d. Encourage the client to share frustrations; validate the client's nonverbal expressions (American Heart Association, 2003). e. Provide the client with opportunities to make decisions about his or her care, whenever appropriate (American Heart Association, 2003). f. Do not force the client to communicate. g. If the client laughs or cries uncontrollably, change the subject or activity.	4. Communication is the core of all human relations. Impaired ability to communicate spontaneously is frustrating and embarrassing. Nursing actions should focus on decreasing the tension and conveying an understanding of how difficult the situation must be for the client.

(continued on page 243)

Interventions	Rationales
5. Make every effort to understand the client's communication efforts: a. Listen attentively. b. Repeat the client's message back to him or her to ensure understanding. c. Ignore inappropriate word usage; do not correct mistakes. d. Do not pretend you understand; if you do not, ask the client to repeat. e. Try to anticipate some needs (e.g., Do you need something to drink?).	5. Nurse and family members should make every attempt to understand the client. Each success, regardless of how minor, decreases frustration and increases motivation (American Heart Association, 2003).
6. Teach the client techniques to improve speech: a. Instruct the client to speak slowly and in short phrases (American Heart Association, 2003). b. Initially ask questions that the client can answer with a "yes" or "no" (American Heart Association, 2003). c. With improvement, allow the client to complete some phrases (e.g., "This is a _____."). d. As the client is able, encourage her or him to share feelings and concerns.	6. Deliberate actions can be taken to improve speech. As the client's speech improves, her or his confidence will increase and she or he will make more attempts at speaking.
7. Use strategies to improve the client's comprehension: a. Gain the client's attention before speaking; call him or her by name. b. Practice consistent speech patterns: • Speak slowly. • Use common words and use the same words consistently for a task. • Repeat or rephrase when indicated. c. Use touch and behavior to communicate calmness. d. Add other nonverbal methods of communication: • Point or use flash cards for basic needs. • Use pantomime. • Use paper/pen or spelling board. • Display the most effective methods at the client's bedside.	7. Improving the client's comprehension can help to decrease frustration and increase trust. Clients with aphasia can correctly interpret tone of voice.
8. Refer to the Parkinson Disease care plan for further strategies to manage dysarthria.	

Documentation

Progress notes
    Dialogues
    Method to use (care plan)

High Risk for Injury Related to Visual Field, Motor, or Perception Deficits

NOC Risk Control, Safety Status: Falls Occurrence

Goal

The client will relate no injuries.

Indicators

• Identify factors that increase the risk for injury.
• Demonstrate safety measures to prevent injury.
• Request assistance when needed.

Fall Prevention, Environmental Management: Safety, Health
Education, Surveillance: Safety, Risk Identification

Interventions	Rationales

1. Take steps to reduce environmental hazards:
   a. Orient the client to his or her surroundings.
   b. Instruct the client to use a call bell to summon assistance. Post high-risk status at bedside.
   c. Keep the bed in a low position with all side rails up.
   d. Keep paths to the bathroom obstacle-free.
   e. Provide adequate lighting in all areas.
   f. Provide a night light.
   g. Ensure that a light switch is accessible next to the bed.
	1. Emphasizing safety can help reduce injuries (American Heart Association, 2007c).

2. If decreased tactile sensitivity is a problem, teach the client to do the following (American Heart Association, 2007c):
   a. Carefully assess the temperature of the bath water and heating pads prior to use; measure with a thermometer, if possible.
   b. Assess the client's extremities daily for undetected injuries.
   c. Keep feet warm and dry and skin softened with emollient lotion (e.g., lanolin or mineral oil).
	2. Post-CVA sensory impairment can interfere with the client's perception of temperature and injuries (American Heart Association, 2007c).

3. Take steps to reduce risks associated with assistive devices:
   a. Assess for proper use of devices.
   b. Assess devices for fit and condition.
   c. Consult with a physical therapist for gait training.
   d. Instruct the client to wear shoes with nonskid soles.
	3. Improper use or fit of assistive devices can cause straining or falls (American Heart Association, 2007c).

4. Teach the client and family to maximize safety and independence at home (American Heart Association, 2007c):
   a. Eliminate throw rugs, clutter and litter, and highly-polished floors.
   b. Provide nonslip surfaces in bathtub or shower by applying traction tapes.
   c. Provide hand grips in the bathroom.
   d. Provide railings in hallways and on stairs.
   e. Remove protruding objects (e.g., coat hooks, shelves, and light fixtures) from stairway walls.
	4. A client with mobility problems needs such safety devices installed and hazards eliminated to aid in activities of daily living (American Heart Association, 2007c).

Documentation

Discharge summary record
   Client teaching

Impaired Physical Mobility Related to Decreased Motor Function of (Specify) Secondary to Damage to Upper Motor Neurons

NOC Ambulation, Joint Movement: Active Mobility Level

Goal

The client will report an increase in strength and endurance of limbs.

Indicators

- Demonstrate the use of adaptive devices to increase mobility.
- Use safety measures to minimize potential for injury.
- Describe rationale for interventions.
- Demonstrate measures to increase mobility.

NIC Exercise Therapy: Joint Mobility, Exercise Promotion: Strength Training, Exercise Therapy: Ambulation, Positioning, Teaching: Prescribed Activity/Exercise, Teaching Assistive Device, Teaching: Strategy

Interventions	Rationales
1. Teach the client to perform active range-of-motion (ROM) exercises on unaffected limbs at least four times a day, if possible.	1. Active ROM increases muscle mass, tone, and strength, and improves cardiac and respiratory functioning.
2. Perform passive ROM on affected limbs three to four times daily. Do the exercises slowly to allow the muscles time to relax, and support the extremity above and below the joint to prevent strain on joints and tissues. Stop at the point when pain or resistance is met.	2. A voluntary muscle will lose tone and strength and become shortened from reduced range of motion or lack of exercise (American Stroke Association, 2001).
3. When the client is in bed, take steps to maintain alignment: a. Use a footboard. b. Avoid prolonged periods of sitting or lying in the same position. c. Change position of shoulder joints every 2 to 4 hours. d. Use a small pillow or no pillow when in Fowler's position. e. Support hand and wrist in natural alignment. f. If the client is supine or prone, place a rolled towel or small pillow under the lumbar curvature or the end of the rib cage. g. Place a trochanter roll or sand bags alongside the client's hips and upper thighs. h. If the client is in the lateral position, place pillow(s) to support the leg from groin to foot and a pillow to flex the shoulder and elbow slightly; if needed, support the lower foot in dorsal flexion with a sandbag. i. Use hand–wrist splints.	3. Prolonged immobility and impaired neurosensory function can cause permanent contractures (American Stroke Association, 2001). a. This measure helps prevent foot drop. b. This measure prevents hip flexion contractures. c. This measure prevents shoulder contractures. d. This measure prevents flexion contracture of the neck. e. This measure prevents dependent edema and flexion contracture of the wrist. f. This measure prevents flexion or hyperflexion of lumbar curvature. g. This measure prevents external rotation of femurs and hip. h. These measures prevent internal rotation and adduction of the femurs and hip, internal rotation and adduction of the shoulder, and foot drop. i. These splints prevent flexion or extension contractures of fingers and abduction of the thumb.
4. Provide progressive mobilization (Schwamm, Pancioli, Acker, Goldstein, Zorowitz et al., 2005): a. Maintain the head of the client's bed at least at a 30-degree angle, unless contraindicated. b. Assist the client slowly from the lying to the sitting position and allow the client to dangle her or his legs over the side of the bed for a few minutes before standing up. c. Initially limit the time out of bed to 15 minutes three times a day. d. Increase the time out of bed by 15-minute increments, as tolerated. e. Progress to ambulation with or without assistive devices. f. If the client cannot walk, assist him or her out of bed to a wheelchair or chair. g. Encourage short, frequent walks (at least three times daily), with assistance if unsteady. h. Increase the length of walks each day.	4. Prolonged bed rest or decreased blood volume can cause a sudden drop in blood pressure (orthostatic hypotension) as blood returns to peripheral circulation. Gradual progression to increased activity reduces fatigue and increases endurance.
5. Gradually help the client progress from active ROM to functional activities, as indicated (Schwamm et al., 2005).	5. Incorporating ROM exercises into the client's daily routine encourages their regular performance.

Documentation

Flow records
> Intake and output
> Incontinent episodes

Functional Incontinence Related to Inability or Difficulty in Reaching Toilet Secondary to Decreased Mobility or Motivation

NOC Tissue Integrity: Skin and Mucous Membranes, Urinary Continence, Urinary Elimination

Goal

The client will report no or fewer episodes of incontinence.

Indicators

- Remove or minimize environmental barriers at home.
- Use proper adaptive equipment to assist with voiding, transfers, and dressing.
- Describe causative factors for incontinence.

NIC Perineal Care, Urinary Incontinence Care, Prompted Voiding, Urinary Habit Training, Urinary Elimination Management, Teaching: Procedure/Treatment

Interventions	Rationales
1. Assess environment for barriers to the client's bathroom access.	1. Barriers can delay access to the toilet and cause incontinence if the client cannot delay urination.
2. Provide grab rails and a raised toilet seat, if necessary.	2. These devices can promote independence and reduce toileting difficulties.
3. If the client requires assistance, provide ready access to a call bell and respond promptly when summoned.	3. A few seconds' delay in reaching the bathroom can make the difference between continence and incontinence.
4. Encourage the client to wear pajamas or ordinary clothes.	4. Wearing normal clothing or nightwear helps to simulate the home environment where incontinence may not occur. A hospital gown may reinforce incontinence.
5. For a client with incontinence, provide bladder training (American Heart Association, 2007a): a. Offer toileting reminders every 2 hours after meals and before bedtime. b. Provide verbal instruction for toileting activities. c. Praise success and good attempts.	5. A client with incontinence and/or cognitive deficit needs constant verbal cues and reminders to establish a routine and reduce incontinence (American Heart Association, 2007a; American Stroke Association, 2001)
6. Maintain optimal hydration (2000 to 2500 mL/day unless contraindicated). Space fluids every 2 hours.	6. Dehydration can prevent the sensation of a full bladder and can contribute to loss of bladder tone. Spacing fluids helps to promote regular bladder filling and emptying.
7. Minimize intake of coffee, tea, colas, and grapefruit juice.	7. These beverages act as diuretics, which can cause urgency.

Documentation

Flow records
> Range of motion exercises
> Progress in activities and ambulation

Impaired Swallowing Related to Muscle Paralysis or Paresis Secondary to Damage to Upper Motor Neurons

NOC Aspiration Control, Swallowing Status

Goal

The client will report improved ability to swallow.

Indicators

- Describe causative factors when known.
- Describe rationale and procedures for treatment.

NIC Aspiration Precautions, Swallowing Therapy, Surveillance, Referral, Positioning

Interventions	Rationales
1. Consult with speech pathologist for evaluation and a specific plan regarding speech and swallowing (American Heart Association, 2003, 2007a).	1. The speech pathologist has the expertise needed to perform the dysphagia evaluation.
2. Establish a visual method to communicate to staff at bedside that the client is dysphagic.	2. The risk of aspiration can be reduced if all staff are alerted.
3. Plan meals for when the client is well-rested; ensure that reliable suction equipment is on hand during meals. Discontinue feeding if client is tired.	3. Fatigue can increase the risk of aspiration.
4. If indicated, use modified supraglottic swallow technique: a. Position the head of the bed in semi- or high Fowler's position, with the client's neck flexed forward slightly and chin tilted down. b. Use cutout cup (remove and round out ⅓ of side of foam cup). c. Take bolus of food and have the client hold it in the strongest side of her or his mouth for one to two seconds, then immediately flex the neck with the chin tucked against the chest. d. Then, have the client swallow as many times as needed, without breathing. e. When client's mouth is emptied, have them raise chin and clear throat. f. Avoid straws.	4. Supraglottic swallow technique: a. This position uses the force of gravity to aid downward motion of food and decreases risk of aspiration. b. This prevents neck extension, which opens the client's airway and decreases risk of aspiration. c e. This maneuver triggers the protective mechanisms of epiglottis movement, laryngeal elevation, and vocal cord adduction (closure). f. Straws hasten transit time and increase the risk of aspiration (National Institute of Neurological Disorders and Stroke, 2000).
5. Offer high viscous foods first at meal (e.g., mashed bananas, mashed potatoes, gelatin, and gravy).	5. Post-CVA clients may have slowed peristalsis. Viscous foods increase peristaltic pump action.
6. Offer thick liquids (e.g., milk shakes, slushes, nectars, or cream soups).	6. Thicker fluids have a slower transit time and allow more time to trigger the swallow reflex (National Institute of Neurological Disorders and Stroke, 2000).
7. Establish a goal for fluid intake.	7. These clients are at risk for dehydration because of self-imposed fluid restrictions related to fear of choking.

(continued on page 248)

Interventions	Rationales

8. If the client drools, use a quick-stretch stimulation just before each meal and toward the end of the meal.
  a. Digitally apply short, rapid, downward strokes to the edge of the client's bottom lip, particularly on the affected side.
  b. Use a cold washcloth over finger for added stimulation.
	8. This maneuver stimulates the orbicularis oris muscle to facilitate labial adduction. Damage to VII cranial nerves causes this motor impairment.

9. If a bolus of food is pocketed in the affected side, teach the client to use his or her tongue to transfer food, or apply external digital pressure to his or her cheek to help remove the trapped bolus.	9. Poor tongue control with impaired oral sensation allows food into the affected side.

10. For a client with cognitive deficits, do the following:
  a. Divide eating tasks into the smallest steps possible.
  b. Describe and point out food.
  c. Provide a verbal command for each step.
  d. Progress slowly, limit conversation.
  e. Continue verbal assistance at each meal, as needed.
  f. Provide several small meals to accommodate short attention span.
  g. Provide a written checklist for other staff.
	10. A confused client needs repetitive, simple instructions.

Documentation

Flow records
  Intake of foods and fluids
Progress notes
  Swallowing difficulties

Unilateral Neglect Related to (Specify Site) Secondary to Right Hemispheric Brain Damage

NOC Body Image, Body Positioning: Self-Initiated, Self-Care: Activities of Daily Living (ADLs)

Goal

The client will demonstrate an ability to scan the visual field to compensate for loss of function or sensation in affected limb(s).

Indicators

• Describe the deficit and the rationale for treatments.
• Identify safety hazards in the environment.

NIC Unilateral Neglect Management, Self-Care Assistance

Interventions	Rationales

1. Initially adapt the client's environment:
  a. Place the call light, telephone, and bedside stand on the unaffected side.
  b. Always approach the client from the center or midline.
	1. This will minimize sensory deprivation initially; however, attempts should be made to have the client attend to both sides (American Stroke Association, 2001).

2. Orient the client to the environment and teach him or her to recognize the forgotten field (e.g., place the telephone out of client's visual field).	2. These reminders can help the client to adapt to the environment.

(continued on page 249)

Interventions	Rationales

3. Provide a simplified, uncluttered environment:
  a. Provide a moment between activities.
  b. Provide concrete cues such as, "You are on your side facing the wall."
	3.
	  a. Rapid movements can precipitate anxiety.
	  b. Cues can help with adjustment to position changes.

4. Reassure the client that the problem is a result of CVA.	4. Clients know that something is wrong, but may attribute it to being "disturbed."

5. Teach the client to:
  a. Stroke the affected side.
  b. Watch the body part as she or he strokes.
  c. Vary tactile stimulation (e.g., warm, cold, rough, soft).
	5. Tactile stimulation of the affected parts promotes their reintegration into the whole body.

6. Teach the client to scan the entire environment, turning the head to compensate for visual field cuts. Remind the client to scan when ambulating.	6. Scanning can help to prevent injury and increase awareness of entire space.

7. Teach the client to:
  a. Wear an arm sling when upright.
  b. Position the arm on a lapboard.
  c. Use a Plexiglas lapboard to view the affected leg.
  d. Recognize the danger of sources of cold and heat and moving machinery to the affected limb(s).
	7. Decreased sensation or motor function increases vulnerability to injury.

8. For self-care, instruct the client to
  a. Attend to the affected side first.
  b. Use adaptive equipment as needed.
  c. Always check the affected limb(s) during activities of daily living (ADLs).
	8. The client may need specific reminders to prevent her or him from ignoring nonfunctioning body parts.

Documentation

Progress notes
  Presence of neglect
Discharge summary record
  Client teaching
  Response to teaching

High Risk for Ineffective Therapeutic Regimen Management Related to Altered Ability to Maintain Self at Home Secondary to Sensory/Motor/Cognitive Deficits and Lack of Knowledge of Caregivers of Home Care, Reality Orientation, Bowel/Bladder Program, Skin Care, and Signs and Symptoms of Complications, and Community Resources

NOC Compliance Behavior, Knowledge: Treatment Regimen, Participation in Health Care Decisions, Treatment Behavior: Illness and Injury, Anticipatory Guidance, Health Education, Risk Managment, Learning Facilitation

Goals

The goals for this diagnosis represent those associated with discharge planning.

NIC Anticipatory Guidance, Risk Identification, Learning Facilitation, Health Education, Teaching: Procedure/Treatment, Health System Guidance

Interventions	Rationales
1. Teach about the condition, its cause, and treatments (Schwamm et al., 2005).	1. Understanding can reinforce the need to comply with the treatment regimen (Schwamm et al., 2005).
2. Identify controllable risk factors: a. Hypertension b. Smoking c. Obesity d. High-fat diet e. High-sodium diet f. Sedentary life style	2. Focusing on factors that can be controlled can improve compliance, increase self-esteem, and reduce feelings of helplessness. a. Hypertension with increased peripheral resistance damages the intima of blood vessels, contributing to arteriosclerosis. b. Smoking produces tachycardia, raises blood pressure, and constricts blood vessels. c. Obesity increases cardiac workload. d. A high-fat diet may increase arteriosclerosis and plaque formation. e. Sodium controls water distribution throughout the body. A gain in sodium causes a gain in water, thus increasing the circulating volume. f. Participation in walking and sports has been shown to reduce stroke risk by 20%–29% (Rosamond, Flegal, Friday, Furie, Go, et al., 2007), and maintain normal glycemic ranges (Sacco, Adams, Albers, Alberts, Benavente et al., 2006).
3. Explain signs and symptoms of complications, and stress the need for prompt reporting: a. Development of or increase in weakness, lethargy, dysphagia, aphasia, vision problems, confusion b. Seizures	3. These signs and symptoms may indicate increasing ICP or cerebral tissue hypoxia.
4. Discuss with the client's family the anticipated stressors associated with CVA and its treatment: a. Financial b. Changes in role responsibilities c. Dependency (Refer to Chapter 4, The Ill Adult: Issues and Responses, for information regarding the effects of chronic illness on families.) d. Caregiver responsibilities (Refer to Caregiver Role Strain in the Index for specific interventions.): • Assess for signs and symptoms of depression and treat accordingly.	4. Serious illness of a family member can cause disruption of family functioning. • Post-stroke depression affects two-thirds of clients (Eslinger, 2002). Post-stroke depression has negative effects on functional recovery; pharmacological treatment of depression can counterbalance this effect (Gainotti, 2001). Post-stroke clients may have periods of being emotionally labile (American Heart Association, 2007b).
5. Provide information about or initiate referrals to community resources [e.g., counselors, home health agencies, American Heart Association, American Stroke Association, and National Stroke Association (Schwamm et al., 2005)].	5. Such resources can provide needed assistance with home management and help to minimize the potentially destructive effects on the client and family (American Stroke Association, 2004; Schwamm et al., 2005).
6. Educate the client and his or her family about potential complications associated with thrombolytic therapy (Smith, Johnston, & Easton, 2005) a. Generalized bleeding and hemorrhage b. Hemorrhagic stroke	6. The client and family must be prepared for unforeseen complications related to treatment (Smith et al., 2005).

Documentation

Discharge summary record
  Client teaching
  Outcome achievement or status
  Referrals if indicated
For a Care Map on cerebrovascular accident (stroke), visit http://thePoint.lww.com

Guillain-Barré Syndrome

Guillain-Barré syndrome (GBS) is an acute (though it can also become a chronic syndrome) inflammatory, immune-mediated, demyelinating polyneuropathy of the peripheral nervous system, affecting 1.5–2 individuals per 100,000 people. GBS affects mainly the Schwann cell, which synthesizes and maintains the peripheral nerve myelin sheath. Its etiology is unclear, but it is believed to be an autoimmune response to a viral infection. However, studies suggest that macrophages penetrate the basement membrane and strip normal myelin from intact peripheral nerve axons, causing the characteristic signs and symptoms of GBS. The ventral (motor) root axons of the anterior horn cells, which innervate voluntary skeletal muscles, are primarily involved. Dorsal (sensory) root axons of the posterior horn are not as affected (Baird, Keen, & Swearingen, 2005; Hickey, 2003). The syndrome affects all age groups, races, and both sexes; has presented in all countries; and is considered a nonseasonal syndrome. Statistics show that 5% of clients will die of respiratory–cardiovascular complications, 20% will suffer irreversible distal paresthesia (glove and stocking anesthesia), and 75% will "recover with little or no" residual deficits. The pathophysiologic findings are multiple and varied, including inflammation, demyelinization of the peripheral nerves, loss of granular bodies, and degeneration of the basement membrane of the Schwann cell, resulting in an ascending symmetric flaccid paralysis and loss of cranial nerve functions (Hickey, 2003). Recovery of neurologic function depends on the proliferation of Schwann cells and remyelination of axons (Baird, Keen, & Swearingen, 2005). The four different variants of GBS reflect the degree of peripheral nerve involvement: ascending GBS, descending GBS, Miller-Fisher variant and pure motor GBS (Hickey, 2003). Another term for GBS is chronic idiopathic demyelinating polyneuropathy (CIDP).

Time Frame
Initial diagnosis: 1 year

DIAGNOSTIC CLUSTER*

Collaborative Problems

PC: Acute Respiratory Failure (ARF)
PC: Autonomic Nervous System Failure (Autonomic Dysreflexia)
PC: Peripheral Nervous System Failure
PC: Deep Vein Thrombus
PC: Decreased Cardiac Output
PC: Pneumonia

Nursing Diagnoses	Refer to
High Risk for Ineffective Airway Clearance related to impaired ability to cough	Thoracic Surgery
High Risk for Impaired Skin Integrity related to immobility, incontinence, sensory-motor deficits	Immobility
Impaired Swallowing related to swallowing/chewing problems secondary to cranial nerve impairment	Cerebrovascular Accident [Stroke]
Activity Intolerance related to fatigue and difficulties in performing activities of daily living	Chronic Obstructive Pulmonary Disease
Powerlessness related to the unpredictable nature of the condition	Chronic Obstructive Pulmonary Disease
High Risk for Self-Care Deficits related to flaccid paralysis, paresis, and fatigue	Immobility

(continued on page 252)

251

Nursing Diagnoses	Refer to
High Risk for Deficient Diversional Activity related to inability to perform usual job-related/recreational-related activities	Paralytic ileus
High Risk for Interrupted Family Process related to nature of disorder, role disturbances, and uncertain future	
High Risk for Ineffective Therapeutic Regimen Management related to lack of knowledge of condition, treatments required, stress management, signs and symptoms of complications, and availability of community resources	

✳ This medical condition was not included in the validation study.

Discharge Criteria

Before discharge the client or family will:

1. Relate intent to discuss fears and concerns with family/trusted friends after discharge.
2. Relate necessity of continuation of therapeutic programs.
3. Identify strategies to increase independence.
4. Relate safety precautions to prevent falls/injury.
5. Identify signs and symptoms that must be reported to a health care professional.

Collaborative Problems

Potential Complication: Acute Respiratory Failure (ARF)

Potential Complication: Autonomic Nervous System Failure (Autonomic Dysreflexia)

Potential Complication: Peripheral Nervous System Failure

Potential Complication: Deep Vein Thrombus

Potential Complication: Decreased Cardiac Output

Nursing Goal

The nurse will detect early signs/symptoms of (a) acute respiratory failure, (b) autonomic nervous system dysfunction, (c) cranial nerve dysfunction, (d) deep vein thrombus, and (e) decreased cardiac output, and collaboratively intervenes to stabilize the client.

Indicators

- Respiration 16–20 breaths/min (a)
- Oxygen saturation (pulse oximetry) >95% (a)
- Serum pH 7.35–7.45 (a)
- Serum PCO_2 35–45 mmHg (a)
- Cardiac normal sinus rhythm (a)
- Bowel sounds present (b)
- Alert, oriented (a)
- Cranial nerves II–XXII intact (c)
- Urine output >5 mL/kg/h (a)
- Dry, warm skin (b)
- Positive Homans sign (d)
- Fever (d)
- Pain in calf (d)

- Calf tenderness (d)
- Hypotension systolic <80 mmHg, or a 5–10 mmHg ___ with every assessment (e)
- Restlessness (e)
- Confusion (e)
- Dizziness (e)

Interventions	Rationales
1. Monitor for signs and symptoms of pneumonia and acute respiratory failure (ARF) to assist with breathing.	1. Ventilation may become necessary as acute Guillain-Barré progresses, due to increased damage to the phrenic and intercostal nerves.
a. Auscultate breath sounds.	a. Auscultating breath sounds assesses the adequacy of air flow and detects the presence of adventitious sounds (see Mechanical Ventilation for more information).
b. Assess for secretions: • Encourage the client to deep breathe and cough. • Position the client on alternate sides to assist movement of secretions. • Suction if client is unable to manage secretions. • Reassure client by maintaining a calm environment.	b. When the respiratory muscles fatigue, cough becomes ineffective, leading to the accumulation of mucus and the formation of mucous plugs in the airway. This accumulation of secretions causes alveolar collapse, leading to acute respiratory failure.
c. Assess O_2 saturation via pulse oximetry.	c. Pulse oximetry provides ongoing data on O_2 saturation.
d. Assess blood gases: • Monitor for signs of decreased respiratory functions, pH, $PaCO_2$, O_2 saturation, and HCO_3.	d. An increase in the $PaCO_2$ levels indicates hypoventilation and signifies that the client requires intubation to avoid acute respiratory failure.
e. Explain the necessity of intubation to the client and family.	e. Intubation is initiated to relieve shortness of breath to avoid acute respiratory failure, aspiration, and pneumonia.
f. Provide assurance and encouragement for the client.	f. This will reduce fear of the disease process. Most Guillain-Barré clients had been healthy, active individuals who suddenly became victims of dependency.
g. Report to the physician changes regarding: • Respiratory status and reduced vital capacity and arterial blood gases • Neurologic status • GI status	g. Early recognition enables prompt intervention to prevent further complications.
2. Monitor signs and symptoms of autonomic nervous system dysfunction: a. Blood pressure variations and cardiac dysrhythmias	2. Signs and symptoms of autonomic nervous system dysfunction: a. The vagal nerve involvement causes hypertension, postural hypotension, bradycardia, sinus tachycardia, and diaphoresis.
b. Cardiac monitor to evaluate cardiac status	b. Client may experience chest discomfort.
c. Urinary retention	c. Urinary retention is associated with autonomic nervous system dysfunction.
d. Watch carefully for activities that precipitate autonomic dysreflexia, such as: position changes, vigorous coughing, straining with bowel movements, and suctioning (Baird, Keen, & Swearingen, 2005). e. constipation (Baird, Keen, & Swearingen, 2005).	
3. Monitor signs and symptoms of cranial nerve dysfunction: a. Assess the following:	3. Demyelination of the efferent fibers of the spinal and cranial nerve creates a delay in conduction, resulting in motor weakness or loss of conduction, producing paralysis (Hickey, 2003). • Involvement of this cranial nerve will decrease the client's ability to wrinkle her or his forehead and close her or his eyes; the client will present a flat affect (Hickey, 2003).

(continued on page 254)

Interventions	Rationales
• Cranial nerve VII • Cranial nerve XI	• With involvement of this cranial nerve, the client will be unable to turn his or her head and will have drooping shoulders (Hickey, 2003).
• Cranial nerve V	• Involvement of this cranial nerve will cause the client to lose sensation in the face, forehead, and temples, and to have difficulty chewing (Hickey, 2003).
• Cranial nerves III, IV, and VI	• Involvement of these cranial nerves will cause the client to have visual problems: ptosis, diplopia, and deviations in upward and outward movement of the eyeballs (Hickey, 2003).
• Cranial nerves IX, X, and XII	• Involvement of these cranial nerves will cause the client to have problems with coughing, swallowing, and with the gag mechanism (Hickey, 2003).

 Related Physician-Prescribed Interventions

Medications. Steroids, antidysrhythmics (beta blocker, atropine)
Diagnostic Studies. Electrophysiologic studies (EPS), spinal tap
Therapies. EKG monitoring, plasmapheresis, mechanical ventilation

Documentation

Flow records
   Vital signs
   Intake and output
   Neurologic assessment findings
Progress notes
   Changes in respiratory status
   Response to interventions
   Neurologic changes

Nursing Diagnoses

High Risk for Deficient Diversional Activity Related to the Inability to Perform Usual Job-Related/Recreational Activities

NOC Leisure Participation, Social Involvement

Goal

The client will report more satisfaction with activity level.

Indicators

• Report participation in activity each day.
• Relate methods of coping with feelings caused by boredom.

NIC Recreation Therapy, Socialization Enhancement, Self-Esteem Enhancement

Interventions	Rationales

1. Identify the client's fears:
  a. Provide an environment conducive to verbalization of fears.
  b. Be a good listener.
  c. Provide accurate answers to questions.
	1. The rapid onset of GBS causes the disease to equally affect the mind and spirit. Feelings of dependency may develop, with the constant fear of permanent paralysis or disability.

2. Identify the client's vocation:
  a. Student
  b. Clerical
  c. Laborer
  d. Professional
  e. Retired
	2. Using the client's previous work environment as a source of stimulation in performing self-care activities promotes an attitude of wellness and reduces the anxiety of dependency.

3. Encourage visitors.	3. Visitors provide socialization. Have a select former GBS client visit with the client for emotional support.
4. Discuss interests and hobbies.	4. Discussion will help in identifying recreational activities.

5. Use variations in the physical environment and daily routines to increase mental stimulation:
  a. Select a room with a view for the client.
  b. Provide a variety of reading material.
  c. Provide reading stand, if necessary.
  d. Obtain talking books.
  e. Encourage participation in board games with visitors.
  f. Use video tapes and games.
  g. Encourage family and friends to bring in pictures and small prized items. Allow the client the choice of the arrangement of items.
  h. Change hygiene routines two or three times a week.
  i. Allow and encourage the client to dress in street clothes.
  j. Allow trips to the hospital cafeteria with family and friends. Allow trips on hospital grounds with family, friends, and volunteers when conditions are considered safe for the above activities.
  k. Encourage family and friends to bring the client's favorite foods.
  l. When the client is able to perform any vocational skills, encourage the use of laptop computers and preparation of reports. Continue studies of the client's physical tolerance and mental needs.
	5. Change reduces boredom.

6. Encourage the client to participate in open discussions with nursing staff and visitors concerning experiences, activities, and events of interest.	6. Discussions will give the client opportunities to be involved in various matters beyond self-concerns.

Documentation

Progress notes
Participation in self-care activities

High Risk for Interrupted Family Process Related to Nature of Disorder, Role Disturbances, and Uncertain Future

NOC Family Coping, Family Normalization, Parenting, Family Environment: Internal

Goal

Family members will maintain a functional system of mutual support.

Indicators

- Frequently verbalize feelings to professional nurse and to one another.
- Identify appropriate external resources available.

NIC Family Involvement Promotion, Coping Enhancement, Family Integrity Promotion, Family Therapy, Counseling, Referral

Interventions	Rationales
1. Provide family members with accurate, simply stated information regarding the condition.	1. Anxiety and stressful states produced by hospitalization impair the client's ability to process information effectively. Simple, brief explanations can relay valuable information effectively.
2. Identify the family's perception of the client's condition.	2. Evaluate each family member's learning level and provide teaching at this level of understanding.
3. Observe the dynamics of client–family interactions: a. Need to visit b. Effects of visit on client c. Family interactions d. Physical contact	3. These observations provide vital information regarding family roles, interrelationships, and the quality and amount of support family members are able to provide each other. Family members may need nursing permission to have physical contact with the client because of fear that they may "hurt" the client.
4. Observe and determine the family's coping skills: a. Assist the family with rethinking role responsibilities at home, redistributing tasks, and setting priorities.	4. The rapid onset of the illness may create the necessity of role changes that place a family in a high-stress situation.
5. Assess emotional responses to stressors of hospitalization: a. Explain procedures. b. Explain therapies.	5. An understanding of the multiple procedures and therapies involved with the diagnosis of the client's condition will relieve the family's fears and enhance cooperation.
6. Encourage family members to reorganize their schedules to meet their own physical and psychological needs: a. Encourage calls to the nursing unit or client for condition reports. b. Encourage select friends to visit. c. Adjust visiting hours to accommodate the family's schedules. d. Provide information on living accommodations near the hospital.	6. Family members who ignore their own health requirements are prone to becoming ill, which may reduce their effectiveness as support persons. A family member who falls ill may cause the client to have feelings of guilt.
7. Observe and promote family strengths: a. Gradually involve family members in the physical care of the client. b. Show your appreciation of the family involvement.	7. Allowing involvement of family members with care will maintain a supportive family structure and strengthen the family unit.
8. Address the client's financial concerns and responsibilities: a. Provide an environment for the client to verbalize his or her concerns. b. Initiate a referral to Social Services for assistance.	8. The sudden lack of income can be overwhelming, causing excessive mental anguish and slowing progress with goal-setting.

High Risk for Ineffective Therapeutic Regimen Management Related to Lack of Knowledge of Condition, Treatments Required, Stress Management, Signs and Symptoms of Complications, and Availability of Community Resources

NOC Compliance Behavior, Knowledge: Treatment Regimen, Participation in Health Care Decisions, Treatment Behavior: Illness or Injury

Goals

Refer to discharge criteria.

NIC Anticipatory Guidance, Learning Facilitation, Risk Identification, Health Education, Teaching: Procedure/Treatment, Health System Guidance

Interventions	Rationales
1. Teach the client and his or her family the basic pathology of the client's condition.	1. Understanding can improve compliance and reduce the family unit's frustrations.
2. Assist the client in identifying realistic short-term goals.	2. Preparation of the client to set realistic goals for recovery will reduce feelings of depression if goals are not attainable.
3. Teach the client the value of continued strengthening–stretching exercise programs. Consult Physical Therapy.	3. Exercise will recondition all muscle groups (NINDS, 2007).
4. Teach the client energy conservation techniques: a. Schedule planned rest periods. b. Exercise consistent with tolerance levels.	4. Energy conservation can reduce fatigue (NINDS, 2007).
5. Teach care of alterations in body functions: a. Bowel and bladder functions: Encourage an intake of fluids to 2000 mL every day unless contraindicated. b. Nutritional requirements: Provide a diet high in calories and protein. c. Self-care deficits, if necessary: Areas of concern: • Dressing • Grooming • Safe ambulation	5. Bodily care teachings: a. These are required to prevent constipation resulting from reduced peristalsis and activity. b. Protein and calories are required to rebuild muscle mass. c. Encourage maximum client self-care with ADL activities for purpose of strengthening muscles and increasing independence.
6. Initiate a referral to rehabilitation services.	6. Client will require outpatient or home care for postdischarge therapies.
7. Explain signs and symptoms that must be reported to a health care professional: a. Productive cough b. Difficulty with urination or odor to urine c. Prolonged constipation d. Increased weakness or fatigue e. Weight loss	7. Early interventions will minimize complications of the condition.
8. Provide information and literature to assist the client and family to manage at home. Refer to following resources: a. Guillain-Barré Syndrome Foundation provides emotional and educational support to clients and their families. b. Home health agency c. Case manager referral	8. When the client and her or his family receive community support, they are able to cope more effectively with home management. a. The mainstay of treatment is supportive care. Guillain-Barré Syndrome Foundation, P.O. Box 262, Wynnewood, PA 19096

Documentation

Discharge summary record
   Client teaching
   Outcome achievement or status
   Referrals if indicated

Multiple Sclerosis

Multiple sclerosis (MS) is the most common autoimmune, inflammatory demyelinating disease of the central nervous system (CNS) (Olek, 2007b). It is characterized by acute exacerbations or gradual worsening of neurologic functions and disability (Ben-Zacharia, 2001). MS affects some 300,000 Americans yearly, 75% of whom are female. The disease is a leading cause of disability among young adults and typically strikes during young adulthood, with peak incidence between 20 and 40 years of age (Olek, 2007a).

MRI studies have shown clear evidence that central to the disease process is the gradual destruction of the myelin sheath surrounding nerve cells by autoreactive T-cells (Olek, 2007c). This stripping of nerve fibers interferes with nerve conduction, which leads to various degrees of paralysis and to the other symptoms of the disease (Glaser, 2000).

MS can profoundly affect the client's quality of life. With its disabling effects and chronic and unforeseeable features, MS brings about a series of changes in the client's life (Landoni, 2000).

There are four categories of MS: relapsing-remitting (80% of all cases), secondary progressive, progressive-relapsing, and primary progressive (Hickey, 2003). In people with MS, the range of main symptoms includes the loss of mobility and spasticity, pain, tremors, abnormal eye movements, paroxysmal symptoms, bladder and bowel dysfunction, sexual disturbances, fatigue, cognitive impairment, sexual dysfunction, seizures, optic neuritis, vertigo, and depression (Clanet, 2000; Olek, 2007a; Olek, 2007c).

Time Frame
Initial diagnosis
Recurrent acute exacerbations

▪▪▪▪▪▪ DIAGNOSTIC CLUSTER*

Collaborative Problems	Refer to
PC: Urinary Tract Infection	
PC: Renal Insufficiency	
PC: Pneumonia	Cerebrovascular Accident [Stroke]

Nursing Diagnoses	Refer to
High Risk for Disturbed Self-Concept related to the effects of prolonged debilitating condition on life style and on achieving developmental tasks and uncertain prognosis	
Impaired Comfort related to demyelinated areas of the sensory tract	
High Risk for Injury related to visual disturbances, vertigo, and altered gait	

(continued on page 259)

Nursing Diagnoses	Refer to
Interrupted Family Processes related to nature of disorder, role disturbances, and uncertain future	
High Risk for Ineffective Therapeutic Regimen Management related to lack of knowledge of condition, treatments, prevention of infection, stress management, aggravating factors, signs and symptoms of complications, and community resources	
Impaired Swallowing related to cerebellar lesions	Cerebrovascular Accident [Stroke]
Impaired Verbal Communication related to dysarthria secondary to ataxia of the muscles of speech	Parkinson Disease
Fatigue related to extremity weakness, spasticity, fear of injury, and stressors	Inflammatory Joint Disease
Urinary Retention related to sensorimotor deficits	Neurogenic Bladder
Incontinence (specify) related to poor sphincter control and spastic bladder	
Powerlessness related to the unpredictable nature of condition (remission/exacerbation)	Chronic Obstructive Pulmonary Disease
Related Care Plans	
Immobility or Unconsciousness Corticosteroid Therapy	

* This medical condition was not included in the validation study.

Discharge Criteria

Before discharge, the client and family will

1. Relate an intent to share concerns with other family members or trusted friend(s).
2. Identify one strategy to increase independence.
3. Describe actions that can reduce the risk of exacerbation.
4. Identify signs and symptoms that must be reported to a health care professional.

Collaborative Problems

Potential Complication: Urinary Tract Infections
Potential Complication: Renal Insufficiency

Nursing Goal

The nurse will detect early signs/symptoms of (a) urinary tract infections and (b) renal insufficiency, and collaboratively intervene to stabilize the client.

Indicators

- Temperature 98–99.5°F (a)
- Urine specific gravity 0.005–0.030 (b)
- Urine output >5 mL/kg/h (b)
- Clear urine (a, b)

- Blood urea nitrogen 5–25 mg/hr (b)
- Creatinine (b)
  - Male: 0.6–1.5 mg/dL
  - Female 0.6–1.1 mg/dL
  - Potassium 3.5–5.0 mEq/L (b)
- Phosphate 1.8%–2% mEq/L (b)
- Urine creatinine clearance (b)
  - Male 95–135 mL/min
  - Female 85–125 mL/min

Interventions	Rationales
1. Monitor for signs and symptoms of urinary tract infection:	1. MS exacerbation can be precipitated by any infection (Olek, 2007c). MS can cause urinary retention owing to lesions of the afferent pathways from the bladder. Resulting urine stasis contributes to growth of microorganisms. Also, corticosteroid therapy reduces the effectiveness of WBCs against infection.
a. Chills, fever	a. Bacteria can act as a pyrogen by raising the hypothalamic thermostat through the production of endogenous pyrogen that may mediate through prostaglandins. Chills can occur when the temperature setpoint of the hypothalamus changes rapidly.
b. Costovertebral angle (CVA) pain (a dull, constant backache below the 12th rib)	b. CVA pain results from distention of the renal capsule.
c. Leukocytosis	c. Leukocytosis reflects an increase in WBCs to fight infection through phagocytosis.
d. Foul odor or pus in urine	d. Bacteria change the odor and pH of urine.
e. Dysuria, frequent urination	e. Bacteria irritate bladder tissue, causing spasms and frequent urination.
2. Monitor for early signs and symptoms of renal insufficiency: a. Sustained elevated urine specific gravity b. Elevated urine sodium levels	2. Repeated infections can alter renal function. a,b. Decreased ability of the renal tubules to reabsorb electrolytes causes increased urine sodium levels and increased specific gravity.
c. Sustained insufficient urine output (30 mL/h) d. Elevated blood pressure	c,d. Decreased glomerular filtration rate eventually causes sustained insufficient urine output (<30 mL/m), and stimulates renin production that raises the blood pressure in the body's attempt to increase blood flow to the kidneys.
e. Increasing blood urea nitrogen (BUN) and pressure serum creatinine, phosphate, and potassium; and decreased creatinine clearance	e. Decreased excretion of urea potassium and creatinine in the urine results in elevated BUN potassium and creatinine levels. The kidneys' inability to excrete hydrogen ions, phosphates, sulfates, and ketone bodies causes increased levels of acidosis.
3. Instruct client to: a. Drink a minimum of six to eight glasses of fluids per day.	3. a. Dilute urine reduces the incidence of bacterial growth that otherwise would lead to infection
b. Empty bladder completely using Credé technique or self-catheterization (see Credé and Clean Intermittent Self-Catheterization techniques in Neurogenic Bladder care plan).	b. Reduces the incidence of urinary stasis.
c. Wipe from front to back, especially after a bowel movement. d. Avoid undergarments made of synthetic materials.	c. Reduces the introduction of inappropriate bacteria to the urinary tract.
e. Empty bladder before and after intercourse. f. Change wet or soiled undergarments frequently in situations of dribbling or incontinence.	e,f. Reduces the incidence of urinary stasis.

(continued on page 261)

Interventions	Rationales
g. Identify and notify the physician of urinary tract infection (UTI) signs and symptoms: • Foul-smelling urine • Increased frequency and urge to urinate • Change in color—dark yellow • Change in consistency—cloudy, sediment, or flecks of blood	

 ### Related Physician-Prescribed Treatments

Medications. Muscle relaxants, vitamin B, tricyclic antidepressants, selective serotonin uptake inhibitor (SSRI), corticosteroids, immunosuppressives, bulk-forming laxatives, antibiotics, Betaseron, beta blockers, Vitamin C (1000 mg four times/day), Avonex, glatiramer, spasmolytic (Urispas or Ditropan), urinary tract antiseptics (Macrodantin or Hiprex), cholinesterase inhibitors, analgesics, amantadine, methylphenidate, modafinil, pro-erectile medications

Intravenous Therapy. Adrenocorticotropic hormone (ACTH), intravenous immunoglobin (IVIG)

Laboratory Studies. Electrophoresis, white blood count, gamma globulin levels, serum antimyelin antibodies

Diagnostic Studies. EEG, MRI, CT scan of the brain, lumbar puncture, urinary retention study, evoked potential studies, electrophoresis, cerebrospinal fluid analysis

Therapies. Dependent on deficits (e.g., urinary and motor); dependent on bladder emptying problems (Credé technique, clean intermittent self-catheterization [CISC], indwelling Foley catheter, and suprapubic cystotomy), intrathecal muscle relaxants, physiotherapy, immunosuppressive therapy (total lymphoid radiation), plasma exchange, hematopoietic stem cell transplantation (HSCT)

Documentation

Flow records
Intake and output
Urine specific gravity

Nursing Diagnoses

High Risk for Disturbed Self-Concept Related to the Effects of Prolonged Debilitating Uncertain Prognosis Condition on Life Style and on Achieving Developmental Tasks

 Quality of Life, Depression Level, Self-Esteem, Coping

Goal

The client will report an improved sense of well-being and increased satisfaction with relationships, life style, and with him- or herself.

Indicators

• Acknowledge changes in body structure and function.
• Communicate feelings about disability.
• Participate in self-care.

NIC Hope Instillation, Mood Management, Values Clarification, Counseling, Referral, Support Group, Coping Enhancement

Interventions	Rationales
1. Contact the client frequently and treat her or him with warm, positive regard.	1. Frequent contact by the caregiver indicates acceptance and may facilitate trust. The client may be hesitant to approach the staff because of negative self-concept.
2. Encourage the client to express feelings and thoughts about the following: a. Condition b. Progress c. Prognosis d. Effects on life style e. Support system f. Treatments	2. Encouraging the client to share feelings can provide a safe outlet for fears and frustrations and can increase self-awareness.
3. Provide reliable information and clarify any misconceptions.	3. Misconceptions can needlessly increase anxiety and damage self-concept.
4. Help the client to identify positive attributes, hopefulness, and possible new opportunities. Explore new techniques to increase hopefulness, such as relaxation techniques, exercise programs, and religious and social activities (Glaser, 2000).	4. The client may tend to focus only on the change in self-image and not on the positive characteristics that contribute to the whole concept of self. The nurse must reinforce these positive aspects and encourage the client to reincorporate them into his or her new self-concept.
5. Assist with hygiene and grooming, as needed.	5. Participation in self-care and planning can aid in positive coping (Hickey, 2003).
6. Encourage visitors.	6. Frequent visits by family and significant others can help the client feel that she or he is still a worthwhile, acceptable person. This should promote a positive self-concept.
7. Help the client identify strategies to increase independence and maintain role responsibilities such as the following: a. Prioritizing activities b. Getting assistance with less valued or most fatiguing activities (e.g., shopping and housekeeping) c. Using energy conservation techniques. (Refer to the nursing diagnosis Fatigue in the Inflammatory Joint Disease care plan for specific strategies.) Refer the MS client to an occupational therapist. d. Using mobility aids and assistive devices, as needed	7. Occupational Therapy helps people with disabilities remain as independent as possible. Clients are taught to use special equipment and adapt to their home, workplace, or vehicle for greater safety and comfort (Hickey, 2003).
8. Discuss ways that the client can provide support to his or her family and significant others: a. Actively listening to their problems b. Attempting to decrease the focus on disabilities (Refer to Chapter 4, the Ill Adult: Issues and Responses, for more information.)	8. The nurse can help the client learn how to balance relationships and preserve the family system.
9. Allow the client's family and other support persons to share their feelings regarding the diagnoses and actual or anticipated effects.	9. Multiple sclerosis can have a big impact on families. They may have to share the financial burden, tackle additional chores, and help the person with MS deal with illness emotionally (National Multiple Sclerosis Society, 2002).

(continued on page 263)

Interventions	Rationales
10. Assess for signs of negative response to changes in appearance: a. Refusal to discuss loss b. Denial of changes c. Decreased self-care ability d. Social isolation e. Refusal to discuss the future	10. These signs may indicate that the client is at high risk for unsuccessful adjustment.
11. Refer an at-risk client for professional counseling	11. Follow-up therapy may be indicated to assist with adjustment.

Documentation

Progress notes
Present emotional status
Interventions
Response to interventions

Impaired Comfort Related to Demyelinated Areas of the Sensory Tract

NOC Symptom Control

Goals

- The client will relate improvement of pain and an increase in daily activities as evidenced by (specify).
- The client's family and significant others will support the management plan.

Indicators

- Participate in developing, carrying out, and evaluating the pain management plan.
- Report an improved sense of well-being and increased satisfaction with relationships, life style, and with him- or herself.

NIC Pruritus Management, Fever Treatment, Environmental Management: Comfort

Interventions	Rationales
1. Acknowledge the existence of the client's pain.	1. This establishes a trusting relationship (Glaser, 2000).
2. Identify the location, nature, intensity, and duration of pain. 3. Assist the client in identifying pain patterns (situations and factors that precipitate or intensify the pain).	2,3. Pain has a pervasive impact on role, mood, capacity to work and rest, and interpersonal relationships. Optimal therapy treatment involves a commitment to the goals of controlled pain and improved quality of life (Hickey, 2003).
4. Collaborate with pain management specialists to develop appropriate cutaneous, affective, and cognitive treatment modalities (Hickey, 2003). 5. Collaborate with other care providers to establish a management plan (Hickey, 2003).	4,5. Team collaboration will establish an individualized and comprehensive pain management plan.
6. Review pain management options with the client (Hickey, 2003).	6–9. Understanding the pain management plan and options will empower the client to make her or his own choices, which allows for greater acceptance.

(continued on page 264)

Interventions	Rationales
7. Teach the client, family, and significant others about the nature of the pain.	
8. Provide guidance regarding anticipated life style changes.	
9. Provide opportunities for the client to verbalize feelings related to the chronicity of pain.	

Documentation

Progress notes
Present description of client's pattern of pain
Interventions
Client's response to interventions
Discharge summary record
Client/family teaching
Outcome achievement or status
Referrals, if indicated

High Risk for Injury Related to Visual Disturbances, Vertigo, and Altered Gait

NOC Risk Control

Goal

The client will relate fewer injuries.

Indicators

- Relate the intent to use safety measures to prevent injury.
- Relate the intent to practice selected prevention measures.

NIC Fall Prevention, Environmental Management: Safety, Health Education, Surveillance: Safety, Risk Identification

Interventions	Rationales
1. Identify the type of visual disturbance the client is experiencing (diplopia, nystagmus, optic neuritis, or blurred vision).	1–4. Identifying the types of visual disturbances and options available will allow the client to take the necessary precautions. Optic neuritis is a common presenting symptom of MS; 90% of clients regain normal vision within 2–6 months (Olek, 2007c).
2. Explain the options available (i.e., eye patch for diplopia, rest for fatigue-related disturbances, or environmental precautions for the visually impaired.)	
3. Reassure the client that blindness seldom occurs, and some of these disturbances frequently remit.	
4. Refer the client to the Association for the Blind.	

Documentation

Progress notes
Present visual disturbances
Interventions
Client's response to interventions
Discharge summary record

Client teaching
Outcome achievement or status
Referrals if indicated

Interrupted Family Processes Related to Nature of Disorder, Role Disturbances, and Uncertain Future

NOC Family Coping, Family Normalization, Family Environment: Internal, Parenting

Goal

Family members will maintain a functional system of mutual support.

Indicators

• Frequently verbalize feelings to professional nurse and each other.
• Identify appropriate external resources available.

NIC Family Involvement Promotion, Coping Enhancement, Family Integrity Promotion, Family Therapy, Counseling, Referral

Interventions	Rationales
1. Convey an understanding of the situation and its impact on the family.	1. Communicating understanding and a sense of caring and concern facilitates trust and strengthens the nurse's relationships with the client and family.
2. Explore the family members' perceptions of the situation. Encourage verbalization of feelings such as guilt, anger, and blame.	2. Verbalization can provide opportunities for clarification and validation of feelings and concerns; this contributes to family unity.
3. Determine if present coping mechanisms are effective.	3. Illness of a family member may cause great changes, putting the family at high risk for maladaptation. Multiple sclerosis also involves the family: relatives must revise plans and projects made before the illness (Landoni, 2000; Hickey, 2003).
4. Take steps to promote family strengths: a. Acknowledge the assistance of family members. b. Involve the family in the client's care. c. To prevent burnout, encourage family members to take time away from care-giving. d. Encourage humor. (Refer to Chapter 4, The Ill Adult: Issues and Responses, for more information.)	4. This can help to maintain the existing family structure and its function as a supportive unit.
5. Assist the family to reorganize roles at home, set new priorities, and redistribute responsibilities.	5. Planning and prioritizing can help maintain family integrity and reduce stress (Hickey, 2003).
6. Prepare the family for signs of depression, anxiety, anger, and dependency in the client and other family members.	6. Anticipatory guidance can alert members to potential problems before they occur. This enables prompt intervention at early signs. Depression is the most common manifestation of MS secondary to the stress of coping with a chronic, incurable disease (Olek, 2007a).
7. Encourage the family to call on its social network (e.g., friends, relatives, church members) for emotional and other support. Refer the family to receive psychological support.	7. Outside assistance may help reduce the perception that the family must "go it alone." Psychological support could help relatives with the emotions associated with care-giving. Support will also give them a listening space for their distresses and fears (Landoni, 2000).

(continued on page 266)

Interventions	Rationales
8. Identify dysfunctional coping mechanisms: a. Substance abuse b. Continued denial c. Exploitation of one or more family members d. Separation or avoidance (Glaser, 2000) Refer for counseling as necessary.	8. A family with a history of unsuccessful coping may need additional resources. A family with unresolved conflicts prior to diagnosis is at high risk.
9. Direct to community agencies and other sources of assistance (e.g., financial, housekeeping, or direct care), as needed.	9. The family may need assistance to help with management at home.

Documentation

Progress notes
Present family functioning
Interventions
Family's response to interventions
Discharge summary record
Referrals, if indicated

High Risk for Ineffective Therapeutic Regimen Management Related to Lack of Knowledge of Condition, Treatments, Prevention of Infection, Stress Management, Aggravating Factors, Signs and Symptoms of Complications, and Community Resources

NOC Compliance Behavior, Knowledge: Treatment Regimen, Participation in Health Care Decisions, Treatment Behavior: Illness or Injury

Goals

The goals for this diagnosis represent those associated with discharge planning. Refer to the discharge criteria.

NIC Anticipatory Guidance, Learning Facilitation, Risk Identification, Health Education, Teaching: Procedure/Treatment, Health System Guidance

Interventions	Rationales
1. Assist in formulating and accepting realistic short- and long-term goals.	1. Mutual goal-setting reinforces the client's role in improving his or her quality of life.
2. Teach about the diagnosis and management techniques, including alternative methods.	2. Understanding can help to improve compliance and reduce exacerbations.
3. Discuss the importance of strengthening and stretching exercises for the arms, legs, and facial and respiratory muscles. Consult with a physical therapist (Glaser, 2000; Hickey, 2003).	3. Exercise can prevent underused muscles from becoming weak. Facial and respiratory muscle exercises can improve speech deficits (Glaser, 2000). Although motor function loss is permanent, range-of-motion and muscle-strengthening exercises help maintain intact function (Hickey, 2003).

(continued on page 267)

Interventions	Rationales

4. Discuss the factors known to trigger exacerbation (Hickey, 2003):
  a. Undue fatigue or excessive exertion
  b. Overheating or excessive chilling or cold exposure
  c. Infections
  d. Hot environments/hot baths
  e. Fever
  f. Emotional stress
  g. Pregnancy
  h. Cigarette smoking
  i. Alcohol use
	4. This information gives the client insight into aspects of the condition that can be controlled; this may promote a sense of control and encourage compliance. As body temperature rises above the normal range, it blocks conduction across demyelinated regions in the brain and can worsen MS (Glaser, 1999).

5. Teach energy conservation techniques. (Refer to the nursing diagnosis Fatigue in the Inflammatory Joint Disease care plan for more information.)	5. Energy conservation can prevent fatigue.
6. Instruct a pregnant client or one contemplating pregnancy to consult a physician about the problems associated with pregnancy (Hickey, 2003).	6. Pregnancy is associated with onset and exacerbations of MS.

7. Explain the hazards of infection and ways to reduce the risk:
  a. Avoid contact with infected persons.
  b. Receive immunization against influenza and streptococcal pneumonia, if advised.
  c. Cleanse all equipment and utensils well.
 	
  d. Eat a well-balanced diet and get sufficient rest.
 	
  e. Drink 2000 mL of fluids daily, unless contraindicated by renal insufficiency.
	7. Minor infections can cause serious problems in a client with MS.
	  a. This precaution reduces the risk of cross-infection.
	  b. Immunization confers protection against these infections.
	  c. Proper cleansing removes microorganisms and secretions that are media for microorganism growth.
	  d. Adequate nutrition and rest promote overall good health and increase resistance to infection.
	  e. Adequate hydration prevents concentrated urine with high levels of bacteria.

8. Teach the importance of constructive stress management and reduction (Hickey, 2003); explain measures such as the following:
  a. Progressive relaxation techniques
  b. Self-coaching
  c. Thought-stopping
  d. Assertiveness techniques
  e. Guided imagery
    If possible, refer to community resources for specific courses or assistance.
	8. Managing stress helps the client to cope and adapt to changes caused by MS (Hickey, 2003). Approaches to stress management include massage therapy, exercise programs, and involvement in religious and social activities (Glaser, 2000).

9. Teach the effects of MS on bowel function and the techniques to prevent constipation or incontinence. (Refer to appropriate nursing diagnoses in the Immobility or Unconsciousness care plan for specific interventions.)	9. Clients rate constipation and fecal incontinence as having a major impact on their lives (Wiesel, 2000). Preparing the client for these bowel symptoms helps him or her to handle them. Constipation results from decreased immobility, upper and lower motor neuron impairment (Olek, 2007c), and decreased fluid and fiber intake. Bowel incontinence is caused by lesions of the efferent pathways of the corticospinal tract, resulting in loss of sphincter control. Constipation is more common than fecal incontinence (Olek, 2007c).
10. Explore with the client and her or his partner current and previous sexual patterns and partner problems that may interfere with sexual activity: a. Low self-esteem	10. Libido is negatively influenced by stress, fatigue, and low self-esteem. Ejaculatory disorders and erectile dysfunction (Olek, 2007c) result from lesions in the pyramidal tracts of the spinal cord.

(continued on page 268)

Interventions	Rationales
b. Fatigue c. Ejaculatory disorders d. Thigh muscle spasms e. Fear of bowel or bladder incontinence	Many people with multiple sclerosis are able to enjoy a completely normal sex life. Others may have some problems. Communicating openly and being flexible about sexual expression are often the keys to enjoyment (Hickey, 2003).
11. Discuss options available for sexual enjoyment: a. Medication management b. Phosphodiesterase type-5 inhibitor (Viagra, Levitra), prostaglandins, or penile prosthetics c. Positioning	11. Options for sexual enjoyment a. The client may be taking medications that interfere with the normal sexual response (i.e., some antihypertensives, antidepressants, or tranquilizers), or may need the appropriate medication relating to the specific MS problem (i.e., spasticity or leg spasms can be reduced by timing antispastic medications to maximize effectiveness during sexual activity). b. Client may be experiencing insufficient erections secondary to MS lesions. c. Proper positions may reduce spasticity problems. d. Women may have difficulty achieving orgasm (Olek, 2007c).
12. Refer the client and family to appropriate health care professionals (neurologist, urologist, or counselor). 13. Refer to a counselor for continued therapy.	12,13. The client may need follow-up therapy.
14. Explain the signs and symptoms that must be reported to a health care professional: a. Worsening of symptoms (e.g., weakness, spasticity, visual disturbances) b. Temperature elevation c. Change in urination patterns or cloudy, foul-smelling urine d. Productive cough with cloudy greenish sputum e. Cessation of menses	14. Early detection enables prompt intervention to minimize complications. a. Worsening symptoms may herald an exacerbation. b–d. These symptoms may indicate infection (urinary tract or pulmonary). e. Cessation of menses may indicate pregnancy, which can exacerbate MS.
15. Provide information and materials to assist the client and family to maintain goals and manage at home from sources such as the following: a. Multiple Sclerosis Society b. Home health agencies c. American Red Cross d. Individual/family counselors e. Jimmie Heuga Center	15. A client who feels well-supported can cope more effectively with the multiple stressors associated with chronic debilitating disease.

Documentation

Discharge summary record
Client teaching
Outcome achievement or status
Referrals if indicated
Refer to website http://thePoint.lww.com for critical paths for this condition.

Myasthenia Gravis

Myasthenia gravis (MG) is a chronic, unpredictable autoimmune disease that is characterized by the destruction of acetylcholine (ACh) receptors, resulting in a decreased number of ACh receptor sites at the neuromuscular junctions. This prevents ACh molecules from attaching to receptor molecules in muscle cells and stimulating muscle contraction, thus producing muscle weakness and excessive fatigue (Lewis, Heitkemper, Dirksen, O'Brien, Giddens et al., 2004). The disease affects voluntary skeletal muscles in single or multiple groups, particularly the generalized muscle groups affecting respiration, speech, chewing, and swallowing (Hickey, 2003; Lewis et al., 2004).

The thymus gland, which lies in the upper chest area beneath the breastbone, plays an important role in the development of the immune system in early life. Its cells form a part of the body's normal immune system. The gland is somewhat large in infants, grows gradually until puberty, and then gets smaller and is replaced by fat with age. In adults with myasthenia gravis, the thymus gland is abnormal. It contains certain clusters of immune cells indicative of lymphoid hyperplasia—a condition usually found only in the spleen and lymph nodes during an active immune response. Some individuals with myasthenia gravis develop thymomas or tumors of the thymus gland. Generally thymomas are benign, but they can become malignant.

The relationship between the thymus gland and MG is not fully understood. Studies have shown how scientists believe the thymus gland may give incorrect instructions to developing immune cells, ultimately resulting in autoimmunity and the production of the ACh receptor antibodies, thereby setting the stage for the attack on neuromuscular transmission (Hickey, 2003; Lewis et al., 2004; MGFA, 2007).

A thymectomy is beneficial in 60%–70% of clients with MG by providing relief of symptoms. The prevalence rate is 14 per 100,000 in the United States. MG can occur at any age, but most commonly occurs between the ages of 10 and 65 (Lewis et al., 2004). The peak age of onset of MG is between 20 to 30 years for women and 40 to 60 years for men. MG is three times more common in women; however, after 60 years of age, the incidence is similar for both sexes (Lewis et al., 2004).

The onset of MG is usually gradual, although rapid onset has been reported in association with respiratory infections or emotional upsets. The course of the illness is extremely variable (Hickey, 2003). Exacerbations of MG, commonly referred to as Myasthenic Crisis, involve an acute exacerbation of muscle weakness triggered by infection, emotional stress, ultraviolet light, surgery, pregnancy, and overdose of—or inadequate—drugs (Lewis et al., 2004; MGFA, 2007; NINDS, 2007).

Time Frame
Initial diagnosis
Acute exacerbations
Remissions

 DIAGNOSTIC CLUSTER*

Collaborative Problems

PC: Respiratory Insufficiency
PC: Myasthenic/Cholinergic Crisis
PC: Aspiration

Nursing Diagnoses	Refer to
High Risk for Ineffective Airway Clearance related to impaired ability to cough	Chronic Obstructive Pulmonary Disease
High Risk for Impaired Swallowing related to cerebellar dysfunction	Cerebrovascular Accident [Stroke]
High Risk for Injury related to visual disturbances, unsteady gait, weakness	Cerebrovascular Accident [Stroke]
High Risk for Impaired Verbal Communications related to involvement of muscles for speech	Parkinson

(continued on page 270)

Nursing Diagnoses	Refer to
High Risk for Impaired Skin Integrity related to immobility	Immobility
High Risk for Activity Intolerance related to fatigue and difficulty in performing activities of daily living	Pressure Sores
High Risk for Powerlessness related to the unpredictable nature of the condition (remissions/exacerbations)	Cerebrovascular Accident [Stroke]
High Risk for Ineffective Therapeutic Regimen Management related to insufficient knowledge of condition, treatments, prevention of infections, stress management, aggravating factors, signs and symptoms of complications, and community resources	Chronic Obstructive Pulmonary Disease

✱ This medical condition was not included in the validation study.

Discharge Criteria

Before discharge the client or family will:

1. Relate intent to share concerns with other family members or a trusted friend.
2. Relate the side effects of the prescribed medications as well as the critical rationale for taking their correct doses (Lewis et al., 2004).
3. Identify strategies to reduce stress.
4. Identify signs and symptoms that must be reported to a health care professional.
5. Describe long-term management of the disease.
6. State the value of wearing a Med-Alert bracelet.
7. Receive information on and referral to the local chapter of the Myasthenia Gravis Foundation (www.myasthenia.org)

Collaborative Problems

Potential Complication: Respiratory Insufficiency
Potential Complication: Myasthenic/Cholinergic Crisis
Potential Complication: Aspiration

Nursing Goal

The nurse will detect early signs/symptoms of (a) respiratory insufficiency, (b) myasthenic/cholinergic crisis, and (c) aspiration, and collaboratively intervene to stabilize the client.

Indicators

- Respiration 16–20 breaths/min (a)
- Clear breath sounds with no adventitious sounds (a, c)
- Vital capacity 4600 mL (a)
- Expiratory reserve volume 1100 mL (a)
- Total lung capacity 5800 mL (a)
- Intact cough-gag reflexes (b, c)
- Heart rate 60–100 beats/min (a, b)
- Intact muscle strength (b)
- Dry, warm skin (a, b)
- BP >90/60, <140–90 mmHg (a, b)
- No nausea/vomiting (b, c)
- No muscle twitching/cramping (b)
- No continual coughing with swallowing (Lewis et al., 2004) (c)

Interventions	Rationales
1. Monitor for signs and symptoms of respiratory distress: a. Monitor for changes in respiratory status: • Respiratory rate increase • Change in respiratory pattern • Change in breath sounds • Serial vital capacity measurements b. Monitor for increased pulse rate. c. Elevate head of bed 30–40 degrees.	1. The most dangerous aspect of MG is weakened muscle contraction and the resultant ineffective inspiration. The client's first complaint may be dyspnea at rest (Baird, Keen & Swearingen, 2005) a. Antibodies to acetylcholine receptors at muscle sites block nerve transmission to the striated muscles, specifically the intercostal muscles and diaphragm, that control respiratory functions (Baird, Keen, & Swearingen, 2005; Bhardwaj, Mirski, & Ulatowski, 2004). b. This sign indicates difficulty with air exchange. c. Elevation will enhance diaphragmatic movement.
2. Assess ability to clear airway: a. Cough-gag reflexes b. Suction secretions as necessary every ½ to 1 hour. c. Postural drainage d. Position client side to side. e. Coughing while attempting to drink fluids or swallowing own saliva (Baird, Keen, & Swearingen, 2005)	2. Ability to clear airway: a. The absence or presence of reflexes denotes weakness of muscle groups innervated by the 10 cranial nerves originating in the brain stem. These are the muscles necessary for chewing, swallowing, eye movement, neck movement, and facial expression (Hickey, 2003; Lewis et al., 2004). b. If the person cannot manage secretions, intubation may be necessary to control secretion or support ventilation. c. To mobilize secretions d. To reduce pooling of secretions and prevent aspiration and pneumonia
3. Assess communication ability: a. Anxiety and panic: • Provide a calm, reassuring environment. • Provide explanations for treatment. b. Increased muscle weakness involving speech. • Listen to client and repeat requests for accuracy. • Ask questions that require yes or no answers. • Ask client to move fingers or toes, or give yes or no answer.	3. Weakness in facial muscles can affect facial expression, phonation, and articulation. A normal smile may look like a snarl, and speech may become slurred (Hickey, 2003). a. To reduce anxiety and promote easier respiration b. Establish a method of communication to reduce anxiety or panic.
4. Monitor the client response to a Tensilon test (edrophonium chloride).	4. This medication is administered intravenously, providing a differentiated diagnosis of myasthenia gravis/cholinergic crisis. A positive Tensilon test equals an increase in muscle strength 30–90 seconds after administration, suggesting the diagnosis of a myasthenia gravis (Torpy, 2005).
5. Report to the physician changes in respiratory status, swallowing ability, and speech.	5. To adjust treatment
6. Monitor for signs and symptoms of myasthenic/cholinergic crisis:	6. Myasthenic crises result from inadequate amounts of acetylcholine (ACh) due to disease progression or undermedication. Cholinergic crises can result from excessive amounts of ACh from overmedication with anticholinesterase drugs. These are often difficult to distinguish clinically.

(continued on page 272)

Interventions	Rationales
a. Monitor for • Restlessness, anxiety • Dyspnea • Generalized muscle weakness • Increased bronchial secretions/sweating • Difficulty swallowing/speaking • Bradycardia/tachycardia • Hypotension/hypertension	a. Refer to rationale above.
7. Monitor for: a. Nausea and vomiting b. Diarrhea and abdominal cramping c. Sweating d. Increased salivation/bronchial secretions e. Tachycardia/bradycardia/hypotension f. Increased muscle weakness g. Increased fatigue h. Bronchial relaxation (collapse) i. Muscle twitching/cramping	7. These symptoms are adverse effects of cholinergic drugs. The anticholinesterase medication that helps to improve acetylcholine effects at the neuromuscular junctions and helps to control symptoms, also has an effect on the autonomic nervous system. Acetylcholine activates muscarinic receptors that have an effect on smooth muscles, cardiac muscles, and granular tissue. Acetylcholine activates nicotinic receptors, which involves the functioning of the skeletal muscles and the ganglion cells (Lehne, 2004; NINDS, 2007).
8. Assess for diplopia (double vision): a. Alternate patching of eyes for short periods.	8. An eye patch will relieve double vision and provide comfort and ability to do self-care.
9. Assess for ptosis: a. Tape eyes open for short intervals. b. Use artificial tears to prevent corneal damage. c. Use sunglasses to reduce photophobia.	9. To provide comfort and avoid eye injuries (Hickey, 2003).

 Related Physician-Prescribed Interventions

Medications. Mestinon (pyridostigmine bromide), Prostigmin (neostigmine bromide), Mytelase (ambenonium chloride), corticosteroids, immunosuppressants (azathioprine, cyclophosphamide, intravenous immunoglobulin [IVIG]).

Diagnostic Studies. Electrophysiologic studies (electromyogram), nerve conduction studies, Tensilon (edrophonium chloride), chest x-ray, swallowing video, acetylcholine receptor antibodies (found in 86% of MG clients), striatal antibody (found in 80% MG clients)

Therapies. Plasmapheresis, tracheotomy, thymectomy, mechanical ventilation

Documentation

Vital signs
Neurologic
Progress notes
   Change in status
   Response to interventions

Nursing Diagnoses

High Risk for Ineffective Therapeutic Regimen Management Related to Insufficient Knowledge of Condition, Treatments, Prevention of Infections, Stress Management, Aggravating Factors, Signs and Symptoms of Complications, and Community Resources

NOC Compliance Behavior, Knowledge: Treatment Regimen, Participation in Health Care Decisions, Treatment Behavior: Illness or Injury

Goals

The goals for this diagnosis represent those associated with discharge planning. Refer to the discharge criteria.

NIC Anticipatory Guidance, Learning Facilitation, Risk Identification, Health Education, Teaching: Procedure/Treatment, Health System Guidance

Interventions	Rationales
1. Determine the client's and his or her family's level of learning. Then explain to them the diagnosis and long-term management of the disease, using methods appropriate to their level of learning.	1. The client and his or her family must have a good understanding of this chronic disease process to enable them to recognize symptoms leading to complications.
2. Teach the client the signs and symptoms of myasthenic crisis as distinguished from those of cholinergic crisis: a. Myasthenic crisis: • Increased blood pressure • Tachycardia • Restlessness • Apprehension • Increased bronchial secretions, lacrimation, and sweating • Generalized muscle weakness • Absent cough reflex • Dyspnea • Difficulty swallowing • Difficulty speaking b. Cholinergic crisis: • Decreased blood pressure • Bradycardia • Restlessness • Apprehension • Increased bronchial secretions, lacrimation, and sweating • Generalized muscle weakness • Fasciculations • Dyspnea • Difficulty swallowing • Difficulty speaking • Blurred vision • Nausea and vomiting • Abdominal cramps and diarrhea	2. A myasthenic crisis results from an *insufficiency* of acetylcholine, usually induced by a change or withdrawal of medications. Cholinergic crises result from *excessive* amounts of acetylcholine, usually from overmedication with anticholinesterase medication. The client needs to know the symptoms of overdose and underdose of his or her medications.
3. Teach incompatibility of medications: a. Quinine—also found in tonics. b. Alcohol—speeds drugs' absorption and should be consumed 1 hour after taking anticholinesterase medications. c. Aminoglycoside antibiotics are to be used with caution. d. Other medications known to aggravate MG are morphine, diuretics, procainamide, and beta blockers (Lehne, 2004; MGFA, 2007; NINDS, 2007).	3. The client and her or his family need to know that these medications will aggravate the disease. Other medical professionals may unknowingly order these medications.
4. Teach medication administration: a. Correct time—1 hour before meals b. Accurate dosage c. Advise the client to keep a medication diary to determine peak medication function.	4. The exact time of an accurate medication dosage coincides with increases in energy demands. Taking medications before meals is essential to provide muscle strength for chewing food.

(continued on page 274)

Interventions	Rationales

5. Teach how to manage diplopia and ptosis:
    a. Use eye patch; alternate eye every 2 to 4 hours.
 	
    b. Use lubricating eye drops.
	5.
	    a. Eye patch will relieve double vision and provide the client with comfort and some ability to care for him- or herself (Hickey, 2003; Torpy, 2005).
	    b. Eye drops will prevent corneal abrasions (Hickey, 2003; Torpy, 2005).

6. Teach energy conservation.	6. Rest periods should be scheduled when medication peaks are low. The client should learn to space tasks. Teach the family the importance of vital rest periods and planning activities.

7. Teach stress management strategies:
    a. Use of relaxation tapes
    b. Guided imagery
    c. Referral to community resource for stress management course
	7. Uncontrolled stress factors can lead to an acute exacerbation of the disease.

8. Inform the client of factors that are known to trigger exacerbations:
    a. Excessive weakness
    b. Increased stressors
    c. Upper respiratory infection
    d. Exposure to ultraviolet light
    e. Surgery
    f. Pregnancy
    g. Hot and cold temperatures
	8. This information can provide the client with insight of the disease and promote a sense of personal control. If the client is pregnant or considering a pregnancy, she should consult with her physician as the course of pregnancy with MG is unpredictable, and she will require close observation.

9. Explain signs and symptoms that must be reported to a health care professional:
    a. Increased muscle weakness
    b. Progressive symptoms of visual disturbance. Difficulty breathing, chewing and swallowing, and sweating
    c. Productive cough
	9. Early intervention can minimize pending complications. These symptoms can be warnings of a crisis.

10. Teach chewing and swallowing techniques:
    a. When eating, sit in an upright position with head bent slightly forward.
    b. Wear a soft cervical collar for neck support while eating.
 	
    c. Limit hot food intake.
    d. Refer to Impaired Swallowing—CVA care plan for specific teaching to prevent aspiration.
	10.
	    a. This position will create a gravity force for the downward motion of food.
	    b. A collar will help support the neck and head and reduce fatigue.
	    c. Hot foods tend to increase muscle weakness.

11. Provide information and literature to assist the client and her or his family to manage long-term goals at home. Resources are as follows:
    a. Myasthenia Gravis Foundation (www.myasthenia.org)
    b. Home health agency
    c. Case manager referral
	11. The client and family who receive community support will cope more effectively with this progressive chronic disease.

Documentation

Discharge summary record
    Client teaching while ensuring the client and family members understand the education given to them.
    Outcome achievement or status
    Referrals if indicated

Neurogenic Bladder

A neurogenic bladder is any bladder disturbance attributable to the motor or sensory pathways in the central or peripheral nervous systems that have input to the bladder (Hickey, 2003). Lapides and Diokno (1976) classified neurogenic bladders into five groups to help pinpoint the underlying pathologic process: autonomous, reflex, motor paralytic, sensory paralytic, and uninhibited neurogenic bladders (Hickey, 2003).

An *autonomous* neurogenic bladder results from destruction of the *bladder center in the sacral spinal cord* at or below T12–L1 (Hickey, 2003). The client feels no conscious sensation to void and has no micturition reflex; the bladder empties irregularly.

A *reflex* neurogenic bladder occurs with damage between the sacral spinal cord and the cerebral cortex, above T12–L1 (Hickey, 2003). The client has no sensation to void and cannot void volitionally. The uninhibited detrusor contractions may be poorly sustained with inefficient bladder emptying. If the micturition reflex arc is intact, reflex voiding can occur. If there is detrusor-sphincter dyssynergy, there will be increased bladder pressure and high residual urine.

A *motor paralytic* neurogenic bladder occurs when there is damage in the anterior horn cells of the S2–S4 ventral roots (Hickey, 2003) and the motor side of the micturition reflex arc is damaged. The client has intact sensation, but experiences partial or complete loss of motor function. Bladder capacity may increase, with a large residual urine. There may be overflow incontinence.

A *sensory paralytic* neurogenic bladder occurs when the dorsal roots of S2–S4 or the sensory pathways to the cerebral cortex are damaged (Hickey, 2003). The client loses sensation, but can void volitionally. Bladder capacity may increase, with subsequent overflow incontinence.

An *uninhibited* neurogenic bladder results from damage to the *bladder center in the cerebral cortex*. The client has limited sensation of bladder distention, but has no ability to inhibit urination. Urgency results from the short time between limited sensation to void and the uninhibited bladder contraction. The bladder usually empties completely.

 Time Frame
Secondary diagnosis (hospitalization not usual for neurogenic bladder)

■■■■■ DIAGNOSTIC CLUSTER*

Collaborative Problems

PC: Renal Calculi
PC: Vesicoureteral Reflux
PC: Urinary Tract Infection
PC: Renal Failure/Hydronephrosis/Multiple Sclerosis

Nursing Diagnoses	Refer to
Overflow Incontinence related to chronically overfilled bladder with loss of sensation of bladder distention	
Overflow Incontinence related to detrusor–sphincter dyssynergy (DSD)	
Reflex Incontinence related to absence of sensation to void and loss of ability to inhibit bladder contraction	
High Risk for Infection related to retention of urine or introduction of urinary catheter	
Urge Incontinence related to inability to inhibit urination after urge is perceived	
High Risk for Loneliness related to embarrassment from incontinence in front of others and fear of odor from urine	

(continued on page 276)

Nursing Diagnoses	Refer to
High Risk for Ineffective Therapeutic Regimen Management related to insufficient knowledge of etiology of incontinence, management, bladder retraining programs, signs and symptoms of complications, and community resources	
High Risk for Dysreflexia related to reflex stimulation of sympathetic nervous system secondary to loss of autonomic control	Spinal Cord Injury
High Risk for Impaired Skin Integrity related to constant irritation from urine	Pressure Ulcers

✱ This medical condition was not included in the validation study.

Discharge Criteria

Before discharge, the client or family will

1. Identify measures to reduce incontinence.
2. Relate the intent to discuss fears and concerns with family after discharge.
3. Relate signs and symptoms that must be reported to a health care professional.
4. Demonstrate correct self-catheterization technique.
5. Relate the intent to continue exercises and fluid intake program at home.

Collaborative Problems

Potential Complication: Renal Calculi

Potential Complication: Urinary Tract Infection

Nursing Goal

The nurse will detect early signs/symptoms of (a) renal calculi and (b) urinary tract infections and collaboratively intervene to stabilize the client.

Indicators

- Temperature 98–99.5°F (a, b)
- Urine specific gravity 0.005–0.030 (a, b)
- Urine output >5 mL/kg/h (a, b)
- Clear urine (a, b)
- Prealbumin 20–50 mg/dL (a, b)
- No flank pain (a, b)

Interventions	Rationales
1. Monitor for signs and symptoms of renal calculi:	1. Urinary stasis and infection increase the risk of renal calculi because of increased precipitants in the urine. Stones remain a major source of morbidity in clients with neurogenic bladder.
a. Acute flank pain	a,b. Stones can cause severe pain owing to obstruction and ureter spasms, or CVA pain due to distention of the renal capsule.
b. CVA (costovertebral angle) pain (a dull, constant backache below the 12th rib)	
c. Hematuria	c. The abrasive action of the stone can sever small blood vessels.
d. Nausea and vomiting	d. Afferent stimuli in the renal capsule may cause pylorospasm of the smooth muscle of the GI tract.

(continued on page 277)

Interventions	Rationales
2. Monitor for signs of urinary tract infection: 　a. Change in urine color, odor, volume 　b. Fever 　c. Increased urgency, frequency, or incontinence	2. UTIs, especially if frequent or chronic, will place a person at risk for upper urinary tract disease, as well as sclerosis of ureters, causing increased renal pressure.
3. Monitor for urinary retention by paying attention to output vs. intake amounts.	3. Urine retention, especially associated with high pressure, can cause reflux at the vesicoureteral junction, with potential hydronephrosis.

 Related Physician-Prescribed Interventions

Medications. Antimuscarinics, terazosin, alpha-adrenergic stimulators, phenoxybenzamine, pseudo-ephedrine, dicyclomine, flavoxate, imipramine, propantheline, methantheline, oral and transdermal oxybutynin, gabapentin, botulinum toxin A
Diagnostic Studies. Voiding cystourethrogram
Therapies. Corrective surgery

Documentation

Flow records
　Urine output and characteristics
　Intake and output
Progress notes
　Complaints of pain, nausea, vomiting
　Urination pattern
　Complaints of change in urinary status

Nursing Diagnoses

Overflow Incontinence Related to Chronically Overfilled Bladder with Loss of Sensation of Bladder Distention

 Tissue Integrity, Urinary Continence

Goal

The client will achieve a state of dryness that is personally satisfactory.

Indicators

• Empty the bladder using Credé's or Valsalva maneuver with a residual urine of less than 50 mL, if indicated.
• Void voluntarily.

 Urinary Incontinence Care, Urinary Habit Training, Urinary Elimination Management

Interventions	Rationales
1. Teach the client methods to empty the bladder. 　a. Credé's maneuver: 　　• Place the hands (either flat or in fists) just below the umbilical area, one hand on top of the other. 　　• Firmly press down and in toward the pelvic arch. 　　• Repeat six or seven times until no more urine is expelled. 　　• Wait several minutes, then repeat again to ensure complete emptying.	1. 　a. In many clients, Credé's maneuver can help to empty the bladder. This maneuver is inappropriate, however, if the urinary sphincters are chronically contracted. In this case, pressing the bladder can force urine up the ureters as well as through the urethra. Reflux of urine into the renal pelvis may result in renal infection.

(continued on page 278)

Interventions	Rationales
b. Valsalva maneuver (bearing down): • Lean forward on thighs. • Contract abdominal muscles, if possible, and strain or bear down while holding the breath. • Hold until urine flow stops; wait one minute, then repeat. • Continue until no more urine is expelled. c. Clean intermittent self-catheterization (CISC), used alone or in combination with the above methods. (Refer to the nursing diagnosis High Risk for Ineffective Therapeutic Regimen Management in this care plan for specific teaching points.) d. A baseline cystometrogram (CMG) may be warranted.	b. Valsalva maneuver contracts the abdominal muscles, which manually compresses the bladder. c. CISC prevents overdistention, helps to maintain detrusor muscle tone, and ensures complete bladder emptying. CISC may be used initially to determine residual urine following Credé's maneuver or tapping. As residual urine decreases, catheterization may be tapered. CISC may recondition the voiding reflex in some clients. d. Discuss diagnostic testing CMG to help plan and evaluate a bladder program.

Documentation

Flow records
    Fluid intake
    Voiding patterns (amount, time, method used)
Discharge summary record
    Client teaching
    Outcome achievement or status

Overflow Incontinence Related to Detrusor–Sphincter Dyssynergy (DSD)

NOC   See Functional Incontinence

Goal

Refer to Goals for Overflow Incontinence Related to Chronically Overfilled Bladder with Loss of Sensation of Bladder Distention.

NIC   See also Functional Incontinence, Urinary Bladder Training

Interventions	Rationales
1. Cutaneous triggering by suprapubic tapping (see under Reflex Incontinence)	
2. The anal stretch maneuver (see under Reflex Incontinence)	
3. Intermittent catheterization (see under Urinary Retention related to chronically overfilled bladder)	

Documentation

Flow records
    Fluid intake
    Urine output
    Amount from IC immediately after voiding
Discharge summary record
    Client teaching
    Outcome achievement or status

Reflex Incontinence Related to Absence of Sensation to Void and Loss of Ability to Inhibit Bladder Contraction

NOC See Functional Incontinence

Goal

The client will report a state of dryness that is personally satisfactory.

Indicators

- Have a residual urine volume of less that 50 mL.
- Use triggering mechanisms to initiate reflex voiding.

NIC See also Functional Incontinence, Pelvic Muscle Exercise, Weight Management

Interventions	Rationales
1. Ensure adequate fluid intake (at least 2000 mL/day unless contraindicated).	1. Adequate fluid intake prevents concentrated urine that can irritate the bladder and cause increased bladder instability.
2. Consult with the physician about prescribing medication to relax the bladder (e.g., anticholinergics).	2. Anticholinergic medications can eliminate hyperirritable and uninhibited bladder contractions and allow successful bladder retraining.
3. Teach techniques to trigger reflex voiding. a. Place client in half-sitting position. b. Tap on bladder wall at a rate of seven to eight times in five seconds for ½ minute. c. Tell the client to contract abdominal muscles.	3. a,b. Stimulating the reflex arc relaxes the internal sphincter of the bladder and allows urination. Stimulating the bladder wall or cutaneous sites (e.g., suprapubic, pubic) can trigger the reflex arc. c. Contraction of abdominal muscles compresses the bladder to empty it.
4. Cutaneous triggering by suprapubic tapping: • Assume a half-sitting position. • Using the fingers of one hand, aim tapping directly at the bladder wall; tap at a rate of seven or eight times every 5 seconds for a total of 50 taps. • Shift the site of tapping over the bladder to find the most effective site. • Continue stimulation until a good stream starts. • Wait about 1 minute, then repeat stimulation until the bladder is empty. (One or two series of stimulations without urination indicates bladder emptying.) If tapping is ineffective, perform each of the following for 2 to 3 minutes each: • Stroke the glans penis. • Lightly punch the abdomen above the inguinal ligaments. • Stroke the inner thigh.	4. External cutaneous stimulation can stimulate the voiding reflex.
5. The anal stretch maneuver: • Sit on the commode or toilet, leaning forward on the thighs. • Insert one or two lubricated fingers into the anus, to the anal sphincter. • Spread fingers apart or pull in the posterior direction to stretch the anal sphincter. • Bear down and void while performing the Valsalva maneuver. • Relax then repeat the procedure until the bladder is empty.	5. Anal sphincter stimulation can stimulate the voiding reflex.

(continued on page 280)

Interventions	Rationales

6. Teach measures to help reduce detrusor activity:
  a. Resist voiding for as long as possible.
  b. Drink sufficient fluid to distend the bladder.
  c. Time fluid intake so that detrusor activity is restricted to waking hours.
	6. To increase comfort associated with voiding, the client must condition the voiding reflex by ingesting adequate fluids and inhibiting bladder contractions. Frequent toileting causes chronic low-volume voiding and increases detrusor activity. Resisting the urge to void may increase voiding intervals and reduce detrusor muscle activity.

7. Encourage the client to void or trigger at least every 3 hours.	7. A regular voiding pattern can prevent incontinent episodes and urinary tract infections (Lemke, Kasprowicz, & Worral, 2005).
8. Manage incontinence with CISC and incontinence products, whichever are most appropriate for the client and caregiver. External urine collection devices may be used if urodynamic studies show complete bladder emptying. Protect skin.	8. Loss of both the sensation to void and the ability to inhibit contractions makes bladder retraining impossible. CISC, often in conjunction with medications, is then the procedure of choice for managing incontinence. Incontinence is a factor in skin breakouts.

Documentation

Flow records
  Fluid intake
  Voiding patterns (amount, time, method used)
Discharge summary record
  Client teaching
  Outcome achievement or status

High Risk for Infection Related to Retention of Urine or Introduction of Urinary Catheter

NOC Infection Status, Wound Healing: Primary Intention, Immune Status

Goal

The client will be free of bladder infection.

Indicators

• Urine is clear.
• Temperature is between 98–99.5°F.
• Demonstrate techniques to prevent infection.

NIC Infection Control, Wound Care, Incision Site Care, Health Education

Interventions	Rationales
1. Ensure adequate fluid intake (at least 2000 mL/day, unless contraindicated).	1. Dilute urine helps to prevent infection and bladder irritation.

2. Eliminate residual urine by aiding urine outflow through methods such as the following (Lemke et al., 2005):
  a. Credé maneuver
  b. Suprapubic tapping
  c. Multiple voiding
  d. Valsalva maneuver
  e. Intermittent catheterization
	2. Bacteria multiply rapidly in stagnant urine retained in the bladder. Moreover, overdistention hinders blood flow to the bladder wall, increasing the susceptibility to infection from bacterial growth. Regular, complete bladder emptying greatly reduces the risk of infection.

(continued on page 281)

Interventions	Rationales
3. Consult with the physician for medication to relieve detrusor sphincter dyssynergia (DSD).	3. DSD is associated with large amounts of residual urine.
4. Administer vitamin C and cranberry tablets, as ordered.	4. Acidic urine deters the growth of most bacteria implicated in cystitis.
5. Monitor residual urine (should be no more than 50 mL).	5. Careful monitoring detects problems early, enabling prompt intervention to prevent urine stasis.
6. Test an uncontaminated urine sample for bacteria.	6. A bacteria count over 10^5/mL of urine suggests infection, when pyuria is present. Some physicians may not want to treat until the client has symptoms.
7. Maintain sterile technique for intermittent catheterization while the client is hospitalized (Lemke et al., 2005); clean technique is used at home (Lemke et al., 2005).	7. The most common cause of infection is bacteria introduced by a caregiver who did not wash hands adequately between clients.
8. Avoid using an indwelling catheter unless it is indicated by a client's individual situation (e.g., inability to perform CISC due to immobility).	8. Indwelling catheters are associated with urinary tract infection related to the catheter sliding in and out of the urethra, which introduces pathogens.

Documentation

Flow records
    Urine characteristics
    Temperature
    Elimination pattern (amount, time)
    Urine retention >50 mL

Urge Incontinence Related to Disruption of the Inhibitory Efferent Impulses Secondary to Brain or Spinal Cord Dysfunction

 Tissue Integrity: Skin & Mucous Membranes, Urinary Continence, Urinary Elimination

Goals

The client will report no or fewer episodes of incontinence (specify).

Indicators

• Explain causes of incontinence.
• Describe bladder irritants.

 Perineal Care, Urinary Incontinence Care, Prompted Voiding, Urinary Habit Training, Urinary Elimination Management, Teaching: Procedure/Treatment

Interventions	Rationales

1. Reduce any impediments to voiding routine by providing the following, if necessary:
  a. Velcro straps on clothes
  b. Handrails or mobility aids to bathroom
	1. These measures ensure the client's ability to self-toilet before incontinence occurs. Often, little time exists between onset of the sensation to void and the bladder contraction.

(continued on page 282)

Interventions	Rationales
c. Bedside commode d. Urinal	
2. Assess voiding patterns and develop a schedule of frequent timed voiding.	2. Frequent timed voiding can reduce urgency from bladder overdistention.
3. If incontinence occurs, decrease the time between planned voidings.	3. Bladder capacity may be insufficient to accommodate the urine volume, necessitating more frequent voiding.
4. If indicated, restrict fluid intake during the evening.	4. Evening fluid restrictions may help to prevent enuresis.
5. If needed, teach trigger voiding, external manual compression, or abdominal straining. Refer to nursing diagnosis, Reflex Bladder.	5. A client with an intact reflex arc may be taught parasympathetic stimulation of the detrusor muscle, which will initiate and sustain bladder contractions to aid bladder emptying.

6. Teach pelvic floor exercises (Kegel exercises) to help restore bladder control if the client is a candidate:
  a. Help the client to identify the muscles that start and stop urination.
  b. Instruct the client to try the exercises for 3 to 4 months to strengthen the periurethral tissue.
	6. Useful for some clients with stress incontinence, Kegel exercises strengthen the pelvic floor muscles, which in turn may increase urinary sphincter competence.

7. Reinforce the need for optimal hydration (at least 2000 mL/day, unless contraindicated).	7. Optimal hydration is needed to prevent urinary tract infection and renal calculi.
8. Teach biofeedback if the client is a candidate. (The client must be alert and have a good memory.) The client may be able to learn sphincter control and prevent uninhibited bladder contractions by watching information on a screen as the bladder fills during cystometry, or by hearing movement of the sphincter muscles in action.	8. Effective for some clients with urge incontinence, biofeedback uses behavior modification to habituate the client to recognize and control unwanted bladder spasms.

9. If other measures fail, plan for managing incontinence:
  a. Incontinent males can manage fairly easily by using an external condom drainage system and a leg bag or pubic pressure urinal.
  b. Incontinent females have a more difficult problem. Incontinence pads are frequently used; new external collection devices are being marketed, but are not yet perfected.
	9. If bladder emptying techniques are unsuccessful, other methods of managing incontinence are necessary.

Documentation

Flow records
    Intake
    Voidings (amount, time)
    Method used
    Incontinent episodes
Discharge summary record
    Client teaching

High Risk for Loneliness Related to Embarrassment of Incontinence in Front of Others and Fear of Odor From Urine

NOC Loneliness, Social Involvement

Goals

The client will report decreased feelings of loneliness.

Indicators

• Identify the reasons for feelings of isolation.
• Discuss ways of increasing meaningful relationships.

NIC Socialization Enhancement, Spiritual Support, Behavior Modification: Social Skills, Presence, Anticipatory Guidance

Interventions	Rationales
1. Acknowledge the client's frustration with incontinence.	1. To the client, incontinence may seem like a reversion to an infantile state, in which he or she has no control over body functions and feels ostracized by others. Acknowledging the difficulty of the situation can help to reduce feelings of frustration.
2. Determine the client's eligibility for bladder training, CISC, or other methods to manage incontinence.	2. These measures can increase control and reduce fear of accidents. CISC has a low incidence of UTI compared with Foley indwelling catheters (Webb, Lawson, & Neal, 1990).
3. Teach the client ways to control wetness and odor. Many products make wetting manageable by providing reliable leakage protection and masking odors.	3. Helping the client to manage incontinence encourages socialization.
4. Encourage the client to initially venture out socially for short periods, then to increase the length of social contacts as success at incontinence management increases.	4. Short trips help the client to gradually gain confidence and reduce fears.

Documentation

Progress notes
   Significant dialogue
   Discharge summary record
Client teaching

High Risk for Ineffective Therapeutic Regimen Management Related to Insufficient Knowledge of Etiology of Incontinence, Management, Bladder Retraining Programs, Signs and Symptoms of Complications, and Community Resources

NOC Compliance Behavior, Knowledge: Treatment Regimen, Participation in Health Care Decisions, Treatment Behavior: Illness or Injury

Goals

The goals for this diagnosis represent those associated with discharge planning. Refer to the discharge criteria.

NIC Anticipatory Guidance, Learning Facilitation, Risk Identification, Health Education, Teaching: Procedure/Treatment, Health System Guidance

Interventions	Rationales
1. Teach the client about the condition, its causes, and management.	1. Understanding can encourage compliance with and participation in the treatment regimen.

2. If the client has voluntary control, institute a bladder training program.
  a. Document fluid intake, incontinence episodes, periods of continence, and client behavior on a voiding chart; this provides reinforcement for the client.
  b. Have the client void "by the clock" rather than from an urge.
  c. Ensure that the client assumes an anatomically correct position for voiding attempts.
  d. Ensure privacy.
  e. Encourage use of the toilet 30 minutes before any usual incontinent episodes.
  f. Increase the scheduled time between voidings as the client remains continent for longer periods.
	2. Bladder training, an acceptable treatment for urge incontinence, can help to increase bladder volume and extend the length of time between voidings.

3. Encourage an obese client to lose weight.	3. Obesity places excessive intra-abdominal pressure on the bladder, which can aggravate incontinence.

4. Teach the client about any drugs prescribed for managing incontinence:
  a. Anticholinergics decrease uninhibited bladder contractions.
  b. Smooth muscle relaxants increase bladder capacity.
  c. Alpha-adrenergic agents stimulate the urethral sphincter.
  d. Alpha-blocking agents decrease neural sphincter resistance and help to reduce overflow incontinence.
	4. Understanding the medications' actions may encourage the client's compliance with the therapeutic regimen.

5. Explain possible surgical options, as appropriate:
  a. Artificial urinary sphincters are increasing in popularity for clients with a malfunctioning sphincter or those who have undergone prostatectomy.
  b. Prostate resection often can eliminate overflow incontinence.
  c. Subarachnoid block, sacral rhizotomy, sacral nerve dissection, sphincterectomy, and urinary diversions may benefit spinal cord-injured clients with severe spasticity. The client must have a complete neurological and urodynamic evaluation to identify the appropriate surgical or medical treatment.
	5. The client may be a candidate for surgery to control or cure incontinence.

6. If indicated, teach CISC to the client or caregiver.
  a. In women, follow this procedure:
    • Wash hands thoroughly.
    • Hold the catheter 1½ inches from the tip. With the other hand, separate the labia, using the second and fourth fingers, and locate the urethral meatus with the middle finger. Use this finger as a guide for insertion.
    • Gently insert the catheter into the urethral meatus by slipping the catheter tip just under the middle finger. Advance the catheter in an upward direction.
    • Guide the catheter into the bladder, about one inch past the point at which urine begins to flow.
	6. Intermittent self-catheterization is appropriate for children and adults who are motivated and physically able to perform the procedure. Often, a caregiver may be taught to catheterize the client. CISC stimulates normal voiding, prevents infection, and maintains integrity of the ureterovesical junction. In the hospital, aseptic technique is used because of increased microorganisms in the hospital environment; at home, clean technique is used. CISC entails fewer complications than an indwelling catheter and is the procedure of choice for clients who are unable to empty the bladder completely.

(continued on page 285)

Interventions	Rationales

• Drain the bladder of urine. When urine stops flowing, slowly begin removing the catheter. If urine flow begins again during removal, hold the catheter in position and wait until the flow stops.
• After removal, cleanse the outer surface of the catheter with water and the same soap used to wash hands, then rinse the inside and outside with clear water. Let the catheter dry before storing it in its container. Remember to discard a catheter that becomes too stiff or soft.
b. In men, use the following procedure:
  • Wash hands and prepare the catheter. Generously apply water-soluble lubricant to the catheter tip.
  • Hold the catheter about 1½ inches from the tip. With the other hand, hold the penis straight out from the body.
  • Insert the catheter into the urinary meatus until slight resistance is felt. Then, using gentle but firm pressure, advance the catheter to the bladder, one inch past the point at which urine begins to flow.
  • Drain the bladder of urine. When urine stops flowing, slowly begin removing the catheter. If urine flow begins again during removal, hold the catheter in position and wait until flow stops.
  • After removal, cleanse the outer surface of the catheter with water and the same soap used to wash hands, then rinse the inside and outside with clear water.
  • Dry and store the catheter in its container. Remember to discard a catheter that becomes too stiff or soft.	

7. Teach the client to keep a record of catheterization times, amount of fluid intake and urine output, and any incontinent periods.	7. Accurate record-keeping aids in evaluating status. Teach the client about the dehydrating effects of alcohol.
8. Teach the client to notify the physician of the following: a. Bleeding from urethral opening b. Reactions from medications c. Difficulty inserting catheter d. Dark, bloody, cloudy, or strong-smelling urine e. Pain in the abdomen or back f. Elevated temperature	8. Early reporting enables prompt treatment to prevent serious problems. a. Bleeding may indicate trauma or renal calculi. b. Drug reactions may indicate overdose. c. Difficult catheter insertion may indicate a stricture. d. These urine changes may point to infection. e. Pain may indicate renal calculi. f. Fever may be the first sign of urinary tract infection.
9. Explain available community resources.	9. The client and family may need assistance or more information for home care.
10. Provide AHCPR booklet *Urinary Incontinence in Adults: A Patient's Guide*.	

Documentation

Discharge summary record
   Client teaching
   Outcome achievement or status

Parkinson Disease

Parkinson disease (PD) is a chronic neurodegenerative disease caused by a depletion of dopamine-producing cells in the basal ganglia and includes striatum, globus pallidum, subthalamic nucleus, substantia nigra, and red nucleus. Dopamine is a neurotransmitter that is produced and stored in the substantia nigra and is depleted when substantia nigra cells are damaged. A decrease in dopamine disrupts its inhibitory effects and causes an increase in the excitatory effect of acetylcholine.

The cardinal features of Parkinson disease include resting tremors, bradykinesia, and limb rigidity, which are referred to as the Classic Triad. Other features of PD include diminished postural stability and dystonia (Dewey, Kelley, & Shulman, 2002; Bader & Littlejohns, 2004).

Initial symptoms typically develop after age 50. Onset is insidious, and a diagnosis may not be made for years. People over 60 have a 2–4% risk of developing Parkinson disease, compared with the 1–2% risk in the general population. However, genetics can account for a two-to-threefold increase in the risk of developing PD (Parkinson Disease Foundation, 2007).

Time Frame
Secondary diagnosis (hospitalization not usual)

 DIAGNOSTIC CLUSTER*

Collaborative Problems

PC: Long-Term Levodopa Treatment Syndrome
PC: Dysphasia (leading to malnutrition or aspiration)
PC: Pneumonia
PC: Urinary Tract Infections
PC: Orthostatic Hypotension

Nursing Diagnoses

Impaired Verbal Communication related to dysarthria secondary to ataxia of muscles of speech

Impaired Physical Mobility related to effects of muscle rigidity, tremors, and slowness of movement on activities of daily living

Related Care Plans

Immobility or Unconsciousness
Multiple Sclerosis

∗ This medical condition was not included in the validation study.

Discharge Criteria

Before discharge, the client and family will

1. Relate the intent to share concerns with another family member or a trusted friend.
2. Identify one strategy to increase independence.
3. Describe measures that can reduce the risk of exacerbation.
4. Identify signs and symptoms that must be reported to a health care professional.
5. Make sure the client and his or her family know what community resources are available to them, such as the Parkinson Disease Foundation (http://www.pdf.org).

Collaborative Problems

Potential Complication: Long-Term Levodopa Treatment Syndrome

Potential Complication: Dysphasia (leading to malnutrition or aspiration)

Potential Complication: Pneumonia

Potential Complication: Urinary Tract Infections

Potential Complication: Orthostatic Hypotension

Nursing Goal

The nurse will detect early signs/symptoms of (a) long-term levodopa treatment syndrome, (b) Dysphagia, (c) pneumonia, (d) urinary tract infections, and (e) orthostatic hypotension.

Indicators

- Less or no fluctuations between involuntary movements (tics, tremors, rigidity, and repetitive, bizarre movements) and bradykinesia (slowed movements) (a)
- Intact cough-gag reflexes (b, c)
- Intact muscle strength (b, c)
- No continual coughing with swallowing (b, c)
- Dizziness, lightheadedness, and possible fainting with standing (e)
- Sudden decrease in blood pressure when sitting or standing (e)
- Headaches (e)
- Respiration 16–20 breaths/min (a, b)
- Respiration relaxed and rhythmic (b, c)
- Breath sound present all lobes (b, c)
- No rales or wheezing (b, c)
- Blurred or dimmed vision (possibly to the point of momentary blindness) (e)
- Extremity numbness or tingling (e)
- Frequent urination (d)
- Nocturia (d)
- Pain on voiding (burning) (d)
- Fever (d)

Interventions	Rationales
1. Explain long-term levodopa treatment syndrome to the client and family.	1. This syndrome occurs 2 to 6 years after beginning treatment and is characterized by a deterioration of levodopa efficacy (Lehne, 2004).
2. Explain symptoms of the syndrome (on-off syndrome): a. Fluctuates between being symptom-free and severe Parkinson symptoms. b. Symptoms may last minutes or hours.	2. This syndrome is believed to be caused by altered sensitivity of dopamine receptors or to serum level changes in levodopa (Lehne, 2004).
3. Encourage the client to discuss with the physician the possibility of a "drug holiday."	3. Some physicians advocate from 1 to 2 days to 10–14 days of a drug holiday in a hospital setting to permit resensitization of dopamine receptors.
4. Evaluate knowledge of dietary precautions: a. The need to avoid foods high in pyridoxine (e.g., B_6 vitamins, pork, beef, liver, bananas, ham, and egg yolks) b. Advise the client to divide daily protein intake into equal amounts over the entire day. c. After taking levodopa, wait 45 minutes before eating. If nausea develops, the client may take the dosage with food. d. The need to have a diet high in fiber and fluid (unless contraindicated)	4. a. Pyridoxine accelerates the breakdown of levodopa to dopamine before it reaches the brain. b,c. Protein competes with levodopa for transport to the brain. Levodopa is best absorbed on an empty stomach. However, it may cause nausea, and should then be taken with food. d. Constipation and nausea are side effects of levodopa (Lehne, 2004).
5. Observe for psychiatric disturbances: a. Visual hallucinations	5. Drug-related psychiatric disturbances can occur in 30% of treated clients. Disturbances include hallucinations; confused, delusional, abnormal dreams; and sleep disturbances.

(continued on page 288)

Interventions	Rationales
b. Sleep disturbances	b. Sleep disorders may be treated medically after sleep apnea is ruled out.
c. Depression	c. Depression in Parkinson is associated with advancing disease severity, recent disease deterioration, and occurrence of falls (Lewis et al., 2004).
d. Confusion	d. Confusion, although less common, is also a side effect of levodopa (Lehne, 2004).

6. Prevent complications leading to exacerbation of symptoms. Refer to index under following subjects:
  a. High risk for aspiration
 	
  b. Impaired swallowing
 	
  c. Disuse syndrome
  d. Thrombophlebitis
  e. Avoid alcohol
	6.
	
	  a. Swallowing disorders are common in Parkinson disease and may cause dehydration, weight loss, aspiration pneumonia, and airway obstruction.
	  b. A barium swallow study is useful for identifying the swallowing disorder (Kee, 2005).
	
	  e. Alcohol may antagonize the effects of levodopa.

7. Monitor client for signs and symptoms of infection.
  a. Chills and fever
  b. Leukocytosis
  c. Bacteria and pus in urine
  d. Dysuria and frequency
  e. Bladder distention
  f. Urine overflow (30–60 mL of urine every 15–30 minutes)	

8. Monitor for signs and symptoms of respiratory distress, and position to assist with breathing.
  a. Auscultate breath sounds.
  b. Assess for secretions:
    • Encourage the client to breathe deep and cough.
    • Position client side to side to assist movement of secretions.
    • Suction if client is unable to manage secretions.
    • Reassure client by maintaining a calm environment.
  c. Assess O_2 saturation via pulse oximetry.	

9. Ventilation may become necessary as Parkinson disease progresses, due to decreased muscle tone and mobility
  a. Auscultating breath sounds assesses adequacy of air flow and detects the presence of adventitious sounds (see Mechanical Ventilation for more information).
  b. When the respiratory muscles fatigue, cough becomes ineffective, leading to the accumulation of mucus and formation of mucous plugs in the airway. This accumulation of secretions causes alveolar collapse leading to acute respiratory failure.
  c. Pulse oximetry provides ongoing data on O_2 saturation.
  d. An increase in the $PaCO_2$ levels indicates hypoventilation and that the client requires intubation to avoid acute respiratory distress.
  e. Intubation is initiated to relieve shortness of breath to avoid acute respiratory failure, aspiration, and pneumonia.
  f. Early recognition enables prompt intervention to prevent further complications.	

10. Monitor for signs and symptoms of orthostatic hypotension and assist client with ambulation.	

(continued on page 289)

Interventions	Rationales
• Assist client to sit and stand slowly • Assist client when transferring to bed/chair • Make sure client has clear pathway if blurred vision and or momentary blindness occurs.	
11. Instruct client to march on spot to maintain adequate blood pressure and cerebral perfusion with standing and bending (Hickey 2003).	

 ### Related Physician-Prescribed Interventions

Medications. Dopaminergic agonists, dopaminergics, catechol-o-methyltransferase inhibitors
Intravenous Therapy. None
Laboratory Studies. Stereotaxic neurosurgery, urine dopamine levels
Diagnostic Studies. Autologous tissue transplantation, CT scan or MRI (to rule out other disorders)
Therapies. Fetal tissue transplantation, physical therapy, deep brain stimulation

Documentation

Progress notes
Changes in symptoms

Nursing Diagnoses

Impaired Verbal Communication Related to Dysarthria Secondary to Ataxia of Muscles of Speech

NOC Communication: Expressive Ability

Goal

The client will demonstrate improved ability to express self.

Indicator

• Demonstrate techniques and exercises to improve speech and strengthen muscles.

NIC Active Listening, Communication Enhancement: Speech Deficit

Interventions	Rationales
1. Explain the disorder's effects on speech.	1. Understanding may promote compliance with speech improvement exercises.
2. Explain the benefits of daily speech improvement exercises.	2. Daily exercises help to improve the efficiency of speech musculature and increase rate, volume, and articulation.
3. Refer the client to a speech pathologist to design an individualized speech program, as recommended by the American Parkinson's Disease Association. Support the client in efforts to: a. Practice in front of a mirror.	3. These exercises improve muscle tone and control and speech clarity. a. Practicing in front of a mirror allows the client to see and evaluate lip and tongue movements.

(continued on page 290)

Interventions	Rationales
b. Do exercises to improve voice loudness.	b. These exercises increase air intake, and improve control over inhalation and exhalation during speech.
c. Do exercises to improve voice variation: "I will" (softly) "I will" (a little louder) "I will" (much louder) • Say a sentence several times and stress a word. Change the word each time. For example, use the following sentence: *I* don't want that blue hat. I *don't* want that blue hat. I don't *want* that blue hat. I don't want *that* blue hat. I don't want *blue* hat. I don't want that blue *hat*. • Practice asking questions and giving answers. Raise the voice after a question, lower it with an answer.	c. These exercises enhance speech intelligibility.
d. Practice tongue exercises several times: • Stick tongue out as far as you can; hold; relax. • Stick tongue out and move it slowly from one side of the mouth to the other. • Stretch tongue to chin and then to nose. • Stick tongue out, then pull it in as fast as you can. • Move tongue in a circle around the lips as quickly as you can.	d. These exercises strengthen the tongue and increase its range of motion to improve articulation.
e. Practice lip and jaw exercises; repeat several times: • Open and close mouth slowly; close lips completely. Do it again, this time as fast as you can. • Close lips and press together tightly for a few seconds. • Stretch lips into a wide smile—hold—relax. • Pucker lips—hold—relax. • Pucker—hold—smile—hold. • Say "ma-ma-ma-ma" as fast as you can.	e. These exercises strengthen the lips and increase their range of movement for the formation of speech sounds.
f. Do exercises to slow the speaking rate: • Say words in syllables: pos-si-bil-i-ty pa-ci-fic hor-ri-ble • Say phrases in syllables: when-ev-er pos-si-ble fam-i-ly bus-i-ness	f. These exercises help to improve deliberate word-by-word pronunciation.
g. Practice varying facial expression: Using a mirror, make faces (e.g., smile, frown, laugh, grin, whistle, puff out cheeks).	g. Parkinson disease causes limited movement of facial muscles, which produces a masklike facies; these exercises help to overcome this effect.
h. Read the newspaper out loud. Determine how many words you can speak in one breath before the volume decreases.	h. This helps the client learn to maintain volume for each syllable and final consonant sounds.
4. Refer the client to American Parkinson Disease Association 135 Parkinson Avenue Staten Island, NY 10305-1425 apda@apdaparkinson.org http://www.apdaparkinson.org Tel: 718-981-8001; 1-800-223-2732 (Parkinson's Disease Foundation)	4. The client requires additional instruction.

Documentation

Discharge summary record
Assessment of speech

Exercises taught
Outcome achievement or status
Referrals, if indicated

Impaired Physical Mobility Related to Effects of Muscle Rigidity, Tremors, and Slowness of Movement on Activities of Daily Living

NOC Ambulation: Walking, Joint Movement: Active Mobility Level

Goal

The client will describe measures to increase mobility.

Indicators

- Demonstrate exercises to improve mobility.
- Demonstrate a wide-base gait with arm swinging.
- Identify one strategy to increase independence.
- Relate intent to exercise at home.

NIC Exercise Therapy: Joint Mobility, Exercise Promotion: Strength Training, Exercise Therapy: Ambulation, Positioning, Teaching: Prescribed Activity/Exercise

Interventions	Rationales
1. Explain the causes of the symptoms.	1. The client's understanding may help to promote compliance with an exercise program at home.
2. Teach the client to walk erect while looking at the horizon, with feet separated and arms swinging normally.	2. Conscious efforts to simulate normal gait and posture can improve mobility and minimize loss of balance.
3. Instruct the client to exercise three to five times a week.	3. Exercise has been proven to delay disability; ameliorate diseases; and fortify strength, balance, flexibility, and endurance, even in older clients who are frail or have a medical condition (Bader & Littlejohns, 2004). Specific benefits include the following: a. Increased muscle strength b. Improved coordination and dexterity c. Reduced rigidity d. Help prevent contractures e. Improved flexibility f. Enhanced peristalsis g. Improved cardiovascular endurance h. Increased ability to tolerate stress i. A sense of control, reducing feelings of powerlessness j. Slows osteoporosis k. Reduces LDL cholesterol l. Reduces systolic BP, raises HDL cholesterol
4. Consult with a primary care provider for a specific exercise program. Teach that an exercise program should include the following: a. Warm-up for 10 minutes. b. Exercise for 15 to 40 minutes.	4. An exercise program of range of motion and aerobic exercise (tailored to the person's ability) can help to preserve muscle strength and coordination (NINDS, 2007). a. Warmup stretches muscles, which helps to prevent injury. b. The workout conditions the heart and tones other muscles. Walking, dancing, swimming, and riding a stationary bike are examples.

(continued on page 292)

Interventions	Rationales
c. Cool down for 10 minutes.	c. Cooling down serves to promote excretion of body wastes from the exercise and to gradually reduce the heart rate.
d. Lower body, torso, upper body, and head exercises	d. A range of exercises ensures that all affected muscle areas are exercised.
e. Relaxation exercises	e. Relaxation exercises provide some control over the anxiety associated with fear of "freezing" or falling.
f. Explain that short bouts of physical activity are also beneficial.	f. Exercise programs should begin with low intensity activities, and gradually intensify (Parkinson's Disease Foundation, 2007).
5. Stress to the client that compliance with the exercise program is ultimately his or her choice.	5. Promoting the client's feelings of control and self-determination may improve compliance with the exercise program.
6. Include family members or significant others in teaching sessions; stress that they are not to "police" the client's compliance.	6. Support from family members and significant others can encourage the client to comply with the exercise program (Lewis et al., 2004).
7. Refer to a physical therapist or reference material for specific exercise guidelines.	7. Physical or occupational therapy as well as some alternative therapies may help clients deal with disability, provide palliation, or reduce stress (Lewis et al., 2004).
8. Discuss strategies to maintain as much independence as possible. 9. Discuss the importance of accomplishing tasks and planning events to look forward to.	8,9. Parkinson disease seems to advance more slowly in people who remain involved in their pre-Parkinson activities or who find new activities to amuse them and engage their interests (Parkinson's Disease Foundation, 2007).
10. Refer to the Fatigue nursing diagnosis in the index for additional interventions.	

Documentation

Discharge summary record
Assessment of mobility
Exercises taught
Outcome achievement or status
Referrals, if indicated
Refer to website http://thePoint.lww.com for critical paths for this condition.

Seizure Disorders

Seizure disorders constitute a chronic syndrome in which a neurologic dysfunction in cerebral tissue produces recurrent paroxysmal episodes, which are referred to as seizures. A seizure is defined as an uncontrolled electrical discharge of neurons in the brain that interrupts normal functions, such as: disturbances of behavior, mood, sensation, perception, movement, and/or muscle tone.

Seizures are often symptoms of an underlying illness. They may be idiopathic, arising from an unknown cause; or cryptogenic, arising from a presumed cause that is unknown or ill defined (Bader & Littlejohns, 2004). The disorder is thought to be an electrical disturbance in cerebral nerve cells that causes them to produce abnormal, repetitive electrical charges.

Seizures are diagnosed as epileptic or reactive. Epilepsy is a chronic neurologic condition, usually with an underlying condition (as permanent brain injury) that affects the delicate systems which govern how electrical energy behaves in the brain, making the brain susceptible to recurring seizures (Lewis et al., 2004; Epilepsy Foundation, 2007). Reactive seizures are single or multiple seizures resulting from a transient systemic problem (e.g., fever, infection, alcohol withdrawal, tumors, stroke, and toxic or metabolic disturbances).

The International League Against Epilepsy has established a system of seizure classification by grouping them under different categories. This system is based on classifying *unprovoked, recurring* seizures into different types. Firstly, *partial* (or *focal*) seizures are distinguished as either *simple* or *complex*. Secondly, *generalized seizures* are classified into the following categories: (a) absence, (b) myoclonic, (c) tonic-clonic, (d) tonic, and (e) atonic seizures (International League Against Epilepsy, 2007).

 Time Frame
Initial diagnosis
Recurrent acute episodes

▪▪▪▪▪ DIAGNOSTIC CLUSTER

Collaborative Problems

✳ PC: Status Epilepticus
✳ PC: Severe Multiple Injuries

Nursing Diagnoses

▲ High Risk for Ineffective Airway Clearance related to relaxation of tongue and gag reflexes secondary to disruption in muscle innervation

Anxiety related to fear of embarrassment secondary to having a seizure in public

△ High Risk for Ineffective Therapeutic Regimen Management related to insufficient knowledge of condition, medication, and care during seizures, environmental hazards, and community resources

▲ This diagnosis was reported to be monitored for or managed frequently (75%–100%).
△ This diagnosis was reported to be monitored for or managed often (50%–74%).
✳ This diagnosis was not included in the validation study.

Discharge Criteria

Before discharge, the client or family will

1. State the intent to wear medical identification.
2. Relate activities to be avoided.
3. Relate the importance of complying with the prescribed medication regimen.
4. Relate the side effects of prescribed medications.
5. State situations that increase the possibility of a seizure.
6. State signs and symptoms that must be reported to a health care professional.
7. Ensure that the client and her or his family are aware of community resources for epilepsy, such as: http://www.ilae-epilepsy.org/ and, http://www.epilepsyfoundation.org.
8. Make sure that the client has understood all required follow-up appointments prior to discharge.

Collaborative Problems

Potential Complication: Status Epilepticus

Potential Complication: Aspiration

Potential Complication: Severe Injury or Even Death (from trauma suffered during a seizure)

Nursing Goal

The nurse will detect early signs/symptoms of (a) status epilepticus, (b) aspiration, and (c) injury, and collaboratively intervene to stabilize the client.

Indicators

- Respiration 16–20 breaths/min (a, b)
- Heart rate 60–100 beats/min (a, b, c)
- BP >90/60, <140/90 mmHg (a, c)
- No seizure activity (a, b, c)
- Serum pH 7.35–7.45 (a)
- Serum PCO_2 35–45 mmHg (a, b)
- Pulse oximetry (SaO_2) >95 (a, b)
- Sustained decreased level of consciousness (c)
- Respiratory distress (b, c)
- Hemorrhage (internal and external) (c)
- Bony deformities (c)
- Reactive pupils (c)

Interventions	Rationales

1. If the client continues to have generalized convulsions, notify the physician and initiate protocol:
  a. Clear the client's airway as soon as safely possible.
  b. Do not attempt to open the client's mouth to insert something in it.
  c. Do not try to restrain the client. Ensure that the area around client is safe; remove any obstructive objects, and pad the area where possible, to decrease the chances of injury.
  d. Suction as needed.
  e. Administer oxygen via a nasal catheter.
  f. Initiate an intravenous line.
	1. Status epilepticus is a convulsive or generalized tonic-clonic continuous seizure that lasts >30 minutes, or consists of two consecutive seizures without mental clearing in between. It is a medical emergency that requires prompt and appropriate intervention. Maintenance of adequate vital function with attention to airway, breathing, and circulation; prevention of systemic complications; and rapid termination of seizures must be coupled with investigating and treating any underlying cause (Baird, Keen, & Swearingen, 2005; Bader & Littlejohns, 2004).

2. Monitor for signs/symptoms of underlying cause:
  • Abrupt cessation of antiepileptic medication
  • Increased intracranial pressure
  • Metabolic disorders
  • Infectious process
	2. The underlying cause must be diagnosed and corrected for the seizures to be controlled (Baird, Keen, & Swearingen, 2005; Bader & Littlejohns, 2004).

 ### Related Physician-Prescribed Interventions

Medications. Antiepileptic drugs (Lehne, 2004)
Intravenous Therapy. Diazepam, lorazepam, glucose solution (IV) or fosphenytoin (IV)
Laboratory Studies. Drug levels (Tegretol, Dilantin); complete blood cell count (CBC); electrolytes; blood urea nitrogen (BUN); calcium; magnesium; fasting blood glucose; urinalysis
Diagnostic Studies. EEG; ECG; CT scan; cerebrospinal fluid examination; pulse oximetry; MRI

Documentation

Progress notes
  Abnormal findings
  Interventions
  Response
Seizure activity flow sheet

Nursing Diagnoses

High Risk for Ineffective Airway Clearance Related to Relaxation of Tongue and Gag Reflexes Secondary to Disruption in Muscle Innervation

NOC Aspiration Control, Respiratory Status

Goal

The client will demonstrate continued airway patency.

Indicator

• The family will describe and demonstrate interventions to maintain a patent airway during seizures.

NIC Cough Enhancement, Airway Suctioning, Positioning, Energy Management

Interventions	Rationales

1. During a seizure, do the following:
  a. Provide privacy, if possible, and stay with the client.
  b. Ease the client to the floor, if possible.
  c. Roll the person on his or her side, if possible.
  d. Remove anything that may cause injury.
  e. Loosen any restraining clothing.
  f. Allow the client to proceed with seizure; do not restrain him or her, as this could cause injury.
  g. If it is safe to do so, clear the airway (nose and mouth), so breathing is not obstructed.
  h. Never put anything in the client's mouth.
  i. If the seizure lasts for more than 5 minutes, call 911 (Epilepsy Foundation, 2007).
	1. These measures can help reduce injury and embarrassment (Epilepsy Foundation, 2007).

2. Observe the seizure and document its characteristics:
  a. Onset and duration
  b. Preseizure events (e.g., visual, auditory, olfactory, or tactile stimuli)
  c. Part of the client's body where the seizure started, including initial movement
  d. Eyes open or closed, pupil size
  e. Body parts involved, type of movements
  f. Involuntary motor activities (e.g., lip smacking or repeated swallowing)
  g. Incontinence (fecal or urinary)
  h. Loss of consciousness
  i. Post-seizure ability to speak, sleep, confusion, weakness, paralysis
	2. This information gives clues to the location of the epileptogenic focus in the brain and is useful in guiding treatment (Epilepsy Foundation, 2007).

3. If the client reports an aura, have him or her lie down.	3. A recumbent position can prevent injuries from a fall.
4. Teach family members or significant others how to respond to the client during a seizure.	4. Others can be taught measures to prevent airway obstruction and injury.

Documentation

Progress notes
  Description of seizures
Discharge summary record
  Client teaching

Anxiety Related to Fear of Embarrassment Secondary to Having a Seizure in Public

NOC Anxiety Level, Coping, Impulse Control

Goal

The client will relate an increase in psychological and physiologic comfort.

Indicators

- Use effective coping mechanisms.
- Describe his or her anxiety and perceptions.

NIC Anxiety Reduction, Impulse Control Training, Anticipatory Guidance

Interventions	Rationales
1. Allow opportunities for the client to share concerns regarding seizures in public.	1. Stigma associated with epilepsy is a huge concern for people living with epilepsy. A client with epilepsy may tend to separate him- or herself from family, friends, and society (Lewis et al., 2004)
2. Provide support and validate that client's concerns are normal.	2. Possible losses related to epilepsy are loss of control, independence, employment, self-confidence, transportation, family, and friends. When a person feels listened to and understood, his or her loss is validated and normalized (Lewis et al., 2004).
3. Assist the client in identifying activities that are pleasurable and nonhazardous.	3. Fear of injury may contribute to isolation.
4. Stress the importance of adhering to the treatment plan.	4. Adherence to the medication regimen can help to prevent or reduce seizure episodes.
5. Discuss sharing the diagnosis with family members, friends, coworkers, and social contacts.	5. Open dialogue with others forewarns them of possible seizures; this can reduce the shock of witnessing a seizure and possibly enable assistive action.
6. Discuss situations through which the client can meet others in a similar situation: a. Support groups b. Epilepsy Foundation of America	6. Sharing with others in a similar situation may give the client a more realistic view of the seizure disorder and of societal perception of it (Epilepsy Foundation, 2007).

Documentation

Progress notes
    Client's concerns
    Interaction with client

High Risk for Ineffective Therapeutic Regimen Management Related to Insufficient Knowledge of Condition, Medications, Care during Seizures, Environmental Hazards, and Community Resources

NOC Compliance Behavior, Knowledge: Treatment Regimen, Participation in Health Care Decisions, Treatment Behavior: Illness or Injury

Goals

The goals for this diagnosis represent those associated with discharge planning. Refer to the discharge criteria.

NIC Anticipatory Guidance, Learning Facilitation, Risk Identification, Health Education, Health System Guidance

Interventions	Rationales
1. Teach the client and her or his family about seizure disorders and treatment; correct any misconceptions.	1. The client and family's understanding of seizure disorders and the prescribed treatment regimen strongly influences compliance with the regimen.

2. If the client is on medication therapy, teach the following information:
  a. Never discontinue a drug abruptly
  b. Side effects and signs of toxicity
 	
  c. The need to have drug blood levels monitored
 	
  d. The need for periodic complete blood counts, if indicated
 	
  e. The effects of diphenylhydantoin (Dilantin), if ordered, on gingival tissue and the need for regular dental examinations
	2. Certain precautions must be emphasized to ensure safe, effective drug therapy:
	  a. Abrupt discontinuation can precipitate status epilepticus.
	  b. Early identification of problems enables prompt intervention to prevent serious complications.
	  c. Drug blood levels provide a guide for adjusting drug dosage.
	  d. Long-term use of some anticonvulsive drugs, such as hydantoins (e.g., phenytoin [Dilantin]), can cause blood dyscrasias.
	  e. Long-term phenytoin therapy can cause gingival hyperplasia.

3. Provide information regarding situations that increase the risk of seizure (Bader & Littlejohns, 2004).
  a. Alcohol ingestion
  b. Excessive caffeine intake
  c. Excessive fatigue or stress
  d. Febrile illness
  e. Poorly adjusted television screen
  f. Sedentary activity level
  g. Lack of sleep
  h. Hypoglycemia
  i. Constipation
  j. Diarrhea
	3. Certain situations have been identified as increasing seizure episodes, although the actual mechanisms behind them are unknown (Bader & Littlejohns, 2004).

4. Discuss why certain activities are hazardous and should be avoided:
  a. Swimming alone
  b. Driving (unless seizure-free for 1 to 3 years, depending on state)
  c. Operating potentially hazardous machinery
  d. Mountain climbing
  e. Occupations in which the client could be injured or cause injury to others
	4. Generally a client prone to seizures should avoid any activity that could place him, her, or others in danger should a seizure occur. Teach the client how to recognize the warning signals of a seizure and what to do to minimize injury (Lewis et al., 2004; Bader & Littlejohns, 2004).

5. Provide opportunities for the client and significant others to express their feelings alone and with each other.	5. Witnessing a seizure is terrifying for others and embarrassing for the client prone to them. This shame and humiliation contributes to anxiety, depression, hostility, and secrecy. Family members also may experience these feelings. Frank discussions may reduce feelings of shame and isolation.
6. Refer the client and family to community resources and reference material for assistance with management (e.g., Epilepsy Foundation of America, counseling, occupational rehabilitation).	6. Such resources may provide additional information and support.

Documentation

Discharge summary record
    Client teaching
    Outcome achievement or status
    Referrals if indicated
Refer to website http://thePoint.lww.com for critical paths for this condition.

Spinal Cord Injury

Spinal cord injury (SCI) results from compression, tearing, laceration, or ischemia of the spinal cord resulting in permanent or temporary loss of normal sensory, motor, or autonomic function. Neurological function may be further compromised by spinal cord edema. General factors that affect morbidity and mortality after SCI include age at the time of SCI, level of injury, and neurological grade (quantifies SCI based on the number of muscle groups affected, the degree of motor weakness, and the presence of sensory impairment) (Bader & Littlejohns, 2004, Lewis et al., 2004). The consequences of spinal cord injury depend on the location and extent of cord injury. The severity of cord injury is classified according to the American Spinal Injury Association (ASIA) Scale.

 Time Frame
Initial acute episode (post-intensive care, prerehabilitation)
Secondary diagnosis

▪▪▪▪▪ DIAGNOSTIC CLUSTER

Collaborative Problems	Refer to
△ PC: Fracture Dislocation	
▲ PC: Hypoxemia	
△ PC: Paralytic Ileus	
△ PC: Urinary Retention	
PC: Pyelonephritis	
△ PC: Renal Insufficiency	
△ PC: Gastrointestinal (GI) Bleeding	
△ PC: Electrolyte Imbalance	Acute Renal Failure
▲ PC: Thrombophlebitis	Fractures
▲ PC: Autonomic Dysreflexia	
▲ PC: Spinal Shock	
▲ PC: Neurogenic Shock	
▲ PC: Respiratory Failure	
▲ PC: Cardiovascular Insufficiency	

Nursing Diagnoses	Refer to
▲ Anxiety related to perceived effects of injury on life style and unknown future	
▲ Grieving related to loss of body function and its effects on life style	
△ High Risk for Disturbed Self-Concept related to effects of disability on achieving developmental tasks and life style	
△ Bowel Incontinence: Reflexic related to lack of voluntary sphincter control secondary to spinal cord injury above the eleventh thoracic vertebra (T11)	
△ Bowel Incontinence: Areflexic related to lack of voluntary sphincter control secondary to spinal cord injury involving sacral reflex arc (S2–S4)	
△ High Risk for Autonomic Dysreflexia related to reflex stimulation of sympathetic nervous system secondary to loss of autonomic control	

(continued on page 299)

Nursing Diagnoses	Refer to
△ Interrupted Family Processes related to adjustment requirements, role disturbances, and uncertain future	
△ High Risk for Ineffective Sexuality Pattern related to physiologic, sensory, and psychological effects of disability on sexuality or function	
△ High Risk for Ineffective Therapeutic Regimen Management related to insufficient knowledge of the effects of altered skin, bowel, bladder, respiratory, thermoregulation, and sexual function and their management; signs and symptoms of complications; follow-up care; and community resources	
▲ Self-Care Deficit related to sensorimotor deficits secondary to level of spinal cord injury	Immobility or Unconsciousness

Related Care Plans

Immobility or Unconsciousness
Pressure Ulcer
Neurogenic Bladder
Tracheostomy

▲ This diagnosis was reported to be monitored for or managed frequently (75%–100%).
△ This diagnosis was reported to be monitored for or managed often (50%–74%).

Discharge Planning

Before discharge, the client or family will

1. Describe the effects of the injury on functioning, and methods of home management.
2. Express feelings regarding the effects of the injury on life style.
3. Relate an intent to share feelings with significant others after discharge.
4. State signs and symptoms that must be reported to a health care professional.
5. Identify a plan for rehabilitation and follow-up care.
6. Identify available community resources.

Collaborative Problems

Potential Complication: Fracture Dislocation

Potential Complication: Hypoxemia

Potential Complication: Electrolyte Imbalance

Potential Complication: Paralytic Ileus

Potential Complication: Urinary Retention

Potential Complication: Pyelonephritis

Potential Complication: Renal Insufficiency

Potential Complication: Gastrointestinal (GI) Bleeding

Potential Complication: Autonomic Dysreflexia

Potential Complication: Spinal Shock
Potential Complication: Neurogenic Shock
Potential Complication: Respiratory Failure
Potential Complication: Cardiovascular Insufficiency

Nursing Goal

The nurse will monitor for early signs/symptoms of (a) fracture dislocation, (b) cardiovascular, (c) respiratory, (d) metabolic, (e) renal, and (f) gastrointestinal dysfunction, (g) autonomic dysreflexia, (h) spinal shock, (i) neurogenic shock, (j) respiratory failure, and (k) cardiovascular insufficiency, and collaboratively intervene to stabilize client.

Indicators

- Correct alignment of cord (a)
- Heart rate 60–100 beats/min (b, c, i, j, k)
- BP <140/90, >90/60 mmHg (b, c, i, j, k)
- Lung sounds clear, no adventitious sounds (b, j)
- Temperature 98–99.5°F (c)
- Serum pH 7.35–7.45 (b, c)
- Serum PCO_2 35–45 mmHg (b, c)
- Oxygen saturation (pulse oximeter) >95% (b, c, j)
- Alert, oriented (b, c, d, g, h, i, j, k)
- Urine output >5 mL/kg/h (b, c, e, g, k)
- Prealbumin 16–40 m/µ/mL (e)
- Urine specific gravity 1.005–1.030 (b, e)
- Urine sodium 130–200 mEq/24h (e)
- Blood urea nitrogen 5–25 mg/dL (e)
- Serum electrolytes (refer to laboratory range for normal) (e)
- 24-hour creatinine clearance (e)
  - Male: 95–135 mL/min
  - Female: 85–125 mL/min
- Negative stool for occult blood (f)
- Hemoglobin (b)
  - Male: 14–18 g/dL
  - Female: 12–16 g/dL
- Dry, cool to warm skin (g, h, i, k)
- Throbbing headache (g, j)
- Blurred vision (g)
- Nausea (g, h, i, j, k)
- Chest pain (g, k)
- Respiration 12–20 breaths/min (g, j, k)

Interventions	Rationales
1. Maintain immobilization with skeletal traction (e.g., tongs, calipers, collar or halo vest); ensure that ropes and weights hang freely. Check the orthopedic frame and traction daily (e.g., secure nuts/bolts).	1. Skeletal traction stabilizes the vertebral column to prevent further spinal cord injury and to allow reduction and immobilization of the vertebral column into correct alignment by constant traction force. Once traction is in place, pain is diminished by separating and aligning the injured vertebrae and reducing spasms (Hickey, 2003).

(continued on page 301)

Interventions	Rationales
2. Turn the client every 2 hours around the clock while on bed rest with skeletal traction. Use the triple log-rolling technique with a fourth person to stabilize weights during turning (Hickey, 2003).	2. A change of position helps maintain skin integrity, decrease lower extremity spasms, and mobilize secretions. Log-rolling helps to maintain spinal alignment during turning.
3. If traction disconnects or fails, stabilize the head, neck, and shoulders with a cervical collar, hands, or sand bags.	3. Stabilization of the injured area is vital to prevent misalignment and further damage.

4. Monitor for spinal shock:
  a. Decreased blood pressure
  b. Decreased heart rate
  c. Absent reflexes below injury
  d. Decreased cardiac output
  e. Decreased PO_2 (if injury at cervical or thoracic level)
  f. Increased PCO_2 (if injury at cervical or thoracic level)
	4. Sudden depression of reflex activity in the spinal cord causes complete paralysis of muscle innervated by that part of the cord (Hickey, 2003; Baird, Keen, & Swearingen, 2005).

5. Monitor for complications of neurovascular injury:
  a. Bradycardia
 	
  b. Hypotension, orthostatic hypotension
 	
  c. Hypothermia/Hyperthermia
 	
  d. Hypoglycemia
 	
  e. Deep vein thrombosis (DVT) (swelling, warmth, redness of lower extremities) (filters are not standard of care for SCI with DVT)
	5.
	  a. Cardiac function is altered because of vagal stimulation, which has no sympathetic control (unopposed parasympathetic response).
	  b. Sympathetic blockage causes vasodilation, with resulting decreased venous return. With time and conditioning, the client can tolerate low BP with no symptoms (Bader & Littlejohns, 2004).
	  c. Temperature regulation is highly dependent on an intact sympathetic nervous system. High level SCI clients are unable to adapt to environmental temperature changes because of their inability to shiver or vasoconstrict cutaneous blood vessels. Hyperthermia can occur with increased environmental temperatures or in response to infection. The client loses the ability to sweat (Baird, Keen, & Swearingen, 2005); this phenomenon is called poikilothermia.
	  d. In quadriplegics, insulin-induced hypoglycemia does not raise levels of plasma adrenaline or noradrenaline that would cause clinical manifestations of anxiety, tremulousness, hunger, sweating, tachycardia, and a rise in systolic blood pressure. Therefore, in these clients, sedation and a drop in systolic blood pressure are the only symptoms (Bader & Littlejohns, 2004).
	  e. Pooling of blood coupled with immobility greatly increases the risk of vascular stasis. DVT may result in pulmonary embolus. Sequential compression boots and prophylactic heparin are usually indicated (Hickey, 2003).

6. Monitor for signs of hypoxemia:
 	
  a. Abnormal arterial blood gases (ABGs) (pH <7.35 and PCO_2 >46 mmHg)
  b. Increased and irregular heart rate
  c. Increased respiratory rate, followed by decreased rate
 	
  d. Changes in mentation
	6. Spinal cord injuries can impair the muscles of respiration depending on the level of injury (e.g., diaphragm [C3–C5], intercostals [T1–T7], accessory muscles [C2–C7], and abdominal muscles [T6–T12]) (Bader & Littlejohns, 2004).
	  a. ABG analysis helps to evaluate gas exchange in the lungs.
	
	  b,c. Respiratory acidosis results from excessive CO_2 retention. A client with respiratory acidosis initially exhibits increased heart rate and respiration in an attempt to correct decreased circulating oxygen; then, client begins to breathe more slowly and with prolonged expiration.
	  d. Altered mentation may indicate cerebral tissue hypoxia.

(continued on page 302)

Interventions	Rationales
e. Decreased urine output (<30 mL/h) f. Cool, pale, or cyanotic skin	e,f. The compensatory response to decreased circulating oxygen is to increase heart and respiratory rates and to decrease circulation to the kidneys (resulting in decreased urine output) and to the extremities (resulting in diminished pulses and skin changes).
7. Administer low-flow (2 L/min) oxygen through a cannula, as needed.	7. Supplemental oxygen therapy increases circulating oxygen. Higher flow rates increase CO_2 retention. Use of a nasal cannula rather than a mask minimizes feelings of suffocation (Wagner, Johnson, & Kidd, 2006).
8. Assess the client's ability to cough and use accessory muscles. Suction as needed. Perform assisted coughing techniques to aid in moving secretions to the upper airways.	8. Lost innervation of intercostal muscles (T1–T7) and abdominal muscles (T6–T12) destroys the ability to cough and deep breathe effectively (Bader & Littlejohns, 2004).
9. Auscultate lung fields regularly.	9. Auscultation can detect accumulation of retained secretions and asymmetric breath sounds that may indicate pneumonia and pneumothorax.
10. Monitor serial vital capacities.	10. Ascending edema of the spinal cord can cause respiratory difficulty, requiring immediate intervention (Hickey, 2003).
11. Monitor for signs of paralytic ileus: a. Decreased or absent bowel sounds b. Abdominal distention	11. Gastric dilatation and ileus can result from depressed reflexes, and hypoxia is a late sign of spinal shock (Bader & Littlejohns, 2004; Baird, Keen, & Swearingen, 2005).
12. Monitor for signs of urinary retention: a. Bladder distention b. Decreased urine output	12. Urinary retention is caused by bladder atony and contraction of the urinary sphincter during spinal shock. Bladder distention can lead to urinary reflux, pyelonephritis, stone formation, renal insufficiency, and dysreflexia (Bader & Littlejohns, 2004).
13. Monitor for signs and symptoms of pyelonephritis: a. Fever, chills b. Costovertebral angle pain (CVA), if sensation is intact at this level; otherwise, vague, referred pain c. Leukocytosis d. Bacteria, pus, and nitrites in urine e. Dysuria, frequency	13. Urinary tract infections can be caused by urinary stasis (Bader & Littlejohns, 2004). a. Bacteria can act as a pyrogen by raising the hypothalamic thermostat through the production of endogenous pyrogen that may mediate through prostaglandins. Chills can occur when the temperature setpoint of the hypothalamus rapidly changes. b. CVA pain results from distention of the renal capsule. c. Leukocytosis reflects an increase in WBCs to fight infection through phagocytosis. d. Bacteria changes urine's odor and pH because of increased nitrites, a byproduct of bacteria. e. Bacteria irritate bladder tissue, causing spasms and frequency.
14. Monitor for early signs and symptoms of renal insufficiency: a. Sustained elevated urine specific gravity b. Elevated urine sodium level c. Sustained insufficient urine output (<30 mL/h) d. Elevated blood pressure e. Elevated blood urea nitrogen (BUN); serum creatinine, potassium, phosphorus, and prealbumin; and creatinine clearance	14. Repeated infections can alter renal function (Bader & Littlejohns, 2004). a,b. Decreased ability of the renal tubules to reabsorb electrolytes causes increased urine sodium levels and increased specific gravity. c,d. Decreased glomerular filtration rate eventually causes insufficient urine output and stimulates renin production, which raises blood pressure in an attempt to increase blood flow to the kidneys. e. Decreased excretion of urea and creatinine in the urine results in elevated BUN and creatinine levels.

(continued on page 303)

Interventions	Rationales
15. Monitor intake and output.	15. Intake and output measurements help to evaluate hydration status.

16. Monitor for signs and symptoms of GI bleeding:
  a. Shoulder pain (referred pain)
  b. Frank or occult blood in stool
  c. Hemoptysis
  d. Nausea and vomiting
  e. Drop in hemoglobin
  f. Increased gastric pH
	16. GI bleeding can result from irritation of gastric mucosa as a side effect of corticosteroids or from a stress ulcer caused by vagal stimulation, which produces gastric hyperacidity (Hickey, 2003).
	Also monitor laboratory test results for signs and symptoms of pancreatitis.

17. Provide range of motion to all extremities. 18. Consult physical therapist and occupational therapist.	17,18. Range of motion of all extremities can reduce new bone formation around joints of paralyzed limbs (Hickey, 2003).

19. Monitor for signs and symptoms of cardiovascular insufficiency:
  a. Heart rate: 60–100 beats/min
  b. Blood pressure: <140/90–>90/60 mmHg
  c. Urine output >30 mL/h (0.5–1.0 mL/kg/h)
  d. alert, orientated
  e. dry, warm skin
  f. chest pain, tightness
  g. clear breath sounds in all lobes	

 Related Physician-Prescribed Interventions

Medications. Muscle relaxants; stool softeners, laxatives, suppositories; anticholinergic drugs; etidronate disodium (Didronel); alpha-adrenergic antagonists; methylprednisolone; heparin (subcutaneous); antibiotics; low-molecular weight heparins (LMWH)

Intravenous Therapy. IV steroid therapy initially postinjury, IV fluids during spinal shock phase, IV water antagonists during spinal shock phase (to prevent GI bleeding)

Laboratory Studies. Renal function studies, urodynamic studies, arterial blood gases, joint x-ray films, serum alkaline phosphatase, bone scans, erythrocyte sedimentation rate, antibiotic-resistant organisms (ARO) cultures

Diagnostic Studies. Spinal x-ray films, magnetic resonance imaging (MRI), computed tomography (CT) scan, pulmonary function studies

Therapies. Immobilization devices, myelograms, alternating pressure beds, ultrasound (lower extremities), antiembolic stockings, physical therapy, speech therapy, indwelling catheterization, laminectomy, occupational therapy, spinal fusion, psychological services

Documentation

Flow records
Vital signs
Intake and output
Respiratory assessment
Abdominal assessment (bowel sounds, distention)
Stool and emesis assessment (blood)
Traction (type, weights)
Vital capacity
Muscle testing
Progress notes
Change in status

Interventions
Response to interventions

Nursing Diagnoses

Anxiety Related to Perceived Effects of Injury on Life Style and Unknown Future

NOC Anxiety Level, Coping, Impulse Control

Goal

The client will relate increased psychologic and physiologic comfort.

Indicators

• Share feelings and fears.
• Discuss feelings with significant others.

NIC Anxiety Reduction, Impulse Control Training, Anticipatory Guidance

Interventions	Rationales
1. Provide opportunities for the client to share feelings and concerns. Maintain a calm, relaxed atmosphere; convey a nonjudgmental attitude; and listen attentively. Identify the client's support systems and coping mechanisms and suggest alternatives, as necessary.	1. Sharing feelings openly facilitates trust and helps reduce anxiety (Lewis et al., 2004).
2. Explain the following: a. The need for frequent assessments b. Diagnostic tests c. The consequences of spinal shock (flaccid paralysis and absent reflexes) d. Treatment	2. Accurate descriptions of expected sensations and procedures help to ease anxiety and fear (Lewis et al., 2004).
3. Attempt to provide consistency with staff assignments.	3. Familiarity may increase opportunities for sharing and provide stability and security.
4. Provide opportunities for family members or significant others to share their concerns.	4. Exploration gives the nurse opportunities to correct misinformation and to validate the situation as difficult and frightening.
5. Identify a client at risk for unsuccessful adjustment; look for the following characteristics: a. Poor ego strength b. Ineffective problem-solving strategies c. Lack of motivation d. External focus of control e. Poor health f. Unsatisfactory preinjury sex life g. Lack of positive support systems h. Unstable economic status i. Rejection of counseling j. Poor goal directions	5. A client's successful adjustment is influenced by such factors as previous coping success, achievement of developmental tasks before the injury, the extent to which the disability interferes with goal-directed activity, sense of control, and realistic perception of the situation by self and support persons (NSCIA, 2007; Lewis et al., 2004).
6. Refer high-risk clients to appropriate agencies.	6. Cognitive aspects of depression are less amenable to pharmacologic strategies and warrant psychologic interventions (Lewis et al., 2004).

Documentation

Progress notes
Present emotional status
Interventions
Client's and/or family's response to interventions

Grieving Related to Loss of Body Function and Its Effects on Life Style

This diagnosis is not currently on the NANDA list but has been added for clarity and usefulness.

NOC Anxiety Self-Control, Coping, Impulse Self-Control

Goal

The client will express grief.

Indicators

• Describe the meaning of loss.
• Report an intent to discuss feelings with significant others.

NIC Family Support, Grief Work Facilitation, Coping Enhancement, Anticipatory Guidance, Emotional Support, Anxiety Reduction

Interventions	Rationales
1. Provide opportunities for the client and family members to ventilate feelings, discuss the loss openly, and explore the personal meaning of the loss. Explain that grief is a common and healthy reaction.	1. Loss may give rise to feelings of powerlessness, anger, profound sadness, and other grief responses. Open, honest discussions can help the client and family members to accept and cope with the situation and their responses to it.
2. Encourage use of positive coping strategies that have proved successful in the past.	2. Positive coping strategies aid acceptance and problem-solving.
3. Encourage the client to express positive self-attributes.	3. Focusing on positive attributes increases self-acceptance and acceptance of the loss.
4. Implement measures to support the family and promote cohesiveness: a. Help them acknowledge and accept losses. b. Explain the grieving process. c. Encourage verbalization of feelings. d. Allow family members to participate in client care.	4. Family cohesiveness is important to client support.
5. Promote grief work with each response: a. Denial: • Encourage acceptance of the situation; do not reinforce denial by giving false reassurance. • Promote hope through assurances of care, comfort, and support. • Explain the use of denial by one family member to other members. • Do not push a client to move past denial until he or she is emotionally ready.	5. Grieving involves profound emotional responses; interventions depend on the particular response.

(continued on page 306)

Interventions	Rationales

b. Isolation:
  * Convey acceptance by encouraging expressions of grief.
  * Promote open, honest communication to encourage sharing.
  * Reinforce the client's self-worth by providing for privacy, when desired.
  * Encourage socialization as feasible (e.g., support groups, church activities).
c. Depression:
  * Reinforce the client's self-esteem.
  * Employ empathetic sharing and acknowledge grief.
  * Identify the degree of depression and develop appropriate strategies.
d. Anger:
  * Explain to other family members that anger represents an attempt to control the environment and stems from frustration at the inability to control the disease.
  * Encourage verbalization of anger.
e. Guilt:
  * Acknowledge the person's expressed self-image.
  * Encourage identification of the relationship's positive aspects.
  * Avoid arguing and participating in the person's system of thinking, "I should have . . ." and, "I shouldn't have. . . ."
f. Fear:
  * Focus on the present and maintain a safe and secure environment.
  * Help the client explore reasons for and meanings of the fears.
g. Rejection:
  * Provide reassurance by explaining what is happening.
  * Explain this response to other family members.
h. Hysteria:
  * Reduce environmental stressors (e.g., limit personnel).
  * Provide a safe, private area in which to express grief.

Documentation

Progress notes
Present emotional status
Interventions
Response to nursing interventions

High Risk for Disturbed Self-Concept Related to Effects of Disability on Achieving Developmental Tasks and Life Style

NOC Quality of Life, Depression Level, Self-Esteem, Coping

Goal

The client will demonstrate positive coping skills.

Indicators

* Acknowledge changes in body structure and function.
* Communicate feelings about disability
* Participate in self-care.

NIC Hope Instillation, Mood Management, Values Clarification, Counseling, Referral, Referral Support Group, Coping Enhancement

Interventions	Rationales
1. Contact client frequently and treat him or her with warm, positive regard.	1. Frequent contact by the caregiver indicates acceptance and may facilitate trust. The client may be hesitant to approach the staff because of negative self-concept (Wagner, Johnson, & Kidd, 2006).
2. Encourage client to express feelings and thoughts about the following: a. Condition b. Progress c. Prognosis d. Effects on life style e. Support system f. Treatments	2. Encouraging the client to share feelings can provide a safe outlet for fears and frustrations, and can increase self-awareness (Wagner, Johnson, & Kidd, 2006).
3. Provide reliable information and clarify any misconceptions.	3. Misconceptions can needlessly increase anxiety and damage self-concept. Answer all questions honestly.
4. Help client to identify positive attributes and possible new opportunities.	4. Client may tend to focus only on the change in self-image and not on the positive characteristics that contribute to the whole concept of self. The nurse must reinforce these positive aspects and encourage the client to reincorporate them into a new self-concept (Wagner, Johnson, & Kidd, 2006).
5. Assist with hygiene and grooming, as needed.	5. Participation in self-care and planning can aid positive coping.
6. Encourage visitors.	6. Frequent visits by support persons can help the client feel that he or she is still a worthwhile, acceptable person; this should promote a positive self-concept.
7. Help client to identify strategies to increase independence and maintain role responsibilities: a. Prioritizing activities b. Using mobility aids and assistive devices, as needed.	7. A strong component of self-concept is the ability to perform functions expected of one's role, thus decreasing dependency and reducing the need for others' involvement.
8. Prepare significant others for the physical and emotional changes.	8. Others can give support more freely and more realistically if they are prepared (Wagner, Johnson, & Kidd, 2006).
9. Discuss with members of the client's support system the importance of communicating the client's value and importance to them.	9. This will enhance self-esteem and promote adjustment (Lewis et al., 2004).
10. Allow the client's support persons to share their feelings regarding the diagnoses and actual or anticipated effects.	10. Spinal cord injury can negatively affect support persons financially, socially, and emotionally.
11. Assess for signs of negative response to changes in appearance: a. Refusal to discuss loss b. Denial of changes c. Decreased self-care ability d. Social isolation e. Refusal to discuss future	11. These signs may indicate that the client is at high risk for unsuccessful adjustment.
12. Refer an at-risk client for professional counseling.	12. Follow-up therapy may be indicated to assist with adjustment.

Documentation

Progress notes
Present emotional status
Interventions
    Response to interventions

High Risk for Autonomic Dysreflexia Related to Reflex Stimulation of Sympathetic Nervous System Below the Level of Cord Injury Secondary to Loss of Autonomic Control

NOC Neurological Status, Neurological Status: Autonomic, Vital Signs Status

Goal

The client and family will prevent or respond to early signs/symptoms of dysreflexia.

Indicators

- State the factors that cause autonomic dysreflexia.
- Describe the treatment for autonomic dysreflexia.
- Relate when emergency treatment is indicated.

NIC Dysreflexia Management, Vital Signs Monitoring, Emergency Care, Medication Administration

Interventions	Rationales

1. Monitor for signs and symptoms of dysreflexia:
  a. Paroxysmal hypertension (sudden periodic elevated blood pressure: systolic pressure >140 mmHg, diastolic >90 mmHg)
  b. Bradycardia or tachycardia
  c. Diaphoresis
  d. Red splotches on skin above the level of injury
  e. Pallor below the level of injury
  f. Headache
	1. Spasms of the pelvic viscera and arterioles cause vasoconstriction below the level of injury, producing hypertension and pallor. Afferent impulses triggered by high blood pressure cause vagal stimulation, resulting in bradycardia. Baroreceptors in the aortic arch and carotid sinus respond to the hypertension, triggering superficial vasodilation, flushing, diaphoresis, and headache (above the level of cord injury) (Bader & Littlejohns, 2004).

2. If signs of dysreflexia occur, raise the head of the bed, loosen constrictive clothing or restraints, and remove noxious stimuli as follows:
  a. Bladder distention:
    • Check for distended bladder
    • If catheterized, check the catheter for kinks or compression; empty collection bag; irrigate very slowly with only 30 mL of saline solution instilled; replace the catheter if it will not drain.
    • If not catheterized, insert a catheter using dibucaine hydrochloride ointment (Nupercaine). Then remove the 500 mL clamp for 15 minutes; repeat until the bladder is drained. The client may have bladder spasm secondary to urinary tract infection. *NOTE:* Send urine culture before giving Nupercaine.
  b. Fecal impaction:
    • First, apply Nupercaine to the anus and about one inch into the rectum. Wait five to 10 minutes before removing stool.
	2. These interventions aim to reduce cerebral hypertension and induce orthostatic hypotension (Bader & Littlejohns, 2004).
	
	  a. Bladder distention is the most common cause of dysreflexia. Bladder distention can trigger dysreflexia by stimulating sensory receptors. Nupercaine ointment reduces tissue stimulation. Too rapid removal of urine can result in compensatory hypotension.
	
	  b. Fecal impaction prevents stimulation of sensory receptors. It is the second most common cause.

(continued on page 309)

Interventions	Rationales
• Gently check the rectum with a well-lubricated gloved finger. • Insert a rectal suppository, or gently remove the impaction. c. Skin stimulation: Spray the skin lesion triggering dysreflexia with a topical anesthetic agent.	c. Dysreflexia can be triggered by stimulation (e.g., of the glans penis or skin lesions).
3. Continue to monitor blood pressure every three to five minutes.	3. Failure to reverse severe hypertension can result in status epilepticus, cerebrovascular accident, and death (Bader & Littlejohns, 2004; Baird, Keen, & Swearingen, 2005; Wagner, Johnson, & Kidd, 2006).
4. Immediately consult the physician for pharmacological treatment if symptoms or noxious stimuli are not eliminated. Continue to search for cause (e.g., pulmonary embolus).	4. Use an antihypertensive agent with rapid onset and short duration while the causes of autonomic dysreflexia are investigated. Nifedipine and nitrates are the most commonly used agents. The nifedipine used should be in the immediate-release form; sublingual nifedipine may lead to erratic absorption. Other drugs used to treat AD with severe symptoms include hydralazine, mecamylamine, diazoxide, and phenoxybenzamine. If 2% nitroglycerin ointment is used, 1″ may be applied to the skin above the level of the SCI. For monitored settings, the use of IV drip of sodium nitroprusside can be used. Nitropaste is used. Blood pressure is monitored.
5. Initiate health teaching and referrals, as indicated: a. Teach signs and symptoms and treatment of dysreflexia. b. Teach when immediate medical intervention is warranted. c. Explain what situations can trigger dysreflexia (e.g., menstrual cycle, sexual activity, bladder or bowel routines). d. Teach the client to watch for early signs and to intervene immediately. c. Teach the client to observe for early signs of bladder infections and skin lesions (e.g., pressure ulcers or ingrown toenails). f. Advise the client to consult with the physician for long-term pharmacologic management if the client is very vulnerable to dysreflexia. g. The unit should have a protocol and an emergency medication tray for autonomic dysreflexia.	5. Good teaching can help the client and family to successfully prevent or treat dysreflexia at home.

Documentation

Progress notes
    Episodes of autonomic dysreflexia (cause, treatment, response)
Discharge summary record
Client teaching

Interrupted Family Processes Related to Adjustment Requirements, Role Disturbance, and Uncertain Future

NOC Family Coping, Family Normalization, Parenting Performance

Goal

The client and family members will demonstrate or report a functional system of mutual support.

Indicators

- Verbalize feelings regarding the situation.
- Identify signs of family dysfunction.
- Identify appropriate resources to seek when needed.

NIC   Family Involvement Promotion, Coping Enhancement, Family Integrity Promotion, Family Therapy, Counseling, Referral

Interventions	Rationales
1. Convey an understanding of the situation and its impact on the family.	1. Communicating understanding and a sense of caring and concern facilitates trust and strengthens the nurse's relationship with the client and family.
2. Explore family members' perceptions of the situation. Encourage verbalization of feelings such as guilt, anger, helplessness and blame.	2. Verbalization can provide opportunities for clarification and validation of feelings and concerns. This contributes to family unity.
3. Determine if present coping mechanisms are effective.	3. Illness of a family member may cause great changes, which puts the family at high risk for maladaptation.
4. Take steps to promote family strengths: a. Acknowledge the assistance of family members. b. Involve them in the client's care. c. To prevent burnout, encourage time away from care-giving. d. Encourage humor. (Refer to Chapter 4, The Ill Adult: Issues and Responses, for more information.)	4. This can help to maintain the existing family structure and its function as a supportive unit (Wagner, Johnson, & Kidd, 2006; Baird, Keen, & Swearingen, 2005).
5. Assist the family to reorganize roles at home, set new priorities, and redistribute responsibilities.	5. Planning and prioritizing can help to maintain family integrity and reduce stress.
6. Prepare the family for signs of depression, anxiety, anger, and dependency in the client and other family members.	6. Anticipatory guidance can alert members to potential problems before they occur. This enables prompt intervention at early signs.
7. Encourage the family to call on its social network (e.g., friends, relatives, church members) for emotional and other support.	7. Outside assistance may help to reduce the perception that the family must "go it alone."
8. Identify dysfunctional coping mechanisms, such as the following: a. Substance abuse b. Continued denial c. Exploitation of one or more family members d. Separation or avoidance Refer for counseling as necessary.	8. A family with a history of unsuccessful coping may need additional resources. A family with unresolved conflicts prior to diagnosis is at high risk (Wagner, Johnson, & Kidd, 2006; Baird, Keen, & Swearingen, 2005).
9. Provide health education and specific information regarding injury, treatments, procedures, and illness symptoms.	9. Thorough education for the family is necessary to assist in maintaining the client's health and to manage the effects of the disability (Lewis et al., 2004).
10. Direct to community agencies and other sources of assistance (e.g., financial, housekeeping, or direct care), as needed.	10. The family may need assistance to help with management at home.

Documentation

Progress notes
   Present family functioning
   Interventions
     Family's response to interventions
Discharge summary record
   Referrals if indicated

High Risk for Ineffective Sexuality Pattern Related to Physiologic, Sensory, and Psychological Effects of Disability on Sexuality or Function

NOC Body Image, Self-Esteem, Role Performance, Sexual Identity: Acceptance

Goal

The client will report satisfying sexual activity.

Indicators

- Discuss own feelings and partner's concerns regarding sexual functioning.
- Verbalize intention to discuss concerns with partner before discharge.
- Be knowledgeable of alternative means of sexual satisfaction.

NIC Behavior Management: Sexual, Counseling, Sexual Counseling, Emotional Support, Active Listening, Teaching: Sexuality

Interventions	Rationales
1. Initiate a discussion regarding concerns associated with sexuality and sexual function. Use the "PLISSIT" model: P-permission, L-limited I-information, S-pecific, Suggestions, I-intensive, T-therapy/treatment.	1. Many clients are reluctant to discuss sexual matters; initiating discussions demonstrates your empathy and concern (Lewis et al., 2004).
2. Provide accurate information on the effect of the cord injury on sexual functioning.	2. Accurate information can prevent false hope or give real hope, as appropriate.
3. Reaffirm the need for frank discussion between sexual partners.	3. Both partners have fears and concerns about sexual activity. Repressing these feelings affects the relationship negatively.
4. Explain how the client and partner can use role-playing to bring concerns about sex out in the open.	4. Role-playing helps a person gain insight by placing self in the position of another and allows more spontaneous sharing of fears and concerns.
5. Discuss alternate means of sexual satisfaction for the client and partner (e.g., vibrators, touching, oral-genital techniques, and body massage); consider past sexual experiences before suggesting specific techniques.	5. The client and partner can experience sexual satisfaction and gratification through various alternatives to intercourse (Lewis et al., 2004).
6. Encourage the client to consult with others with spinal cord injuries for an exchange of information; refer the client to pertinent literature and organizations.	6. Interacting with others in a similar situation can help to reduce feelings of isolation, provide information on alternative sexual practices, and allow frank sharing of problems and concerns.
7. Provide information on managing bowel and bladder programs prior to sexual intercourse.	7. Performing bowel and bladder routines before sex activities decreases incontinence episodes (Lewis et al., 2004).

(continued on page 312)

Interventions	Rationales
8. Refer the client and partner to a certified sex or mental health professional, if desired.	8. Certain sexual problems require continuing therapy and the advanced knowledge of therapists.
9. Explore birth control options.	9. Because of the risk of thrombophlebitis with the "pill," oral contraceptives are not a good option for an SCI woman.

Documentation

Progress notes
   Dialogues
Discharge summary record
   Referrals, if indicated

Bowel Incontinence: Reflexic Related to Lack of Voluntary Sphincter Control Secondary to Spinal Cord Injury Above the Eleventh Thoracic Vertebra (T11)

NOC Bowel Continence, Tissue Integrity: Skin & Mucous Membranes, Bowel Elimination

Goal

The client will evacuate a soft-formed stool every other day or every third day.

NIC Bowel Incontinence Care, Bowel Training, Bowel Management, Skin Surveillance

Interventions	Rationales
1. Assess previous bowel elimination patterns, diet, and life style.	1. This assessment enables the nurse to plan a bowel program to meet the client's habits and needs.
2. Determine present neurologic and physiologic status and functional levels.	2. Establishing an appropriate bowel program in accordance with the client's functional level and ability helps to reduce frustration.
3. Plan a consistent, appropriate time for elimination. Institute a daily bowel program for five days or until a pattern develops, then an alternate-day program (morning or evening).	3. A routine evacuation schedule decreases or eliminates the chance of involuntary stool passage.
4. Provide privacy and a nonstressful environment.	4. Privacy decreases anxiety and promotes self-image and -esteem.
5. Position in an upright or sitting position, if functionally able. If not functionally able (quadriplegic, tetraplegic), position in left side-lying position; use digital stimulation—gloves, lubricant, or index finger (adults) (Bader & Littlejohns, 2004).	5. Upright positioning facilitates movement of stool by enlisting the aid of gravity and by aiding emptying of the descending colon into the sigmoid colon.
6. For a functionally able client, use assistive devices (e.g., dil stick, digital stimulator, raised commode seat, lubricant and gloves). as appropriate.	6. A digital stimulator and dil stick stimulate the rectal sphincter and lower colon, initiating peristalsis for movement of fecal material.

(continued on page 313)

Interventions	Rationales
7. For a client with upper extremity mobility and abdominal musculature innervation, teach bowel elimination facilitation techniques, as appropriate: a. Valsalva maneuver b. Forward bends c. Sitting push-ups d. Abdominal massage in clockwise manner.	7. These techniques increase intra-abdominal pressure to facilitate passage of stool at evacuation time. a. Do not teach Valsalva maneuver if the client has a cardiac problem (Wagner, Johnson, & Kidd, 2006).
8. Assist with or provide equipment needed for hygiene measures, as necessary.	8. Good hygiene helps to prevent skin breakdown.
9. Maintain an elimination record or a flow sheet of the bowel schedule that includes time, stool characteristics, assistive method(s) used, and number of involuntary stools, if any.	9. Ongoing documentation of elimination schedule and results provides data helpful to bowel program management.
10. Provide reassurance and protection from embarrassment while establishing the bowel program.	10. Reassurance decreases anxiety and promotes self-esteem.
11. Initiate a nutritional consultation; provide a diet high in fluids and fibers. Monitor fluid intake and output.	11. Frequency and consistency of stool are related to fluid and food intake. Fiber increases fecal bulk and enhances water absorption into stool. Adequate dietary fiber and fluid intake promotes firm but soft, well-formed stools and decreases the risk of hard, dry, constipated stools.
12. Provide physical activity and exercise appropriate to the client's functional ability and endurance.	12. Physical activity promotes peristalsis, aids digestion, and facilitates elimination.
13. Teach appropriate use of stool softeners, laxatives, and suppositories; explain the hazards of enemas.	13. Laxatives upset a bowel program because they cause much of the bowel to empty and can cause unscheduled bowel movements. With constant laxative use, the colon loses tone and bowel retraining becomes difficult. Chronic use of bowel aids can lead to irregular stool consistency, which interferes with the scheduled bowel program and bowel management. Stool softeners may not be necessary if diet and fluid intake are adequate. Enemas lead to overstretching of the bowel and loss of bowel tone, contributing to further constipation.
14. Explain the signs and symptoms of fecal impaction and constipation.	14. Fecal impaction and constipation may lead to autonomic dysreflexia in a client with injury at T7 or higher, owing to bowel overdistention. Chronic constipation can lead to overdistention of the bowel with further loss of bowel tone. Unrelieved constipation may result in fecal impaction. Early intervention in diet and fluid intake and in bowel evacuation methods and schedules helps to prevent constipation, further loss of bowel tone, and fecal impaction.
15. Initiate teaching of a bowel program as soon as the client is able to sit up in a wheelchair for 2 to 4 hours. If the client is functionally able, encourage independence with the bowel program; if client is quadriplegic, with limited hand function, incorporate assistive devices or attendant care, as needed.	15. Teaching bowel management techniques, bowel complications, and the impact of diet, fluids, and exercise on elimination can help to promote independent functioning or help the client to instruct others on specific care measures that promote adequate elimination and prevent complications.

Documentation

Flow records
   Stool results (time, method used, involuntary stools)

Discharge summary record
Client teaching
Outcome achievement or status

Bowel Incontinence: Areflexia Related to Lack of Voluntary Sphincter Secondary to Spinal Cord Injury Involving Sacral Reflex Arc (S2–S4)

NOC Bowel Continence, Tissue Integrity: Skin & Mucous Membranes, Bowel Elimination

Goal

The client will evacuate a firm, formed stool every day.

Indicator

• Relate bowel elimination techniques.

NIC Bowel Incontinence Care, Bowel Training, Bowel Management, Skin Surveillance

Interventions	Rationales
1. Assess previous bowel elimination patterns, diet, and life style.	1. This assessment enables the nurse to plan a bowel program to meet the client's habits and needs.
2. Determine present neurologic and physiologic statuses and functional levels.	2. Establishing an appropriate bowel program in accordance with the client's functional level and ability helps to reduce frustration.
3. Plan a consistent, appropriate time for elimination. Institute a *daily* bowel program.	3. A routine evacuation schedule decreases or eliminates the chance of involuntary stool passage. Evacuating any stool in rectum before periods of activity can prevent accidents. A major evacuation should be performed daily (Wagner, Johnson, & Kidd, 2006; Baird, Keen, & Swearingen, 2005).
4. Provide privacy and a nonstressful environment.	4. Privacy decreases anxiety and promotes self-image and -esteem.
5. Position in an upright or sitting position as soon as client's condition warrants.	5. Upright positioning facilitates movement of stool by enlisting the aid of gravity and by aiding emptying of the descending colon into the sigmoid colon.
6. Digitally (manually) empty the rectum with a gloved and well-lubricated finger.	6. Techniques used to trigger a stimulus–response reflex, such as digital stimulation or suppository administration, are not effective with an areflexic bowel because of the absence of the sacral reflex arc.
7. Teach bowel elimination facilitation techniques: a. Valsalva maneuver b. Forward bends c. Sitting push-ups d. Abdominal massage in clockwise manner	7. These techniques increase intra-abdominal pressure to facilitate stool passage at evacuation time. Upper-extremity function should be intact with this level of lesion, and thus the client can assume responsibility for the procedure. a. Do not teach Valsalva maneuver if client has a cardiac problem (Wagner, Johnson, & Kidd, 2006).
8. Assist with or provide equipment needed for hygiene measures, as necessary.	8. Good hygiene helps to prevent skin breakdown.

(continued on page 315)

Interventions	Rationales
9. Maintain an elimination record or a flow sheet of the bowel schedule that includes time, stool characteristics, assistive method(s) used, and number of involuntary stools, if any.	9. Ongoing documentation of elimination schedule and results provides data helpful to bowel program management.
10. Provide reassurance and protection from embarrassment while establishing the bowel program.	10. Reassurance decreases anxiety and promotes self-esteem.
11. Initiate a nutritional consultation; provide a diet high in fluids and fibers. Monitor fluid intake and output.	11. Frequency and consistency of stool are related to fluid and food intake. Fiber increases fecal bulk and enhances water absorption into the stool. Adequate dietary fiber and fluid intake promotes firm but soft, well-formed stools and decreases the risk of hard, dry, constipated stools.
12. Provide physical activity and exercise appropriate to the client's functional ability and endurance.	12. Physical activity promotes peristalsis, aids digestion, and facilitates elimination.
13. Teach appropriate use of stool softeners and laxatives; explain the hazards of enemas.	13. Laxatives upset a bowel program because they cause much of the bowel to empty and can cause unscheduled bowel movements. With constant laxative use, the colon loses tone and bowel retraining becomes difficult. Chronic use of bowel aids can lead to inconsistent stool consistency, which interferes with the scheduled bowel program and bowel management. Stool softeners may not be necessary if diet and fluid intake are adequate. Enemas lead to over-stretching of the bowel and loss of bowel tone, contributing to further constipation.
14. Explain the signs and symptoms of fecal impaction and constipation.	14. Bowel motility is decreased in lower motor neuron (LMN) cord damage; decreased stool movement through the colon can result in increased fluid absorption from stool, resulting in hard, dry stools and constipation. Unrelieved constipation may result in fecal impaction. Early intervention in diet and fluid intake and in bowel evacuation methods and schedules helps to prevent constipation, further loss of bowel tone, and fecal impaction.
15. Initiate teaching of a bowel program when the client is mobile (wheelchair or ambulation). Encourage independence with the bowel program.	15. Teaching bowel management techniques, bowel complications, and the impact of diet, fluids, and exercise on elimination can help to promote independent functioning, or help the client to instruct others in specific care measures that promote adequate elimination and prevent complications.

Documentation

Flow records
    Consistency of stool
    Amount of stool
    Time of evacuation
    Time and number of involuntary stools if any
    Any leakage of stool from rectum
    Bowel sounds
    Intake and output
    Assistive devices, if any
Progress notes
    Unsatisfactory results/toleration of procedure
    Evidence of hemorrhoids, bleeding, abnormal sacral skin appearance

Discharge summary record
Client teaching

High Risk for Ineffective Therapeutic Regimen Management Related to Insufficient Knowledge of the Effects of Altered Skin, Bowel, Bladder, Respiratory, Thermoregulatory, and Sexual Function and Their Management; Signs and Symptoms of Complications; Follow-up Care; and Community Resources

NOC Compliance Behavior, Knowledge: Treatment Regimen, Participation in Health Care Decisions, Treatment Behavior: Illness or Injury

Goals

The goals for this diagnosis represent those associated with discharge planning. Refer to the discharge criteria.

NIC Anticipatory Guidance, Learning Facilitation, Risk Identification, Health Education, Teaching: Procedure/Treatment, Health System Guidance

Interventions	Rationales
1. Explain the effects of injury on bowel, bladder, thermoregulation, respiratory system, and integumentary functions.	1. This information may encourage the client and family to comply with the therapeutic regimen.
2. Assist in formulating and accepting realistic short- and long-term goals.	2. Mutual goal-setting reinforces the client's sense of control over her or his life.
3. Evaluate the client's and family member's or significant other's ability to perform the following: a. Skin care and assessment b. Bowel program c. Bladder program d. Proper positioning e. Transfer techniques f. Application of abdominal binder, antiembolic hose, splints, and protectors g. Range-of-motion exercises (active and passive) h. Assisted coughing techniques	3. These skills are essential to an effective home management program.
4. Reinforce teaching about dysreflexia and its treatment.	4. Reinforcement promotes feelings of competency and confidence.
5. Explain the reasons for temperature fluctuations and risks of hypothermia and hyperthermia.	5. Interruption in the sympathetic system disrupts the vasoconstriction or vasodilatation response to temperature changes. Also, diaphoresis is absent below the level of cord injury. As a result, the client's body assumes the temperature of the environment (poikilothermia).
6. Explain the importance of a well-balanced diet with caloric intake appropriate for activity level.	6. A well-balanced diet is needed to maintain tissue integrity, prevent complications (e.g., skin problems, infection, osteoporosis), and prevent weight gain.

(continued on page 317)

Interventions	Rationales
7. Instruct client to report the following: a. Cloudy, foul-smelling urine b. Unresolved signs of dysreflexia c. Fever, chills d. Green, purulent, or rust-colored sputum e. Nausea and vomiting f. Persistent skin lesion or irritation g. Swelling and redness of lower extremities h. Increased restriction of movement i. Unsatisfactory bowel or bladder results	7. Early detection of complications enables prompt interventions to prevent debilitating results. Complications can include infections (urinary tract, respiratory, or GI), thrombophlebitis, pressure ulcers, contractures, and dysreflexia.
8. Emphasize the need to participate in the scheduled rehabilitation plan.	8. With training and assistance, most spinal cord-injured clients can attain some degree of independence in activities of daily living.
9. Initiate a referral for assistance with home care (e.g., community nurses, social service).	9. Regardless of the success experienced in the hospital, the client and family need assistance with adjustment postdischarge.
10. Provide information on self-help sessions and hand out printed material, such as the following: a. National Spinal Cord Injury Association, 1 Church Street, Suite 600, Rockville, MD 20850, 1-800-962-9629 b. *Yes, You Can! A Guide To Self-Care for Persons with Spinal Cord Injury* Paralyzed Veterans of America (National Headquarters), 801 Eighteenth Street, N.W., Washington, DC 20006, 1-800-424-8200 c. Spinal Network, P.O. Box 4162, Boulder, CO 80306, 1-800-338-5412	10. Specialized organizations and resources can provide timely information on a variety of related issues or problems.

Documentation

Discharge summary record
    Client teaching
    Outcome achievement or status
    Referrals, if indicated

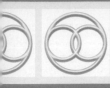

Sickle Cell Disease

Sickle cell disease (SCD) is an incurable genetic disorder affecting approximately 1 of every 375 African Americans. The term *sickle cell disease* actually represents a group of disorders characterized by the production of hemoglobin S (Hb S). Under certain conditions, this hemoglobin leads to anemia and acute and chronic tissue damage secondary to the "sickling"—that is, turning into the sickle form—of the abnormal red cells. Hemoglobin S molecules tend to bond to one another and to hemoglobin A, forming long aggregates or tactoids. These aggregates increase the viscosity of blood, causing stasis in blood flow. The low oxygen tension concentration of Hb S causes the cells to assume a sickle rather than a biconcave shape. This hemoglobin damages erythrocyte membranes, leading to erythrocyte rupture and chronic hemolytic anemia (Porth, 2005).

Symptoms of sickle cell anemia result from thrombosis and infarction, leading to vascular occlusion by the "sickled" cells and the hemolytic anemia. These episodes are called *sickle cell crises*. The incidence of sickle cell crises varies among clients. Some report an incident once a year, whereas others report more than one each month.

In the United States the disease is primarily seen among African Americans, but may also be found among people of Mediterranean, Caribbean, South and Central American, and East Indian descent (U.S. Department of Health, 1992). This chronic disease leaves its victims not only debilitated, but also with a shortened life span. Presently the disease has no cure, but some options are available for altering its course.

Clients can carry the sickle cell trait but not have the disease. These asymptomatic people have reported some sickling symptoms in low oxygen (e.g., unpressurized airplanes, high altitudes, scuba diving).

 Time Frame
Acute sickling crisis

■■■■■■ DIAGNOSTIC CLUSTER

Collaborative Problems

△ PC: Acute Chest Syndrome
△ PC: Infection
✳ PC: Anemia
✳ Vaso-occlusive Crisis
✳ Aplastic Crisis
✳ PC: Leg Ulcers
✳ PC: Neurologic Dysfunction
✳ PC: Splenic Dysfunction
✳ Avascular Necrosis of Femoral/Humeral Heads
✳ Priapism

Nursing Diagnoses

▲ Acute Pain related to viscous blood and tissue hypoxia

△ High Risk for Ineffective Therapeutic Regimen Management related to insufficient knowledge of disease process, risk factors for sickling crisis, pain management, signs and symptoms of complications, genetic counseling, and family planning services

✳ Powerlessness related to future development of complications of SCD (refer to Diabetes Mellitus)

▲ This diagnosis was reported to be monitored for or managed frequently (75%–100%).
△ This diagnosis was reported to be monitored for or managed often (50%–74%).
✳ This diagnosis was not included in the validation study.

Discharge Criteria

Before discharge, the client or family will

1. Identify precipitating factors of present crisis, if possible.
2. Plan one change in life style to reduce crisis or to improve health.
3. Describe signs and symptoms that must be reported to a health care professional.
4. Describe necessary health maintenance and follow-up care.

Collaborative Problems

Potential Complication: Anemia

Potential Complication: Sickle Cell Crisis

Potential Complication: Acute Chest Syndrome

Potential Complication: Infection

Potential Complication: Leg Ulcers

Potential Complication: Neurologic Dysfunction

Potential Complication: Splenic Dysfunction

Potential Complication: Osteonecrosis

Nursing Goal

The nurse will detect early signs and symptoms of (a) anemia, (b) vaso-occlusive crisis, (c) acute chest syndrome, (d) aplastic anemia, (e) infection, (f) leg ulcers, (g) neurologic dysfunction, (h) splenic dysfunction, (i) priapism, and (j) osteonecrosis (femoral/humeral heads) and collaboratively intervene to stabilize client.

Indicators

- Hemoglobin (a, b, d)
  - Males: 13–18 gm/dL
  - Females: 12–16 gm/dL
- Hematocrit (a, b, d)
  - Males: 42%–50%
  - Females: 40%–48%
- Red blood cells (a, b, d)
  - Males: 4.6–5.9 million/mm³
  - Females: 4.2–5.4 million/mm³
- Platelets 150,000–400,000/mm³ (e)
- White blood cells 4,300–10,800/mm³ (e)
- Oxygen saturation >95% (a, b, c, d)
- No or minimal bone pain (b, e, j)
- No or minimal abdominal pain (b, e, h)
- No or minimal chest pain (c)
- No or minimal fatigue (a, b, e)
- Pinkish, ruddy, brownish, or olive skin tones (a, b)
- No or minimal headache (b, g)
- Clear, oriented (b, g)
- Clear speech (b, g)
- Pulse rate 60–100 beats/min (a, b, c, g, h)
- Respirations 16–20 breaths/min (b, c, e, g)
- BP >90/60, <140/90 mmHg (a, b, c, g, h)
- Temperature 98–99.5°F (b, a, e, f, j)
- Urine output >5 mL/kg/h (b, c, h)
- Urine specific gravity 1.005–1.030 (b, c, h)
- Flaccid penis (i)

Interventions	Rationales

1. Monitor for signs and symptoms of anemia.
  a. Lethargy
  b. Weakness
  c. Fatigue
  d. Increased pallor
  e. Dyspnea on exertion
	1. Because anemia is common with most of these clients, low hemoglobins are relatively tolerated; therefore, changes should be described in reference to a client's baseline or acute symptoms (Porth, 2005).

2. Monitor laboratory values, including complete blood cell count (CBC) with reticulocyte count.	2. Elevated reticulocytes (normal level about 1%) indicate active erythropoiesis. Lack of elevation with anemia may represent a problem (Porth, 2005).

3. Monitor for vaso-occlusive crisis:
  a. Abdominal pain
  b. Chest pain
  c. Bones, joints
	3. Sickle cells block capillaries and cause pain by infarction.

4. Obtain:
  a. Chest x-ray
  b. Abdominal x-ray
  c. CBC with differential
  d. Electrolytes
  e. BUN (blood urea nitrogen)
  f. Liver function test
	4. Other causes of pain (e.g., appendicitis) must be ruled out first.

5. Monitor:
  a. Oxygen saturation with pulse oximetry
 	
  b. Hydration status (urine output, specific gravity)
 	
  c. Level of consciousness
	5.
	  a. O_2 should be administered only if oxygen saturation is less than 95%.
	  b. Increased hydration is needed to mobilize clustered cells and improve tissue perfusion.
	  c. Glasgow Coma Scale can be used to detect cerebral infarction.

6. Aggressively hydrate client (1.5 × maintenance volume). Avoid IV therapy, if possible.	6. Hydration can disrupt the clustered cells and improve hypoxemia.

7. Monitor for signs and symptoms of acute chest syndrome:
  a. Fever
  b. Acute chest pain
  c. Cough
	7. Acute chest syndrome is the term used to represent this group of symptoms, namely, acute pleuritic chest pain, fever, leukocytosis, and infiltrates on chest x-ray seen in SCD. This represents a medical emergency and may be caused by "sickling" leading to pulmonary infarction (Porth, 2005).

8. Teach client how to use incentive spirometer and its importance.	8. Incentive spirometry has been shown to help prevent acute chest syndrome.

9. Monitor for signs and symptoms of infection:
  a. Fever
  b. Pain
  c. Chills
  d. Increased white blood cells
	9. Bacterial infection is one major cause of morbidity and mortality. Decreased functioning of the spleen (asplenia) results from sickle cell anemia. The loss of the spleen's ability to filter and to destroy various infectious organisms increases the risk of infection.

10. Monitor for aplastic crisis:
  a. CBC with differential
  b. Pallor
  c. Tachycardia
	10. With infection (e.g., Parvovirus B19), production of RBCs pauses temporarily, causing even more severe acute anemia (Newcombe, 2002).

(continued on page 321)

Interventions	Rationales
11. Monitor for signs and symptoms of leg ulcers: 　a. Hyperpigmentation 　b. Skin wrinkling 　c. Pruritus, tenderness	11. Leg ulcers can occur in 50%–75% of older children and adults with sickle cell anemia. Minor leg trauma can result in localized edema and compression of the tissue around the injury. Capillary blood flow is decreased, causing increased arterial pressure. This increased pressure causes some arterial blood carrying oxygen to the tissue to be redirected to the veins without reaching the injured area. Skin grafting may be needed (Waterbury, 2003).
12. Monitor for changes in neurologic function: 　a. Speech disturbances 　b. Sudden headache 　c. Numbness, tingling	12. Cerebral infarction and intracranial hemorrhage are complications of SCD. Occlusion of nutrient arteries to major cerebral arteries causes progressive wall damage and eventual occlusion of the major vessel. Intracerebral hemorrhage may be secondary to hypoxic necrosis of vessel walls (Porth, 2005).
13. Monitor for splenic dysfunction.	13. The spleen is responsible for filtering blood to remove old bacteria. Sluggish circulation and increased viscosity of sickle cells causes splenic blockage. The spleen's normal acidic and anoxic environment stimulates sickling, which increases blood flow obstruction.
14. Monitor for splenic sequestration crisis: 　a. Sudden onset of lassitude 　b. Very pale, listless 　c. Rapid pulse 　d. Shallow respirations 　e. Low blood pressure	14. Increased blood obstruction from the spleen together with rapid sickling can cause sudden pooling of blood into the spleen. This causes intravascular hypovolemia and hypoxia, progressing to shock.
15. Intervene for priapism. 　a. Provide analgesics, sedation. 　b. Maintain hydration. 　c. Apply ice packs to penis. 　d. Prepare for needle aspiration of blood from corpora cavernosa. 　e. Prepare for surgical intervention if previous interventions are unsuccessful.	15. Sickle cells impairing blood flow cause priapism (involuntary, prolonged, abnormal, and painful erection). Persistent stasis priapism not resolved in 24–48 hours can cause permanent erectile dysfunction (Waterbury, 2003). 　a. Sedation may cause tissue relaxation and improve perfusion. 　b. Hydration can mobilize cluster cells. 　c. Icing can reduce edema and improve perfusion. 　d. Removal of clustered sickle cells can improve circulation. 　e. Shunting by incision of dorsal arteries of penis may be needed to prevent tissue necrosis.
16. Monitor for osteonecrosis and instruct client to report any of the following: 　a. Bone pain (hip, leg) 　b. Fever 　c. Limited movement	16. Osteonecrosis is death of tissue from decreased circulation secondary to clustered sickle cells. Symptomatic osteonecrosis of the femoral head is a rapidly progressive disease that requires an orthopedic surgical consultation (Hernigou, Bachir, & Galacteros, 2003).

 ## Related Physician-Prescribed Interventions

Medications. Anti-sickling agents, analgesics, folic acid, hydroxyurea

Intravenous Therapy. Exchange transfusions

Laboratory Studies. CBC, liver function tests, hemoglobin electrophoresis, serum iron, erythrocyte sedimentation rate, arterial blood gases, peripheral blood smear

Diagnostic Studies. Depend on complications (e.g., CVA, Head CT, MRI)

Therapies. Depend on complications, bone marrow/stem cell transplantation, recombinant human erythropoietin (r-HuEPO), L-arginine therapy, steroid therapy

Documentation

Flow records
    Skin assessment
    Neurologic
    Vital signs
Progress notes
    Abnormal findings
    Interventions
    Evaluation

Nursing Diagnoses

Acute Pain Related to Viscous Blood and Tissue Hypoxia

NOC Comfort Level, Pain Control

Goal

The client will report decreased pain after pain-relief measures.

Indicators

- Relate factors that increase pain.
- Relate factors that can precipitate pain.

NIC Pain Management, Medication Management, Emotional Support, Teaching: Individual, Heat/Cold Application, Simple Massage

Interventions	Rationales
1. Explore with client if the painful episode is "typical" or "unusual."	1. Most clients have a distinctive, unique pattern of pain. Changes may indicate another complication (e.g., infection, abdominal surgical emergency).
2. Assess for any signs of infection (e.g., respiratory, urinary, vaginal).	2. Painful events often occur with infection.
3. Aggressively manage acute pain episodes. Consult with physician or advanced practice nurse.	3. The pain of SCD, like the pain of cancer, should be treated based on client's tolerance and discretion (Waterbury, 2003).
4. Provide narcotic analgesic every 2 hours (not PRN). Consider client-controlled analgesic.	4. People with sickle cells metabolize narcotics rapidly (Waterbury, 2003).
5. Provide an initial bolus dose of a narcotic analgesic (e.g., morphine) followed by continuous low-dose narcotic or dosing at fixed intervals.	5. A continuous serum level of narcotic is needed to control pain (Jenkins, 2002).
6. Avoid meperidine (Demerol).	6. Meperidine contains the metabolite normeperide that the kidney must excrete; increased levels are associated with increased seizures (Jenkins, 2002).
7. After the acute pain crisis, taper narcotics.	7. This will help to minimize physical dependence (Jenkins, 2002).

(continued on page 323)

Interventions	Rationales
8. Discuss complementary therapies and provide community sources if desired for: • Relaxation techniques, massage, yoga • Acupuncture, biofeedback • Music therapy • Prayer • Herbal remedies • Transcutaneous Electric Nerve Stimulation (TENS)	8. These can be useful adjuncts to a pain management program.
9. Refer to High Risk for Ineffective Therapeutic Regimen Management of Chronic Pain postdischarge.	9. Using an objective scoring system helps to evaluate a subjective experience.
10. Assess level of pain using a 0 to 10 scale before and after analgesics. 11. Evaluate whether or not pain is decreasing.	10,11. The pain of sickling should decrease. A decrease in the pain score of 2 or more points is an indication to reduce the narcotic analgesic (Ballas & Delengowski, 1993).

Documentation

Medication administration record
    Type, route, and dosage of all medications
Progress notes
    Status of pain
    Degree of relief from pain-relief measures

High Risk for Ineffective Therapeutic Regimen Management Related to Insufficient Knowledge of Disease Process, Risk Factors for Sickling Crisis, Pain Management, Signs and Symptoms of Complications, Genetic Counseling, and Family Planning Services

NOC Compliance Behavior, Knowledge: Treatment Regimen, Participation in Health Care Decisions, Treatment Behavior: Illness or Injury

Goals

The goals for this diagnosis represent those associated with discharge planning. Refer to the discharge criteria.

NIC Anticipatory Guidance, Risk Identification, Health Education, Learning Facilitation

Interventions	Rationales
1. Review present situation, disease process, and treatment.	1. Even though the client has had the disease since childhood, the nurse should evaluate present knowledge.

2. Discuss precipitating factors.
  a. High altitude (more than 7000 feet above sea level)
  b. Unpressurized aircraft
  c. Dehydration (e.g., diaphoresis, diarrhea, vomiting)
  d. Strenuous physical activity
  e. Cold temperatures (e.g., iced liquids)
	2.
	  a,b. Decreased oxygen tension can cause red blood cells to sickle.
	  c,d. Any situation that causes dehydration or increases blood viscosity can precipitate sickling.
	  e. Cold causes peripheral vasoconstriction, which slows circulation.

(continued on page 324)

Interventions	Rationales
f. Infection (e.g., respiratory, urinary, vaginal) g. Ingestion of alcohol h. Cigarette smoking	f. The exact mechanism is unknown. g. Alcohol use promotes dehydration. h. Nicotine interferes with oxygen exchange.
3. Emphasize the need to drink at least 16 cups (8 oz) of fluid daily and to increase to 24–32 cups during a painful crisis or when at risk for dehydration.	3. Dehydration must be prevented to prevent a sickling crisis (Marchiondo & Thompson, 1996).
4. Discuss the importance of maintaining optimal health. a. Regular health care professional examinations (e.g., ophthalmic, general) b. Good nutrition c. Stress reduction methods d. Dental hygiene e. Immunization	4. Adhering to a health maintenance plan can reduce risk factors that contribute to crisis.
5. Explain the importance of an eye examination every 6 to 12 months.	5. SCD can cause retinopathy by plugging small retinal vessels and causing neovascularization (Porth, 2005).
6. Explain the susceptibility to infection.	6. Certain organisms (e.g., salmonella) thrive in diminished oxygen status. Phagocytosis, which is dependent on oxygen, is inhibited with SCD (Porth, 2005).
7. Stress the importance of reporting signs and symptoms of infection early. a. Persistent cough b. Fever c. Foul-smelling vaginal drainage d. Cloudy, reddish, or foul-smelling urine e. Increased redness of wound f. Purulent drainage	7. Early recognition and treatment may prevent a crisis.
8. After crisis, help the client identify some warning signs that occur days or hours before a crisis.	8. Most clients with SCD experience a prodromal stage (a gradual buildup of symptoms for days before a crisis). More commonly, however, symptoms begin less than 1 hour before a crisis (Newcombe, 2002).
9. Instruct the client to provide prompt treatment of cuts, insect bites, and the like.	9. Decreased peripheral circulation increases the risk of infection.
10. Instruct to report: a. Any acute illness b. Severe joint or bone pain c. Chest pain d. Abdominal pain e. Headaches, dizziness f. Gastric distress	10. These symptoms may indicate vaso-occlusion in varied sites from sickling. Some illnesses may predispose a client to dehydration.
11. Provide access to training for new coping strategies: a. Relaxation breathing b. Imagery c. Calming self statements d. Mental counting technique e. Focus on physical surroundings f. Reinterpretation of pain sensations	11. Individuals who practice selected coping strategies during pain episodes tend to have less need for ER management (Gil, Carson, Sedway, et al., 2000).

(continued on page 3

Interventions	Rationales
12. Advise client to practice coping strategies daily, regardless of pain level.	12. Practice is needed to improve efficiency of the strategy when it is needed (Gil et al., 2000).
13. Explore the client's knowledge regarding the genetic aspects of the disease. Refer to appropriate resource (e.g., genetic counseling).	13. This disease is hereditary. The incidence of offspring inheriting SCD is related to parents as carriers or noncarriers of the hemoglobin genotype AS.
14. Explore with the client the effects of SCD on family, roles, occupation, and personal goals.	14. Clients with SCD tend to experience it personally and have witnessed its effects on others. This chronic disease regularly challenges client and family functioning. Adults are at risk for poor psychological adjustment.
15. Refer to community support groups and appropriate agencies (e.g., Sickle Cell Disease Association of America [www.sicklecelldisease.org], American Sickle Cell Anemia Association [www.ascaa.org]).	15. Successful coping is promoted by witnessing others successfully coping, and others believing that they will be successful (Bandura, 1982).

Documentation

Discharge summary record
    Client teaching
    Outcome achievement
    Referrals if indicated

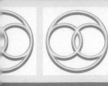

Pressure Ulcers

Pressure ulcers are localized areas of cellular necrosis that tend to occur from prolonged compression of soft tissue between a bony prominence and a firm surface—most commonly as a result of immobility. Injury ranges from nonblanchable erythema of intact skin to deep ulceration extending to the bone. Extrinsic factors that exert mechanical force on soft tissue include pressure, shear, friction, and maceration. Intrinsic factors that determine susceptibility to tissue breakdown include malnutrition, anemia, loss of sensation, impaired mobility, advanced age, decreased mental status, incontinence, and infection. Extrinsic and intrinsic factors interact to produce ischemia and necrosis of soft tissue in susceptible persons (Agency for Health Care Policy Research [AHCPR], 1994; Berlowitz, 2007a; Maklebust & Sieggreen, 2001).

 Time Frame
Secondary diagnosis

▪▪▪▪▪▪ DIAGNOSTIC CLUSTER

Collaborative Problems

▲ PC: Sepsis

Nursing Diagnoses	Refer to
▲ Impaired Tissue Integrity related to mechanical destruction of tissue secondary to pressure, shear, or friction	
▲ Impaired Physical Mobility related to imposed restrictions, deconditioned status, loss of motor control, or altered mental status	
▲ Imbalanced Nutrition: Less Than Body Requirements related to insufficient oral intake	Thermal Injury
▲ High Risk for Infection related to exposure of ulcer base to fecal/urinary drainage	
△ High Risk for Ineffective Therapeutic Regimen Management related to insufficient knowledge of etiology, prevention, treatment, and home care	

Related Nursing Care Plan

Immobility or Unconsciousness

▲ This diagnosis was reported to be monitored for or managed frequently (75%–100%).
△ This diagnosis was reported to be monitored for or managed often (50%–74%).

Discharge Criteria

Before discharge, the client or family will

1. Identify factors that contribute to ulcer development.
2. Demonstrate the ability to perform skills necessary to prevent and treat pressure ulcers.
3. State the intent to continue prevention and treatment strategies at home (e.g., activity, nutrition).

Collaborative Problems

Potential Complication: Sepsis

Nursing Goal

The nurse will monitor for signs/symptoms of sepsis and collaboratively intervene to stabilize the client.

Indicators

- Temperature 98–99.5°F
- Heart rate 60–100 beats/min
- Blood pressure >90/60, <140/90 mmHg
- Respiration 16–20 breaths/min
- Urine output >5 mL/kg/h
- Clear urine
- Negative blood culture
- White blood count 4300–10,800 cells/mm³
- Oriented, alert

Interventions	Rationales
1. Monitor for signs and symptoms of sepsis: a. Temperature >101°F or <98.6°F b. Tachycardia (>90 beats/min) and tachypnea (>20 breaths/min) c. Pale, cool skin d. Decreased urine output e. WBCs and bacteria in urine f. Positive blood culture g. Elevated white blood count >12,000 cells/mm³ or decreased WBC <4000 cells/mm³ h. Confusion, changes in mentation	1. Gram-positive and gram-negative organisms can invade open wounds; debilitated clients are more vulnerable. Response to sepsis results in massive vasodilation with hypovolemia, resulting in tissue hypoxia and decreased renal function and cardiac output. This, in turn triggers a compensatory response of increased heart rate and respirations to correct hypoxia and acidosis. Bacteria in urine or blood indicate infection. h. These may be the only signs in older adults.

 ### Related Physician-Prescribed Interventions

Medications. Topical or oral antibiotics, proteolytic enzymes, pharmacologic therapy (depending on laboratory results, analgesics)

Intravenous Therapy. Intravenous antibiotics

Laboratory Studies. Tissue cultures, blood cultures

Therapies. Topical skin barriers; wound care; pressure-relief systems (air-fluidized bed, low-air-loss bed, kinetic bed); ulcer care; folic acid; thiamine, topical growth factors, electrotherapy, negative pressure wound therapy (e.g., wound vac), radiant heat bandages, normothermic wound therapy, ultrasound, hyperbaric oxygen (HBO) therapy, infrared and ultraviolet light therapy, hydrotherapy, debridement (chemical, manual, or surgical) and surgical interventions (e.g., grafting).

Documentation

Flow records
 Vital signs

Nursing Diagnoses

Impaired Tissue Integrity Related to Mechanical Destruction of Tissue Secondary to Pressure, Shear, or Friction

NOC Tissue Integrity: Skin & Mucous Membranes

Goal

The client will demonstrate progressive healing of tissue.

Indicators

- Participate in risk assessment.
- Express willingness to participate in prevention of pressure ulcers.
- Describe etiology and prevention measures.
- Explain rationale for interventions.

NIC   Teaching: Individual, Surveillance

Interventions	Rationales
1. Apply pressure ulcer prevention principles:	1. Principles of pressure ulcer prevention include reducing or rotating pressure on soft tissue. If pressure on soft tissue exceeds intracapillary pressure (approximately 32 mmHg), capillary occlusion and resulting hypoxia can cause tissue damage.
a. Encourage range-of-motion (ROM) exercise and weight-bearing mobility when possible.	a,b. Exercise and mobility increase blood flow to all areas.
b. Promote optimal mobility (AHCPR, 1994; Berlowitz, 2007a). (Refer to the Impaired Mobility care plan for more information.)	
c. Keep the bed as flat as possible (lower than 30 degrees) and support feet with a footboard (AHCPR, 1994; Berlowitz, 2007b).	c. These measures help prevent shear, the pressure created when two adjacent tissue layers move in opposition. If a bony prominence slides across the subcutaneous tissue, the subepidermal capillaries may become bent and pinched, resulting in decreased tissue perfusion.
d. Avoid using a knee gatch.	d. A knee gatch may promote blood pooling and decrease circulation in the lower extremities.
e. Use foam blocks or pillows to provide a bridging effect to support the body above and below the high-risk or ulcerated area; this prevents the affected area from touching the bed surface (Berlowitz, 2007b). Do not use foam donuts or inflatable rings (AHCPR, 1994; Crewe, 1987; National Pressure Ulcer Advisory Panel, 2001a, 2001b).	e. This measure helps to distribute pressure to a larger area.
f. Alternate or reduce pressure on the skin surface with devices such as these (Berlowitz, 2007b; National Pressure Ulcer Advisory Panel, 2001b): • Air mattresses • Low-air-loss beds • Air-fluidized beds • Vascular boots or pillow under calf to suspend heels off the bed surface	f. Foam mattresses (e.g., egg-crate type) are for comfort; they generally do not provide adequate pressure relief. Special air mattresses and air beds redistribute the body weight evenly across the body surface (Berlowitz, 2007b; Maklebust & Sieggreen, 2001).
g. Use sufficient personnel to lift the client up in bed or chair without sliding or pulling the skin surface. Use long sleeves or stockings to reduce friction on elbows and heels.	g. Proper transfer technique reduces friction forces that can rub away or abrade skin.
h. Instruct a sitting client to lift him- or herself using the chair arms every 10 minutes, if possible, or assist the client in rising up off the chair every 10–20 minutes, depending on risk factors present (National Pressure Ulcer Advisory Panel, 2001a).	h. This measure allows periodic reperfusion of ischemic areas.
i. Do not elevate the client's legs unless the calves are supported. Support the client's calves and align the hip and knee bone while helping him or her to sit on a chair, to avoid shifting weight to the ischial tuberosities.	i. Supporting the calves reduces pressure over the ischial tuberosities (AHCPR, 1994).

(continued on page 329)

Interventions	Rationales
j. Pad the chair with a pressure-relieving device (Berlowitz, 2007b).	j. Ischial tuberosities are prime areas for pressure ulcer development. Air cushions provide better pressure relief than foam cushions.
k. Inspect other areas at risk for developing ulcers with each position change: • Ears • Elbows • Occiput • Trochanter • Heels • Ischia • Sacrum • Scapula • Scrotum	k. A client with one pressure ulcer is at increased risk for developing others.
l. When positioned on side, the client should be placed at a 30-degree angle (Berlowitz, 2007b).	l. This reduces pressure on greater trochanter (Berlowitz, 2007b).
m. Consider physical therapy for immobilized clients (Berlowitz, 2007b).	m. Clients may benefit from physical therapy to improve mobility (Berlowitz, 2007b).
2. Observe for erythema and blanching and palpate surrounding area for warmth and tissue sponginess with each position change.	2. Warmth and sponginess are signs of tissue damage.
3. Compensate for sensory deficits: a. Inspect the client's skin every 2 hours for signs of injury. b. Teach the client and family members to inspect the skin frequently. Show the client how to use a mirror to inspect hard-to-see areas.	3. a. An immobilized client may have impaired sensation; this interferes with the ability to perceive pain from skin damage. b. Regular skin inspection enables early detection of damage. The client's involvement promotes responsibility for self-care.
4. Identify the stage of pressure ulcer development (Berlowitz, 2007a; National Pressure Ulcer Advisory Panel, 2007b). Take photographs of the wound/s as aids in tracking changes (Berlowitz, 2007b). a. Stage I: nonblanchable erythema of intact skin b. Stage II: ulceration of epidermis or dermis not involving underlying subcutaneous fat (partial thickness) (National Pressure Ulcer Advisory Panel, 2007b) c. Stage III: ulceration involving subcutaneous fat or fascia (full-thickness) (National Pressure Ulcer Advisory Panel, 2007b) d. Stage IV: extensive ulceration penetrating muscle and bone (full-thickness with exposed bone, tendon, or muscle) (National Pressure Ulcer Advisory Panel, 2007b) e. Unstageable: Full-thickness tissue loss with the wound bed covered with slough (green, yellow, tan, gray, or brown) and/or eschar (tan, black, or brown). Wound cannot be staged without debridement and cleaning (National Pressure Ulcer Advisory Panel, 2007b). f. Suspected Deep Tissue Injury: Localized purple- or maroon-colored, intact skin or blood-filled blister due to damage of underlying tissue from pressure and/or shear. The affected area may be painful, firm, mushy, boggy, cooler, or warmer than surrounding areas (National Pressure Ulcer Advisory Panel, 2007b). May be difficult to detect in dark skin tones (Berlowitz, 2007a).	4. Staging is a standardized communication tool that denotes the anatomic depth of tissue involvement and amount of tissue loss (Berlowitz, 2007a; National Pressure Ulcer Advisory Panel, 2007b).

(continued on page 330)

Interventions	Rationales
5. Reduce or eliminate factors that contribute to extension of existing pressure ulcers: a. Wash the area surrounding the ulcer gently with a mild soap, rinse area thoroughly to remove soap, and pat dry. b. Avoid vigorous massage of any reddened areas. c. Institute one or a combination of the following barrier products (National Pressure Ulcer Advisory Panel, 2001a): • Apply a thin coat of liquid copolymer skin sealant. • Cover area with a moisture-permeable film dressing. • Cover area with a hydroactive wafer barrier and secure with strips of one-inch microscope tape; leave in place for 4–5 days.	5. Mechanical or chemical forces contribute to pressure ulcer deterioration. a. Soap is an irritant and dries skin. b. Vigorous massage angulates and tears the vessels. Massaging over reddened areas might break capillaries and traumatize skin (Berlowitz, 2007b; Maklebust & Sieggreen, 2001). c. Healthy skin should be protected.
6. Devise a plan for treating pressure ulcers using moist-wound healing principles, as follows: a. Avoid breaking blisters. b. Flush ulcer base with sterile saline solution. If it is infected, use forceful irrigation. c. Avoid using wound cleaners and topical antiseptics (Agency for Health Care Policy and Research [AHCPR], 1992). d. Consult with a surgeon or wound specialist to debride necrotic tissue chemically, mechanically, or surgically (Berlowitz, 2007b). e. Cover pressure ulcers that have broken skin with a dressing that maintains a moist environment over the ulcer base (e.g., film dressing, hydrocolloid wafer dressing, absorption dressing, moist gauze dressing) (Berlowitz, 2007b). f. Avoid drying agents (e.g., heat lamps, Maalox, Milk of Magnesia). g. Stable (dry, adherent, intact, without erythema or movement) eschar on heels should not be removed (National Pressure Ulcer Advisory Panel, 2007b).	6. When wounds are semi-occluded and the wounds' surface remains moist, epidermal cells migrate more rapidly over the surface (Maklebust & Sieggreen, 2001). a. Blisters indicate stage II pressure ulcers; the fluid contained in the blister provides an environment for formation of granulation tissue. b. Irrigation with normal saline solution may aid in removing dead cells and reducing bacterial count. Forceful irrigation should not be used in the presence of granulation tissue and new epithelium. c. These products may be cytotoxic to tissue. d. A necrotic tissue promotes bacterial growth and does not heal until the necrotic tissue is removed (Berlowitz, 2007b). e. Moist wounds heal faster (AHCPR, 1994). f. Heat creates an increased oxygen demand. Heat lamps are contraindicated in pressure ulcers, as the lamps increase the oxygen demand to tissue that is already stressed (Maklebust & Sieggreen, 2001). g. Stable eschar serves as a natural biological cover for wound (National Pressure Ulcer Advisory Panel, 2007b).
7. Consult with a nurse specialist or physician for treatment of deep or infected pressure ulcers.	7. Expert consultation may be needed for more specific interventions. a. Notify interdisciplinary team of the wound.
8. Determine the client's nutritional status. Consult with a nutritionist.	8. Wound healing requires increased protein and CHO intake to prevent weight loss and promote healing (Dudek, 2005).

Documentation

Flow records
Staging (National Pressure Ulcer Advisory Panel, 2001b)
   Size of ulcer base (length, width, depth)

Wound bed characteristics: granulation, epithelialization, necrotic tissue, undermined areas, sinus tracts, drainage, surrounding erythema, induration

Pain

Treatment

Healing response

Unsatisfactory response

Impaired Physical Mobility Related to Imposed Restrictions, Deconditioned Status, Loss of Motor Control, or Altered Mental Status

NOC Ambulation, Joint Movement, Passive, Active, Mobility Level

Goal

The client will demonstrate increased mobility as (specify).

Indicators

- Shift body weight at least every 2 hours.
- Demonstrate reduced interface pressure and redistribution over the ulcer to less than 32 mmHg.
- Show intact skin without nonblanchable erythema.

NIC Exercise Therapy: Joint Mobility, Exercise Promotion: Strength Training, Exercise Therapy: Ambulation, Positioning, Teaching: Prescribed Activity/Exercise

Interventions	Rationales
1. Encourage the highest level of mobility. Provide devices such as overhead or partial side rails, if possible, to facilitate independent movement (AHCPR, 1994). Consider physical therapy to improve mobility (Berlowitz, 2007b).	1. Regular movement relieves constant pressure over a bony prominence (Berlowitz, 2007b).
2. Promote optimal circulation while in bed. a. If the client cannot turn self, reposition every two hours. Use a "turn clock" to indicate the appropriate position for each full-body turn (Berlowitz, 2007b; Maklebust & Sieggreen, 2001). b. Make minor shifts in body position between full turns. c. Examine bony prominences with each repositioning. If reddened areas do not fade within 30 minutes after repositioning, turn the client more frequently. d. Position the client in a 30-degree, laterally inclined position. Do *not* use high Fowler's position (AHCPR, 1994; Berlowitz, 2007b). e. Use a pressure-relief device to augment the turning schedule. f. Do not use foam donuts or rubber rings (AHCPR, 1994). g. Pay particular attention to the heels. h. *Do not* vigorously massage reddened areas (Berlowitz, 2007b).	2. a. Intermittent pressure relief lets blood reenter capillaries that compression had deprived of blood and oxygen. b. Minor shifts in body weight aid reperfusion of compressed areas. c. Reactive hyperemia may be insufficient to compensate for local ischemia. d. This position relieves pressure over the trochanter and sacrum simultaneously (Berlowitz, 2007b). High Fowler's position increases sacral shear. e. Pressure-reducing devices may increase the time intervals between necessary repositioning. f. These devices compress the surrounding vasculature, increasing the area of ischemia. g. Studies demonstrate that the heels are extremely vulnerable to breakdown because of the high concentration of body weight over their relatively small surface. h. Vigorous massage can angulate and break capillaries (AHCPR, 1994; Berlowitz, 2007b)

Documentation

Flow record
 Degree of mobility
 Frequency of repositioning
 Actual body position (e.g., left side, supine, right side, prone, 30-degree laterally inclined on left or right)
 Pressure relief devices used
Progress notes
 Abnormal local tissue response to repositioning

High Risk for Infection Related to Exposure of Ulcer Base to Fecal/Urinary Drainage

NOC Infection Severity, Wound Healing: Primary Intention, Immune Status

Goal

The client will report risk factors associated with infection, and the precautions needed.

Indicators

- Demonstrate meticulous hand-washing and skin hygiene technique by the time of discharge.
- Describe methods of infection transmission.
- Describe the influence of nutrition on infection prevention.

NIC Infection Control, Wound Care, Incision Site Care, Health Education

Interventions	Rationales
1. Teach the importance of good skin hygiene. Use emollients if skin is dry, but do not leave skin "wet" from too much lotion or cream.	1. Dry skin is susceptible to cracking and infection. Excessive emollient use can lead to maceration.
2. Protect the skin from exposure to urine/feces a. Cleanse the skin thoroughly after each incontinent episode, using a liquid soap that does not alter skin pH. b. Collect feces and urine in an appropriate containment device (e.g., condom catheter, fecal incontinence pouch, polymer-filled incontinent pads), or apply a skin sealant, cream, or emollient to act as a barrier to urine and feces.	2. Contact with urine and stool can cause skin maceration. Feces may be more ulcerogenic than urine, owing to bacteria and toxins in stool. Incontinent clients are five times at greater risk for pressure ulcers (Berlowitz, 2007a).
3. Consider using occlusive dressings on clean superficial ulcers, but never on deep ulcers.	3. Occlusive dressings protect superficial wounds from urine and feces, but can trap bacteria in deep wounds.
4. Ensure meticulous hand-washing to prevent infection transmission.	4. Improper hand-washing by caregivers is the primary source of infection transmission in hospitalized clients.
5. Use good technique during all dressing changes.	5. Good technique reduces the entry of pathogenic organisms into the wound.
6. Flush the ulcer base with sterile saline solution.	6. Infection produces necrotic debris with secretions that provide an excellent medium for microorganism growth. Flushing helps to remove necrotic debris and dilutes the bacterial count. An infected partial-thickness wound may progress to wound sepsis with increasing necrosis, then eventually to a full-thickness lesion.

(continued on page 333)

Interventions	Rationales
7. Use new gloves for each dressing change on a client with multiple pressure ulcers (AHCPR, 1994).	7. Each ulcer may be contaminated with different organisms; this measure helps to prevent cross-infection.
8. Monitor for signs of local wound infection (e.g., purulent drainage, cellulitis).	8. Infected ulcers require additional interventions.
9. Monitor stages of healing (Berlowitz, 2007a).	9. Healing progresses as follows (Berlowitz, 2007a): a. Granulation b. Wound contraction c. Reepithelialization d. Scar formation Reverse staging is not appropriate to describe healing (Berlowitz, 2007a; National Pressure Ulcer Advisory Panel, 2000, 2001b, 2007b).

Documentation

Flow records
  Skin condition (e.g., redness, maceration, denuded areas)
  Amount and frequency of incontinence
  Skin care and hygiene measures
  Containment devices used
Progress notes
  Change in skin condition

High Risk for Ineffective Therapeutic Regimen Management Related to Insufficient Knowledge of Etiology, Prevention, Treatment, and Home Care

NOC Compliance Behavior, Knowledge: Treatment Regimen, Participation in Health Care Decisions, Treatment Behavior: Illness or Injury

Goals

The goals for this diagnosis represent those associated with discharge planning. Refer to the discharge criteria.

NIC Anticipatory Guidance, Risk Identification, Learning Facilitation, Learning Readiness Enhancement

Interventions	Rationales
1. Teach the client measures to prevent pressure ulcers (AHCPR, 1992; National Pressure Ulcer Advisory Panel, 2001a): a. Adequate nutrition b. Mobility c. Turning and pressure relief d. Small shifts in body weight e. Active and passive range of motion f. Skin care g. Skin protection from urine and feces h. Recognition of tissue damage	1. Preventing pressure ulcers is much easier than treating them.

(continued on page 334)

Interventions	Rationales

2. Teach the client methods of treating pressure ulcers (National Pressure Ulcer Advisory Panel, 2001b):
  a. Use of pressure ulcer prevention principles
  b. Wound care specific to each ulcer
  c. How to evaluate effectiveness of current treatment
	2. These specific instructions help the client and family learn to promote healing and prevent infection.

3. Ask family members to determine the amount of assistance they need in caring for the client.	3. This assessment is required to determine if the family can provide necessary care and assistance.
4. Determine equipment and supply needs (e.g., pressure relief devices, wheelchair cushion, dressings). Consult with social services, if necessary, for assistance in obtaining needed equipment and supplies.	4. Equipment and supplies should be arranged for before discharge.
5. If appropriate, refer the client and family to a home health agency for ongoing assessment and evaluation of complex care.	5. Ongoing assessment and teaching may be necessary to sustain the complex level of care.
6. Encourage available caregivers to share the chores of client care.	6. Role fatigue and burnout may occur when one person devotes an inordinate amount of time to care-giving. Periodic relief or assistance can help to prevent this situation.
7. Stress the need to continue wound care and maintain adequate nutrition at home. (Refer to the nursing diagnoses Impaired Tissue Integrity in this care plan and Imbalanced Nutrition in the Thermal Injury care plan for specific information.)	7. Strategies must be continued at home for complete healing to occur.

Documentation

Discharge summary record
  Client teaching
  Outcome achievement or status
  Referrals, if indicated

Thermal Injuries

Thermal injuries, or burns, are classified according to cause as thermal (e.g., fire, steam, hot liquids), chemical (e.g., acid, oven cleaners), electrical, or radiation (e.g., sun, x-rays). The risk of injury and precise cause are often related to the victim's age, occupation, and recreational activities. The burning agent, intensity and duration to exposure, location and depth of burn, percentage of body exposure, age of the client, and pre-injury health are factors in determining injury severity and outcome (Baird, Keen, & Swearingen, 2005; Singh, Devgan, Bhat, & Milner, 2007).

Burn injuries are categorized based on depth and extent (size of injury), the longer and more intense the exposure to the burning agent, the greater the depth of injury. A burn is medically described as either a partial-thickness or full-thickness injury, relative to the layer(s) of skin and tissues involved (Singh et al., 2007). Partial-thickness injuries are further differentiated into superficial and deep partial-thickness burns. *Superficial injury,* commonly referred to as "first-degree" burn (e.g., sunburn), damages only the epidermis. These burns typically heal within 3–5 days without permanent scarring. *Partial-thickness injury,* also called a "second-degree" burn, involves varying levels of the dermis which contain structures essential to skin function (e.g., sweat and sebaceous glands, hair follicles, sensory and motor nerves, and capillary network). These burns heal within 14–21 days or longer, depending on the depth.

Full-thickness injury, a "third-degree" burn, exposes the poorly vascularized fat layer, which contains adipose tissue, roots of sweat glands, and hair follicles; this injury destroys all epidermal elements. This class of injury may heal by granulation and migration of healthy epithelium from the wound margins (small wound only). If the wound requires more that 2–3 weeks to heal, surgical excision and skin grafting may be required to improve functional and cosmetic outcomes. Some clinicians may also subdivide full-thickness injuries and include a description of "fourth-degree" burns. These injuries are the deepest and require excision, possibly amputation of extremities, and skin grafting to heal (Baird, Keen, & Swearingen, 2005; Singh et al., 2007; Namias, 2007). Injuries related to thermal injuries in the United States range from 1.4 to 2 million annually and, of those, approximately 70,000 require hospitalization (Singh et al., 2007).

This care plan focuses on the period of hospitalization after emergency treatment on admission and before admission to a rehabilitation unit.

 Time Frame
Acute episode (post emergency room)

■■■■■■ DIAGNOSTIC CLUSTER

Collaborative Problems

* ✳ PC: Hypoxia
* ▲ PC: Hypovolemia/Shock
* ▲ PC: Electrolyte Imbalance
* △ PC: Metabolic Acidosis
* ✳ PC: Compartment Syndrome
* △ PC: Paralytic Ileus
* △ PC: Curling Ulcer
* △ PC: Renal Insufficiency
* △ PC: Negative Nitrogen Balance
* ✳ PC: Cellulitis/Infection
* ▲ PC: Graft Rejection
* ▲ PC: Sepsis

Nursing Diagnoses	Refer to
▲ Anxiety related to sudden injury, treatments, uncertainty of outcome, and pain	
▲ Acute pain related to thermal injury treatments and immobility	
▲ High Risk for Imbalanced Nutrition: Less than Body Requirements related to increased protein, calorie, and vitamin requirements for wound healing and decreased intake secondary to pain, decreased mobility and activity, and possibly nausea and vomiting	
△ High Risk for Disturbed Self-Concept related to effects of burn on appearance, increased dependence on others, and disruption of life style and role responsibilities	
△ Deficient Diversional Activity related to prolonged hospitalization, physical limitations, and monotony of confinement	

(continued on page 336)

Nursing Diagnoses	Refer to
✻ Impaired Physical Mobility related to painful burn wounds	
△ High Risk for Ineffective Therapeutic Regimen Management related to insufficient knowledge of wound care, healed skin care, nutritional requirements, management of pain and itching, burn prevention, and follow-up care	
△ Disuse Syndrome related to effects of immobility and pain on muscle and joint function	
△ Self-Care Deficit (specify) related to impaired range-of-motion ability secondary to pain	
▲ High Risk for Infection related to loss of protective layer secondary to thermal injury	Pressure Ulcers
Related Care Plan	
Immobility or Unconsciousness	

▲ This diagnosis was reported to be monitored for or managed frequently (75%–100%).
△ This diagnosis was reported to be monitored for or managed often (50%–74%).
✻ This diagnosis was not included in the validation study.

Discharge Criteria

Before discharge, the client or family will

1. Relate an intent to discuss feelings and concerns with significant others after discharge.
2. Relate the need to comply with the prescribed dietary and daily exercise program and the consequences of noncompliance.
3. Demonstrate correct wound care.
4. Describe methods to decrease the risk of infection.
5. State the signs and symptoms that must be reported to a health care professional.
6. Relate an intent to adhere to the follow-up schedule.
7. Describe community resources available for assistance at home.

Collaborative Problems

Potential Complication: Hypoxia

Potential Complication: Hypovolemia/Shock

Potential Complication: Electrolyte Imbalance

Potential Complication: Metabolic Acidosis

Potential Complication: Compartment Syndrome

Potential Complication: Paralytic Ileus

Potential Complication: Curling Ulcer

Potential Complication: Renal Insufficiency

Potential Complication: Negative Nitrogen Balance

Potential Complication: Cellulitis/Infection

Potential Complication: Graft Rejection
Potential Complication: Sepsis

Nursing Goal

The nurse will detect early signs and symptoms of (a) hypoxia, (b) inhalation injury, (c) hypovolemia/shock, (d) electrolyte imbalances, (e) metabolic acidosis, (f) compartment syndrome, (g) paralytic ileus, (h) Curling ulcer, (i) renal insufficiency, (j) negative nitrogen balance, (k) cellulites/infection, (l) graft rejection, (m) sepsis, and (n) thromboembolism, and collaboratively intervene to stabilize the client.

Indicators

- Temperature 98–99.5°F (k, m)
- Respiratory rate 16–20 breaths/min (a, b, c, e, m)
- Normal breath sounds, no adventitious sounds (a, b, c)
- Normal, relaxed, quiet, even breathing (a, b, c)
- Peripheral pulses full, bounding (c, f)
- Pulse 60–100 beats/min (a, b, c, m)
- Blood pressure >90/60, <140/90 mmHg (a, b, c)
- SAO$_2$ arterial oxygen saturation (pulse oximetry) >95% (a, b, c, d, e, m)
- PaCO$_2$ arterial carbon dioxide 35–45 mmHg (a, b, c, d, e, m)
- Serum pH 7.35–7.45 (a, b, c, d, e, m)
- Serum carboxyhemoglobin (e)
  Adult values: *Non-Smoker:* <2.5% of hemoglobin
  Smoker: 4%–5% saturation of hemoglobin
  Heavy smoker: 5%–12% saturation of hemoglobin
  Toxic: >15% saturation of hemoglobin
  Child values: Similar to adult non-smoker (Kee, 2004, p. 81; Fraser, Mullany, & Traber, 2007)
- EKG—normal sinus rhythm (d)
- Warm, dry skin (a, c)
- Pinkish, ruddy-brownish, or olive skin tones (c, f)
- Calm, oriented (a, b, c)
- No nausea or vomiting (c, d, e, g)
- No headache or dizziness (d, e)
- No hoarseness or voice changes (b)
- No bloody, purulent, or sooty sputum (b, k)
- Urine output >5 mL/kg/h (a, c, e, i, j, n)
- Urine specific gravity 1.005–1.030 (a, c, e, i, j, n)
- Pale yellow urine (i)
- Blood urea nitrogen 5–25 mg/dL (could be slightly higher for elderly clients); urea nitrogen/creatinine ratio: 10:1–20:1; averages: 15:1 (Kee, 2005, p. 71–72) (i)
- Serum pre-albumin 20–50 mg/dL (i)
- Red blood cells (a)
  - Male 4.6–5.9 million/mm^3
  - Female 4.2–5.4 million/mm^3
- White blood count 4300–10,800 mm^3 (k, m)
- Serum potassium 3.5–5.0 mEq/L (d, i)
- Creatinine clearance (i)
  - Male 95–135 mL/mm
  - Female 85–125 mL/mm
  - Slightly decreased values than adults in elderly clients, due to decreased glomerular filtration rate (GFR) caused by reduction renal plasma flow. Urine creatinine: 1–2 g/24 hour (Kee, 2005, p. 113).
- Serum sodium 135–145 mEq/L (d, i)
- No extremity edema (k, n, f, m, n)
- Capillary refill <3 seconds (c, f, m, n)
- Bowel sounds present in all quadrants (g)
- Stool occult blood negative (h)
- Wounds without increased redness or purulent drainage (k, l, m)

- Negative Homans sign (n)
- No calf tenderness, unusual warmth or redness (n)
- Usual weight (j)
- No complaints of paresthesia, tingling (f)
- No pain with stretching of toes/fingers (f)

Interventions	Rationales
1. Assess and monitor respiratory function: breath sounds, rate and rhythm of respiration, and hemoglobin. Initiate pulse oximetry.	1. Three separate oxygenation complications are associated with smoke inhalation: carbon monoxide poisoning, laryngeal swelling and upper airway obstruction, and chemical pneumonia (Fraser, Mullany, & Traber, 2007).

2. Assess for risk factors of inhalation injury:
  a. Facial burns
  b. Singed eyebrows/nasal hair
  c. History of confinement in burning environment
  d. Bloody or sooty sputum
  e. Hoarseness, voice change, dry cough, stridor
  f. Labored or rapid breathing
	2. Inhalation injury produces the inflammatory response, which leads to erythema, edema, possible de-epithelialization of the respiratory mucosa, and increased secretions, possibly resulting in respiratory compromise. This can cause pulmonary edema, atelectasis, pneumonia, and adult respiratory distress syndrome.

3. Monitor arterial blood gases and carboxyhemoglobin.
 	
4. Monitor for signs and symptoms of the following:
  a. Carbon monoxide poisoning
    • Headache, dizziness
    • Nausea, vomiting
    • Dyspnea
    • Cherry-red skin
  b. Upper airway obstruction
    • Increased respiratory rate
    • Decreased depth of breathing
    • Hoarseness
  c. Chemical pneumonitis
    • Increased pH
    • Decreased partial pressure of carbon dioxide
    • Increased respiratory rate
	3,4. High levels of carbon monoxide lower the oxygen-carrying capacity of hemoglobin molecules (Fraser, Mullany, & Traber, 2007).

5. Encourage turning, deep breathing, and coughing every two hours. Percuss and suction the client, as needed.	5. Inhalation injury raises mucus production because of irritation of airway mucosa. In lower airway injury, the inactivation of cilia weakens the ability to clear secretions. Also, inactivation of surfactant can lead to alveolar collapse and atelectasis (Fraser, Mullany, & Traber, 2007; Baird, Keen, & Swearingen, 2005).
6. Consider positioning the client, based on chest x-ray results, to maximize oxygenation.	6. The position of the client should be dependent on the need to perfuse alveoli or enhance bronchial drainage.

7. Monitor for signs of pulmonary infection.
  a. Chest x-ray results
  b. Sputum production: color and amount
  c. Temperature, white blood cell count, and sputum culture reports
	7. Inhalation injury alters the client's defense mechanism, placing him or her at risk for infection. Elevated bands are an early indication of infection. Chest x-ray results and sputum are monitored for changes indicating infection (Fraser, Mullany, & Traber, 2007; Baird, Keen, & Swearingen, 2005).

8. Monitor trends in peak airway pressure when the client is intubated and mechanically ventilated.	8. Elevated peak airway pressures that do not decrease after suctioning may be an early indication of pulmonary edema or adult respiratory distress syndrome.

(continued on page 339)

Interventions	Rationales
9. Calculate fluid resuscitation for the first 24 hours, using the formula used by the facility (e.g., Evans, Brooke, Monafo, Parkland, and Consensus Formula).	9. Because fluid requirements vary for each client, it is necessary to calculate an estimated volume to assist in the administration of fluids and the evaluation of fluid status and burn injury (Baird, Keen, & Swearingen, 2005).
10. Monitor intake and output: a. Maintain urine output at 0.5–1 mL/kg/h. b. Maintain and adjust intravenous fluid rates according to orders and urine output. c. Monitor urine color.	10. Urine output is the best indicator of adequate fluid resuscitation. Intravenous fluid rates may need to be adjusted frequently throughout the first 24 hours to achieve a urine output at 0.5–1 mL/kg/h and perfuse the kidneys. Burn injury causes vasoconstriction of the renal artery. Port wine-colored urine is an indication of cell degradation products and myoglobin in the urine. Intravenous fluids need to be increased to prevent precipitation in the renal tubules and acute tubular necrosis (usually to maintain urine output >250 mL/h while the myoglobin is present in the urine) (Baird, Keen, & Swearingen, 2005; Freiburg et al., 2007).
11. Monitor for signs and symptoms of hypovolemia/shock: a. Urine output <5 mL/kg/h b. Increasing pulse rate with a low, normal, or slightly decreased blood pressure c. Restlessness, agitation, and change in mentation d. Increasing respiratory rate e. Diminished peripheral pulses f. Cool, pale, or mottled skin g. Decreased serum pH h. Elevated hematocrit	11. In the immediate period after the burn, the body releases large amounts of vasoactive substances, which increases capillary permeability. Serum, proteins, and electrolytes leak into damaged and normal tissue, resulting in severe hypovolemia and edema (a phenomenon known as *third spacing*). Circulating blood volume can be reduced by 50%. Capillary integrity is generally reestablished at any time from 12–48 hours postburn. The compensatory response to decreased circulatory volume is to increase blood oxygen by increasing heart and respiratory rates and decreasing circulation to the extremities (manifested by decreased pulses and cool skin). Diminished cerebral oxygenation can cause changes in mentation (Bhardwaj, Mirski, & Ulatowski, 2004).
12. Encourage oral fluids (e.g., juices or Gatorade), as long as the client can tolerate.	12. Clients with smaller-percentage burns (generally <25% partial thickness [PT] and full-thickness [FT]) can often be resuscitated orally (Baird, Keen, & Swearingen, 2005).
13. During the first 48–72 hours, avoid raising the body's free water through drinking.	13. Free water is hypotonic. As a result of the fluid shifts, excess free water tends to move into the cell, causing cellular swelling and death (Baird, Keen, & Swearingen, 2005).
14. Obtain daily weights. Ensure accuracy by weighing the client after dressing change or hydrotherapy, when dressings are dry. If a litter scale or specialty bed weight is obtained, use the same number of linens each time. Remove all extremity splints for weight.	14. Accurate daily weights provide data to aid in determining fluid status (Maghsoudi, Adyani, & Ahmadian, 2007).
15. Monitor fluid status continuously. Assess mucous membranes, peripheral pulses, color, and temperature of unburned areas, wound and nasogastric drainage.	15. The burn patient is at risk for fluid imbalance throughout hospitalization, because of large open wounds and numerous surgical procedures to achieve wound coverage (Wagner, Johnson, & Kidd, 2006).
16. Monitor laboratory study results: electrolytes, glucose, arterial blood gases, blood urea nitrogen (BUN), serum prealbumin, hematocrit, hemoglobin, carboxyhemoglobin, red blood cell count, and white blood count.	16. A major burn affects all body systems either through direct burn damage or through compensatory mechanisms that attempt to maintain homeostasis. All body-system functioning must be assessed frequently for status and response to treatment.

(continued on page 340)

Interventions	Rationales

17. Monitor for signs and symptoms of electrolyte imbalances:
  a. Hyperkalemia (serum potassium >5.5 mEq/L):
    • Irregular pulse or dysrhythmias such as premature ventricular contractions
    • Weakness or paralysis
    • Muscle irritability
    • Paresthesias
    • Nausea, abdominal cramps, or diarrhea
  b. Hypokalemia:
    • Dysrhythmias, such as premature contractions or tachyarrhythmias
    • Muscle weakness progressing to muscle paralysis
    • Electrocardiogram changes, such as T-wave inversion, ST depression
 	
  c. Hyponatremia (serum sodium <135 mEq/L):
    • Lethargy, coma
    • Weakness
    • Abdominal pain
    • Muscle twitching and convulsions
	17.
	  a,b. During the emergent period, damaged cells release potassium into the circulation. In addition, sodium potassium pump activity is altered due to hypoxia. If fluid resuscitation is inadequate or renal blood flow is compromised, serum potassium levels rise. However, once fluid resuscitation is adequate, potassium will be excreted in the urine, with a subsequent decrease in serum potassium. Generally, a hypokalemia is seen more often because of increased awareness of adequate fluid resuscitation. Fluctuations in potassium affect neuromuscular transmission and can cause such complications as cardiac dysrhythmias and reduced action of the gastrointestinal (GI) smooth muscles (Baird, Keen, & Swearingen, 2005; Freiburg et al., 2007).
	  c. Sodium losses result from denuded skin areas and the shift into interstitial spaces during periods of increased capillary permeability. Cellular edema, caused by osmosis, produces changes in sensorium, weakness, and muscle cramps (Baird, Keen, & Swearingen, 2005; Freiburg et al., 2007).

18. Monitor for signs and symptoms of metabolic acidosis:
  a. Decreased serum pH and negative base excess
  b. Rapid, shallow respirations
  c. Behavioral changes and drowsiness
  d. Headache
  e. Nausea and vomiting
	18. Metabolic acidosis can result from fixed acids released from damaged cells, hyperkalemia, or reduced renal tubular function. Excessive ketone bodies cause headaches, nausea, abdominal pain, and vomiting. Respiratory rate and depth increase in an attempt to increase excretion of carbon dioxide and reduce acidosis. Acidosis affects the central nervous system and can increase neuromuscular irritability (Edelman et al., 2007).

19. Monitor for signs and symptoms of compartment syndrome in extremities with circumferential burns (Namias, 2007; Baird, Keen, & Swearingen, 2005):
  a. Diminishing pulses—if hands and fingers are burned, assess palmar arch pulse and pulses along medial or lateral aspect of fingers
  b. Coolness, pallor
  c. Mottled or cyanotic skin
  d. Pressure resulting from significant edema
  e. Pain with passive stretch movement of toes or fingers
  f. Delayed capillary refill >3 seconds
  g. Numbness of peripheral pulses
	19. The tight, leathery eschar of a full-thickness burn, together with the increasing interstitial edema resulting from third spacing and fluid resuscitation, place an extremity with a circumferential injury at risk for neurovascular compromise. An escharotomy (a linear incision down through the eschar of a full-thickness burn until punctate bleeding is reached) or fasciotomy is the surgical procedure necessary to restore circulation.

20. Elevate affected extremities at heart level, or leave in a neutral position.	20. Edema impairs circulation; however, if the extremity is elevated above heart level, this may decrease arterial blood flow. In a partial-thickness burn, edema may diminish blood flow and thus increase the depth of the burn wound (Singh et al., 2007).
21. Monitor with Doppler ultrasound hourly.	21. Doppler assessments will detect early changes in circulation.

22. Assess and monitor escharotomy sites:
  a. Return of adequate pulse
  b. Normal capillary refill, color, and skin temperature
  c. Bleeding
	22. A successful escharotomy will produce immediate return of pulses. Escharotomies are most often performed during the emergent period, when circulating volume is diminished and there is minimal bleeding from the site. However, when volume is restored, bleeding may increase (Namias, 2007).

(continued on page 341)

Interventions	Rationales
23. Encourage active range-of-motion exercises and self-care activities, if appropriate for the client.	23. Activity enhances mobilization of fluid and minimizes edema.
24. Monitor for nausea and vomiting.	24. During the emergent period, nausea and vomiting may develop because of gastric dilation as a result of hypoperfusion to the GI tract. Treatment involves not giving the client anything by mouth and inserting a nasogastric tube (Baird, Keen, & Swearingen, 2005).
25. Monitor for signs and symptoms of paralytic ileus: a. Nausea and vomiting b. Absent bowel sounds c. Abdominal distention	25. Hypoperfusion of the GI tract can also lead to paralytic ileus and is especially associated with a major burn. Treatment involves inserting a nasogastric tube and ensuring adequate fluid resuscitation (Baird, Keen, & Swearingen, 2005; Wagner, Johnson, & Kidd, 2006).
26. If there are no bowel sounds, initiate insertion of a NG tube.	26. This reduces gastric distention and prevents vomiting.
27. Monitor for signs and symptoms of Curling ulcer: a. Blood in vomitus or nasogastric drainage b. Tarry stools c. Pain d. gastric pH > 5.0 (Baird, Keen, & Swearingen, 2005).	27. Curling ulcer is an acute peptic ulcer of the duodenum resulting as a complication from severe burns, when reduced plasma volume leads to sloughing of the gastric mucosa. Curling ulcers have a higher incidence of perforation and hemorrhage than other forms of ulcers. A combination of therapies, including enteral feeding with added antacids such as H_2-receptor antagonists or, more recently, proton pump inhibitors such as omeprazole, have made Curling ulcer a rare complication (Purdue, 2007).
28. Monitor for early signs and symptoms of renal insufficiency (Wagner, Johnsons, & Kidd, 2006): a. Sustained elevated urine specific gravity b. Elevated urine sodium c. Sustained insufficient urine output (<5 mL/kg/h) d. Elevated BUN, serum creatinine, potassium, phosphorus, ammonia; and decreased creatinine clearance	28. Decreased renal blood flow results from hypotension and secretion of antidiuretic hormone and aldosterone. In addition, nephrons can be blocked by free hemoglobin increased by red blood cell destruction (Baird, Keen, & Swearingen, 2005). a,b. Decreased ability of the renal tubules to reabsorb electrolytes results in increased urine sodium levels and urine specific gravity. c. Decreased glomerular filtration rate eventually leads to insufficient urine output. d. These changes result from decreased excretion of urea and creatinine in urine.
29. Monitor for signs of negative nitrogen balance: a. Weight loss b. 24-hour urine nitrogen balance below zero	29. Burns produce a hypermetabolic response due to greater heat loss from wounds and a rise in beta-adrenergic activity, causing a need for additional nutrients to prevent nitrogen deficiency (Baird, Keen, & Swearingen, 2005; Namias, 2007).
30. Institute daily calorie counts when the client is able to tolerate a diet.	30. An accurate calorie and protein intake can be calculated to ensure that the client is meeting nutritional requirements (Baird, Keen, & Swearingen, 2005; Namias, 2007).
31. Offer high-protein, high-calorie snacks at regular intervals. Determine the client's food preferences and eating patterns before injury.	31. Because the burn client's appetite often decreases because of inactivity, it is difficult to meet nutritional requirements at mealtime alone (Baird, Keen, & Swearingen, 2005; Namias, 2007).

(continued on page 342)

Interventions	Rationales
32. Consult with the physician on the need for total parenteral nutrition on tube feedings.	32. When a client sustains a major burn injury, total parenteral nutrition is instituted within 2–4 days, when the client's fluid and electrolytes are stabilized. Often, duodenal feeding tubes are used until the client can to take in adequate protein and calories orally.
33. Monitor for signs and symptoms of wound infection and cellulitis: a. Increased thick, yellow, or green drainage b. Foul-smelling drainage c. Spotty, black areas underneath eschar d. Soft, sloughing eschar e. Increased swelling f. Increased redness around periphery of wound	33. Initially, large amounts of serum drainage are expected from a burn wound. About 4–5 days postburn, normal drainage consists of moderate amounts of yellow drainage. It is also normal to observe a small amount of erythema at the edge of the wound; however, when this increases in intensity and width, cellulitis may have developed. Cellulitis is caused by streptococcus, which will dissolve an autograft.
34. Provide hydrotherapy and dressing changes daily or b.i.d. (twice a day), depending on the status of the wounds: a. Premedicate client. b. Assess wounds. c. Cleanse with antiseptic soap. d. Debride loose eschar or debris. e. Apply antimicrobial cream, synthetic dressing, and so forth, as ordered by the physician.	34. Initially, burn wounds are cleansed twice daily until drainage decreases and the wound begins to heal. Also, antimicrobial cream is generally applied to all burn wounds initially. When drainage decreases and the wound begins to heal, a synthetic dressing may be applied. Various synthetic and biosynthetic dressings are used as autograft dressings; the selection often depends on physician preference.
35. Monitor for signs of graft loss or infection: a. Sloughing b. Continued pale white-yellow or gray appearance c. No blanching or capillary refill d. Increased drainage	35. Autografts (skin taken from the client's own body) are used to provide permanent wound coverage. Skin substitutes (biologic or synthetic) are used until autograft is possible (Purdue, 2007; Singh et al., 2007).
36. Teach the client to do the following: a. Avoid movement of a grafted area, especially if the graft is over a joint. b. Avoid pressure on the graft. c. Elevate the involved body part. d. Turn in the bed carefully to avoid shearing of graft.	36. Excessive movement and pressure may interfere with revascularization. Elevation facilitates venous return and minimizes edema.
37. Provide donor site care according to type of dressing.	37. Donor site care may vary depending on the dressing. The donor site is a partial-thickness wound and generally takes about 10–14 days to heal.
38. Monitor for signs and symptoms of sepsis (Baird, Keen, & Swearingen, 2005; Graf & Janssens, 2007). a. Temperature <100.4°F (38°C) or <96.8°F (36°C) b. Heart rate <90 beats/min c. Respiratory rate >20 breaths/min or $PaCO_2$ <32 torr (<4.3 kPa) d. White blood cell (WBC) count >10,000 cells/mm³, <3000 cells/mm³, or >10% immature (band) forms (Graf & Janssens, 2007).	38. The skin provides a physical barrier that protects the body from infection. When a burn injury occurs, organisms invade open wounds. Also, the burn injury alters the immune response. Bacteria in urine, sputum, or blood indicates infection. Sepsis results in massive vasodilation with hypovolemia; this leads to tissue hypoxia and results in decreased renal function and cardiac output. The compensatory response of increased heart rate and respiration attempts to correct hypoxia and acidosis.
39. Monitor for signs and symptoms of thromboembolism:	39. Hypovolemia increases blood viscosity because of hemoconcentration. Immobility reduces vasomotor tone, resulting in decreased venous return with peripheral blood pooling (Baird, Keen, & Swearingen, 2005; Freiburg et al., 2007).

(continued on page 343)

Interventions	Rationales
a. Positive Homans sign (dorsiflexion of the foot causes pain) b. Calf tenderness, unusual warmth, or redness c. Low-grade fever d. Extremity edema	a. Positive Homans sign indicates insufficient circulation. b,c. These signs and symptoms point to inflammation.
40. Encourage the client to do leg exercises. Discourage placing pillows under the knees, use of a knee gatch, crossing the legs, and prolonged sitting.	40. These measures help to increase venous return and prevent venous stasis (Baird, Keen, & Swearingen, 2005; Namias, 2007).
41. Have the client ambulate as soon as possible with at least five minutes of walking each waking hour. Avoid prolonged sitting on a chair with legs dependent.	41. Walking contracts the leg muscles, stimulates the venous pump, and reduces stasis (Baird, Keen, & Swearingen, 2005; Namias, 2007).

Related Physician-Prescribed Interventions

Medications. Antacids, antibiotics, histamine inhibitors
Intravenous Therapy. Hyperalimentation; replacement therapy (fluids, electrolytes, plasma, and albumin); blood products
Laboratory Studies. Complete blood count, serum glucose, WBC count, serum prealbumin, serum electrolytes, alkaline phosphatase, wound cultures
Diagnostic Studies. Serial chest x-ray films
Therapies. Pressure-relief beds; grafts (autograft, biologic, synthetic); whirlpool; analgesics; topical agents (silver sulfadiazine, mafenide acetate, silver nitrate); blood cultures; sputum cultures; urine cultures; serum osmolarity; urine osmolarity; BUN; stools for occult blood; wound care/dressings; debridement; autografts

Documentation

Flow records
   Vital signs
   Respiratory assessment
   Weight (daily)
   Edema (sites, amount)
   Urine specific gravity
   Intake and output (calories, amounts)
   Occult blood tests
   Bowel sounds
Progress notes
   Complaints of nausea, vomiting, muscle cramps
   Changes in behavior or sensorium
   Treatments
   Condition of graft and donor sites (appearance, evidence of epithelialization, exudates, odor)

Nursing Diagnoses

Anxiety Related to Sudden Injury, Treatment, Uncertainty of Outcome, and Pain

NOC Anxiety Self-Control, Coping, Impulse Self-Control

Goal

The client will report reduced anxiety to a mild/moderate level.

Indicators

- Effectively communicate feelings regarding injuries.
- Describes usual patterns of coping with stress.

NIC Anxiety Reduction, Impulse Control Training, Anticipatory Guidance

Interventions	Rationales
1. Help the client to reduce anxiety: a. Provide constant comfort and reassurance. b. Stay with the client as much as possible. c. Speak in a calm, soothing voice. d. Identify and support effective coping mechanisms. e. Convey your understanding and empathy. f. Encourage the client to verbalize fears and concerns.	1. An anxious client has a narrowed perceptual field and a diminished ability to learn. He or she may experience muscle tension, pain, and sleep disturbances, and may be disposed to overreact to situations. Anxiety tends to feed on itself and can catch the client in a widening spiral of tension and physical and emotional pain; thus, anxiety reduction is essential to effective client care (Lewis et al., 2004).
2. If anxiety is mild to moderate, take the opportunity to teach the client about procedures.	2. Accurate information about what to expect may help to reduce anxiety associated with the unknown.
3. Encourage family and friends to verbalize their fears and concerns to staff. Prepare them for their initial visit by discussing the client's appearance and any invasive lines or other care measures they may see.	3. Discussions help clarify misconceptions and allow sharing. Descriptions of what to expect help to prevent a shocked response that may trigger anxiety in the client.
4. Encourage the use of relaxation techniques.	4. Relaxation exercises provide control over the body's response to stress and can help reduce anxiety.
5. Notify the physician immediately if anxiety reaches the severe or panic level.	5. Severe or panic anxiety can lead to injury or other problems, and makes learning and compliance with treatment impossible.

Documentation

Progress notes
Present emotional status
Response to nursing interventions

Acute Pain Related to Thermal Injury Treatments and Immobility

NOC Comfort Level, Pain Control

Goal

The client will report progressive reduction of pain and relief after pain relief measures.

Indicators

- Relate factors that increase pain.
- Relate effective interventions.

NIC Pain Management, Medication Management, Emotional Support, Teaching: Individual, Heat/Cold Application, Simple Massage

Interventions	Rationales
1. Convey that you acknowledge and accept the client's pain.	1. A client who feels that he or she must convince skeptical caregivers of the seriousness of his or her pain becomes more anxious, further intensifying the pain.
2. Provide accurate information: a. Explain the cause of pain, if known; if not, then direct the client and family to the appropriate professional to answers questions, thereby reducing fear and anxiety (Baird, Keen, & Swearingen, 2005; Namias, 2007). b. Explain how long the pain should last, if known. c. If indicated, reassure the client that narcotic addiction is not likely to develop from the pain relief regimen.	2. A client who understands and is prepared for pain by detailed explanations tends to experience less stress—and consequently less pain—than a client who receives vague or no explanations.
3. Provide privacy for the client during acute pain episodes.	3. Privacy reduces embarrassment and anxiety and enables more effective coping.
4. Collaborate with the client to identify effective pain relief measures. This should include a measure to be used during dressing changes: a. Distraction b. Breathing exercises c. Relaxation techniques	4. The client can provide valuable insights into the pain and its relief. Burn pain cannot be resolved entirely until the wound is completely healed. Distraction stimulates the thalamus, midbrain, and brain stem; this increases production of endorphins and alters pain transmission. Distraction techniques have been demonstrated to reduce pain and anxiety during dressing change (Bhardwaj, Mieski, & Ulatowski, 2004). Breathing exercises and relaxation techniques decrease oxygen consumption, respiratory rate, heart rate, and muscle tension that interrupt the cycle of pain–anxiety–muscle tension.
5. Provide optimal pain relief with prescribed analgesics, while ensuring that the client's respiratory function is not compromised if she or he is not on a ventilator (Lehne, 2004). a. Consult with a pharmacist for possible adverse interactions with other medications the client is taking, such as muscle relaxants and tranquilizers. b. Use a preventive approach to pain medication: administer the pain medication before treatment procedures or activity, and instruct the client to request p.r.n. (as-needed) pain medications before pain becomes severe (Lehne, 2004). c. Assess vital signs, especially respiratory rate, before and after administration. d. About ½ hour after administration, assess pain relief.	5. a. Some medications potentiate the effects of narcotics. b. The preventive approach (e.g., every four hours) may reduce the total 24-hour drug dose as compared with the p.r.n. approach and may reduce the client's anxiety associated with having to ask for and wait for p.r.n. medications (Lehne, 2004). c. Narcotics depress the brain's respiratory center. d. Response to analgesics can vary with stress levels, fatigue, and pain intensity.
6. Explain the prescribed burn wound care and its advantages and disadvantages: a. Open method—no dressings, with frequent reapplication of ointment. *Advantages:* no dressings, hastened eschar separation reduces infection. *Disadvantages:* requires frequent reapplication; increased heat loss. b. Semiclosed method—dressings, with antimicrobials changed once or twice a day. *Advantages:* dressing removal debrides wounds; heat loss is reduced; wounds are not always visible. *Disadvantages:* dressing changes are required; debridement is painful. c. Closed method—occlusive dressings not changed for up to 72 hours. *Advantages:* fewer dressing changes; others the same as the semiclosed method. *Disadvantages:* wounds cannot be inspected daily; dressings can be too tight or too loose.	6. Explaining the method and its advantages and disadvantages can help the client to recognize and report any problems or complications.

(continued on page 346)

Interventions	Rationales

7. Take steps to reduce pain during dressing changes:
 	
  a. Administer analgesics 30 minutes before treatment. Consider additional intravenous boluses during treatment, if needed.
  b. Encourage the client to use relaxation or distraction techniques.
  c. Regulate the amount of debridement or staple removal to be done with each dressing change.
  d. Inform the client when a process will be painful.
  e. Handle carefully wounds that are healing.
  f. Moisten adherent dressings on skin graft or healing wounds with decreased drainage.
  g. Use heat lights if the client's body temperature allows.
  h. Encourage the client to become involved in wound care, when appropriate.
	7. Dressing changes are painful because of manipulation of wounds, exposure to air, and associated debridement.
	  a. Early administration allows full drug effects during the dressing change.
	
	  b. Refer to rationale for Intervention 4.
	
	  c. This will prevent excessive pain in one session.
	
	  d. Fear of unknown can increase anxiety and pain.
	  e. Healing wounds have increased sensitivity.
	  f. These wounds do not require debridement with dressing removal. Wet dressings facilitate removal and reduce discomfort and bleeding.
	
	  h. Client involvement gives the client a sense of control.

8. Reduce exposure time during treatments.	8. Loss of insulating skin surface increases heat loss. Exposure of wound surface to air often causes the burning sensation.
9. Collaborate with the client to evaluate the effectiveness of medication and non-pharmacologic measures to minimize pain during hydrotherapy.	9. The client's participation enhances cooperation and success.

Documentation

Medication administration record
    Type, dosage, schedule, and route of all medications administered
Progress notes
    Pain relief measures
    Unsatisfactory pain relief from these measures

High Risk for Imbalanced Nutrition: Less Than Body Requirements Related to Increased Protein, Calorie, and Vitamin Requirements for Wound Healing and Decreased Intake Secondary to Pain, Decreased Mobility and Activity, and Possibly Nausea and Vomiting

NOC Nutritional Status

Goal

The client will resume ingesting the daily nutritional requirements.

Indicators

- Select from the four basic food groups.
- Consume 2000 to 3000 mL of fluids each day.
- Consume adequate vitamins, minerals, and fiber.
- Maintain or gain weight.
- Maintain high-protein, moderate-carbohydrate diet (due to high metabolic activity and increased protein, catabolism related to burn injury results in dramatic increases in energy requirements and nutritional needs).

NIC Nutrition Management, Nutritional Monitoring, Teaching: Prescribed Diet

Interventions	Rationales
1. Discuss the nutritional requirements and dietary sources.	1. Major complications of trauma and sepsis increase the metabolic rate from 10%–50%. In the presence of insufficient protein, the body breaks down its own endogenous protein stores (Baird, Keen, & Swearingen, 2005; Namias, 2007).
a. Calories a day: 2500–3000; a client may require enteral feeding (other than oral) if they are unable to tolerate the high protein and caloric diet required to maintain the accelerated metabolic activity (Baird, Keen, & Swearingen, 2005).	a,b. Increased caloric and protein intake is needed to enhance the body's protein-sparing capacity.
b. Protein: 100–125 g; sources: dairy, meat, poultry, fish, and legumes	
c. B-complex vitamins; sources: meat, nuts, and fortified cereals	c. B-complex vitamins are required for metabolism of CHO, fat, and protein.
d. Vitamin C: 75–300 mg; sources: green vegetables and citrus fruits	d. Vitamin C is essential for collagen formation and wound healing.
e. Phosphorus, magnesium, and vitamin D; sources: multivitamins	e. These nutrients are required for healing.
2. Consult with a nutritionist to establish daily caloric and food type requirements.	2. Meeting a burn client's special nutritional needs requires expert consultation.
3. Determine the client's food preferences and eating patterns before the injury. Collaborate with the client to establish a mutually acceptable nutrition plan, if appropriate.	3. Knowledge of the client's eating habits prior to injury and her or his input and acceptance of the meal plan will increase success in meeting nutritional requirements.
4. Explain the causes of anorexia and nausea.	4. Pain, fatigue, analgesics, and immobility can contribute to anorexia and nausea. Explanations can reduce the anxiety associated with the unknown.
5. Provide rest periods for the client before meals and after therapies such as rehabilitation.	5. Fatigue further diminishes a decreased desire to eat.
6. Offer frequent small feedings (six per day plus snacks) rather than infrequent large meals.	6. Distributing the caloric intake over the day helps increase total intake.
7. Restrict liquids with meals and one hour before and after meals.	7. Overdistending the stomach decreases appetite and intake.
8. Maintain good oral hygiene before and after meals.	8. Accumulation of food particles can contribute to foul odors and taste that diminish the appetite.
9. Arrange to have foods with the highest protein and calorie content served at the times when the client usually feels most like eating.	9. This measure may improve protein and calorie intake.
10. Prevent pain from interfering with eating: a. Plan the care so that painful procedures are not done immediately before meals. b. Provide pain medication ½ hour before meals, or as ordered.	10. Pain causes fatigue, which can reduce appetite.
11. Take steps to prevent nausea and vomiting: a. Frequently provide small amounts of ice chips or cool clear liquid (e.g., dilute tea, Jell-O, water, flat ginger ale, or cola), unless vomiting persists.	11. Control of nausea and vomiting improves nutritional status. a. Frequent intake of small amounts of fluid helps to prevent overdistention.

(continued on page 348)

Interventions	Rationales
b. Eliminate unpleasant sights and odors.	b. This diminishes visual and olfactory stimulation of the vomiting center.
c. Provide good oral care after vomiting.	c. Good oral hygiene can reduce nausea.
d. Encourage deep breathing.	d. Deep breathing can suppress the vomiting reflex.
e. Restrict liquids before meals.	e. Restricting liquids can prevent overdistention.
f. Avoid having the client lie down for at least two hours after meals. A client who must rest should sit or recline so that the head is at least four inches higher than the feet.	f. Sitting reduces gastric pressure.
g. Administer antiemetics before meals, if indicated.	g. Antiemetics prior to meals can prevent nausea and vomiting.
12. Encourage the client to try commercial supplements available in many forms (liquids, powder, pudding); keep switching brands until some are acceptable to the client in taste and consistency.	12. These supplements can substantially increase caloric intake without the need to consume large quantities of food.
13. Teach the client techniques to enhance the nutritional content of food: a. Add powdered milk or egg to milkshakes, gravies, sauces, puddings, cereals, etc. to increase protein and calorie content. b. Add blenderized or baby foods to meat juices or soups. c. Use fortified milk: one cup nonfat dry milk added to one quart fresh milk. d. Use milk, half-and-half, or soy milk instead of water when making soups and sauces. e. Add cheese or diced meat to foods whenever able. f. Spread cream cheese or peanut butter on toast, crackers, and celery sticks. g. Add extra butter or margarine to foods. h. Use mayonnaise instead of salad dressing. i. Add raisins, dates, nuts, and brown sugar to hot and cold cereals. j. Keep snacks readily available.	13. Simple food additives can increase calorie, protein, carbohydrate, and fat intake.
14. If the client still has insufficient nutritional intake, consult with the physician for alternative strategies.	14. The client may require high-protein supplements, tube feedings, or total parenteral nutrition.

Documentation

Flow records
  Weight
  Intake (type, amount)

High Risk for Disturbed Self-Concept Related to Effects of Burn on Appearance, Increased Dependence on Others, and Disruption of Life Style and Role Responsibilities

NOC Quality of Life, Depression Level, Self-Esteem, Coping

Goal

The client will demonstrate healthy adaptation and coping skills.

Indicators

• Communicate his or her feelings about the burns.
• Participate in self-care.

NIC Hope Instillation, Mood Management, Values Clarification, Counseling, Referral, Support Group, Coping Enhancement

Interventions	Rationales
1. Contact the client often and treat him or her with warm, positive regard.	1. Frequent client contact indicates acceptance and may facilitate trust. The client may be hesitant to approach staff because of a poor self-concept.
2. Incorporate emotional support into the technical self-care sessions. Encourage narration, visualization, participation, and exploration.	2. These activities promote exploration of feelings and resolution of emotional conflicts during acquisition of technical skills. Four stages of psychological adjustment have been identified: • *Narration:* The client recounts the injury experience and reveals an understanding of how and why he or she is in this situation. • *Visualization and verbalization:* The person looks at and expresses feelings about the injury. • *Participation:* The person progresses from observer to assistant, then to independent practitioner of the medical aspects of wound care. • *Exploration:* The person begins to explore methods of incorporating appearance changes into his or her life style.
3. Encourage the client to look at burned areas.	3. The client begins the adaptation process by acknowledging the injury and loss.
4. Encourage client to verbalize feelings and perceptions about how the burns have affected their lifestyle. Validate these perceptions by assuring him or her that these responses are normal and appropriate.	4. Validating the client's feelings and perceptions heightens her or his self-awareness and boosts her or his self-concept.
5. Have the client participate in care as much as possible. Provide feedback on progress and reinforce positive behavior and proper techniques.	5. Participation in care can improve the client's self-esteem and sense of control; feedback and reinforcement encourage continued participation.
6. Have the client demonstrate wound care and teach the procedure independently to a support person.	6. Evaluation of a return demonstration helps the nurse to identify any need for further teaching and supervision.
7. Involve family members or significant other(s) in learning wound care.	7. Acceptance by support persons is one of the most important factors in the client's acceptance of body image changes.
8. Encourage the client to verbalize positive self-attributes.	8. Evidence that the client will pursue personal goals and maintain his or her life style reflects positive adjustment.
9. Encourage contact with others on the unit.	9. Such contacts give client the opportunity to test the responses of others to his or her injuries and possible altered appearance.
10. Offer constant verbal encouragement to achieve short-term goals.	10. This enhances the client's level of hope.
11. Identify a client at risk for unsuccessful adjustment; look for these characteristics: a. Poor ego strength b. Ineffective problem-solving ability	11. Successful adjustment to changes in appearance is influenced by factors such as the following: a. Previous successful coping b. Achievement of developmental tasks pre-injury

(continued on page 350)

Interventions	Rationales
c. Learning difficulty	c. Extent to which injury interferes with goal-directed activity
d. Lack of motivation e. External focus of control f. Poor health g. Unsatisfactory pre-injury sex life h. Lack of positive support systems i. Rejection of counseling	d. Sense of control e. Realistic self-perception and realistic perception from support persons
12. Prepare the client for other people's responses to their scars and bandages (e.g., staring, questions) (Acton, 2004). Role play some responses (e.g., when someone is staring, say "how are you today?").	12. Preparing the client for possible reactions increases their personal autonomy and allows them to increase their control of the situation (Acton, 2004).

Documentation

Progress notes
Present emotional status
Interventions
Client's or family's responses to nursing interventions

Deficient Diversional Activity Related to Prolonged Hospitalization, Physical Limitations, and Monotony of Confinement

NOC Leisure Participation, Social Involvement

Goal

The client will engage in a diversional activity.

Indicators

- Relate feelings of boredom and discuss methods of finding diversional activities.
- Relate methods of coping with feelings of anger or depression caused by boredom.

NIC Recreation Therapy, Socialization Enhancement, Self-Esteem Enhancement

Interventions	Rationales
1. Validate the client's boredom.	1. Acknowledgment may increase motivation to increase stimulation.
2. Explore the client's likes and dislikes.	2. Exploration may help to identify possible recreational activities.
3. Vary the client's routine, when possible.	3. Monotony contributes to boredom.
4. Encourage visitors, telephone calls, and letter-writing, if appropriate.	4. Visitors provide social interaction and mental stimulation.
5. To reduce boredom, use various strategies to vary the physical environment and the daily routine: a. Update bulletin boards, change pictures on the walls, rearrange furniture.	5. Creative strategies to vary the environment and daily routine can reduce boredom.

(continued on page 351)

Interventions	Rationales
b. Maintain a pleasant, cheerful environment. Position client near a window, if possible. If appropriate, provide a gold-fish bowl for visual variety. c. Provide a variety of reading materials (or "books on tape" if impairment hinders reading ability) and a television and radio. d. Discourage excessive television watching. e. Plan some "special" activity daily to give the client something to look forward to each day. f. Consider enlisting a volunteer to read to the client or play board games or card games with him or her. g. Encourage the client to devise his or her own strategies to combat boredom.	
6. If feasible, volunteer at an organization (e.g., hospital, cancer society, etc.)	6. Such work provides opportunities to assist others and reduces feelings of dependency and isolation.
7. Encourage the staff and visitors to discuss their experiences	7. Initiating such discussions validates that the client has interests and opinions and also involves the client in subjects beyond personal concerns.

Documentation

Progress notes
Activities
Participation in self-care activities

Impaired Physical Mobility Related to Painful Burn Wounds

NOC Ambulation, Joint Movement, Mobility

Goal

The client will participate in self-care activities.

Indicators

- Experience minimal immobility as a result of the burn injury.
- Adapt physically to the undesirable outcomes of the burn injury.

NIC Exercise Therapy: Joint Mobility, Exercise Promotion: Strength Training, Exercise Therapy: Ambulation, Positioning, Teaching: Prescribed Activity/Exercise

Interventions	Rationales
1. Determine client's preburn level of activity, tolerance, and use of assistive devices.	1. Knowledge of preburn activity allows for reasonable expectations related to the outcome of the program.
2. Collaborate with a physical therapist and occupational therapist to plan an exercise and activity program conducive to increasing range of affected extremities.	2. Consultation allows for expert evaluation and interventions to be reinforced by all team members.

(continued on page 352)

Interventions	Rationales
3. Plan for a team meeting with the client to discuss the exercise and activity program, its purpose, and expectations of therapists, nursing, and client.	3. Knowledge and understanding of the program enhances client cooperation and program effectiveness.
4. Perform passive range-of-motion exercises, as recommended by therapists.	4,6. Burn patients require frequent exercising to remain mobile. Although therapists are primarily responsible for rehabilitation, it is also necessary for nurses to assist with follow-up.
5. Continue splinting of affected extremities, as recommended by therapists. 6. Encourage the client to perform active range-of-motion exercises independently at regular intervals throughout the day.	5. Splinting is required to maintain position of function rather than position of comfort for affected extremity.
7. Apply pressure dressings (Ace wraps or Tubigrip) or pressure garments, as recommended by therapists.	7. Pressure garments are worn when wounds are healed and edema has subsided. These dressings and garments promote collagen breakdown and thus minimize hypertrophic scarring by exerting a controlled amount of pressure over the affected areas. Ace wraps can be used before the wound is healed. Pressure garments must be worn at all times.
8. Encourage self-care activities. Collaborate with the therapist and client to determine methods or devices that would facilitate self-care.	8. Performance of self-care activities builds up the client's self-esteem and helps him or her to achieve improvement and recovery.

High Risk for Ineffective Therapeutic Regimen Management Related to Insufficient Knowledge of Wound Care, Healed Skin Care, Nutritional Requirements, Management of Pain and Itching, Burn Prevention, and Follow-up Care

NOC Compliance Behavior, Knowledge: Treatment Regimen, Participation in Health Care Decisions, Treatment Behavior: Illness or Injury

Goals

The goals for this diagnosis represent those associated with discharge planning. Refer to the discharge criteria.

NIC Anticipatory Guidance, Learning Facilitation, Risk Identification, Health Education, Teaching: Procedure/Treatment, Health System Guidance

Interventions	Rationales
1. Explain the appearance of the burn wound at various stages of healing.	1. Knowledge of the healing process provides the client with reasonable expectations.
2. Instruct and demonstrate wound care to the client and significant others; be clear and simple. Also provide written information.	2. Knowledge and understanding of the process enhances cooperation.

(continued on page 353)

Interventions	Rationales
3. Allow for return demonstration of wound care by the client and significant other.	3. Evaluation of a return demonstration helps the nurse identify the need for further teaching and supervision.

4. Discuss skin care measures:
  a. Apply lubricant (e.g., cocoa butter) frequently to healed and unaffected skin.
  b. Use sunscreen.
 	
  c. Wear loose-fitting cotton garments next to the skin.
  d. Avoid harsh soaps and hot water.
	4. A healing skin is more vulnerable to injury.
	  a. Lubricants relieve pruritus of dry skin (grafted skin areas do not contain sweat or oil glands).
	  b. Burned and grafted skin tans unevenly, and burned skin is more vulnerable to skin cancer.
	  c. Cotton garments reduce itching and abrasion.
	  d. Healed burned skin may be hypersensitive.

5. Instruct the client and family to watch for and report the following:
  a. Change in healed areas
  b. Change in wound drainage or color
  c. Fever or chills
  d. Weight loss
	5. Healing burns are prone to infection and require optimal nutrition.
	  a. Changes may point to infection or graft rejection.
	  b, c. These signs may indicate infection.
	
	  d. Weight loss indicates that intake is insufficient to meet metabolic needs.

6. Describe the action of pressure garments (e.g., Jobst) and the need to wear them 23 hours a day (1 hour to launder).	6. Constant pressure on the wound throughout scar maturation (usually 1 year) can retard scar growth.
7. Explain the importance of continuing range-of-motion exercises at home.	7. As the burn heals, hypertrophic scar tissue formation causes some shortening or contraction. Daily exercise can help reduce severity.
8. Explain the need to maintain adequate nutrition after discharge. (Refer to the nursing diagnosis Imbalanced Nutrition in this care plan for specific instructions.)	8. Burn healing requires increased protein and carbohydrate intake.
9. Describe available community resources (e.g., home care, vocational rehabilitation, financial assistance).	9. Such resources may assist in recovery.

Documentation

Discharge summary record
Client teaching
Outcome achievement or status
Referrals, if indicated

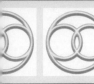

MUSCULOSKELETAL AND CONNECTIVE TISSUE DISORDERS

Fractures

Fractures are breaks in the continuity of a bone. They result from external pressure greater than the bone can absorb. When a fracture displaces a bone, it also damages surrounding structures—muscles, tendons, nerves, and blood vessels.

Traumatic injuries cause most fractures. Pathologic fractures, however, occur even without trauma in bones weakened from excessive demineralization. Fracture incidence peaks in youth and the elderly. Among youth, long bone fractures predominate and are more common among males. After the age of 35, fracture incidence climbs precipitously, as bone density declines (Walker-Bone, Walter, & Cooper, 2002).

 Time Frame
Initial diagnosis

■■■■■ DIAGNOSTIC CLUSTER

Collaborative Problems

▲ PC: Neurovascular Compromise
✱ PC: Compartment Syndrome
▲ PC: Fat Embolism
▲ PC: Hemorrhage/Hematoma Formation
▲ PC: Thromboembolism

Nursing Diagnoses	Refer to
▲ Acute pain related to tissue trauma secondary to fracture	
△ High Risk for Ineffective Therapeutic Regimen Management related to insufficient knowledge of condition, signs and symptoms of complications, activity restrictions	
▲ Self-Care Deficit (specify) related to limitation of movement secondary to fracture	Casts
▲ High Risk for Ineffective Respiratory Function related to immobility secondary to traction or fixation devices	Immobility or Unconsciousness

Related Care Plan

Casts

▲ This diagnosis was reported to be monitored for or managed frequently (75%–100%).
△ This diagnosis was reported to be monitored for or managed often (50%–74%).
✱ This diagnosis was not included in the validation study.

Discharge Criteria

Before discharge, the client or family will

1. Describe necessary precautions during activity.
2. State signs and symptoms that must be reported to a health care professional.
3. Demonstrate the ability to provide self-care or report available assistance at home.

Collaborative Problems

Potential Complication: Neurovascular Compromise

Potential Complication: Compartment Syndrome

Potential Complication: Fat Embolism

Potential Complication: Hemorrhage/Hematoma Formation

Potential Complication: Thromboembolism

Nursing Goal

The nurse will detect early signs and symptoms of (a) neurovascular compromise, (b) compartment syndrome, (c) fat embolism, and (d) cardiovascular alterations, and collaboratively intervene to stabilize the client.

Indicators

- Pedal pulses 2+, equal (a, b, d)
- Capillary refill <3 seconds (a, b, d)
- Warm extremities (a, b, d)
- No complaints of paresthesia, tingling (a, b, d)
- Pain relieved by medications (b)
- Minimal swelling (a, b, d)
- Ability to move toes or fingers (b)
- BP >90/60, <140/90 mmHg (d)
- Pulse 60–100 beats/min (d)
- Respiration 16–20 breaths/min (d)
- Temperature 98–99.5°F (c)
- Oriented, calm, alert (c, d)
- Urine output >5 mL/kg/h (c, d)
- Negative Homans sign (a, b)

Interventions	Rationales
1. Monitor for signs and symptoms of neurovascular compromise, comparing findings on the affected limb to those of the other limb: a. Diminished or absent pedal pulses b. Numbness or tingling c. Capillary refill time >3 seconds d. Pallor, blanching, cyanosis, coolness e. Inability to flex or extend extremity	1. Trauma causes tissue edema and blood loss that reduces tissue perfusion. Inadequate circulation and edema damage peripheral nerves, resulting in decreased sensation, movement, and circulation (Porth, 2005).

2. Monitor for signs of compartment syndrome (Kakar, Firoozabadi, McKean, & Tornetta, 2007; Miller & Askew, 2007).
 	
a. Early signs:
  • Unrelieved or increasing pain
  • Pain with passive stretch of toes or fingers
  • Mottled or cyanotic skin
  • Excessive swelling
  • Poor capillary refill
  • Paresthesia
  • Inability to move toes or fingers
  • Tight, shiny skin
	2. Compartment syndrome is a set of conditions in which increased pressure in a limited space compromises circulation and function. Compartment syndrome occurs with bone fractures when there is increased pressure inside the enclosed osteofacial compartment, eventually compromising perfusion (Harris, Kadir, & Donald, 2006). Some causes of increased pressure are bleeding, edema, traction, and casts. If left untreated, irreversible tissue and nerve damage may result (Miller & Askew, 2007).
	a. Pain and paresthesia indicate compression of nerves and increasing pressure within a muscle compartment. Passive stretching of muscles decreases the muscle compartment, thus increasing pain, as does active contraction (Harris et al., 2006). Poor capillary refill, or mottled or cyanotic skin, indicates obstructed capillary blood flow.

(continued on page 356)

Interventions	Rationales
b. Late signs: • Pallor • Diminished or absent pulse • Cold skin c. Six Ps (Miller & Askew, 2007) • Pain out of proportion to injury • Pain with passive stretch • Pallor • Pulselessness • Paresthesia • Paralysis	b. Arterial occlusion will produce these late signs.
3. Assess peripheral nerve function at least every hour for the first 24 hours: color, temperature, capillary refill, palpation of dorsalis pedis and posterior tibial pulses (Miller & Askew, 2007).	3. Peripheral neurovascular compromise may be the first sign.
4. For injured arms: a. Assess for movement ability: • Hyperextension of thumbs, wrist, and four fingers • Abduction (fanning out of) all fingers • Ability to touch small finger with thumb b. Assess sensation with pressure from a sharp point: • Web space between thumb and index finger • Distal fat pad of small finger • Distal surface of the index finger	4. These specific assessment techniques will detect changes in sensation and movement.
5. For injured legs: a. Assess for movement ability: • Dorsiflex (upward movement) ankle and extend toes at metatarsophalangeal joints • Plantarflex (downward movement) ankle and toes b. Assess sensations with pressure from a sharp point: • Web space between great toe and second toe • Medial and lateral surfaces of the sole (upper third)	5. Crush syndrome (Sahjian & Franks, 2007): a. On inspection and palpation, tense swollen extremity may be detected. • There may be no swelling when there is dehydration and peripheral vasoconstriction from shock • Cool, clammy skin with hypovolemia • Accompanying skin changes; erythema, bullae, vesicles b. Decreased urinary output secondary to rhabdomyolysis • Reduced quantity • Brown colored • Varying degrees of renal failure
6. Instruct the client to report unusual, new, or different sensations (e.g., tingling, numbness, decreased ability to move toes or fingers, "pins/needles," "feels asleep").	6. Early detection of compromise can prevent serious impairment (Harris et al., 2006).
7. Reduce edema or its effects on function: a. Remove jewelry from affected limb. b. Elevate limbs unless contraindicated. c. Move fingers or toes of the affected limb two to four times every hour. d. Apply ice bags around injured site. Place a cloth between ice bag and skin. e. Monitor drainage (characteristics and amount) from wounds or incisional site. f. Maintain patency of the wound drainage system.	7. Edema reduction can deter compartment syndrome.
8. Notify the physician if the following occur (Miller & Askew, 2007): a. Change in sensation b. Change in movement ability	8. A decompressive fasciotomy may be needed (Harris et al., 2006).

(continued on page 357)

Interventions	Rationales
c. Pale, mottled, or cyanotic skin d. Slowed capillary refill (more than 3 seconds). e. Diminished or absent pulse f. Increasing pain or pain not controlled by medication g. Pain with passive stretching of muscle h. Pain increased with elevation	
9. If the preceding signs or symptoms occur, discontinue elevation and ice application.	9. These measures will decrease tissue pressure and restore local blood flow (Harris et al., 2006).
10. Monitor for signs and symptoms of fat embolism (de Feiter et al., 2007; Nucifora et al., 2007; Wong, et al., 2004). a. Tachypnea >30 breaths/min b. Sudden onset of chest pain or dyspnea c. Restlessness, apprehension d. Confusion, stupor, headache, lethargy, convulsions, and coma e. Elevated temperature >103°F f. Increased pulse rate >140 beats/min g. Petechial rash (12–72 hours postoperatively) h. Decreased pO$_2$ and oxygen saturation	10. There are two theories regarding the development of fat emboli. The first is a mechanical theory: A fracture can release bone marrow into the bloodstream, where it forms an embolism that can obstruct circulation (distal, cerebral, or pulmonary). The second theory is biomechanical: It identifies the alteration in the metabolism of circulating lipids as the source of emboli. Symptoms depend on the site of obstruction (Meyer, Pennington, Dewitt, & Schmeling, 2007). a–d,h. These changes are the result of hypoxemia. Fatty acids attract red blood cells and platelets to form microaggregates that impair circulation to vital organs (e.g., brain). Fatty globules passing through the pulmonary vasculature cause a chemical reaction that decreases lung compliance and ventilation/perfusion ratio. Pulmonary symptoms are the earliest signs; central nervous system (CNS) dysfunction occurs in up to 86% of clients, but are almost always reversible (de Feiter et al., 2007). e. Temperature increases are a response to circulating fatty acids. f. Refer to rationales 2a–d. g. This rash is the result of capillary fragility. Common sites are conjunctiva, axilla, chest, neck, and oral mucous membrane. Rash usually resolves within a week (de Feiter et al., 2007).
11. Minimize movement of a fractured extremity for the first three days after the injury.	11. Immobilization minimizes further tissue trauma, reduces the risk of embolism dislodgment, and rhabdomyolysis (Sahjian & Frakes, 2007).
12. Ensure adequate hydration.	12. Optimal hydration will dilute the irritating fatty acids throughout the system.
13. Monitor intake/output, urine color, and specific gravity.	13. These data will reflect hydration status.
14. Monitor for signs and symptoms of hemorrhage/shock: a. Increasing pulse rate with normal or slightly decreased blood pressure b. Urine output <5 mL/kg/h c. Restlessness, agitation, change in mentation d. Increasing respiratory rate e. Diminished peripheral pulses f. Cool, pale, or cyanotic skin g. Thirst	14. Bone is very vascular; blood loss can be substantial, especially with multiple fractures and fractures of the pelvis and femur. The compensatory response to decreased circulatory volume involves increasing blood oxygen by raising heart and respiratory rates, and decreasing circulation to the extremities (marked by decreased pulses, cool skin). Diminished cerebral oxygenation can cause altered mentation.

(continued on page 358)

Interventions	Rationales

15. Monitor for signs and symptoms of thrombophlebitis:
  a. Positive Homans sign (dorsiflexion of the foot causes pain from insufficient circulation)
  b. Calf tenderness, unusual warmth, redness
  c. Low-grade fever
  d. Edema of extremity
	15. Three factors increase the incidence of clot formation: stasis, coagulation abnormalities, and vessel damage. Clients with fractures are immobile and sustain vessel damage from trauma. A decrease in fibrinolytic activity occurs after surgery, beginning 24 hours postoperation with the lowest point on day three.

16. In a leg fracture, encourage exercises of the unaffected leg. Discourage placing pillows under the knees, using a knee gatch, crossing the legs, and prolonged sitting.	16. Leg exercises help to increase venous return; avoiding external pressure helps to prevent venous stasis.
17. Ambulate as soon as possible with at least five minutes of walking each waking hour. Avoid prolonged sitting on a chair with legs dependent.	17. Walking contracts leg muscles, stimulates the venous pump, and reduces stasis.

18. For high-risk clients, consult with physician for use of (Clarke-Pearson et al., 2003; Schiff et al., 2005):
 	
  a. Sequential compression stockings
 	
  b. Low-dose heparin
 	
  c. Low-dose dextran
 	
  d. Enoxiparin
	18. High-risk clients are those over 40-years-old, obese, with multiple trauma, a history of circulation deficits and on estrogen therapy, as well as those who have systemic infection or are cigarette smokers (Schiff et al., 2005). "Higher Risk" patients include those over 60-years-old, those with cancer, and a past history of DVT (Clarke-Pearson et al., 2003). Orthopedic surgery is associated with a very high rate (35%–85%) of venous thromboembolism (VTE) (Schiff et al., 2005).
	  a. These stockings reduce venous stasis by applying a graded degree of compression to the ankle and calf.
	  b. Low-dose heparin reduces blood coagulability by acting as antagonist to thrombin, and prevents the conversion of fibrinogen to fibrin.
	  c. Dextran decreases blood viscosity and reduces platelet aggregation. In addition, clots formed in the presence of dextran are more susceptible to fibrinolysis.
	  d. Enoxiparin affects coagulation by altering the ratio of anti-factor Xa to anti-factor IIa activity (Sanofi-Aventis, 2007).

19. Monitor for heparin-induced thrombocytopenia.	19. Heparin causes platelet sequestration.

 Related Physician-Prescribed Interventions

Medications. Analgesics, anticoagulants, muscle relaxants, platelet aggregation inhibitors
Laboratory Studies. Complete blood count, blood chemistry studies, arterial blood gases
Diagnostic Studies. X-ray examinations, tomograms, bone scans, computed tomography (CT) scan, and MRI
Therapies. Casts; wound care; traction (skin, skeletal); compression stockings; oxygen; surgery (internal fixation)

Documentation

Flow records
  Vital signs
  Pulses, color, warmth, sensation, movement of distal areas
  Intake and output

Progress notes
    Unusual complaints

Nursing Diagnoses

Acute Pain Related to Tissue Trauma Secondary to Fracture

NOC Comfort Level, Pain Control

Goal

The client will report progressive reduction of pain and relief after pain-relief measures.

Indicators

- Relate factors that increase pain.
- Relate interventions that are effective.

NIC Pain Management, Medication Management, Emotional Support, Teaching: Individual, Heat/Cold Application, Simple Massage

Interventions	Rationales
1. Refer to the General Surgery care plan, Appendix II, for general pain relief interventions.	1. Rationale is self-evident.
2. Immobilize the injured part as much as possible, using splints, when indicated.	2. Immobilization reduces pain and displacement.
3. Teach the client to change position slowly.	3. Slow movements decrease muscle spasms.
4. Elevate an injured extremity, unless contraindicated.	4. Elevation reduces edema and the resulting pain from compression.
5. Investigate pain not relieved by pain medications or other relief measures.	5. Unrelenting pain can indicate neurovascular compression from embolism, edema, or bleeding.

Documentation

Medication administration record
    Type, dosage, route of all medications administered
Progress notes
    Unrelieved pain and actions taken

High Risk for Ineffective Therapeutic Regimen Management Related to Insufficient Knowledge of Condition, Signs and Symptoms of Complications, and Activity Restrictions

NOC Compliance Behavior, Knowledge: Treatment Regimen, Participation in Health Care Decisions, Treatment Behavior: Illness or Injury

Goals

The goals for this diagnosis represent those associated with discharge planning. Refer to the discharge criteria.

NIC Risk Identification, Health Education, Teaching: Procedure/Treatment

Interventions	Rationales
1. Teach client to watch for and to report the following immediately: a. Severe pain b. Tingling, numbness c. Skin discoloration d. Cold extremities	1. These signs may indicate neurovascular compression, a condition requiring immediate medical intervention.
2. Explain the risks of infection and the signs of osteomyelitis (Miller & Askew, 2007): a. Chills, high fever b. Rapid pulse c. Malaise d. Painful, tender extremity not relieved with medication, rest, ice, and elevation	2. Bone infections can occur during the first 3 months after fracture.
3. Explain activity restrictions.	3. Resting the affected limb promotes healing.
4. Instruct on proper and safe ambulation techniques, as appropriate (Miller & Askew, 2007).	4. Improper use of assistive devices can cause injuries.
5. Refer to Cast care plan	

Documentation

Discharge summary record
    Client teaching
    Outcome achievement or status

Inflammatory Joint Disease (Rheumatoid Arthritis, Infectious Arthritis, or Septic Arthritis)

Rheumatoid arthritis (RA) is a chronic autoimmune-disabling disease. It presents as a characteristic inflammation with destructive synovitis in multiple diarthrodial joints, and causes pain, swelling, weakness, stiffness, and loss of function in the joints. The etiology is unknown, but research has been able to piece together the factors involved, such as: (1) genetic (inherited) factors, (2) environmental factors (viral or bacterial infection, making the individual susceptible to RA), and (3) hormonal factors, or others. Breastfeeding and contraceptive medication may also aggravate the disease. Research has also shown that RA is associated with a 5–15-year reduction in life expectancy.

The joints involved are usually symmetrically affected, with the small bones of the hands and feet affected first. The disease is characterized by cycles of exacerbations and remission. Extra-articular involvement of rheumatoid arthritis can include muscle atrophy; anemia; osteoporosis; and skin, ocular, vascular, pulmonary, and cardiac symptoms. Because many consequences of arthritis cannot be measured (e.g., functional, social, leisure), the impact of arthritis is often underestimated (Maclean et al., 2000; Lewis et al., 2004; Margaretten et al., 2007).

Septic arthritis (infectious or bacterial arthritis), is an invasion of the joint cavity by microorganisms. Bacteria can travel through the bloodstream from another site of active infection, resulting in hematogenous seeding of the joint. Organisms can also be introduced through trauma or surgical incision. *Staphylococcus aureus* is the most common causative organism, but any bacteria can cause the infection in the immunocompromised client; even nonpathogenic bacteria can be responsible for development of septic arthritis, which causes joint inflammation resulting from a viral, bacterial, or fungal organism invading the synovium and synovial fluid. Inflammation of a joint cavity causes severe pain, erythema, and swelling. Because infection often spreads from a primary site elsewhere in the body, fever or shaking chills often accompany articular manifestations.

Precise diagnosis is made by aspiration of the joint (arthrocentesis) and culture of the synovial fluid. Blood cultures for aerobic and anaerobic organisms should also be obtained. Septic arthritis is a medical emergency that requires prompt diagnosis and treatment to prevent joint destruction (Lewis et al., 2004; Zeller, Lym, & Glass 2007; Arthritis Foundation, 2008).

 Time Frame
Initial diagnosis
Secondary diagnosis

▪▪▪▪▪ DIAGNOSTIC CLUSTER*

Collaborative Problems	Refer to
PC: Septic Arthritis	
PC: Sjögren Syndrome	
PC: Neuropathy	
PC: Anemia, Leukopenia	Inflammatory Bowel Disease
PC: Avascular Necrosis	
PC: Cardiopulmonary Effects	
PC: Diabetes	
PC: Septic Shock	

Nursing Diagnoses	Refer to
Fatigue related to decreased mobility, stiffness	
High Risk for Impaired Oral Mucous Membrane related to effects of medications or Sjögren syndrome	
Disturbed Sleep Pattern related to pain or secondary to fibrositis	
High Risk for Loneliness related to ambulation difficulties and fatigue	
(Specify) Self-Care Deficit related to limitations secondary to disease process	
Ineffective Sexuality Patterns related to pain, fatigue, difficulty in assuming positions, and lack of adequate lubrication (female) secondary to disease process	
Impaired Physical Mobility related to pain and limited joint motion	
Chronic Pain related to inflammation of joints and juxta-articular structures	

(continued on page 362)

Nursing Diagnoses	Refer to
High Risk for Ineffective Therapeutic Regimen Management related to insufficient knowledge of condition, pharmacologic therapy, home care, stress management, and quackery	
Interrupted Family Processes related to difficulty/inability of ill client to assume role responsibilities secondary to fatigue and limited motion	Multiple Sclerosis
Powerlessness related to physical and psychological changes imposed by the disease	Chronic Obstructive Pulmonary Disease

Related Care Plans

Corticosteroid Therapy
Raynaud Disease
Congestive Heart Failure
Diabetes Mellitus

＊ This medical condition was not included in the validation study.

Discharge Criteria

Before discharge, the client or family will

1. Identify components of a standard treatment program for inflammatory arthritis.
2. Relate proper use of medications and other treatment modalities.
3. Identify characteristics common to "quack" cures.
4. Identify factors that restrict self-care and home maintenance.
5. Relate signs and symptoms that must be reported to a health care professional.

Collaborative Problems

Potential Complication: Septic Arthritis

Potential Complication: Sjögren Syndrome

Potential Complication: Neuropathy

Potential Complication: Avascular Necrosis

Potential Complication: Cardiopulmonary Effects (pericarditis, pericardial effusion, cardiomyopathy, pleurisy, pleural effusions, and congestive heart failure)

Potential Complication: Diabetes

Potential Complication: Septic Shock

Nursing Goal

The nurse will detect early signs/symptoms of (a) septic arthritis, (b) Sjögren syndrome, (c) neuropathy, (d) anemia, (e) avascular necrosis, (f) cardiopulmonary effects, (g) diabetes, and (h) septic shock, and collaboratively intervene to stabilize the client.

Indicators

- Temperature 98–99.5°F (a, h)
- No change in usual level of pain (a)
- No change in usual level of fatigue (a)
- Moist mucous membranes (b)

- No c/o paresthesias and numbness (c)
- Hemoglobin (d)
  - Male: 14–18 g/dL
  - Female: 12–16 g/dL
  - WBC 4,300–10,800 cells/mm^3 (a, h)
- Joint pain with weight-bearing (e)
- Limited to no range of movement (e)
- Shortness of breath (f)
- Chest pain (sharp, or relieved by sitting up and forward and worsens by laying down) (f)
- Dry cough (f)
- Fatigue (f)
- Anxiety (f)
- Friction rub with respirations (f)
- Weight loss or gain (f)
- Dizziness (f)
- Refractory hypotension (h)
- Tachypnea (h)
- Hypoglycemia/hyperglycemia (g)
- Continual thirst (g)
- Decreased level of consciousness (f, g, h) (Lewis et al., 2004; Maclean et al., 2000; Margaretten et al., 2007; Wagner, Johnson, & Kidd, 2006; Baird, Keen, & Swearingen, 2005).

Interventions	Rationales
1. Monitor for signs and symptoms of septic arthritis: a. Warm, painful, swollen joints b. Decreased range of motion c. Fever, chills, and fatigue d. White blood cell count <4000 cells/mm^3; >12,000 cells/mm^3 e. Refractory hypotension f. Tachycardia g. Decreased level of consciousness	1. The chronic inflammation of arthritis increases the risk of joints becoming infected by other diseased body parts.
2. Explain the need to splint or support and rest the inflamed joint.	2. Reducing movement can prevent permanent damage to the articular cartilage.
3. Monitor for signs and symptoms of Sjögren syndrome: a. Dry mucous membranes (mouth, vagina) b. Nasal crusting and epistaxis c. Decreased salivary and lacrimal gland secretions d. Nonproductive cough	3. The etiology of this syndrome is unknown. It is characterized by faulty secretion of lacrimal, salivary, gastric, and sweat glands.
4. Monitor for symptoms of neuropathy: a. Paresthesias b. Numbness	4. Swelling and actual joint changes can cause nerve entrapment.
5. Provide and explain the importance of disease-modifying antirheumatic medications. Monitor for adverse effects.	5. Refer to a pharmacological reference for specific information.
6. Monitor for signs and symptoms of avascular necrosis: a. Joint pain increasing over time and unrelieved with analgesia b. Increased limited range of movement and weight-bearing capability	6. Avascular necrosis can occur when the circulation to the bone is impaired (e.g., joint edema).
7. Monitor for signs and symptoms of cardiopulmonary involvement.	

(continued on page 364)

Interventions	Rationales
a. Arrhythmias b. Shortness of breath on exertion or rest c. Rales on auscultation d. Chest pain e. Dry or moist cough f. Friction rub with respirations	
8. Monitor for signs and symptoms of diabetes: a. Continual thirst b. Hypoglycemia/hyperglycemia c. Constant urination	

 Related Physician-Prescribed Interventions

Medications. Acetylsalicylates, immunosuppressives, corticosteroids, etanercept, cyclosporin A, cyclophosphamide, hydroxychloride, hydroxyquine, d-Penicillamine, nonsteroidal anti-inflammatory agents, gold salts, sulfasalazine

Laboratory Studies. WBC count, sedimentation rate, agglutination reactions, rheumatoid factor, immunoglobulins

Diagnostic Studies. X-ray films, radionuclide scans, direct arthroscopy, synovial fluid aspirate, bone scan

Therapies. Physical therapy, aqua therapy

Documentation

Progress notes
  Changes in range of motion
  Complaints

Nursing Diagnoses

Fatigue Related to Decreased Mobility, Stiffness

NOC Activity Tolerance, Endurance, Energy Conservation

Goal

The client will report less fatigue.

Indicators

• Identify daily patterns of fatigue.
• Identify signs and symptoms of increased disease activity that affect activity tolerance.
• Identify principles of energy conservation.

NIC Energy Management, Environmental Management, Mutual Goal Setting, Socialization Enhancement

Interventions	Rationales
1. Discuss the causes of fatigue (Maclean, 2000; Miller-Hoover, 2005): a. Joint pain	1. Clients with rheumatoid arthritis report that their fatigue is related to joint pain. In addition, clients with flare were observed to awaken more often and take longer to walk

(continued on page 365)

Interventions	Rationales
b. Decreased sleep efficiency c. Increased effort required for ADL	and perform activities than non-flare clients and the control group (Arthritis Foundation, 2008; Lewis et al., 2004).
2. Assist in identifying energy patterns; have the client rate his or her fatigue on a scale of 0 to 10 (0 = not tired; 10 = total exhaustion) every hour for a 24-h period.	2. Identifying times of peak energy and exhaustion can aid in planning activities to maximize energy conservation and productivity.
3. Allow the client to express feelings regarding the effects of fatigue on his or her life (Lewis et al., 2004; Maclean et al., 2000): a. Identify difficult activities. b. Identify activities that interfere with role responsibilities. c. Identify frustrations.	3. In many chronic diseases, fatigue is the most common, disruptive, and distressful symptom experienced because it interferes with self-care activities (Margaretten et al., 2007; Chester et al., 2007). Exploring with the client the effects of fatigue on his or her life will help both the nurse and the client to plan interventions.
4. Assist the client to identify strengths, abilities, and interests (Lewis et al., 2004; Maclean et al., 2000): a. Identify the client's values and interests. b. Identify the client's areas of success and usefulness; emphasize past accomplishments. c. Use this information to develop goals with the client. d. Assist the client to identify sources of hope (e.g., relationships, faith, things to accomplish). e. Assist the client to develop realistic short- and long-term goals (progress from simple to complex). The client may use a "goal poster" to indicate type and time for achieving specific goals.	4. Focusing the client on her or his strengths and abilities may provide insight into positive events and minimize overgeneralizing the severity of the disease, which can lead to depression (Lewis et al., 2004).
5. Help the client to schedule and coordinate procedures and activities to accommodate energy patterns. a. Promote participation in a fitness/conditioning program to maximize endurance. 6. Explain the purpose of pacing and prioritization (Lewis et al., 2004): a. Assist the client to identify priorities and to eliminate nonessential activities. b. Plan each day to avoid energy- and time-consuming nonessential decision-making. c. Organize work with items within easy reach. d. Distribute difficult tasks throughout the week. e. Rest before difficult tasks and stop before fatigue ensues.	5,6. The client requires rest periods before or after some activities. Planning can provide for adequate rest and reduce unnecessary energy expenditure.

7. Teach energy conservation techniques (Lewis et al., 2004):
a. Modify the environment:
  • Replace steps with ramps.
  • Install grab rails.
  • Elevate chairs by 3–4 inches.
  • Organize kitchen or work areas.
  • Reduce trips up and down stairs (e.g., put a commode on the first floor).
b. Plan small, frequent meals to decrease energy required for digestion.
c. Take a taxi instead of driving self.
d. Delegate housework (e.g., employ a high school student for a few hours after school).
	7. Such strategies can enable continuation of activities and contribute to positive self-esteem.

(continued on page 366)

Interventions	Rationales
8. Explain the effects of conflict and stress on energy levels, and assist the client to learn effective coping skills (Arthritis Foundation, 2007; Lewis et al., 2008). a. Teach the client the importance of mutuality in sharing concerns. b. Explain the benefits of distraction from negative events. c. Teach the client the value of confronting issues. d. Teach and assist the client with relaxation techniques before anticipated stressful events. Encourage mental imagery to promote positive thought processes. e. Allow the client time to reminisce to gain insight into past experiences. f. Teach the client to maximize aesthetic experiences (e.g., smell of coffee, back rub, or feel the warmth of the sun or a breeze). g. Teach the client to anticipate experiences he or she takes delight in each day (e.g., walking, reading a favorite book, or writing a letter).	8. There are many stressors related to chronic illness (e.g., pain, threats to independence, self-concept, future plans, and fulfillment of roles). Clients who learn self-help responses face definable, manageable adversities by maintaining control of everyday problems (Lewis et al., 2004; Maclean et al., 2000).
9. Teach the client to identify signs and symptoms that indicate increased disease action and to decrease her or his activities accordingly: a. Fever b. Weight loss c. Worsening fatigue d. Increased joint symptoms	9. During periods of increased disease activity, rest requirements increase to 10–12 h/day.

Documentation

Progress notes
    Fatigue pattern assessment
Discharge summary record
    Client teaching

High Risk for Impaired Oral Mucous Membrane Related to Effects of Medications or Sjögren Syndrome

NOC Oral Hygiene

Goal

The client will continue to have intact oral mucous membrane.

Indicators

- Identify factors that contribute to altered oral mucosa.
- Relate the need to report oral ulcers or stomatitis to a health care provider.
- Identify strategies for maintaining moist oral mucosa.
- Relate the need for frequent, regular dental care for Sjögren syndrome sequelae.

NIC Oral Health Restoration, Chemotherapy Management, Oral Health Maintenance

Interventions	Rationales
1. Teach client to inspect the mouth during daily oral hygiene activities and to report ulcers or stomatitis to a health care provider.	1. Early detection of these problems enables prompt intervention to prevent serious complications.
2. Teach the client to drink adequate amounts of nonsugared liquids.	2. Well-hydrated oral tissue is more resistant to breakdown.
3. Teach the client the importance of regular dental care.	3. Secondary Sjögren syndrome can result in excessively dry oral mucosa and predispose the client to tooth decay and gum disease (Sjögren's Syndrome Foundation, 2008).
4. Refer the client to Sjögren's Syndrome Foundation, 6707 Democracy Boulevard, suite 325, Bethesda, MD 20817. **Toll Free:** (800) 475-6473, **Local call:** (301) 530-4420, **Fax:** (301) 530-4415 (Sjögren's Syndrome Foundation, 2008).	4. This organization can provide more detailed information on the condition and its management.

Documentation

Flow records
   Oral assessments
Discharge summary record
   Client teaching
   Outcome achievement or status

Disturbed Sleep Pattern Related to Pain or Secondary to Fibrositis

NOC Rest, Sleep

Goal

The client will report a satisfactory balance of rest and activity.

Indicators

* Describe factors that inhibit sleep.
* Identify techniques to facilitate sleep.
* Demonstrate an optimal balance of activity and rest.

NIC Energy Management, Sleep Enhancement, Environmental Management

Interventions	Rationales
1. Discuss sleep patterns and requirements: a. Explain that they vary with age, activity level, and other factors. b. Discourage comparing sleep habits with others. c. Discourage focusing on hours slept; instead, focus on whether or not the client feels rested and restored after sleep. d. Encourage alternate activities if sleep is difficult (e.g., reading or needle-point).	1. Sleep deprivation results in impaired cognitive functioning (e.g., memory, concentration, and judgment) and perception, reduced emotional control, increased suspicion, irritability, and disorientation. It also lowers the pain threshold and decreases production of catecholamines, corticosteroids, and hormones (Arthritis Foundation, 2008; Lewis et al., 2004).
2. Encourage the client to take a warm bath or shower before bedtime; showering first thing in the morning may be beneficial to reduce morning stiffness.	2. Warm water increases circulation to inflamed joints and relaxes the muscles.

(continued on page 368)

Interventions	Rationales
3. Encourage performance of a bedtime ritual such as hygiene activity, reading, or having a warm drink.	3. A bedtime ritual helps to promote relaxation and prepare for sleep.
4. Initiate pain relief measures before bedtime, if appropriate. (Refer to the nursing diagnosis Chronic Pain in this care plan for more details.)	4. A client with inflammatory joint disease often experiences worsening symptoms at night.

5. Encourage proper positioning of joints:
  a. Pillows for limb position
  b. Cervical pillow
	5. Proper positioning may help to prevent pain during sleep and awakenings.

6. Encourage a balance of activity and rest. a. Encourage afternoon nap as needed to minimize fatigue	6. Regular physical exercise also seems helpful in controlling the symptoms of fibrositis (NIAMS, 2008).
7. Provide for uninterrupted sleep to enable completion of a sleep cycle (e.g., use a fan on low setting to drown out sounds).	7. A sleep cycle has an interval of 70–100 minutes. Most persons need to complete 4–5 cycles each night to feel rested (Arthritis Foundation, 2008).

Documentation

Progress notes
  Sleep patterns
  Reports of feeling rested in the morning

High Risk for Loneliness Related to Ambulation Difficulties and Fatigue

NOC Loneliness Severity, Social Involvement

Goal

The client will report continued satisfactory social patterns.

Indicators

- Identify factors that contribute to isolation.
- Identify strategies to increase social interaction.
- Identify appropriate diversional activities.

NIC Socialization Enhancement, Spiritual Support, Behavior Modification: Social Skills, Presence, Anticipatory Guidance

Interventions	Rationales
1. Encourage the client to share his or her feelings and to evaluate socialization patterns.	1. Only the client can determine whether socialization patterns are satisfactory or unsatisfactory. Some clients like to spend much of their time alone; others do not.

2. Discuss ways to initiate social contacts:
  a. Inviting a neighbor (adult or child) over for coffee or a snack 1 or 2 days a week
  b. Calling friends and relatives weekly
  c. Participating in social clubs (e.g., book discussion groups)
  d. Volunteering at the library, hospital, or other organizations
	2. Preoccupation with one's own life, problems, and responsibilities often prevents a client from socializing regularly with neighbors or relatives. Initiating contacts may be needed to break established patterns of isolation.

(continued on page 369)

Interventions	Rationales
3. Discuss the advantages of using leisure time for personal enrichment (e.g., reading or crafts).	3. Diversional activities can make the client more interesting to others.
4. Discourage excessive TV watching.	4. Other than educational documentaries, TV encourages passive participation and usually does not challenge the intellect.

5. Discuss possible options to increase social activities:
  a. Exercise groups (e.g., YWCA/YMCA)
  b. Senior centers and church groups
  c. Foster grandparent program
  d. Day care centers for the elderly
  e. Retirement communities
  f. House sharing
  g. College classes open to older persons
  h. Pets
  i. Telephone contact
  j. Arthritis support groups
	5. Socialization can promote positive self-esteem and coping.

6. Discuss the effects of disease on the client's body image and self-esteem.	6. Verbalization of fears can lead to a more positive approach in the management of the disease and may promote a positive self-concept.

7. Identify barriers to social contact:
  a. Lack of transportation
  b. Pain
  c. Decreased mobility
	7. Mobility problems commonly hinder socialization, but many associated difficulties can be overcome with planning.

Documentation

Progress notes
  Feelings regarding social contacts
Discharge summary record
  Client teaching
  Response to teaching

(Specify) Self-Care Deficit Related to Limitations Secondary to Disease Process

NOC See Bathing/Hygiene, Feeding, Dressing, Toileting, and/or Instrumental Self-Care Deficit

Goal

The client will demonstrate increased functioning in activities of daily living.

Indicators

• Identify the highest possible level of functioning in the following activities: bathing, dressing, feeding, and toileting.
• Demonstrate ability to use assistive devices.

NIC See Feeding, Bathing, Dressing, Toileting, and/or Instrumental Self-Care Deficit

Interventions	Rationales
1. Refer to occupational therapy for instruction in energy conservation techniques and use of assistive devices.	1. Occupational therapy can provide specific instructions and further assistance.

(continued on page 370)

Interventions	Rationales
2. Provide pain relief before the client undertakes self-care activities. (Refer to the nursing diagnosis Chronic Pain in this care plan for more information.)	2. Unrelieved pain can hinder self-care.
3. Provide privacy and an environment conducive to performance of each activity.	3. A comfortable, secure environment can reduce anxiety and enhance self-care abilities.
4. Schedule activities to provide for adequate rest periods.	4. Exhaustion decreases motivation for self-care activities.

5. Teach the client about the variety of assistive devices available for use in the home:
  a. Bathing:
    • Grip bars in shower and bath
    • Bath seat
    • Washing mitt
    • Long-handled washing appliances
    • Built-up toothbrush
    • Dental floss holder
  b. Dressing:
    • Long-handled zipper device
    • Buttoning device
    • Stocking/sock device
    • Long-handled shoe horns
    • Reacher
    • Elastic shoe strings
  c. Feeding:
    • Built-up utensils
    • Plate guard
    • Straw holder
  d. Toileting:
    • Raised toilet seat
    • Grip handle around toilet
	5. Assistive devices can improve self-care ability and enhance the client's sense of control over his or her life.

6. Explain available self-help reference materials, such as those from the Arthritis Foundation.	6. Promoting self-help promotes self-esteem.
7. Discuss with family members or significant others the changing family processes resulting from the client's illness.	7. Disability associated with inflammatory joint disease can interfere with the client's ability to care for self, family, and home; this disrupts family functioning.
8. Discuss the importance of promoting the client's self-care at an appropriate level.	8. Maximum self-care promotes positive self-esteem and reduces feelings of powerlessness; this can contribute to effective family functioning.

Documentation

Progress notes
    Type of assistance needed

Ineffective Sexuality Patterns Related to Pain, Fatigue, Difficulty in Assuming Position, Lack of Adequate Lubrication (Female) Secondary to Disease Process

NOC Body Image, Self-Esteem, Role Performance, Sexual Identity

Goal

The client will relate the intent to practice strategies to improve sexual functioning.

Indicators

- Identify factors that compromise sexual function.
- Identify strategies and techniques to facilitate and enhance sexual pleasure and expression.

NIC Behavior Management: Sexual, Counseling, Sexual Counseling, Emotional Support, Active Listening, Teaching: Sexuality

Interventions	Rationales
1. Encourage the client or couple to identify alternative sexual behaviors that may be used for sexual expression during periods of increased disease activity (e.g., touching, body massage).	1. Sexual expression is not limited to intercourse but encompasses many means of self-pleasure and giving pleasure to others (Arthritis Foundation, 2008; Lewis et al., 2004).
2. Teach the client or couple positions that minimize pain and joint stress during sexual intercourse (e.g., client on bottom, side-lying. Refer them to the Arthritis Foundation pamphlet *Living and Loving* for more information).	2. Inflammatory joint disease can result in loss of joint motion, owing to damage to both articular and juxta-articular structures (muscle, tendon, ligaments). Positions that lessen strain on the client's joints can enhance sexual pleasure (Arthritis Foundation, 2008).
3. Identify times when sexual activity may be more painful—most commonly in the early morning—and encourage having sex at other times. a. Encourage use of analgesics prior to sexual activity.	3. Inflammatory joint disease is often associated with prolonged morning stiffness.
4. Identify products that can be used to replace or supplement natural vaginal lubrication (e.g., water-soluble lubricants [KY jelly, Surgilube]).	4. Inflammatory joint disease is sometimes associated with Sjögren syndrome, which is characterized by a decreased ability to secrete lubricating fluids (e.g., tears, saliva, or vaginal secretions). Use of a lubricant can decrease pain during intercourse.
5. Discuss the need to plan for sexual activity (e.g., schedule it for a certain time of day or take a hot shower or bath before activity).	5. Planning sexual activity allows the client to prepare beforehand, which can increase pleasure for both the client and partner.

Documentation

Progress notes
   Client teaching
   Discussions

Impaired Physical Mobility Related to Pain and Limited Joint Motion

NOC Ambulation, Joint Movement, Mobility

Goal

The client will maintain and, when possible, increase strength and endurance in limbs.

Indicators

- Describe the rationale for interventions.
- Minimize joint stress and injury.
- Demonstrate correct performance of exercises.

NIC Exercise Therapy: Joint Mobility, Exercise Promotion: Strength Training, Exercise Therapy: Ambulation, Positioning, Teaching: Prescribed Activity/Exercise

Interventions	Rationales
1. Provide pain relief, as necessary. (Refer to the nursing diagnosis Chronic Pain in this care plan for specific interventions.) a. Teach the client the use of orthotic devices and ambulatory aids. b. Teach the client the need to achieve ideal body weight to facilitate mobility.	1. Pain can contribute to decreased mobility.
2. Encourage compliance with a prescribed exercise program, which may include the following exercises: a. Range-of-motion (ROM) b. Muscle strengthening c. Endurance	2. A regular exercise program including ROM, isometrics, and selected aerobic activities can help to maintain integrity of joint function, increase strength, and decrease pain and fatigue (Arthritis Foundation, 2008).
3. Encourage an amount of exercise consistent with the degree of disease activity.	3. During periods of acute inflammation, the client may immobilize the joints in the most comfortable position; this is usually partial flexion. Continued immobilization can result in joint stiffness and muscle weakness (extensor groups) that can quickly lead to contractures and more pain (Arthritis Foundation, 2008; Lewis et al., 2004).
4. Teach the client to perform all the following steps (Arthritis Foundation, 2008; Lewis et al., 2004; Maclean, 2000): a. Warm-up: Before exercising, take a warm bath or shower or use warm soaks or a heating pad on affected areas; then perform gentle stretching. b. Gentle ROM exercises without passive pressure at least once daily. c. Isometric and strengthening exercises: Contract muscle group for a count of eight, then relax for two counts. Repeat 10 times, 3–4 times a day on the quadriceps, abdominal muscles, gluteals, and deltoids. d. Endurance/aerobic exercise: Begin with a 5- to 10-minute period and gradually increase time. Appropriate activities include walking, swimming, and light racquet games (badminton, ping-pong). Inappropriate activities include heavy racquet sports (tennis, squash, racquetball), contact sports (football, hockey), and weightlifting or progressive resistance exercise. e. Cool-down: For 5–10 minutes, progressively slacken movements of extremities or walking pace, as the case may be.	4. a. A warm-up period of local heat or gentle stretching prior to strengthening and endurance exercises allows muscles to gradually become ready for more intense work (Arthritis Foundation, 2008; Lewis et al., 2004). b. Gentle ROM exercise prevents injury to joint tissue (Arthritis Foundation, 2008; Lewis et al., 2004). c. Isometric and other strengthening exercises can improve bodily function (Lewis et al., 2004; Maclean, 2000). d. Exercises that jar or bang joints are contraindicated. e. A cool-down period after more intense exercise allows muscle waste products to be removed, and permits the body to return gradually to its pre-exercise state.
5. If the client complains of postexercise pain persisting longer than 1½–2 hours, instruct him or her to do as follows: a. Decrease repetitions the next day. b. For severe soreness the next day, attempt ROM exercises at least once after local heat application to affected joints.	5. Exhaustion and pain decrease motivation to continue an exercise program.
6. Refer to physical therapy, as necessary.	6. Assistance may be needed for development of in-depth instruction in a physical activity program.
7. Refer to community-based exercise groups for people with arthritis (e.g., Arthritis Foundation Aquatic Exercise).	7. Such a program can provide exercise and socialization. Arthritis Foundation Aquatic Exercise provides warm water therapy.

Documentation

Flow records
> Exercises (type, frequency)

Chronic Pain Related to Inflammation of Joints and Juxta-articular Structures

NOC Comfort Level, Pain: Disruptive Effects, Pain Control, Depression Level

Goal

The client will relate improvement of pain and, when possible, increase daily activities.

Indicators

- Receive validation that pain exists.
- Practice selected noninvasive pain relief measures to manage pain.
- Relate improvement of pain and, when possible, increase daily activities.

NIC Pain Management, Medication Management, Exercise Promotion, Mood Management, Coping Enhancement

Interventions	Rationales
1. Teach the client to differentiate between joint pain and stiffness.	1. When there is joint pain, techniques for joint protection are instituted. When flares are diminished, active ROM exercises are indicated (Arthritis Foundation, 2008).
2. If joints are inflamed, let the client rest and avoid activities that stress joints. Gentle ROM exercises may be tried.	2. ROM exercises can prevent contractures. Inflamed joints are at risk for injury.
3. Apply local heat or cold to affected joints for approximately 20–30 minutes three to four times a day. Avoid temperatures likely to cause skin or tissue damage by checking the temperature of warm soaks or covering a cold/ice pack with a towel. 4. Encourage a warm bath or shower first thing in the morning to reduce morning stiffness.	3,4. Treatment of inflammatory joint pain focuses on the reduction of discomfort and inflammation by the use of local comfort measures, joint rest, and the use of anti-inflammatory or disease-modifying medications.
5. Encourage measures to protect affected joints: a. Perform gentle, active ROM exercises once daily during periods of active inflammation. b. Use larger, stronger joints (e.g., forearm, not fingers). c. Rest 5–10 minutes periodically when trying to complete a task. d. Avoid stooping, bending, or overreaching. e. Change positions frequently; avoid positions of stress on joints. f. Use splints. g. Obtain assistance with ADLs, if necessary. h. Maintain proper body alignment. i. Avoid pillows under the knees to prevent knee and hip flexion deformities. j. Use assistive devices, as necessary.	5. Frequent rest periods take the weight off joints and relieve fatigue. Proper positioning is needed to minimize stress on joints (Arthritis Foundation, 2008; Lewis et al., 2004; Maclean et al., 2000).
6. Encourage the use of adjunctive pain control measures: a. Progressive relaxation b. Transcutaneous electrical nerve stimulation (TENS) c. Biofeedback d. Imagery/music/acupuncture	6. Pain is a subjective, multifactorial experience that can be modified by the use of cognitive and physical techniques to reduce the intensity or perception of pain (Arthritis Foundation, 2008; Lewis et al., 2004; Maclean et al., 2000).

Documentation

Progress notes
    In affected joints: pain, swelling, warmth, erythema
    Pain relief measures
    Response to pain relief measures

High Risk for Ineffective Therapeutic Regimen Management Related to Insufficient Knowledge of Condition, Pharmacologic Therapy, Home Care, Stress Management, and Quackery

NOC Compliance Behavior, Knowledge: Treatment Regimen, Participation in Health Care Decisions, Treatment Behavior: Illness or Injury

Goals

The goals for this diagnosis represent those associated with discharge planning. Refer to the discharge criteria.

NIC Anticipatory Guidance, Learning Facilitation, Risk Identification, Health Education, Teaching: Procedure/Treatment, Health System Guidance

Interventions	Rationales

1. Explain inflammatory arthritis using teaching aids appropriate to the client's and family members' levels of understanding. Explain the following:
  a. Inflammatory process
  b. Joint function and structure
  c. Effects of inflammation on joints and juxta-articular structures
  d. Extra-articular manifestations of the disease process
  e. Chronic nature of the disease
  f. Disease course (remission/exacerbation)
  g. Low incidence of significant or total disability
  h. Components of the standard treatment program:
    • Medications (e.g., aspirin, non-steroida anti-inflammatory drugs, disease-modifying agents, cytotoxic agents, corticosteroids)
    • Local comfort measures
    • Exercise/rest
    • Joint protection/assistive devices
    • Consultation with other disciplines
	1. Inflammatory joint disease is a chronic illness. Education should emphasize a good understanding of the inflammatory process and actions the client can take to manage symptoms and minimize their impact on his or her life.

2. Allow significant others opportunities to share feelings and frustrations, including the need for:
  • Adequate nutrition
  • Regular follow-up care
	2. Persons with RA may be difficult to live with, demanding or manipulative (Arthritis Foundation, 2008; Lewis et al., 2004).

3. Teach the client and family to identify characteristics of quackery:
  a. "Secret" formulas or devices for curing arthritis
  b. Advertisements using "case histories" and "testimonials"
  c. Rejection of standard components of a treatment program
  d. Claims of persecution by the "medical establishment"
	3. An accurate and full understanding of inflammatory joint disease and its treatment lessens the client's susceptibility to quackery.

(continued on page 375)

Interventions	Rationales
4. Teach the client to take prescribed medications properly and to report symptoms of side effects promptly.	4. Adhering to the schedule may help to prevent fluctuating drug blood levels and can reduce side effects. Prompt reporting of side effects enables intervention to prevent serious problems.

5. Explain the proper use of other treatment modalities:
  a. Local heat or cold application
  b. Assistive devices
  c. Exercises
	5. Injury can further decrease mobility and motivation to continue therapies.

6. Explain the relationship of stress to inflammatory diseases. Discuss stress management techniques:
  a. Progressive relaxation
  b. Guided imagery
  c. Regular exercise
	6. Stressful events may be associated with an increase in disease activity. Effective use of stress management techniques can help to minimize the effects of stress on the disease process.

7. Reinforce the importance of routine follow-up care.	7. Follow-up care can identify complications early and help to reduce disabilities from disuse.
8. Refer to appropriate community resources such as The Arthritis Foundation, P.O. Box 7669, Atlanta, GA 30357-0669. Telephone: 800 283 7800 (Arthritis Foundation, 2008).	8. Such resources can provide specific additional information to enhance self-care.

Documentation

Discharge summary record
   Client and family teaching
   Outcome achievement or status
   Referrals, if indicated

Osteomyelitis

Osteomyelitis is a disease in which the bone and surrounding tissues are infected. The infection may result from a blood-borne infection from other sites (e.g., infected tonsils, pressure ulcer, inner ear infection); or may be due to direct bone contamination, as with an open fracture, trauma, or surgery. Osteomyelitis also may develop from vascular insufficiency, such as diabetes mellitus or severe atherosclerosis, or from the presence of indwelling fixation or prosthetic devices. The limited blood supply in the bone makes healing more difficult. Acute osteomyelitis may develop over several days to weeks. Chronic osteomyelitis may occur; there is no definitive time when the infection becomes chronic, but it is considered to take months, or even years, for acute osteomyelitis to blend into chronic osteomyelitis. The hallmark of chronic osteomyelitis is the presence of dead bone, known as sequestrum, and local bone loss; sinus tracts may also be present (Calhoun, Bal, & Yin, 2007; Ladd, Jones, & Otanez, 2003), leading to drainage of pus through the skin (U.S. National Library of Medicine, 2006).

 Time Frame
Initial or secondary diagnosis

▪▪▪▪▪ DIAGNOSTIC CLUSTER*

Collaborative Problems	Refer to
PC: Bone Abscess	
PC: Sepsis	Fractured Hip and Femur

Nursing Diagnoses	Refer to
Pain related to soft-tissue edema secondary to infection	Fractured Hip and Femur
Impaired Physical Mobility related to limited range of motion of affected bone	Fractured Hip and Femur
High Risk for Ineffective Therapeutic Regimen Management related to insufficient knowledge of condition, etiology, course, pharmacologic therapy, nutritional requirements, pain management, and signs and symptoms of complications	

Related Care Plan
Long-Term Venous Access Devices

*This medical condition was not included in the validation study.

Discharge Criteria

Before discharge, the client or family will do the following:

1. Identify factors that contribute to osteomyelitis.
2. Relate the signs and symptoms that must be reported to a health care professional.
3. Verbalize an intent to implement life style changes needed for healing.

Collaborative Problem

Potential Complication: Bone Abscess

Potential Complication: Chronic Osteomyelitis

Potential Complication: Reduced Limb or Joint Function

Potential Complication: Amputation

Nursing Goal

The nurse will monitor for early signs/symptoms of bone abscesses and sepsis, and collaboratively intervene to stabilize the client.

Indicators

- Temperature 98–99.5°F
- Heart rate 60–100 beats/min
- Respiratory rate 16–20 breaths/min
- White blood count >12,000 cells/mm³, <4000 cells/mm³

Interventions	Rationales

1. Monitor (Ladd et al., 2003; Mackowiak, 2007):
  a. Fever and chills
  b. Bone pain (with and without movement)
  c. Increasing tenderness
  d. Warmth
  e. Swelling
  f. Erythema (Merck Manuals Online Medical Library, 2005)
	1. As pus accumulates, the pressure increases, causing ischemia in the bone compartment.

2. Assure that antibiotics are given round the clock.	2. Sustained high therapeutic blood levels of the antibiotic are necessary. Teach the client the importance of taking the antibiotics for the entire course as ordered, usually 4–6 weeks at minimum (Carek et al., 2001).

 Related Physician-Prescribed Interventions

Medications. Intravenous antibiotic therapy, analgesics
Diagnostic Studies. Cultures (blood/wound/stool, urine); sedimentation rate; CBC; urinalysis; prealbumin, total protein; C-reactive protein; radionuclide bone scan; MRI, x-rays, computed tomography scanning, ultrasonography, bone scans, bone marrow scans, bone biopsy
Therapies. Incision and drainage of abscesses; surgical debridement; casting or immobilization of affected bone; hyperbaric oxygen; appropriate physical therapy, plastic surgery, vascular surgery, needle aspiration

Documentation

Flow records
  Vital signs
  Pulses, color, warmth, sensation, and movement of distal areas
Progress notes
  Unusual complaints

Nursing Diagnoses

High Risk for Ineffective Therapeutic Regimen Management Related to Insufficient Knowledge of Condition, Etiology, Course, Pharmacologic Therapy, Nutritional Requirements, Pain Management, and Signs and Symptoms of Complications

NOC Compliance Behavior, Knowledge: Treatment Regimen, Participation in Health Care Decisions, Treatment Behavior: Illness or Injury

Goals

The goals for this diagnosis represent those associated with discharge planning. Refer to the discharge criteria.

NIC Anticipatory Guidance, Risk Identification, Learning Facilitation, Health Education, Health System Guidance

Interventions	Rationales

1. Determine the client's knowledge of condition, prognosis, and treatment.
  a. Review proper handling techniques of pin sites or external fixation, if applicable.
	1. The client's understanding contributes to improved compliance and reduced risk.
	  a. Stress on sites should be avoided.

(continued on page 378)

Interventions	Rationales
b. Instruct the client to avoid tenting the skin around the pin and to avoid application of thick ointment and occlusive dressing on the pin site.	b. Occlusion at pin site can engender growth of microorganisms.

2. Teach the client infection control for drains and wounds:
  a. Use proper aseptic techniques for dressing changes and care of pins/external fixates.
  b. Ensure strict hand-washing before and after wound care.
  c. Use proper techniques for disposal of soiled dressing.
	2. These measures help to prevent the introduction of additional microorganisms into the wound; they also reduce the risk of transmitting infection to others.

3. Discuss nutritional requirements and dietary sources:
 	
  a. Calories per day: 2500–3000
  b. Protein: 100–125 g; sources: dairy, meat, poultry, fish, and legumes
  c. B-complex vitamins; sources: meat, nuts, and fortified cereals
  d. Vitamin C: 75–300 mg; sources: green vegetables and citrus fruits
  e. Phosphorus, magnesium, and vitamin D; sources: multivitamins
	3. Major complications of trauma and sepsis increase the metabolic rate from 10%–50%. In the presence of insufficient protein, the body breaks down its own endogenous protein stores (Porth, 2005).
	  a,b. Increased caloric and protein intake is needed to enhance the body's protein-sparing capacity.
	
	  c. B-complex vitamins are required for metabolism of carbohydrates, fat, and protein.
	  d. Vitamin C is essential for collagen formation and wound healing (Porth, 2005).
	  e. These nutrients are required for healing (Porth, 2005).

4. Explain the need for supplements (e.g., milkshakes and puddings).	4. Supplements may be needed to ensure the daily caloric requirement.
5. Discuss techniques to manage pain. Refer to index under acute or chronic pain.	
6. Teach the client to take the prescribed antibiotics diligently.	6. A variety of microorganisms may cause osteomyelitis. More than one organism may be involved. More and more clients may become immunocompromised, thus increasing the number of unusual pathogens such as fungi and mycobacteria (Carek, Dickerson, & Sack, 2001).

7. Teach the client to monitor and report complications of:
  a. Fever
  b. Increasing pain
  c. Visible bone deformity
  d. Swelling
  e. Exudate
	7. Fever and increasing pain can be indicative of sepsis. Sudden pain in an affected limb can indicate a pathologic fracture.

8. Prepare the client and family for the possibility of exacerbations.	8. Chronic osteomyelitis can occur if bacterial growth takes place in vascular scar tissue, which is impenetrable to antibiotics. Chronic osteomyelitis is most common following open fractures, with direct contamination of the wound.
9. Stress the importance of balancing rest, activity, constructive stress management, and optimal nutrition.	9. Clients can be empowered by giving them choices in managing their health.

Documentation

Discharge summary record
  Client teaching
  Outcome achievement or status

Osteoporosis

In osteoporosis, the rate of bone resorption exceeds the rate of bone formation. As a result, the bones become progressively porous and brittle and are prone to fracture from minimal trauma and even normal stress. Small-framed, non-obese Caucasian women are at greatest risk.

 Time Frame
Secondary diagnosis

■ ■ ■ ■ ■ DIAGNOSTIC CLUSTER*

Collaborative Problems

PC: Fractures
PC: Kyphosis
PC: Paralytic Ileus

Nursing Diagnoses

High Risk for Ineffective Therapeutic Regimen Management related to insufficient knowledge of condition, risk factors, nutritional therapy, and prevention

*This medical condition was not included in the validation study.

Discharge Criteria

Before discharge, the client or family will

1. Relate those risk factors that can be modified or eliminated.
2. Describe dietary modifications.
3. Relate signs and symptoms that must be reported to a health care professional.

Collaborative Problems

Potential Complication: Fractures
Potential Complication: Kyphosis
Potential Complication: Paralytic Ileus

Nursing Goal

The nurse will monitor for signs/symptoms of (a) fractures, (b) kyphosis, and (c) paralytic ileus, and collaboratively intervene to stabilize the client.

Indicators

• No new onset of pain (a, b)
• No changes in height (a, b)
• Bowel sound present (c)

Interventions	Rationales
1. Monitor for signs and symptoms of fractures (vertebral, hip, or wrist): a. Pain in lower back or neck b. Localized tenderness c. Pain radiating to abdomen and flank d. Spasm of paravertebral muscles	1. Bones with high amounts of trabecular tissue (e.g., hip, vertebrae, wrist) are more affected by progressive osteoporosis.

(continued on page 380)

Interventions	Rationales
2. Monitor for kyphosis of dorsal spine, marked by loss of height. Kyphosis is indicated when the distance between the foot and the symphysis pubis exceeds the distance between the head and the symphysis pubis by more than 1 cm.	2. This spinal change can cause height loss of 2.5–15 cm.
3. Monitor for signs and symptoms of paralytic ileus: a. Absent bowel sounds b. Abdominal discomfort and distention	3. Vertebral collapse involving the tenth to the twelfth thoracic vertebrae (T10–T12) can interfere with bowel innervation, resulting in ileus.

 Related Physician-Prescribed Interventions

Medications. Calcium, vitamin D supplements; salmon calcitonin; fluoride; estrogen replacement therapy in conjunction with progesterone; bisphosphonates; selective estrogen-receptor modulators
Laboratory Studies. Serum calcium and phosphate; alkaline phosphatase; hydroxyproline; urine calcium excretion; serum osteocalcin; hematocrit
Diagnostic Studies. Dual-energy x-ray absorptiometry of the spine and hip is the diagnostic method of choice. Include the first four vertebrae and use the lowest score to factor the diagnosis (Porth, 2005). If indicated, add bone scan, x-ray, CT, or MRI (Malabanan, 2008).
Therapies. Braces (vertebral), surgery to repair fractures, kyphoplasty, casting

Documentation

Progress notes
Complaints of pain or discomfort
Flow records
Bowel sounds
Height

Nursing Diagnoses

High Risk for Ineffective Therapeutic Regimen Management Related to Insufficient Knowledge of Condition, Risk Factors, Nutritional Therapy, and Prevention

NOC Compliance Behavior, Knowledge: Treatment Regimen, Participation in Health Care Decisions, Treatment Behavior: Illness or Injury

Goal

The goals for this diagnosis represent those associated with discharge planning. Refer to the discharge criteria.

NIC Anticipatory Guidance, Learning Facilitation, Risk Identification, Health Education

Interventions	Rationales
1. Discuss osteoporosis using teaching aids appropriate to the client's or family's level of understanding (e.g., pictures, slides, models). Explain the following:	1. Various teaching strategies may be necessary to maximize understanding and retention of information.

(continued on page 381)

Interventions	Rationales
a. Loss of bone density	a. Bone mass decreases as a result of decreased bone formation or increased bone resorption. Adults reach peak bone mass at age 35. At that time, women slowly begin to lose bone mass until just after menopause, when their rate of resorption increases rapidly (Sampson, 2002). Genetics, estrogen, and risk factors strongly influence the rate of bone loss. Risk factors include heavy caffeine intake, long-term corticosteroid or heparin use, excessive alcohol consumption, smoking, advanced age, postmenopausal age, Parkinson disease, Cushing disease, anorexia nervosa, scoliosis or rheumatoid arthritis, bilateral oopherectomy, and a history of either excessive exercise or a sedentary life style (Sommers, Johnson, & Beery, 2007).
b. Increased incidence of vertebral, hip, and wrist fractures	b. These bones contain large amounts of porous trabecular tissue, which makes them more susceptible to the effects of osteoporosis. Collectively, those over 45 suffer more than 1.5 million fractures per year. More than half of women over 65 have symptomatic osteoporosis. With postmenopausal osteoporosis, women aged 60–70 are frequent victims of wrist and vertebral fractures. The disease is five times more likely to occur in females than in males. The incidence of hip fractures is expected to exceed 750,000 per year due to osteoporosis, by 2050 (Sommers et al., 2007).

2. Explain the risk factors and which ones can be eliminated or modified (Hansen & Vondracek, 2004):
  a. Postmenopausal predisposition (natural or surgical)
 	
  b. Anorexia nervosa
 	
  c. Hyperthyroidism
 	
  d. COPD
 	
  e. Inflammatory bowel disease
 	
  f. Organ transplantation
 	
  g. Medication regimens such as those including glucocorticoids, anticonvulsants, heparin, coumadin, and methotrexate
 	
  h. Sedentary life style
	2. Focusing on the factors that can be modified can help to decrease feelings of helplessness (Hansen & Vondracek, 2004).
	  a. Decreased plasma estrogen level increases bone sensitivity to the resorptive action of parathyroid hormone.
	  b. Anorexia nervosa results in decreased bone density from poor nutritional intake of calcium and Vitamin D (Porth, 2005).
	  c. Hyperthyroidism has been found to trigger an acceleration of bone turnover (Porth, 2005).
	  d. COPD clients often have a long history of glucocorticoid use and an altered nutritional status (Tschopp et al., 2002).
	  e. Individuals with inflammatory bowel disease tend to be more malnourished (with low levels of Vitamin D), have a slighter build (possibly due to anorexia nervosa), and have decreased sex hormone levels. Coupled with chronic corticosteroid use, these individuals are greatly at risk for developing osteoporosis (Bernstein & Leslie, 2004).
	  f. Whether stem cell or organ recipients, transplant clients are predisposed to osteoporosis due to any combination of necessary therapies, nutritional or hormonal deficiencies, graft-versus-host disease, or prolonged immobilization (Mattano, 2004; Cruz et al., 2002).
	  g. Various medications have been linked to the progression of osteoporosis (e.g., some anti-convulsants, aluminum-containing antacids, thyroid supplements, isoniazid, prolonged heparin therapy, tetracycline, furosemide, and corticosteroids [particularly if dosage exceeds 15 mg/day for more than 2 years]). Corticosteroids affect calcium absorption by interfering with vitamin D metabolism. Discontinuation of therapy does not result in restoration of lost bone mass; however, it does prevent further disease progress.
	  h. Inactivity leads to increased rate of bone resorption.

(continued on page 382)

Interventions	Rationales
i. Thinness, small body frame	i. Thin women typically have less bone mass than obese women. Caucasian women with small skeletal frames are at greatest risk. African-American and Oriental women tend to have more bone mass and, thus, are at less risk.
j. Diet low in calcium and vitamin D and high in phosphorus	j. Insufficient dietary calcium and vitamin D can contribute to decreased bone reformation. High phosphate intake associated with high-protein diets stimulates parathyroid activity and, thus, increases bone resorption.
k. Excessive alcohol ingestion	k. Alcohol impairs calcium absorption in the intestines, increases urinary loss of calcium, and has a possible effect on liver activation of vitamin D.
l. Large quantities of caffeine	l. Early research results provide some evidence that caffeine increases calcium loss in kidneys and intestines.
m. Low sodium fluoride levels	m. Sodium fluoride stimulates osteoblastic activity.
n. Cigarette smoking	n. On average, smokers are thinner than nonsmokers; moreover, female smokers usually experience menopause earlier than nonsmokers.
o. Family history	o. Having a family history of osteoporosis predisposes an individual to developing the disease (Schoen, 2004).
p. Asian women and women of Asian descent	p. Asian women and women of Asian descent are known to have lower bone mineral density than non-Asian women. Osteoporosis is common among this population (Walker, Babbar, Opotowsky, McMahon, Liu, & Bilezikian, 2007).
3. Refer to community resources such as smoking cessation workshops, Alcoholics Anonymous, and the Arthritis Foundation.	3. These resources can provide needed assistance after discharge.
4. Teach the client to monitor for and report signs and symptoms of fracture: a. Sudden severe pain in the lower back, particularly after lifting or bending b. Painful paravertebral muscle spasms c. Gradual vertebral collapse (assessed by changes in height or measurements indicating kyphosis) d. Chronic back pain e. Fatigue f. Constipation	4. Early detection and treatment of fractures can prevent serious tissue damage and disabilities. The mortality rate from hip fractures in the elderly is more than 50%. Those that survive can be left greatly debilitated. The cost of treating osteoporosis-related conditions exceeds $6 billion per year in the United States alone (Sommers et al., 2007).
5. Reinforce explanations for nutritional therapy and consult with a dietitian, when indicated: a. Encourage calcium intake of 1000–1500 mg/day. b. Identity foods high in calcium (e.g., sardines, salmon, tofu, dairy products, and dark green leafy vegetables). c. Monitor for signs and symptoms of lactose intolerance, such as diarrhea, flatulence, and bloating. d. Recommend multivitamin containing 400–800 IU of vitamin D daily (Hansen & Vondracek, 2004). e. Identify food sources of vitamin D (e.g., fortified milk, cereals, egg yolks, liver, and saltwater fish).	5. Nutritional therapy is a critical component of treatment. a. The National Osteoporosis Foundation recommends 1200 mg of calcium per day for individuals up to age 24, 1000 mg for adults, and 1500 mg in postmenopausal women not receiving estrogen replacement (National Institutes of Health [NIH], 2000). Older women need increased intake to compensate for decreased absorption, and premenopausal women should prepare for expected bone resorption by increasing intake. b. Dietary sources provide a good means of increasing calcium intake. c. Increased intake of dairy products may lead to development of lactose intolerance, particularly in older clients. d,e. Vitamin D is necessary for the use and absorption of available calcium and phosphorus. However, excessive vitamin D intake can result in bone loss. Side effects, such as hypercalcemia, hypercalciuria, and kidney stones, can occur (NIH, 2000).

(continued on page 383)

Interventions	Rationales
f. Encourage adequate (not excessive) protein intake of approximately 44 g/day in most clients.	f. Protein intake should not exceed normal recommended requirements because excessive protein can enhance bone loss by causing increased urinary acid and resulting increased calcium excretion.
6. Explain the need for increased physical activity and certain restrictions: a. Encourage exercise that results in movement, pull, and stress on the long bones (e.g., walking, stationary bicycling, and rowing).	6. The greater the degree of immobility, the greater the bone resorption (Kawada et al., 2006). a. Weight-bearing exercise (i.e., walking, jogging, dancing, weightlifting, etc.) fosters both the development and maintenance of bone strength (Schmiege, Aiken, Sander, & Gerend, 2007), and aids in the prevention and treatment of osteoporosis. Caution should be used in choosing activities that carry a low risk of fractures. Activities such as jogging and bicycling over rough roads may increase pressure on weight-bearing vertebrae.
b. Instruct the client to exercise at least three times a week for 30–60 minutes each session, as ability allows.	b. A consistent exercise program stimulates bone formation and slows bone loss. It also provides a secondary benefit of improved neuromuscular conditioning, agility, and decreased likelihood of falls.
c. Discourage flexion exercises of the spine and sudden bending, jarring, and strenuous lifting. Avoid activities that rotate the vertebral spine.	c. These maneuvers increase vertical compression force, increasing the risk of vertebral fractures. Extension or isometric exercises are more appropriate and there is less risk of fractures to fragile vertebrae, as stress on the anterior portion of the vertebral body is minimized.
d. Plan adequate rest periods; lay in supine position for at least 15 minutes when chronic pain increases or at certain intervals during the day. e. Instruct the client in the use of a back brace, corset, or splint, if necessary. f. Encourage family members or other caregivers to provide passive range-of-motion exercises for a client immobilized in bed.	d. Fatigue decreases the motivation to exercise. e. This intervention minimizes the possibility of spontaneous fractures. f. Many studies have demonstrated that prolonged immobilization causes even young persons to experience bone loss (approximately 1% of bone mass per week).
7. Explain the importance of safety precautions, such as the following: a. Supporting the back with a firm mattress, body supports, and good body mechanics. b. Protecting against accidental falls by wearing walking shoes with low heels; removing environmental hazards such as throw rugs, slippery floors, electrical cords in pathways, and poor lighting; and avoiding alcohol, hypnotics, and tranquilizers. c. Using assistive devices as necessary (e.g., a cane or crutches) d. Avoiding any flexion movement, such as stooping, bending, and lifting. Explain that vertebral compression fractures can result from minimal trauma resulting from opening a window, lifting a child, coughing, or stooping.	7. Osteoporosis increases the risk of spontaneous fractures. a. Spontaneous fractures occur most often in the mid- to lower-thoracic and lumbar spine. b. Often, a fall is caused by a spontaneous fracture of the hip. Falling from a standing position can result in a fracture of the proximal femur; falling on an outstretched hand can cause Colles fracture. Even though wrist fractures heal easily, they are significant because they are predictors of hip fractures. c. Assistive devices can decrease the risk of falling. d. Any flexion movement should be eliminated to decrease the risk of fracture.
8. Explain any prescribed medication therapy; stress the importance of adhering to the plan and understanding possible side effects. As appropriate, reinforce the following: a. Calcium supplement: 1500 mg/day (Hansen, 2004) b. Vitamin D supplement: 800 IU/day for treatment, 600–800 IU/day for prevention (Hansen & Vondracek, 2004). (Note: If vitamin D is used in conjunction with calcitriol, plasma calcium levels should be monitored weekly for 4–6 weeks and then less frequently.)	8. Compliance with the medication regimen can slow the progression of osteoporosis. Awareness of possible side effects allows prompt reporting and intervention, to minimize adverse effects. a. Risk of renal calculi can be diminished with increased fluid intake. b. Vitamin D supplements increase utilization of phosphorus and calcium in clients with no exposure to sunlight and with inadequate dietary vitamin intake. Hypercalcemia can result.

(continued on page 384)

Interventions	Rationales
c. Parenteral Salmon Calcitonin: FDA-approved dose is 100 IU/daily. Frequently 100 IU/day, three times a week is used initially; then, after x-ray films and evaluation of serum calcium, dosage may decrease to 50 IU/day q 1–3 days. d. Calcitonin Salmon (Miacalcin): 200 IU daily, intra-nasally.	c,d. Serum calcium levels should be monitored closely because of an increased risk of hypercalcemia with induced hyperparathyroidism. Calcitonin decreases further bone loss at vertebrae and femoral sites. There seems to be some protection from postmenopausal bone loss for women who are not able or willing to take estrogen replacement therapy. This is an expensive therapy that may reduce pain associated with fractures. Initial therapy sometimes produces flushing and nausea.
e. Sodium fluoride: usually 60 mg/day at separate time from calcium administration.	e. Taking calcium with fluoride may interfere with fluoride absorption. Fluoride acts as a stimulator for osteoblasts and increases cancellous bone mass. The dosage seems to be an important factor in preventing fractures, with non-vertebral fractures increasing at higher doses. Lower doses, <50 mg, have a beneficial effect on vertebral fractures; however, the trabecular bone mass of the spine is not increased, as it is at higher doses. This indicates a narrow window for the most therapeutic dose (Arcangelo & Peterson, 2005).
f. Alendronate (Fosamax) orally, 35 or 70 mg, once per week, 10 mg/day. g. Risedronate Sodium (Actonel) orally, dosage and administration dependent on indication. h. Ibandronate Sodium (Boniva) orally, 150 mg once monthly.	f,g,h. Bisphosphonates decrease bone resorption and prevent bone loss. They must be taken on an empty stomach, with clear water. The client must remain in an upright position for 30 minutes following each dose. After 30 minutes, the client may eat, move as needed, and take other medications (Boniva requires 60 minutes). This will improve drug absorption and decrease the potential for esophagitis.
i. Raloxifene (Evista) orally, 60 mg/day.	i. Raloxifene decreases resorption and increases bone mineral density. It may increase menopausal hot flashes and venous stasis. Alert the client to avoid long periods of immobility. It is usually prescribed for women who are unable to tolerate bisphosphonates (Morris, 2005).
j. Teriparatide (Forteo) injectable, 20 mcg/day.	j. Teriparatide is a synthetic form of parathyroid hormone. It stimulates bone growth and increases bone density and is well-tolerated. This drug not only slows the progression of osteoporosis, but in some clients, has been shown to reverse the bone damage caused by the disease (Morris, 2005).
k. Strontium ranelate (Protelos) orally, 2 gm, dilute sachet in glass of water at bedtime, daily (not yet approved for sale in the U.S.).	k. Very popular in Europe, Strontium ranelate purports to decrease bone resorption and increases bone formation, balancing bone turnover. This medication claims to reduce both hip and vertebral fractures in postmenopausal women with osteoporosis.

9. Provide information regarding the National Osteoporosis Foundation, 1232 22nd Street, NW, Washington DC, 20037-1202, (202) 223-2226, website: http://www.nof.org.

Documentation

Discharge summary record
Client teaching
Outcome achievement or status
Referrals, if indicated

Human Immunodeficiency Virus/ Acquired Immunodeficiency Syndrome

An infection caused by the human immunodeficiency virus (HIV), acquired immunodeficiency syndrome (AIDS) was first reported in the United States in 1981. AIDS represents the end-stage of a continuum of HIV infection and its sequelae. Major modes of infection transmission include sexual activity with an infected person and exposure to infected needles or drug paraphernalia, blood, or blood products. A fetus can contract HIV infection from an infected mother perinatally. HIV infects primarily the T4-cell lymphocytes; this interferes with cell-mediated immunity. The clinical consequences of this progressive immune deficiency are opportunistic infections and malignancies. Beginning in the 1990s, the increased number of available medications has slowed the course of HIV dramatically.

 Time Frame
Initial diagnosis
Recurrent acute episodes

■■■■■■ DIAGNOSTIC CLUSTER

Collaborative Problems	Refer to
▲ PC: Opportunistic Infections	
△ PC: Malignancies	
▲ PC: Sepsis	Thermal Injury
△ PC: Myelosuppression	Leukemia
✱ PC: Peripheral Neuropathy	
✱ PC: HIV-Related Nephropathy	

Nursing Diagnoses	Refer to
▲ Risk for Infection Transmission related to the infectious nature of the client's blood and body fluids	
✱ High Risk for Imbalanced Nutrition: Less Than Body Requirements related to HIV infection, opportunistic infections/malignancies associated with AIDS	
✱ High Risk for Ineffective Coping related to situational crisis (i.e., new HIV or AIDS diagnosis, first hospitalization)	
✱ High Risk for Caregiver Role Strain related to AIDS-associated shame/stigma, and uncertainty about course of illness and demands on caregiver	
▲ High Risk for Ineffective Therapeutic Regimen Management related to functional and/or cognitive deficits associated with advanced HIV infection and/or opportunistic events	

(continued on page 386)

385

Nursing Diagnoses	Refer to
▲ High Risk for Ineffective Therapeutic Regimen Management related to insufficient knowledge of HIV, its transmission, prevention, treatment, and community resources	
△ Powerlessness related to unpredictable nature of condition	Chronic Obstructive Pulmonary Disease
△ Anxiety related to perceived effects of illness on life style and unknown future	Cancer: Initial Diagnosis
△ Grieving related to loss of body function and its effects on life style	Cancer: Initial Diagnosis
△ Powerlessness related to change from curative to palliative status	Cancer: Initial Diagnosis
▲ High Risk for Infection related to increased suscep-tibility secondary to compromised immune system	Leukemia
▲ Fatigue related to effects of disease, stress, chronic infections, and nutritional deficiency	Inflammatory Joint Disease
▲ High Risk for Impaired Oral Mucous Membrane related to compromised immune system	Chemotherapy

Related Care Plan

Cancer (End-Stage)

▲ This diagnosis was reported to be monitored for or managed frequently (75%–100%).
△ This diagnosis was reported to be monitored for or managed often (50%–74%).
✳ This diagnosis was not included in the validation study.

Discharge Criteria

Before discharge, the client or family will

1. Relate the implications of the diagnosis.
2. Describe the prescribed medication regimen.
3. Identify modes of HIV transmission.
4. Identify infection-control measures.
5. Describe signs and symptoms that must be reported to a health care professional.
6. Identify available community resources.

Collaborative Problems

Potential Complication: Opportunistic Infections

Potential Complication: Malignancies

Potential Complication: Sepsis

Potential Complication: Avascular Necrosis

Potential Complication: Peripheral Neuropathy

Potential Complication: HIV-Related Nephropathy

Nursing Goal

The nurse will detect early signs and symptoms of (a) opportunistic infections (pneumonia, encephalitis, enteritis, cytomegalovirus, herpes simplex, herpes zoster, stomatitis, esophagitis, meningitis), (b) malignancies, (c) sepsis, (d) avascular necrosis, (e) peripheral neuropathy, and (f) HIV-related nephropathy, and collaboratively intervene to stabilize the client.

Indicators

- Temperature 98–99.5°F (a, c)
- Respirations 16–20 breaths/min (a, c)
- SaO$_2$ arterial oxygen saturation (pulse oximeter >95%) (c)
- PaCO$_2$ arterial carbon dioxide 35–45 mmHg (c)
- Urine output >5 mL/kg/h (c, f)
- No proteinuria (f)
- Creatinine 0.2–0.8 ng/mL (f)
- No hematuria (f)
- Serum albumin 3.5–5 g/dL (f)
- Blood urea nitrogen 10–20mg/dL (f)
- No cough (a)
- Alert, oriented (a)
- No seizures, no headaches (a)
- Regular, formed stools (a)
- No herpetic or zoster lesions (a)
- Swallows with no difficulty (a)
- No change in vision (a)
- No weight loss (b)
- No new lesions (b)
- No bone pain (d)
- No lymphadenopathy (b)
- No leg pain, burning, or paresthesia (e)

Interventions	Rationales
1. Monitor for opportunistic infections:	1. Severe immune deficiencies with CD4 <200% cause opportunistic infections (OI) and malignancies. Antiretroviral therapy has dramatically reduced OIs.
a. Protozoal: • *Pneumocystis carinii* pneumonia (dry, nonproductive cough, fever, dyspnea) • *Toxoplasma gondii* encephalitis (headache, lethargy, seizures) • *Cryptosporidium* enteritis (watery diarrhea, malaise, nausea, abdominal cramps)	a. The most common and serious infection is *Pneumocystis carinii* pneumonia.
b. Viral (CD4 count <50): • Genital herpes simplex, herpes simplex perirectal abscesses (severe pain, bleeding, rectal discharge) • Cytomegalovirus (CMV) retinitis, colitis, pneumonitis, encephalitis, or other organ disease • Progressive multifocal leukoencephalopathy (headache, decreased mentation) • *Varicella zoster*, disseminated (shingles)	b. Herpes simplex is common and painful. The CMV infections are responsible for significant morbidity (e.g., blindness).
c. Fungal: • *Candida albicans* oral, stomatitis, and esophagitis (exudate, complaints of unusual taste in mouth) • *Cryptococcus neoformans* meningitis (fever, headache, blurred vision, stiff neck, confusion)	c. Fungal conditions are chronic, with relapses.

(continued on page 388)

Interventions	Rationales
d. Bacterial (CD4 count <50): • *Mycobacterium avium intracellulare* disseminated • *Mycobacterium tuberculosis* extrapulmonary and pulmonary	d. Bacterial infections frequently affect the pulmonary system.
2. Emphasize the need to report symptoms early. Advise that if the client is severely compromised, some symptoms will not be present (e.g., increased temperature).	2. Early treatment can often prevent serious complications (e.g., septicemia) and increases the chance of a favorable response to treatment.
3. Administer medications for opportunistic infections, as prescribed. Consult a pharmacological reference for specific information (Arcangelo & Peterson, 2005).	3. Some treatments for opportunistic infections are life-long to prevent reoccurrences.
4. Monitor for malignancies: a. Kaposi sarcoma: • Painless, palpable lesions (purplish, pinkish, or red) frequently on trunk, neck, arms, and head • Extracutaneous lesions in GI tract, lymph nodes, buccal mucosa, and lungs b. Lymphoma (non-Hodgkin, Burkitt): • Painless lymphadenopathy (an early site at neck, axilla, inguinal area) • Pruritus, weight loss	4. The malignancies that affect AIDS clients are related to immunosuppression: a. Kaposi sarcoma is cancer of the lymphatic vessel (endothelial wall). It is not skin cancer. b. Non-Hodgkin lymphomas can progress into the bone marrow, liver, spleen, gastrointestinal, and nervous systems.
5. Monitor for signs and symptoms of sepsis: a. Temperature >38°C (100.4°F) or <36°C (96.8°F) b. Decreased urine output c. Tachycardia and tachypnea d. Pale, mottled, cool skin; chills e. Unexplained change in mental status f. Hypoglycemia g. White blood cells (WBCs) and bacteria in urine h. Positive blood culture	5. Gram-positive and gram-negative organisms can invade open wounds, causing septicemia. A debilitated client is at increased risk. Sepsis produces massive vasodilation, resulting in hypovolemia and subsequent tissue hypoxia. Hypoxia leads to decreased renal function and cardiac output, triggering a compensatory response of increased respirations and heart rate in an attempt to correct hypoxia and acidosis. Bacteria in urine or blood indicate infection.
6. Monitor and support use of prescribed prophylactic medication (Dolin, Masur, & Saag, 2003): a. If CD4 <200, Bactrim DS 3× week (Monday, Wednesday, Friday) prophylaxis for *P. carinii* pneumonia b. If CD4 <50 Zithromax 1200 mg every week, prophylaxis for cytomegalovirus (CMV).	6. Prophylactic medications can prevent serious infections that increase morbidity and mortality.

 ## Related Physician-Prescribed Interventions

Medications. Antibiotics, antiretrovirals, antiemetics, antifungals, chemotherapy, antipyretics, nucleoside reverse transcriptase inhibitors (NRTI), antiviral agents, protease inhibitors (PI), antidiarrheals, nonnucleoside reverse transcriptase inhibitors (NNRTI), fusion inhibitors

Intravenous Therapy. Creatinine, hyperalimentation, BUN

Laboratory Studies. Liver function tests, viral load, enzyme-linked immunosorbent assay (ELISA), complete blood count, cultures, T-lymphocyte cells, hepatitis panel, CD4 count, Western blot test, CD8 count, serum protein, genotype, phenotype

Diagnostic Studies. Magnetic resonance imaging (MRI), endoscopy, biopsies, thallium scan, chest x-ray film

Therapies. Nasogastric feeding

Documentation

Flow records
Lesions (number, size, locations)
Respiratory assessment
Neurologic assessment (mentation, orientation, affect)

Mouth assessment
Progress notes
Complaints

Risk for Infection Transmission Related to the Infectious Nature of the Client's Blood and Body Fluids (This diagnosis is not currently on the NANDA list, but has been included for clarity and usefulness.)

NOC Infection Severity, Risk Control, Risk Detection

Goal

The client will take necessary steps to prevent infection transmission.

Indicators

- Describe the factors that contribute to HIV transmission
- Describe how to disinfect infected objects or surfaces

NIC Teaching: Disease Process, Infection Protection

Interventions	Rationales
1. Adhere to universal precautions. Wash hands before and after contact with client in care situation.	1. Universal precautions are to prevent the transmission of blood-borne pathogens from client to caregiver. They are taken with all clients regardless of diagnosis, age, or sexual orientation of the client. The particular precautions taken with each individual client are dependent on the potential of transmission related to the care to be rendered and not to the client's diagnosis. Hand-washing is one of the most important means of preventing the spread of infection.
2. Wear latex gloves when performing procedures involving the client's body fluids, including: blood, semen, vaginal fluids, cerebrospinal fluids, peritoneal fluids, amniotic fluids, synovial fluids, pleural fluids, pericardial fluids, or other body fluids with visible blood (e.g., urine, menses, stool, saliva, etc.). Do not reuse gloves (CDC, 2000).	2. Gloves provide a barrier from contact with infectious secretions and excretions.
3. Wear mask, goggles, or eye shield and gown when there is potential for splash of body fluids during client care (e.g., suctioning, tracheotomy; or care-giving for a client with explosive vomiting or diarrhea) (CDC, 2000).	3. Masks prevent transmission by air isolation of infectious agents, if oral mucosal lesions are present. Gowns prevent soiling of clothes if contact with secretions/excretions is likely.
4. Handle needles, scalpels, and other sharp objects carefully to prevent injury to self or others after use with client. Never recap a needle; make sure to bend or break it; and carefully dispose of used needles and other sharps into a puncture-proof sharps container immediately after use (CDC, 2000).	4. Needle sticks and sharp injuries carry by far the highest risk of transmission of blood-borne pathogens to health care personnel.
5. Immediately and thoroughly wash hands or other skin surfaces that may have been contaminated with blood or other potentially infectious body fluids.	
6. Ensure easy access to an adequate supply of gloves, masks, gowns, and eye shields in all client care areas. Nonlatex gloves and disposable resuscitation equipment should also be available.	6. Allergy to latex among the general population is on the rise.

(continued on page 390)

Interventions	Rationales
7. Ensure comprehensive and current institutional or agency policies that direct the management of employee exposure to client blood and infectious body fluids.	7,8. Policies guiding exposure should be comprehensive, current, and supportive of both the client and the involved employee.
8. Be supportive of colleagues, nursing and otherwise, who have sustained exposure to a client's blood or infectious body fluids. Support includes emotional support and protecting the person's confidentiality as much as possible.	
9. Instruct and provide written material on safer sex guidelines and other risks for transmission that include: a. Correct and consistent use of a latex condom with every act of vaginal, anal, and/or oral intercourse; avoid spermicides with nonoxynol 9 b. Provision for adequate lubrication during intercourse by the use of a water-based lubricant c. Maintenance of a faithful monogamous sexual relationship with partner d. No sex or use of sex toys involving any exchange of blood or body fluids e. Avoidance of high-risk behavior conducive to transmission of blood-borne or sexually transmitted diseases, including: • Sex with multiple partners • Engaging in sexual activity when not sober and on street drugs • Sex or behavior that involves the exchange of blood or body fluids • Needle or straw sharing during drug use, tattooing, body piercing, acupuncture, or other such activities • Rough sexual practices that can lead to breaks in the mucosal lining of the rectum, mouth, or vagina	9. Correct and consistent use of a latex condom with every act of intercourse has been shown to significantly reduce the risk of transmission of sexually transmitted diseases, including HIV. Oil-based lubricants (e.g., Vaseline) and nonoxynol 9 spermicides can degrade latex condoms. Any object contaminated with blood must be cleaned with a bleach solution (one part bleach to 10 parts water).
10. Instruct the client and provide written material on transmission precautions for the home setting, including: a. No sharing of toothbrushes, razors, enema or douche equipment, or other sharp objects b. Prompt and adequate disposal of needles and other sharps into a puncture-proof, locked container c. Proper hand-washing after any contact with the clients' blood or infectious body fluids d. Use of gloves for provision of client care involving contact with his or her blood or body fluids e. Cleaning up blood and body fluid spills by using gloves and paper towel to get up the majority of the spill before disinfecting area with a 1:10 solution of bleach	10. Fear of HIV transmission is a common concern of caregivers of persons with HIV. HIV is rapidly inactivated by exposure to disinfecting agents. Household bleach solution (dilute 1:10 with water) is an inexpensive choice.
11. Provide facts to dispel myths regarding transmission of HIV, including: a. HIV is **not** transmitted by skin-to-skin contact, mosquito bites, swimming pools, clothes, eating utensils, telephones, or toilet seats. b. Closed mouth kissing, sweat, tears, urine, and feces do not transmit HIV. c. HIV cannot be contracted while giving blood.	11. Dispelling myths and correcting misinformation can reduce anxiety and allow others to interact more normally with the client.
12. Provide the client and caregiver with the National CDC AIDS hotline number (1-800-342-AIDS).	12. The hotline provides rapid access to accurate information.

High Risk for Imbalanced Nutrition: Less Than Body Requirements Related to HIV Infection, Opportunistic Infections/Malignancies Associated with AIDS

NOC Nutritional Status

Goal

The client will ingest daily nutritional requirements in accordance with activity level and metabolic needs.

Indicators

- Relate importance of good nutrition.
- Identify deficiencies in daily intake.
- Relate methods to increase appetite.

NIC Nutrition Management, Nutritional Monitoring

Interventions	Rationales
1. Assess the client for weight loss and malnutrition at regular intervals. 2. Consult with a dietitian for nutritional assessment, calorie count, meal planning, and nutritional instruction, as indicated.	1,2. All clients, including HIV asymptomatic, should have a complete nutritional assessment on initial contact, and then regularly with a health professional. The three goals for good nutritional management are as follows: a. Preserve lean body mass. b. Provide adequate levels of all nutrients. c. Minimize symptoms of malabsorption.
3. Instruct the client on the importance of and methods to increase calories and proteins in diet: a. Eat cheese, nuts, peanut butter, milk shakes, and so on between meals and at bedtime. b. Enrich soups, vegetables, or starchy foods with milk or cheese. c. Sweeten toast, cereals, and fruits with sugar, jelly, or honey. d. Use sour cream and heavy cream when possible. e. Eat hard-boiled eggs for snack.	3. Significant weight loss is a common finding among clients with HIV. Early nutritional assessment and institution of corrective measures may slow weight loss and prevent the nutritional complications often seen in the later stages of HIV infection.
4. Assist the client with referrals and necessary coordination to assure consistent supply of nutritional supplements, as indicated.	4. Some states cover the costs of nutritional supplements when a dietitian documents the need. Nutritional supplements are drinks containing several micro- and macronutrients. They are usually recommended when the client is experiencing difficulty gaining or maintaining weight or when food intake declines for whatever reason. Instant breakfast mixed with whole milk is a reasonable cost-effective alternative to commercially made supplements in some instances.
5. Regularly assess for client anorexia and institute measures to increase client appetite, as appropriate: a. Rule out psychologic etiology (e.g., depression, anxiety). b. Suggest small, more frequent meals throughout the day. c. Drink liquids 30 minutes before rather than during meals. d. Offer foods in a pleasant atmosphere, and encourage the presence of family and friends during meals, as possible. e. Consult the physician regarding the use of appetite stimulants, when indicated. f. Avoid serving large quantity of food by providing nutritionally dense foods (e.g., nutritional supplements).	5. Anorexia is a loss or change in appetite with a relative decrease in food intake that, left untreated, will result in a loss of body weight and cell mass. Anorexia can be a direct result of advanced HIV infection, AIDS-associated opportunistic infections or malignancies, or any number of medications used to treat them.

(continued on page 392)

Interventions	Rationales
6. Instruct the client on interventions to manage any contributing factors to weight loss/ and wasting. Contributing factors include: a. Mouth soreness: • Avoid hot and cold foods. • Avoid acid-containing drinks and spicy foods. b. Difficulty swallowing: • Avoid hard-to-swallow, sticky foods (e.g., peanut butter). • Choose soft, moist foods (e.g., oatmeal, pudding). • Dunk toast, crackers, and so forth in soup, milk, or other beverages to moisten them. c. Changes in taste: • Add spices to food (e.g., lemon juice, garlic). d. Nausea and vomiting: • Eat smaller, more frequent meals. • Eat foods low in fat and sugar. • Consult with physician regarding antiemetic medication. e. Diarrhea: • Avoid caffeine and fatty foods. • Drink fruit juices to replace fluids and minerals. • Eat foods low in lactose. • Consult with the physician regarding antidiarrheal medication.	6. • Oral and esophageal candidiasis and pharyngeal and esophageal ulcers are relatively common among those with advanced HIV infection. Candidiasis especially is easily recognizable and treatable. • Changes in taste are not uncommon with medications used to treat HIV infection and opportunistic infections (e.g., AZT and Pentamidine). • Nausea and vomiting may be present secondary to medications or to an organic cause requiring treatment. Persistent vomiting may lead to dehydration, fluid and electrolyte imbalance, and weight loss. • Diarrhea is seen frequently in HIV infection and the opportunistic infection within the AIDS spectrum (e.g., cryptosporidium, CMV). Depending on the etiology, malabsorption, fever, or anorexia may accompany the diarrhea, increasing the likelihood of nutritional deficit.
7. Explain to the client the potential gastrointestinal side effects of his or her medications.	7. Many medications used in treating HIV infection and the opportunistic infections seen in AIDS have possible gastrointestinal side effects. These side effects can potentially limit the client's nutritional intake and nutrient absorption (e.g., *AZT:* nausea and vomiting, altered sense of taste; *didanosine (DDI):* nausea and vomiting, diarrhea; *Trimethoprim-Sulfamethoxazole (TMP-SMX):* anorexia, glucose intolerance, stomatitis).
8. Instruct the client and caregiver on methods to avoid food-borne illness: a. Thoroughly cook meat, fish, and eggs. b. Wash hands before handling foods. c. Maintain foods at a safe temperature. d. Wash fruits and vegetables before consumption. e. Use separate cutting boards for raw and cooked foods. f. Monitor the proper serving of foods in summer (e.g., hot foods are hot, cold are cold).	8. Persons with HIV infection are thought to be especially at risk for food-borne diseases because of immunosuppression.
9. Consult a social worker to evaluate the client for referral to agencies supportive of the nutritional needs of the HIV-infected.	9. Fatigue and weakness seen in advanced HIV disease can prevent the client from adequate meal preparation. Home-delivered meals and food basket delivery are examples of services for HIV+ clients seen in some areas.

Documentation

High Risk for Ineffective Coping Related to Situational Crisis (i.e., New HIV or AIDS Diagnosis, First Hospitalization)

NOC Coping, Self-Esteem, Social Interaction Skills

Goal

The client will make decisions and follow through with appropriate actions to change provocative situations in his or her personal environment.

Indicators

- Verbalize feelings related to emotional state.
- Focus on the present.
- Identify response patterns and the consequences of resulting behavior.
- Identify personal strengths and accept support through the nursing relationship.

NIC Coping Enhancement, Counseling, Emotional Support, Active Listening, Assertiveness Training, Behavior Modification

Interventions	Rationales
1. Encourage the client's expression of anxiety, anger, and fear. Listen attentively and nonjudgmentally.	1. Listening is credited as a helpful strategy to assist clients coping with AIDS. Anger at AIDS-associated prejudice or lack of understanding of others occurs commonly among the HIV-infected.
2. Encourage the client to share her or his feelings regarding the multiple losses associated with AIDS (e.g., friends, community, family structure, and social networks).	2. Complex social issues of morality, sexuality, contagion, and shame are associated with AIDS-related losses and interfere with grieving and coping (Mallison, 1999).
3. Determine the client's past coping strategies and assist him or her to develop coping strategies based on previously successful outcomes and personal strengths.	3. Interventions constructed using the client's personal style and character are likely to be of lasting use to her or him. Previous successes should be built on when possible.
4. Discourage coping mechanisms that are maladaptive or self-defeating (e.g., alcohol, drugs, denial, and compulsive behavior).	4. Substance abuse and destructive denial are behaviors often perceived to provide subjective relief. This relief, however, is usually temporary and ultimately self-defeating.
5. Assist the client with finding meaning in illness, and not assuming the victim role.	5. "Focus should be on living with AIDS, not dying of it. Nurses can rekindle the spark that is needed to discover the meaning and purpose in suffering and even death" (Carson & Green, 1992, p. 217).
6. Encourage and reinforce the client's hopes, as appropriate.	6. "All life is based on hope and when hope is low or absent, people see their lives as finished . . . when professional caretakers see hope in the terminally ill as unrealistic and label it as denial, they lower the quality of the years remaining to the person, or force him or her to turn elsewhere for help" (Hall, 1990, p. 183).
7. Assist the client to identify appropriate support systems (e.g., support group, community resources) and encourage their use.	7. Feelings of alienation and social isolation are common among the HIV-infected. Support groups potentially are able to educate, support, and assist the client to anticipate and deal with the crises inevitable to the client's illness (Mallinson, 1999).
8. Encourage and provide exercise, recreation, diversional activities, and independent activities-of-daily-living (ADLs) performance.	8. Diversional activities can provide opportunities of rest from mental and emotional distress. Maximal independence and participation in activities can increase self-confidence and self-esteem.
9. Instruct the client on stress-management techniques (e.g., distraction, relaxation imagery), as appropriate.	9. Stress reduction techniques can assist the client in dealing with personal fears and anxieties.
10. Assist the client with coordination of care, using advocacy as necessary.	10. The physical demands of chronic infection and the frequent complexity of care arrangements can hinder consistent compliance and follow-up with medical care and counseling. Nurses, by making appropriate referrals for the client, decrease demands on the client and are able to advocate for the client, as indicated.

High Risk for Caregiver Role Strain Related to AIDS-Associated Shame/Stigma, and Uncertainty About the Course of Illness and Demands on the Caregiver

NOC Caregiver Well-Being, Role Performance, Care-giving Endurance Potential, Family Coping, Family Integrity

Goals

The caregiver will relate a plan on how to continue social activities despite care-giving responsibilities.

Indicators

* Identify activities that are important for self.
* Relate intent to enlist the help of at least two people.

NIC Caregiver Support, Respite Care, Coping Enhancement, Family Mobilization, Mutual Goal Setting, Support System Enhancement, Anticipatory Guidance

Interventions	Rationales
1. Explore the meanings and beliefs that caregivers hold regarding the client's HIV infection. 2. Explore the caregivers' prior knowledge of, and current feelings about, the client's sexual behavior or drug use.	1,2. The caregiver's feelings of shame or guilt regarding the client's HIV infection or life style may prohibit optimal care-giving. The caregiver may need help in expressing his or her feelings regarding these traditionally taboo topics (Brown & Powell-Cope, 1991; Powell-Cope & Brown, 1992).
3. Encourage the caregiver's consistent acknowledgment of, and support for, the care-giving role.	3. AIDS caregivers often receive little to no support for their care-giving role. Their fear of discrimination and hatred toward themselves or the client stops them from disclosing their situation. This leads to feelings of isolation (Brown & Powell-Cope, 1991; Powell-Cope & Brown, 1992).
4. Assist the caregiver with anticipating the uncertainty, role changes, and unpredictability of their care-giving role, and course of the HIV infection itself.	4. Uncertainty is a common concern in caregivers of persons with life-threatening illnesses. The ability to anticipate certain events or changes can allay some anxiety for caregivers (Brown & Powell-Cope, 1991).
5. Assist the caregiver with decision-making regarding whom to tell about his or her AIDS care-giving role.	5. Fear of rejection and isolation can make the decision of whom to tell anxiety-provoking and overpowering to AIDS caregivers (Powell-Cope & Brown, 1992).
6. Assist the caregiver with the "staging" method of disclosure of the AIDS care-giving role, as appropriate.	6. Disclosure by "staging" of the information is less anxiety-provoking than full disclosure (e.g., *Stage I:* "My son is sick." *Stage II:* "My son is under a doctor's care and needs to stay with me until he is back on his feet." *Stage III:* "My son has AIDS and needs my help.") (Powell-Cope & Brown, 1992).
7. Provide anticipatory guidance and counseling to AIDS caregivers as they prepare to go public with their care-giving role.	7. The process of "going public" with their AIDS care-giving role is complex and stressful for caregivers planning to do so. Rehearsal of how and when to disclose and how to handle potential responses can minimize the stress on the caregiver (Powell-Cope & Brown, 1992).
8. Reinforce the caregivers' knowledge of HIV transmission, infection-control precautions for the home, and so on. Provide written information on same and be available for questions.	8. Fear of HIV transmission to self and other members of their household is a major concern of AIDS caregivers (Brown & Powell-Cope, 1991).

(continued on page 395)

Interventions	Rationales
9. Instruct the caregiver on the signs and symptoms of burnout, and on stress-reduction techniques.	9. AIDS caregivers are subject to burnout and need help to avoid it, if possible. If burnout is inevitable, caregivers need to be able to identify it at early onset, so as to be able to plan for respite care.
10. Identify and assist—with help of community resources supportive of AIDS caregivers, such as community case management services—AIDS caregivers' support groups, day care, respite care, and the like.	10. AIDS caregivers need support that recognizes their unique needs, and support should be used to reinforce their care-giving.
11. Encourage the caregiver to pursue personal goals during his or her AIDS care-giving.	11. Pursuing personal goals during their care-giving assists caregivers to be able to focus on their own interests and lives. These goals carry on and provide their lives with meaning after the death of the client.
12. Allow the caregiver to express her or his frustration or anger at the health care system and health care professionals, as appropriate.	12. Expressing anger and frustration at health professionals or the health care system after perceived situations involving insensitivity or a lack of understanding is a way for caregivers to express their feelings.

High Risk for Ineffective Therapeutic Regimen Management Related to Functional and/or Cognitive Deficits Associated with Advanced HIV Infection and/or Opportunistic Events

NOC Compliance Behavior, Knowledge: Treatment Regimen, Participation in Health Care Decisions, Treatment Behavior: Illness or Injury

Goals

The goals for this diagnosis represent those associated with discharge planning. Refer to the discharge criteria.

NIC Anticipatory Guidance, Risk Identification, Health Education, Learning Facilitation

Interventions	Rationales
I. *Client-Specific Interventions*	
1. Assist the client in clarifying his or her wishes regarding medical treatment issues and short- and long-term goals in relation to his or her quality of life definition.	1. Effective interventions can be planned and implemented only with the client's full understanding and agreement.
2. Collaborate with the client's primary care provider to simplify the medical regimen and to maximize the client's comfort and symptom management, as possible.	2. Medications with limited or questionable efficacy can sometimes be discontinued without loss of clinical benefit to the client. Other medications may be taken less often in certain circumstances, thus simplifying the overall regimen.
3. Assist client to find health care providers who are accessible, experienced at HIV management, and sensitive to the client's gender, cultural, and life style issues.	3. Clients with HIV-experienced providers live longer and suffer less morbidity overall than do those HIV-infected individuals who receive their care from HIV-inexperienced providers.
4. Educate the client about HIV and opportunistic-illness management and the importance of adherence for maximum clinical benefit.	4. Ongoing client-specific education related to the expected benefits of therapy is basic to any effort to assist their long-term adherence.

(continued on page 396)

Interventions	Rationales
5. Arrange for a comprehensive system of ongoing client assessment of the ability to manage the therapeutic regimen by utilizing an HIV-specific or health care–system case management program.	5. A plan for formal ongoing assessment of the client's ability to manage his or her regimen and evaluation of the adequacy of the interventions is crucial to the regimen's success in the long-term.
6. Assist the client's understanding of the actual or potential effects of the use of denial or substance abuse on his or her ability to maintain the therapeutic regimen. Refer motivated clients for mental health or substance abuse assistance, as indicated.	6. Depression, anxiety, and substance abuse can all interfere with the client's ability to attain his or her health-related goals.
7. Advocate for the client to the insurance carrier for uncovered benefits, using cost-effective rationale, as indicated.	7. A well-reasoned argument using clinical benefit and cost-effectiveness can sometimes convince an insurance carrier to reimburse for a normally uncovered benefit.
8. Consult with the dietitian, social worker, or case manager to evaluate client eligibility for special programs or services according to need (e.g., pharmacy providing overnight drug delivery or state Medicaid program coverage of nutritional supplements).	8. HIV-specific programs and services vary from state to state. A variety of health care professionals may be needed to arrange for a specific service.
9. Refer the client to a social worker or attorney for assistance with power of attorney, living will, or last will and testament arrangements, as indicated.	9. Creating a living will or giving a trusted friend, partner, or family member power of attorney for health care allows the client some confidence that his or her wishes and quality of life definition will be respected in the event that he or she is unable to make care-related decisions.
10. Consult physical therapy, occupational therapy, or rehabilitation specialist for client-functional determination as indicated.	10. Physical medicine and rehabilitation physicians specialize in determining the functional potential of clients. With the input of physical and occupational therapists, they develop plans to maximize that potential.
II. *Family/caregiver specific* (with the consent of the client)	
11. Facilitate family or caregivers' meeting to communicate the client's wishes, evaluate the adequacy of client support, and delegate care tasks.	11. Clear communication of the client's needs and wishes related to their care to those persons directly involved in their care is of the utmost importance.
12. Educate family/caregivers on HIV transmission precautions in the home setting and on specific care tasks required (e.g., medication administration, proper body mechanics for client transfer assistance).	12. Fear of HIV transmission is common among caregivers of clients with HIV infection.
13. Counsel the caregiver on anticipating the client's care requirements and integrating these into the caregiver's life.	13. Uncertainty is a common concern of caregivers of persons with life-threatening illnesses. The ability to anticipate certain events or changes can allay some anxiety for caregivers
14. Refer for personal care services, chore provision grant, or "buddy" services, when indicated and available.	14. A variety of care-giving support services are available, depending on locale and client eligibility.
15. Arrange for client "day care" services when the primary caregiver is employed and other supports are lacking.	15. Balancing care-giving responsibilities with employment can be difficult to impossible for persons caring for someone with cognitive and/or functional deficits. Day care arrangements for the client, if eligible, are available in some areas.
16. Refer caregivers to a respite program, when indicated and available.	16. AIDS caregivers need support that recognizes their unique needs and support should be used to reinforce their care-giving.

(continued on page 397)

Interventions	Rationales
III. *Care environment specific*	
17. Arrange for home nursing services for the client.	17. Most insurance carrier policies cover home nursing services when the client is homebound and requires skilled care.
18. Consult with a social worker or care manager to arrange for client placement at a skilled nursing facility, hospice facility, residential living program, or other program or facility commensurate with the client's wishes or short- and long-term goals.	18. The client's care needs and wishes regarding living situation adequacy in relation to those needs are two essential factors affecting the decision for or against an alternative care setting.

Documentation

Discharge summary record
    Client teaching
    Outcome achievement or status
    Referrals, if indicated

High Risk for Ineffective Therapeutic Regimen Management Related to Insufficient Knowledge of HIV, Its Transmission, Prevention, Treatment, Health Promotion Activities, and Community Resources

NOC Compliance Behavior, Knowledge: Treatment Regimen, Participation in Health Care Decisions, Treatment Behavior: Illness or Injury

Goals

The goals for this diagnosis represent those associated with discharge planning. Refer to the discharge criteria.

NIC Anticipatory Guidance, Risk Identification, Health Education, Learning Facilitation

Interventions	Rationales
1. Teach the client and family the basic pathophysiology of HIV infection and concepts of the immune system.	1. The client's understanding of HIV and its effects on the body is the basis of all further learning.
2. Explain HIV infection treatment including those decisions related to the CD4 level and viral load. These include the initiation of antiretroviral therapy and prophylaxis against certain opportunistic infections (e.g., *Pneumocystis carinii* pneumonia [PCP], *mycobacterium avium complex* [MAC]).	2. Besides the symptoms the client may experience as a result of the progress of HIV infection, his or her CD4 and viral load levels are essential to the initiation of antiretroviral therapy and prophylaxis against such opportunistic infections as PCP (Bartlett & Finkbeiner, 2001).
3. Teach HIV routes of transmission and preventive measures/risk reduction activities.	3. The importance of efforts to prevent HIV transmission to infected persons as well as prevention of reinfection by a resistant strain of HIV or with other STDs, if a person is already infected cannot be overstated!
4. Explain the rationale and intended effects of the treatment program: a. Enhanced immune function b. Limitation of HIV infection c. Prevention of opportunistic events	4. Client agreement with commitment to treatment is tied to her or his understanding of treatment goals.

(continued on page 398)

Interventions	Rationales
5. Teach the client and family the name, action, dose, safe use, potential side effects, and interactions of medications.	5. Many individuals will better adhere to therapy if they understand the intended effect of the individual medications on their bodies.
6. Stress the importance of close adherence to combination antiretroviral therapy to prevent viral resistance to therapy.	6. Combination antiretroviral therapy, taken as directed, offers more effective long-term suppression of HIV infection and prevents the emergence of resistant HIV strains by maintenance of a constant effective level in the bloodstream (Sanford, Sonde, & Gilbert, 1996).
7. Ask the client if he or she ever misses doses. Explain the risks of missing doses of antiretroviral medications. Provide tips to prevent missing doses.	7. Poor adherence to antiretroviral drugs can result in the development of resistant virus to multiple medications—even entire classes, such as protease inhibitors (Murphy, Lu, Martin, Hoffman, & Marelich, 2002).
8. Assist the client to identify techniques to take pills on schedule (Bartlett & Finkbeiner, 2000). a. When brushing teeth (twice a day) b. Alarm watch c. Sectioned pill containers d. When watching favorite television shows e. If you miss a dose, take it when you remember; do not "double up."	8. A decrease of 10% of the total pills taken weekly causes a doubling of HIV (Bangsberg et al., 2000).
9. Encourage the client to inform other persons in same household about his or her condition.	9. Keeping a secret and hiding pills increases the risk of missing doses.
10. Teach health promotion/illness prevention practices (Khalsa, 2005): a. Balanced nutrition b. Stress reduction with effective coping strategies c. Screening, as indicated (e.g., syphilis, sexually transmitted infections, or tuberculosis) d. Age-related screening (e.g., Pap tests, mammograms, colonoscopy, prostrate screening antigen) e. Adequate rest f. Leisure activities that relax and renew	10. a. The link between nutrition and immunologic function is well established (Casey, 1997). b. Stress has been associated with reactivation of herpes simplex infection and malignancy because of its negative effect on the immune system (Flaskerud & Ungrarski, 1999). c,d. Screening allows for early detection of cancer, which can increase successful treatment. e. Adequate and consistent periods of rest and sleep can lessen the effects of stress on the body (Flaskerud & Ungrarski, 1999).
11. Teach practices to prevent non-HIV infections and illnesses (Kaplan, 2002): a. Immunizations (influenza, pneumonococcal, hepatitis A & B, tetanus, pertussis) b. Avoidance of food/water borne illnesses: • Avoid raw or undercooked eggs, meat, fish • Use pasteurized juices and dairy products • Avoid contaminated water • Follow travel food precautions (e.g., raw vegetables, fruits) c. Avoid exposure to TB, varicella, salmonella, Campylobacter, Cryptococcus, and other organisms d. Avoid bat droppings and dust storms e. Use caution in homeless shelters, prisons, and day care facilities f. Avoid ill animals and cat excreta	11. These infections can seriously compromise the health of a person with HIV/AIDS.

(continued on page 399)

Interventions	Rationales
12. Explain the factors that impinge on the attainment of the client's health-related goals: a. Unsafe sexual practices b. Substance abuse c. Tobacco use d. Lack of adherence to therapy	12. a. Sexually transmitted infection further compromises the immune system. b. Heroin, cocaine, alcohol (ETOH), marijuana, and amphetamines are all possible factors in immune suppression. Substance abuse also interferes with adherence to medication regimen (Dolin et al., 2003). c. The detrimental effects of nicotine addiction are well known (e.g., circulatory, respiratory). d. Strict adherence to combination antiretroviral therapy is necessary to prevent subtherapeutic levels of medication conducive to the emergence of viral resistance and consequent disease progression.
13. Provide information and encourage appropriate utilization of community resources supportive of persons living with HIV.	13. There are numerous organizations available locally and nationally for a variety of services and support to clients living with HIV and their caregivers.
14. Include significant other/family participation in all phases of client education (only with the client's consent).	14. Ideally, the involvement of supportive others in the client's education regarding HIV and its treatment reinforces the client's learning and supports the caregiver and caregiver's commitment to the client.
15. Instruct the client on signs and symptoms to report to health care provider: a. Visual changes b. Anorexia/weight loss c. Difficult or painful swallowing d. Persistent or severe diarrhea e. Dyspnea or resistant cough f. Headache/stiff neck g. Fever/chills/night sweats h. Fatigue	15. a. Blurred vision, "floaters," and other visual complaints can signify CMV retinitis of HIV retinopathy. CMV retinitis causes blindness if not treated. b. Anorexia or weight loss can be a sign of disease progression, opportunistic disease, or HIV wasting syndrome. c. Dysphagia or odynophagia are symptomatic of esophageal candidiasis or other GI tract infection or ulceration requiring treatment. d. Besides causing dehydration and electrolyte imbalances, diarrhea in the HIV-infected client can be symptomatic of anything from a food intolerance or medication side effect to an opportunistic pathogen. e. Cough or dyspnea in the HIV-infected client can be a sign of TB, PCP, or other bacterial or opportunistic infection. f. A headache with a stiff neck can be a sign of meningitis, bacterial or otherwise. Persistent headache can indicate a central nervous system malignancy or infection, or sinusitis. g. This combination of signs and symptoms can signify HIV progression or a local systemic infection. h. Fatigue can be the first sign of infection or generalized sepsis even in the absence of other signs and symptoms.

Documentation

Discharge summary record
    Client teaching
    Outcome achievement or status
    Referrals, if indicated

Systemic Lupus Erythematosus

Systemic lupus erythematosus (SLE) is a chronic, multisystem, inflammatory, autoimmune disease of connective tissues. SLE can affect pleural and pericardial membranes, joints, skin, blood cells, and nervous and glomerular tissue. The etiology has not been confirmed, but latent viruses, genetic factors, hormones, and medications have been linked to its onset. The Lupus Foundation of America estimated 500,000–1.5 million people with SLE in 2001. The female preponderance of lupus clients is 10:1, with more occurrences in blacks and Hispanics. Incidence is higher in first-degree relatives. The triggering of abnormal immune function results in the formation of antibodies directed against various components of the body (autoantibodies) (Gill et al., 2003; Ruiz-Irastorza et al., 2001).

 Time Frame
Initial diagnosis
Secondary diagnosis

■■■■■ DIAGNOSTIC CLUSTER*

Collaborative Problems

PC: Sepsis
PC: Polymyositis, Serositis, Pericarditis
PC: Vasculitis
PC: Hematologic Abnormalities
PC: Raynaud Disease
PC: Neuropsychiatric Disorders

Nursing Diagnoses	Refer to
High Risk for Injury related to increased dermal vulnerability secondary to disease process	
High Risk for Ineffective Therapeutic Regimen Management related to insufficient knowledge of condition, rest versus activity requirements, pharmacologic therapy, signs and symptoms of complications, risk factors, and community resources	
Powerlessness related to unpredictable course of disease	Diabetes Mellitus
Fatigue related to decreased mobility joint pain and effects of chronic inflammation	Inflammatory Joint Disease
High Risk for Disturbed Self-Concept related to inability to achieve developmental tasks secondary to disabling condition and changes in appearance	Multiple Sclerosis
Related Care Plan	
Corticosteroid Therapy	

*This medical condition was not included in the validation study.

Discharge Criteria

Before discharge, the client or family will

1. State the intent to share concerns with a trusted friend.

2. Identify components of a standard treatment program.
3. Relate proper use of medications.
4. Describe actions to reduce the risk of exacerbation.
5. Identify signs and symptoms that must be reported to a health care professional.

Collaborative Problems

Potential Complication: Sepsis

Potential Complication: Polymyositis, Serositis, Pericarditis

Potential Complication: Vasculitis

Potential Complication: Hematologic Abnormalities

Potential Complication: Raynaud Disease

Potential Complication: Neuropsychiatric Disorders

Potential Complication: Renal Insufficiency (Refer to Multiple Sclerosis)

Potential Complication: Sjögren Syndrome (Refer to Inflammatory Joint Disease)

Nursing Goal

The nurse will detect early signs and symptoms of: (a) polymyositis, serositis, (b) pericarditis, (c) vasculitis, (d) hematologic abnormalities, (e) Raynaud syndrome, (f) neuropsychiatric disorders, and (g) sepsis, and collaboratively intervene to stabilize the client.

Indicators

* No new complaints of pain (a, b, c, f)
* Blood pressure >90/60 mmHg (c, g)
* Pulse 60–100 beats/min (c, g)
* Respirations 16–20 breaths/min (c, g)
* Temperature 98–99.5°F (c, g)
* Capillary refill <3 seconds (e)
* Liver function tests
  * Alanine aminotransferase (ALT) (c)
  * Aspartate aminotransferase (AST) (c)
  * Bilirubin total D.1–1.2 mg/dL (c)
  * Prothrombin time 9.5–12 seconds (c, d)
  * Partial prothrombin time 20–45 seconds (c, d)
  * Bleeding time 1–9 minutes (c, d)
* Stool for occult blood: negative (c)
* Arterial blood gases
  * Oxygen saturation (SaO_2) 94%–100% (c)
  * Carbon dioxide ($PaCO_2$) 35–45 mmHg (c, g)
  * Serum pH 7.35–7.45 (c)
* Renal function
  * Creatinine 0.7–1.4 mg/dL (c)
  * Blood urea nitrogen 10–20 mg/dL (c)
  * Prealbumin (c)
  * Urine creatinine clearance (c)
  * Complement C4 70–150 mg/dL (c)
  * Complement C3 16–45 mg/dL (c)
* Complete blood count
  * Hemoglobin: Male 13–18 gm/dL; Female 12–16 gm/dL (d)
  * Hematocrit: Male 42%–50%; Female 40%–48% (d)

- Red blood cells: Male 4.6–5.9 million/mm^3; Female 4.2–5.4 million/mm^3 (d)
- White blood cells 5000–10,800/mm^3 (d, g)
- Platelets 100,000–400,000/mm^3 (d)
- No c/o cyanosis, membranes tingling, or pain in fingers/hands (c, e)
- No seizures (c, f)
- Intact sensation and motor function (c, f)
- Clear, oriented (c, f)

Interventions	Rationales

1. Monitor for sepsis (Morton et al., 2006)
  a. Temperature >38°C (100.4°F) or <36°C (96.8°F)
  b. Heart rate >90 beats/min
  c. Respiratory rate >20 breaths/min or PaCO$_2$ <32 torr (<4.3 kPa)
  d. White blood cell count >12,000 cells/mm^3, <4000 cells/mm^3 or >10% immature (band) forms
  e. Site specific cultures
  f. Serum lactic acid level
  g. Decreasing platelet count
	1. Damage to cell membranes can provide sites for gram-positive and gram-negative organisms.

2. Monitor for polymyositis, serositis, and pericarditis:
  a. Tendinitis (pain radiating down an extremity)
  b. Bursitis (pain in shoulder, knee, elbow, or hip)
  c. Pericarditis (pain beneath left clavicle and in the neck and left scapular region; aggravated by movement)
	2. Antibodies are produced that damage the cell membrane constituents, DNA, nucleoprotein, and histones. The resulting inflammation stimulates antigens that in turn stimulate autoantibodies, and the cycle begins anew (Lash & Lusk, 2004).

3. Monitor for the effects of vasculitis:
  a. Hypertension
  b. Peripheral vascular disease
  c. Pericarditis
  d. Hepatomegaly
  e. Splenomegaly
  f. Gastritis
  g. Pneumonitis
  h. Seizures
  i. Renal disease
	3. Excessive autoantibodies combine with antigens to form immune complexes. These complexes are deposited in vascular and tissue surfaces, triggering an inflammatory response and eventually local tissue injury. Thus, SLE can affect any organ system (Porth, 2005).

4. Monitor for hematologic disorders:
  a. Hemolytic anemia
  b. Leukopenia
  c. Lymphopenia
  d. Thrombocytopenia
	4. Antibodies against red blood cells result in hemolytic anemia. Antibodies against platelets result in thrombocytopenia. B-lymphocyte production is regulated by a balance of CD4+ and CD8+ lymphocytes (T cells). This balance is disrupted by SLE (Porth, 2005).

5. Monitor laboratory findings for early signs of vasculitis and hematologic disorders:
  a. Liver function tests
  b. Prothrombin time (PT), partial thromboplastin time (PPT)
  c. Bleeding time
  d. Stool for occult blood
  e. Arterial blood gases
  f. BUN, creatinine, prealbumin
  g. Serum pH
  h. Urine creatinine clearance
  i. Complement C3, complement C4
	5. Inflammation of vessel walls lowers blood supply to major organs, causing necrosis, sclerosis, and dysfunction.

(continued on page 403)

Interventions	Rationales
6. Teach the client to report purpura and ecchymosis.	6. These are manifestations of platelet deficiencies.

7. Monitor for Raynaud syndrome:
  a. Vasospasm of arteries in fingers resulting in pallor, changing to cyanosis, and ending in rubor
  b. Numbness, tingling, and pain in affected digits
	7. In Raynaud syndrome, inflammation and subsequent damage to connective tissue produces vasospasm of arteries and arterioles of the fingers and hands (Porth, 2005).

8. Monitor for neurological disorders:
  a. Seizures
  b. Headaches
  c. Myasthenia gravis
  d. Guillain-Barré syndrome
  e. Polyneuropathy
  f. Cranial neuropathy
  g. Acute confusion
	8. The pathological cause of CNS symptoms is unclear. They are thought to result from acute vasculitis that impedes blood flow, causing clots, hemorrhage, or both. Seizures are usually related to renal failure.

9. Monitor for psychiatric disorders:
  a. Anxiety disorder
  b. Cognitive dysfunction
  c. Mood disorder
  d. Psychosis
	9. The cause of psychiatric disorders in clients with SLE is unknown. They have been associated with triggering the onset of SLE.

10. Refer the client to a mental health specialist.	10. About 20% of affected persons have neuropsychiatric disorders (Gladman, 1996).

 Related Physician-Prescribed Interventions

Medications. Cyclophosphamide, cyclosporine, azathioprine, dobutamine, thalidomide, mycophenolate mofetil, methotrexate, nonsteroidal anti-inflammatory agents, antimalarials, cytotoxic agents, corticosteroids

Laboratory Studies. Complete blood count with differential, complement human C4, antiphospholipid antibodies, complement human C3, anticardiolipin (IgM, IgG), BUN, lupus anticoagulant, serum creatinine, urinalysis, 24-hour urine, creatinine clearance, antinuclear antibody titer (ANA), antibody to double-stranded DNA antigen (anti-ds DNA)

Therapies. Plasmapheresis, stem-cell transplantation, immunoablative therapy, joint replacement

Diagnostic Studies. EEG, chest x-ray, EKG, renal biopsy

Documentation

Flow records
  Vital signs
  Peripheral pulses
Progress notes
  Complaints

Nursing Diagnoses

High Risk for Injury Related to Increased Dermal Vulnerability Secondary to Disease Process

NOC Risk Control

Goal

The client will identify causative factors that may increase disease activity (e.g., sun exposure).

Indicators

- Identify measures to reduce damage to skin by the sun.
- Identify strategies to manage skin damage should it occur.
- Identify signs and symptoms of cellulitis.

NIC Fall Prevention, Environmental Management: Safety, Health Education, Surveillance: Safety, Risk Identification

Interventions	Rationales
1. Explain to the client the relationship between sun exposure and disease activity.	1. Through an unknown mechanism, exposure to ultraviolet light can precipitate an exacerbation of both skin and systemic diseases. The client's understanding of this relationship should encourage him or her to limit sun exposure.

2. Identify strategies to limit sun exposure:
  a. Avoid sun exposure between 10 am–2 pm.
  b. Use sunscreen (15 SPF); reapply after swimming or exercise.
  c. Select lightweight, long-sleeved clothing and wide-brimmed hats.
	2. A client with SLE should make every attempt to minimize sun exposure.

3. Explain the need to avoid fluorescent lighting or a too-hot stove.	3. Like sunlight, fluorescent lighting produces ultraviolet rays.
4. Teach the client to keep skin ulcers clean and skin moist.	4. Skin changes associated with SLE increase the vulnerability to injury. Reducing bacteria on the skin reduces risk of infection. Dry skin is more susceptible to breakdown.

5. Teach the client to recognize signs and symptoms of vasculitis and to report them promptly to a health care professional:
  a. Tenderness
  b. Swelling
  c. Warmth
  d. Redness
	5. Vascular inflammation of the smallest blood vessels, capillaries, and venules can cause occlusion.

Documentation

Flow record
    Skin assessment
Discharge summary record
    Client teaching
    Response to teaching

High Risk for Ineffective Therapeutic Regimen Management Related to Insufficient Knowledge of Condition, Rest Versus Activity Requirements, Pharmacologic Therapy, Signs and Symptoms of Complications, Risk Factors, and Community Resources

NOC Compliance Behavior, Knowledge: Treatment Regimen, Participation in Health Care Decisions, Treatment Behavior: Illness or Injury

Goals

The goals for this diagnosis represent those associated with discharge planning. See the discharge criteria.

NIC Anticipatory Guidance, Risk Identification, Learning Facilitation, Support Group

Interventions	Rationales
1. Explain SLE using teaching aids appropriate to client's and family's levels of understanding. Discuss the following: a. The inflammatory process b. Organ systems at risk of involvement (see Potential Complications in this care plan for more information) c. Chronic nature of disease (remission/exacerbation) d. Components of standard treatment program e. Medications f. Exercise and rest g. Regular follow-up care	1. Understanding may help to improve compliance and reduce exacerbations.
2. Teach the client to take medications properly and to report symptoms of side effects. Drugs prescribed for SLE may include the following: a. Nonsteroidal anti-inflammatory drugs b. Corticosteroids (refer to the Corticosteroid care plan for more information) c. Immunosuppressive agents such as azathioprine (Imuran) and cyclophosphamide (Cytoxan) d. Antimalarial agents such as hydroxychloroquine (Plaquenil)	2. Knowledge of and proper adherence to the medication regimen can help to reduce complications and detect side effects early.
3. Teach the need to balance activity and rest. (Refer to the Inflammatory Joint Disease care plan for specific strategies.)	3. The chronic fatigue associated with SLE necessitates strategies to prevent exhaustion and maintain the highest level of independent functioning (Albano & Wallace, 2001).
4. Teach the need for meticulous, gentle mouth care.	4. Vasculitis can increase the risk of mouth lesions and injury.
5. Teach the client to report signs and symptoms of complications: a. Chest pain and dyspnea b. Fever c. Ecchymoses d. Edema e. Decreased urine output, concentrated urine f. Nausea and vomiting g. Leg cramps	5. Early detection of complications enables prompt interventions to prevent serious tissue damage or dysfunction: a. Chest pain and dyspnea may indicate pericarditis or pleural effusion. b. Fever may point to infection. c. Ecchymoses may indicate a clotting disorder. d. Edema may signal renal or hepatic insufficiency. e. These urine changes may indicate renal insufficiency. f. Nausea and vomiting can indicate GI dysfunction. g. Leg cramps may result from peripheral vascular insufficiency.
6. Explain the relationship of stress and autoimmune disorders. Discuss stress management techniques: a. Progressive relaxation b. Guided imagery c. Regular exercise (e.g., walking, swimming) d. Refer the client to a counselor and psychiatrist, as appropriate	6. Stress may be associated with an increase in disease activity. Stress management techniques can reduce the stress and fatigue associated with unmanaged conflicts (Albano & Wallace, 2001).
7. Discuss complementary therapies that may help to reduce inflammation of joints and tissues (Shirato, 2005). a. Massage, acupuncture b. Chiropractic	7. Studies have shown benefits (Shirato, 2005).

(continued on page 406)

Interventions	Rationales
8. Explain the benefits of some dietary supplements (only at recommended daily doses): a. Vitamin E, vitamin A b. SAM-e fish oils c. Flaxseed	8. a. These vitamins may prevent cell damage (Shirato, 2005). b. These have shown to relieve arthritis pain and reduce side effects of nonsteroidal anti-inflammatory drugs (Shirato, 2005). c. Flaxseed may provide some degree of renal protection (Shirato, 2005).
9. Advise the client to avoid excess calories, protein, fat, zinc, and iron in diet	9. Studies have shown these dietary excesses to aggravate symptoms associated with SLE (Brown, 2000).
10. Refer to appropriate community resources: a. Arthritis Foundation, (800) 283-7800, www.arthritis.org b. Lupus Foundation of America, (800) 558-0121, www.lupus.org c. National Institute of Arthritis and Musculoskeletal and Skin Diseases (NIAMS) Information Clearinghouse, (301) 495-4484	10. Additional self-help information may be very useful for self-care. Provide excellent support and education for the client and family (Albano & Wallace, 2001).

Documentation

Discharge summary record
    Client teaching
    Outcome achievement or status
    Referrals, if indicated

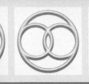

NEOPLASTIC DISORDERS

Cancer: Initial Diagnosis

Cancer involves a disturbance in normal cell growth in which abnormal cells arise from normal cells, reproduce rapidly, and infiltrate tissues, lymph, and blood vessels. The destruction caused by cancer depends on its site, whether or not it metastasizes, its obstructive effects, and its effects on the body's defense system (e.g., nutrition, hematopoiesis). Cancer is classified according to the cell of origin: malignant tumors from epithelial tissue are called *carcinomas* and those from connective tissue are known as *sarcomas*. Treatment varies depending on classification, cancer stage, and other factors.

 Time Frame
Initial diagnosis

▪▪▪▪▪ DIAGNOSTIC CLUSTER

Nursing Diagnoses	Refer to
▲ Anxiety related to unfamiliar hospital environment, uncertainty about outcomes, feelings of helplessness and hopelessness, and insufficient knowledge about cancer and treatment	
△ High Risk for Disturbed Self-Concept related to changes in life style, role responsibilities, and appearance	
▲ Interrupted Family Processes related to fears associated with recent cancer diagnosis, disruptions associated with treatments, financial problems, and uncertain future	
△ Decisional Conflict related to treatment modality choices	
▲ Grieving related to potential loss of body function and the perceived effects of cancer on life style	
△ High Risk for Spiritual Distress related to conflicts centering on the meaning of life, cancer, spiritual beliefs, and death	Cancer: End-Stage

Related Care Plans

Chemotherapy
Radiation Therapy

▲ This diagnosis was reported to be monitored for or managed frequently (75%–100%).
△ This diagnosis was reported to be monitored for or managed often (50%–74%).

Discharge Criteria

Before discharge, the client or family will

1. Relate the intent to share concerns with a trusted confidante.
2. Describe early signs of family dysfunction.

3. Identify signs and symptoms that must be reported to a health care professional.
4. Identify available community resources.

Collaborative Problems

The collaborative problems caused by cancer depend on its site, whether it metastasizes, its obstructive effects, and its effects on the body's defense system (e.g., white blood count, renal insufficiency). For example, cancer of the breast can metastasize to the brain, lung, liver, and bone. In this case, the collaborative problems PC: Increased Intracranial Pressure, PC: Hepatic Insufficiency, PC: Respiratory Insufficiency, and PC: Pathological Fractures would be appropriate. Refer to the index of collaborative problems for specific care plans where those collaborative problems are detailed.

Related Physician-Prescribed Interventions

Medications. Antineoplastics: Vary depending on stage of disease
Intravenous Therapy. None
Laboratory Studies. CBC with differential, liver function tests, renal function tests, blood chemistry, T-helper/T-suppressor ratio, lysozyme, complement C4, complement C3, total acid, urine inorganic phosphorus, urine catecholamines, urine alpha amino nitrogen, serum electrolytes
Selected Markers. Refer to chart below (Griffin-Brown, 2000).
Diagnostic Studies. Magnetic resonance imaging (MRI); varied sites; bone marrow aspiration; bone scan; x-rays (chest, abdomen); liver–spleen scan; bone scan; positron emission tomography (PET) scan; computerized tomography (CT) (chest, abdomen, musculoskeletal, bladder, lung, head, neck); GI barium studies; ultrasound (liver, abdomen, ovary, esophagus, transrectal, transvaginal)

Enzyme	Associated Malignancy
Test Lactate dehydrogenase (LDH)	Lymphoma, seminoma, leukemia, metastatic carcinoma
Prostatic acid phosphatase (PAP)	Metastatic cancer of the prostate, myeloma, lung cancer, osteogenic sarcoma
Placental alkaline phosphatase (PLAP)	Seminoma, lung, ovary, uterus
Neuron-specific enolase (NSE)	Small-cell lung cancer, neuroendocrine tumors, neuroblastoma, medullary thyroid cancer
Creatine kinase-BB (CK-BB)	Breast, colon, ovary, prostate cancers; small-cell lung cancer
Terminal deoxynucleotidyl transferase (TdT)	Lymphoblastic malignancy
Hormones Parathyroid hormone (PTH)	Ectopic hyperparathyroidism from cancer of the kidney, lung (squamous cell), pancreas, ovary, myeloma
Calcitonin	Medullary thyroid, small-cell lung cancer, breast cancer, and carcinoid
Adrenocorticotropic hormone (ACTH)	Lung, prostate, gastrointestinal cancers, neuroendocrine tumors
Antidiuretic hormone (ADH)	Small-cell lung cancer, adenocarcinomas
Human chorionic gonadotropin, beta subunit (B-HCG)	Germ cell tumors of testicle and ovary; ectopic production in cancer of stomach, pancreas, lung, colon, liver

(continued on page 409)

Enzyme	Associated Malignancy
Metabolic Products 5-Hydroxyindoleacetic acid (5-HIAA)	Carcinoid, lung
Vanillylmandelic acid (VMA)	Neuroblastoma

Proteins
Protein electrophoresis (urine-Bence Jones)
   IgG
   IgA
   IgM
   IgD
Beta-2 microglobulin
	Myeloma, lymphoma (serum-immunoglobulins)

Antigens Alpha-fetoprotein (AFP)	Nonseminomatous germ cell testicular cancer, choriocarcinoma, gonadal teratoblastoma in children, cancer of the pancreas, colon, lung, stomach, biliary system, liver
Carcinoembryonic antigen (CEA)	Cancer of the colon–rectum, stomach, pancreas, prostate, lungs, breast
Prostate-specific antigen (PSA)	Prostate cancer
Tissue polypeptide antigen (TPA)	Breast, colon, lung, pancreas cancer
CA-125	Ovary (epithelial), pancreas, breast, colon, lung, liver cancer
CA-a9-9	Pancreas, colon, gastric cancer
CA-15-3	Breast cancer
CA-27-29	Breast cancer
CA-72-4	Gastric cancer
Others Lipid-associated sialic acid (LASA)	Leukemia, lymphoma, melanoma, most solid tumors
Chromosome rearrangements (deletion, translocation)	Melanoma, small-cell lung, renal, testicular cancers, liposarcoma, neuroblastoma, lymphoma, leukemia, and others
Amplified oncogenes (MYC)	Neuroblastoma, small-cell lung cancer, lymphoma, breast cancer
EP1B-B	Glioblastoma, squamous cell carcinomas, breast, gastric, esophagus cancers
C-ERB-B2 (HER-2)	Breast and ovarian cancers, adenocarcinomas

Nursing Diagnoses

Anxiety Related to Unfamiliar Hospital Environment, Uncertainty about Outcomes, Feelings of Helplessness and Hopelessness, and Insufficient Knowledge about Cancer and Treatment

NOC Anxiety Self-Control

Goal

The client will report increased psychologic comfort.

Indicators

- Share concerns regarding the cancer diagnosis.
- Identify one strategy that reduces anxiety.

NIC Anxiety Reduction, Anticipatory Guidance

Interventions	Rationales
1. Provide opportunities for the client and family members to share feelings (anger, guilt, loss, and pain): a. Initiate frequent contacts and provide an atmosphere that promotes calm and relaxation. b. Convey a nonjudgmental attitude and listen attentively. c. Explore own feelings and behaviors.	1. Frequent contact by caregiver indicates acceptance and may facilitate trust. The client may be hesitant to approach the staff because of negative self-concept. The nurse should not make assumptions about a client's or family member's reaction; validating the client's particular fears and concerns helps to increase awareness. The nurse should be aware of how the client and family are reacting and how their reactions are influencing the nurse's feeling and behavior (Barsevick, Much, & Sweeney, 2000).
2. Encourage an open discussion of cancer, including experiences of others and potential for a cure or control of the disease.	2. The nurse who can talk openly about life after a cancer diagnosis offers encouragement and hope.
3. Explain hospital routines and reinforce the physician's explanations of scheduled tests and proposed treatment plan. Focus on what the client can expect.	3. Accurate descriptions of sensations and procedures help to ease anxiety and fear associated with the unknown (Christman & Kirchoff, 1992).
4. Identify those at risk for unsuccessful adjustment: a. Poor ego strength b. Ineffective problem-solving ability c. Poor motivation d. External focus of control e. Poor overall health f. Lack of positive support systems g. Unstable economic status h. Rejection of counseling (Shipes, 1987)	4. A client identified as high-risk may need referrals for counseling. Successful adjustment is influenced by factors such as previous coping success, achievement of developmental tasks, extent to which the disorder and treatment interfere with goal-directed activity, sense of self-determination and control, and realistic perception of the disorder.
5. Convey a sense of hope.	5. Clients who are reacting to a new cancer diagnosis must begin with hope. Hope is necessary to cope with the rigors of treatment (Barsevick, Much, & Sweeney, 2000).
6. Promote physical activity and exercise. Assist the client to determine the level of activity advisable.	6. Physical activity provides diversion and a sense of normalcy. Clients who exercise may improve their quality of life.

Documentation

Progress notes
Present emotional status
Interventions utilized
Response to interventions

High Risk for Disturbed Self-Concept Related to Changes in Life Style, Role Responsibilities, and Appearance

NOC Quality of Life, Depression Level, Coping, Self-Esteem

Goal

The client will relate the intent to continue previous life style as much as possible.

Indicators

• Communicate feelings about possible changes.
• Participate in self-care.

NIC Hope Instillation, Counseling, Coping Enhancement

Interventions	Rationales
1. Contact the client frequently and treat him or her with warm, positive regard.	1. Frequent contact by the caregiver indicates acceptance and may facilitate trust. The client may be hesitant to approach the staff because of negative self-concept.
2. Encourage the client to express feelings and thoughts about the following: a. Condition b. Progress c. Prognosis d. Effects on life style e. Support system f. Treatments	2. Encouraging the client to share feelings can provide a safe outlet for fears and frustration and can increase self-awareness.
3. Provide reliable information and clarify any misconceptions.	3. Misconceptions can needlessly increase anxiety and damage self-concept.
4. Help the client to identify positive attributes and possible new opportunities.	4. The client may tend to focus only on the change in self-image and not on the positive characteristics that contribute to the whole concept of self. The nurse must reinforce these positive aspects and encourage the client to reincorporate them into his or her new self-concept.
5. Assist with hygiene and grooming, as needed.	5. Participation in self-care and planning can aid positive coping.
6. Encourage visitors.	6. Frequent visits by support persons can help the client feel that she or he is still a worthwhile, acceptable person; this should promote a positive self-concept.
7. Help the client to identify strategies to increase independence and maintain role responsibilities: a. Prioritizing activities b. Getting assistance with less valued or most fatiguing activities (e.g., shopping, housekeeping) c. Using energy conservation techniques (Refer to the nursing diagnosis Fatigue in the Inflammatory Joint Disease care plan for specific strategies.) d. Using mobility aids and assistive devices, as needed	7. A strong component of self-concept is the ability to perform functions expected of one's role, thus decreasing dependency and reducing the need for other people's involvement.

(continued on page 412)

Interventions	Rationales
8. Discuss ways that the client can help his or her family/support persons: a. Actively listening to their problems b. Attempting to minimize the focus on disabilities (Refer to Chapter 4, The Ill Adult: Issues and Responses, for more information.) c. Help the client to identify ways of integrating the cancer experience into her or his life, rather than allowing cancer to take it over.	8. The nurse can help the client learn how to balance relationships and preserve the family system. The experience of cancer is different for everyone. What is vitally important to one person may be inconsequential to another (Stevens, 1992).
9. Help the client to identify potential opportunities for self-growth through living with cancer: a. Living and getting the most out of each day b. Value of relationships c. Grow in knowledge, personal strength, and understanding d. Spiritual and moral development	9. Experiences with cancer can provide the client with opportunities to reevaluate his or her life and to focus on personal priorities. The possibility of death promotes a reorientation of values (da Costa Vargens & Bertero, 2007). Many cancer clients have a sense of self-perceived burden regarding their families (Simmons, 2007).
10. Allow the client's family and support persons to share their feelings regarding the diagnosis and actual or anticipated effects (anger, rage, depression, or guilt).	10. Cancer can have a negative impact on the client's family financially, socially, and emotionally (da Costa Vargens & Bertero, 2007). All family members are affected by a cancer diagnosis, including children. This stressor on the children must be addressed; support groups are available (Su & Ryan-Wenger, 2007).
11. Assess for signs of negative response to changes in appearance: a. Refusal to discuss loss b. Denial of changes c. Decreased self-care ability d. Social isolation e. Refusal to discuss future	11. A client at high risk for unsuccessful adjustment should be identified for additional interventions or referrals. There is a 20%–47% documented range of poor adjustment and co-morbid psychiatric disorders (Carlson & Bultz, 2003).
12. Assist with management of alopecia as necessary: a. Explain when the client should expect to begin to lose hair (usually within 2–3 weeks of initiation of therapy) and when hair would begin to regrow (usually 4–6 weeks after discontinuation of therapy). b. Suggest cutting long hair to minimize fallout. c. Suggest resources for wigs and hairpieces. d. Discuss measures to reduce hair loss in low-dose therapy (e.g., wash hair only twice a week, use a mild shampoo, or avoid brushing). e. Encourage good grooming, hygiene, and other measures to enhance appearance (e.g., makeup, manicures, and new clothes).	12. Embarrassment from alopecia can contribute to isolation and negative self-concept (da Costa Vargens & Bertero, 2007).
13. Discuss possible emotional reactions—sadness, depression, and displaced anger. Encourage verbalization of feelings.	13. Changes in appearance often initiate the grieving process (da Costa Vargens & Bertero, 2007).
14. Discuss the advantages and disadvantages of scalp tourniquets and ice caps to prevent hair loss. The advantages are that they provide some control over hair loss and may reduce hair loss, especially in low-dose chemotherapy or radiation therapy. The disadvantages include possible micrometastasis to scalp not protected by chemotherapy, discomfort, and high cost.	14. Understanding advantages and disadvantages allows the client to make an informed decision regarding these treatments.
15. Refer an at-risk client for professional counseling.	15. Some clients may need follow-up therapy to aid with effective adjustment.

Documentation

Progress notes
Present emotional status
Interventions
Response to interventions

Interrupted Family Processes Related to Fears Associated with Recent Cancer Diagnosis, Disruptions Associated with Treatments, Financial Problems, and Uncertain Future

NOC Family Coping, Family Normalization, Parenting Performance

Goal

The family will maintain a functional system of mutual support.

Indicators

• Verbalize feelings regarding the diagnosis and prognosis.
• Identify signs of family dysfunction.
• Identify appropriate resources to seek, when needed.

NIC Family Involvement Promotion, Coping Enhancement, Family Integrity Promotion

Interventions	Rationales
1. Convey an understanding of the situation and its impact on the family.	1. Communicating understanding and a sense of caring and concern facilitates trust and strengthens the nurse's relationship with the client and family.
2. Explore family members' perceptions of the situation: a. The mistaken belief that cancer is contagious and can be "caught." b. Concerns about the hereditary nature of cancer c. Guilt d. Anger/depression e. Revulsion at the client's appearance f. Concerns about care-giving ability g. Worry about death h. Financial problems i. Feeling alone; lack of family support j. Concerns k. Shock	2. Verbalization can provide an opportunity for clarification and validation of feelings and concerns; this contributes to family unity. Spouses report increased anxiety prior to discharge from hospital and anger at the client for egocentricity during home-care period.
3. Determine if present coping mechanisms are effective.	3. If needed, refer families to community resources (e.g., counseling).
4. Take steps to promote family strengths: a. Acknowledge assistance of family members. b. Involve the family in client care. c. Encourage time away from care-giving to prevent burnout. d. Encourage humor. e. Encourage communication. (Refer to Chapter 4, The Ill Adult: Issues and Responses for more information.)	4. This can help to maintain the existing family structure and its function as a supportive unit. Cancer challenges one's values and beliefs; this can result in changed cognitive, affective, and behavioral responses.
5. Assist the family to reorganize roles at home, set new priorities, and redistribute responsibilities.	5. Planning and prioritizing can help to maintain family integrity and reduce stress.

(continued on page 415)

Interventions	Rationales
6. Prepare the family for signs of stress, depression, anxiety, anger, and dependency in the client and other family members.	6. Anticipatory guidance can alert members to potential problems before they occur, enabling prompt intervention at early signs.
7. Encourage the family to call on its social network (e.g., friends, relatives, church members) for emotional and other support.	7. Outside assistance may help to reduce the perception that the family must "go it alone."
8. Encourage open communication between significant others.	8. Family members are reluctant to discuss distressing information or their feelings with the client.
9. Identify dysfunctional coping mechanisms: a. Substance abuse b. Continued denial c. Exploitation of one or more family members d. Separation or avoidance. Refer for counseling, as necessary.	9. A family with a history of unsuccessful coping may need additional resources. A family with unresolved conflicts before diagnosis is at high risk.
10. Direct to community agencies and other sources of assistance (e.g., financial, housekeeping, direct care, childcare), as needed.	10. The family may need assistance with management at home.

Documentation

Progress notes
Present family functioning
Interventions
Response to interventions
Discharge summary record
Referrals if indicated

Decisional Conflict Related to Treatment Modality Choices

NOC Decision-Making, Information Processing, Participation in Health Care Decisions

Goal

The client and family members will

1. Relate the advantages and disadvantages of choices.
2. Share their fears and concerns regarding a decision.
3. Make an informed choice.

NIC Decision-Making Support, Learning Facilitation, Health System Guidance, Patient Rights Protection

Interventions	Rationales
1. Provide, reinforce, and clarify information about the diagnosis, treatment options, and alternative therapies.	1. The client and family need specific and accurate information to make an informed decision. Cancer gives a sense of being out of control. Exploration of all options may help the client to regain a sense of control (Thome, Dykes, Gunnars, & Hallberg, 2003).

(continued on page 415)

Interventions	Rationales
2. Give the client and family members opportunities to share feelings and concerns regarding the decision.	2. Conflict is more intense when the decision has potentially negative impacts or when conflicting opinions exist. Anxiety and fear have a negative impact on decision-making ability. Providing opportunities to share feelings and concerns can help to reduce anxiety (Thome et al., 2003).
3. Ensure that the client and family clearly understand what is involved in each treatment alternative.	3. Informed decisions support a person's right to self-determination. Clients must be prepared for the emotional and physical problems they will face.
4. Assure the client that he or she does not have to abide by decisions that others make, but can choose for him- or herself, as appropriate. Discourage family members and others from undermining the client's confidence in his or her decision-making ability.	4. Each client has the right to make his or her own decisions and to expect respect from others (Thome et al., 2003).
5. Provide as much time as possible for decision-making.	5. Effective and informed decision-making requires time to consider all alternatives thoroughly.
6. If indicated, encourage the client to seek a second professional opinion.	6. A second opinion can confirm information and validate options.

Documentation

Progress notes
Dialogues

Grieving Related to Potential Loss of Body Function and the Perceived Effects of Cancer on Life Style

NOC Coping, Family Coping, Psychosocial Adjustment: Life Change

Goal

The client and family members will

1. Express grief.
2. Describe the personal meaning of the loss.
3. Report an intent to discuss his or her feelings with significant others.

NIC Family Support, Grief Work Facilitation, Coping Enhancement, Anticipatory Guidance, Emotional Support

Interventions	Rationales
1. Provide opportunities for the client and family members to express feelings, discuss the loss openly, and explore the personal meaning of the loss. Explain that grief is a common and healthy reaction.	1. A cancer diagnosis typically gives rise to feelings of powerlessness, anger, profound sadness, and other grief responses. Open and honest discussions can help the client and family members accept and cope with the situation and their responses to it.
2. Encourage the use of positive coping strategies that have proved successful in the past.	2. Positive coping strategies aid in acceptance and problem-solving.

(continued on page 416)

Interventions	Rationales
3. Encourage the client to express positive self-attributes.	3. Focusing on positive attributes increases self-acceptance and acceptance of the diagnosis.
4. Implement measures to support the family and promote cohesiveness: a. Help family members acknowledge their losses. b. Explain the grieving process. c. Encourage the client to verbalize her or his feelings. d. Allow participation in care to promote comfort. e. Encourage discussing the significance of family relationships.	4. Family cohesiveness is important in client support.

5. Promote grief work with each response:
a. Denial:
  • Encourage acceptance of the situation; do not reinforce denial by giving false reassurance.
  • Promote hope through assurances of care, comfort, and support.
  • Explain the use of denial by one family member to other members.
  • Do not push a client to move past denial until he or she is emotionally ready.
b. Isolation:
  • Convey acceptance by encouraging expressions of grief.
  • Promote open, honest communication to encourage sharing.
  • Reinforce the client's self-worth by providing privacy, when desired.
  • Encourage socialization, as feasible (e.g., support groups, church activities).
c. Depression:
  • Reinforce the client's self-esteem.
  • Employ empathetic sharing and acknowledge grief.
  • Identify the degree of depression and develop appropriate strategies.
d. Anger:
  • Explain to other family members that anger represents an attempt to control the environment; it stems from frustration at the inability to control the disease.
  • Encourage verbalization of anger.
e. Guilt:
  • Acknowledge the client's expressed self-image.
  • Encourage identification of the relationship's positive aspects.
  • Avoid arguing and participating in the client's system of "I should have . . ." and "I shouldn't have. . . ."
f. Fear:
  • Focus on the present and maintain a safe and secure environment.
  • Help the client explore reasons for and meanings of the fears.
g. Rejection:
  • Provide reassurance by explaining what is happening.
  • Explain this response to other family members.
h. Hysteria:
  • Reduce environmental stressors (e.g., limit personnel).
  • Provide a safe, private area in which to express grief.
	5. Grieving involves profound emotional responses; interventions depend on the particular response.

(continued on page 417)

Interventions	Rationales
6. Act as a guide to the client through the grief experience by understanding her or his needs and providing help where needed (Bushkin, 1993).	6,7. It is important to realize that clients with cancer often have their own realities that may differ from the nurse's view (Yates, 1993).
7. Validate and reflect impressions with the client.	

Documentation

Progress notes
Present emotional status
Interventions
Response to nursing interventions

Cancer: End-Stage

Cancer is a group of more than 200 diseases characterized by uncontrolled and unregulated growth of cells. It can occur in persons of all ages and all ethnicities and is a major health problem (Lewis et al., 2004). Approximately 400,000 people in the United States die of cancer each year. Cancer that treatment cannot control metastasizes to adjacent organs and structures or spreads through the blood and lymphatics to a distant site, such as the liver, brain, or bones. For example, a client with end-stage colon cancer may have a tumor in the colon causing bowel obstruction. Metastasis to the liver causes ascites, edema, and clotting problems; metastasis to the lung promotes respiratory alterations.

End-stage cancer with metastasis can result in many structural and functional problems, depending on the body area(s) or system(s) affected. Potential complications also depend on the affected site. Only those specific to end-stage cancer are discussed in this care plan. In addition, the client and his or her significant others face multiple challenges of pain, loss, and decreased functioning.

 Time Frame
Terminal stage (care in home, hospital, long-term care facility, or hospice)

■ ■■■■■ DIAGNOSTIC CLUSTER*

Collaborative Problems	Refer to
PC: Hypercalcemia	
PC: Cachexia	
PC: Malignant Effusions	
PC: Narcotic Toxicity	
PC: Pathologic Fractures	
PC: Spinal Cord Compression	
PC: Superior Vena Cava Syndrome	
PC: Intracerebral Metastasis	Cerebrovascular Accident (Stroke)
PC: Myelosuppression	Chemotherapy
PC: Bowel Obstruction	
PC: Hepatotoxicity	
PC: Increased Intracranial Pressure	
PC: Cardiotoxicity	

(continued on page 418)

Nursing Diagnoses	Refer to
Acute and/or Chronic Pain related to direct tumor involvement and/or associated with cancer therapy (surgery, radiation, chemotherapy)	
Grieving related to terminal illness, impending death, functional losses, and withdrawal of, or from, others	
Powerlessness related to change from curative to palliative status	
Hopelessness related to overwhelming functional losses or impending death	
High Risk for Spiritual Distress related to fear of death, overwhelming grief, belief system conflicts, and unresolved relationship conflicts	
High Risk for Ineffective Therapeutic Regimen Management related to insufficient knowledge of home-care, pain management, signs and symptoms of complications, and community resources available	
Imbalanced Nutrition: Less Than Body Requirements related to decreased oral intake, increased metabolic demands of tumor, and altered lipid metabolism	Chemotherapy
Constipation related to decreased dietary fiber intake, decreased intestinal mobility secondary to narcotic medications and inactivity	Immobility or Unconsciousness
Pruritus related to dry skin secondary to dehydration or accumulation of bile salts secondary to biliary duct obstruction	Hepatitis (Viral)
Ineffective Airway Clearance related to decreased ability to expectorate secretions secondary to weakness, increased viscosity, and pain	Pneumonia
Disuse Syndrome related to pain, weakness, fatigue, and edema	Immobility or Unconsciousness
High Risk for Injury related to weakness, fatigue secondary to anemia, electrolyte imbalances, or somnolence secondary to medications or disease process	Cerebrovascular Accident (Stroke)
Self-Care Deficit related to fatigue, weakness, sedation, pain, and decreased sensory-perceptual capacity	Immobility or Unconsciousness
Disturbed Self-Concept related to dependence on others to meet basic needs	Multiple Sclerosis
Interrupted Family Processes related to change to terminal status, unresolved relationship conflicts, and concerns regarding coping and managing home-care	Multiple Sclerosis

(continued on page 419)

*This medical condition was not included in the validation study.

Discharge Criteria

Before discharge, the client or family will

1. Relate the intent to share feelings with a trusted friend.
2. Relate strategies to manage discomfort.
3. Identify personal strengths.
4. Identify community resources available for assistance.
5. Describe signs and symptoms of complication that must be reported to a health care professional.
6. Identify two sources of spiritual comfort.

Collaborative Problems

Potential Complication: Hypercalcemia

Potential Complication: Cachexia

Potential Complication: Malignant Effusions

Potential Complication: Narcotic Toxicity

Potential Complication: Pathologic Fractures

Potential Complication: Spinal Cord Compression

Potential Complication: Superior Vena Cava Syndrome

Potential Complication: Bowel Obstruction

Potential Complication: Hepatotoxicity

Potential Complication: Increased Intracranial Pressure (secondary to chemotherapy)

Potential Complication: Cardiotoxicity (secondary to chemotherapy)

Nursing Goal

The nurse will detect early signs and symptoms of (a) hypercalcemia, (b) cachexia, (c) malignant effusions (pleural ascites pericardial), (d) narcotic toxicity, (e) pathologic fractures, (f) spinal cord compression, (g) superior vena cava syndrome, (h) bowel obstruction, (i) hepatotoxicity, (j) increased intracranial pressure, and (k) cardiotoxicity, and collaboratively intervene to stabilize the client.

Indicators

- Alert, oriented (a, d, g, i, j)
- EKG: normal sinus rhythm (a, k)
- No seizures (a, j)
- No nausea or vomiting (a, h, i, j)
- No significant weight gain or loss (b)
- No edema (b, c, e, g, k)
- No anorexia or early satiety (b, c)
- Pulse 60–100 beats/min (b, d, k)
- Respirations 16–20 breaths/min (b, d)
- Easy, rhythmic breathing (b, c, d)
- No pleuritic pain (b)

- Full breath sounds in all quadrants (b, c)
- No increase in abdominal girth (c)
- No visual changes (g)
- No hoarseness or stridor (g)
- No bone pain (e)
- Full range of motion (e)
- No visible bone deformity (e)
- No sensory or motor losses (f)
- No neck or back pain (f)
- Normal bowel movements (f, h)
- No venous distention (c, g)
- Serum magnesium 1.3–2.4 mEq/L (c)
- Serum sodium 135–145 mEq/L (c)
- Serum potassium 3.8–5 mEq/L (c)
- Serum calcium 8.5–10.5 mg/dL (a, c)
- Serum albumin 3.5–5 g/dL (c)
- Serum prealbumin 20–50 g/dL (c)
- Serum protein 6–8 g/dL (c)
- Partial thromboplastin time (PTT) 20–45 sec (c)
- Hemoglobin (c)
  - Male: 13–18 g/dL
  - Female: 12–16 g/dL
- Hematocrit (c)
  - Male: 42%–50%
  - Female: 40%–48%
- Platelets 100,000–400,000/mm^3 (c)
- Blood urea nitrogen (BUN) 10–20 mg/dL (could be slightly higher for elderly clients); Urea nitrogen/creatinine ratio: 10:1–20:1; averages: 15:1 (Kee, 2005, p. 71–72) (c)
- Alanine aminotransferase (ALT) 7–40 U/mL (c, i)
- Aspartate aminotransferase (AST) 10–40 U/mL (c, i)
- Cardiac ejection fraction >55% (Boron & Boulpaep, 2005).

Interventions	Rationales

1. Monitor for signs and symptoms of hypercalcemia:
   a. Altered mental status
   b. Dysrhythmias (shortened QT interval and widened T wave) (ECG interpretation, 2006)
   c. Numbness or tingling in fingers and toes
   d. Muscle cramps
   e. Seizures
   f. Nausea/vomiting
   g. Depression (Wagner, Johnson, & Kidd, 2006)
   h. Pancreatitis (Wagner, Johnson, & Kidd, 2006)
   i. Constipation (Wagner, Johnson, & Kidd, 2006)
   j. Increased urination (Wagner, Johnson, & Kidd, 2006)
	1. Hypercalcemia (serum calcium >11 mg/dL) is a common complication of end-stage cancer. It occurs most often in multiple myeloma, lung cancer, head and neck cancer, breast cancer, and metastatic bone cancer, owing to disturbed calcium reabsorption (Lewis, Heitkemper, Dirksen et al., 2004).

2. Monitor for signs/symptoms of cachexia:
   a. Weight loss
   b. Early satiety
   c. Edema
   d. Anorexia
	2. A client with advanced cancer has an abnormal sugar tolerance with resistance or decreased sensitivity to insulin; this inhibits cell nourishment. Cachexia results from the increased metabolic demands of the tumor, altered lipid metabolism, and anorexia. Impaired carbohydrate metabolism causes increased metabolism of fats and protein, which can lead to negative nitrogen balance, especially in the presence of metabolic acidosis. Nutritional deficiencies are associated with development of pressure sores, impaired cellular and hormonal immunity, higher risk for infection, apathy, and depression (Lewis, Heitkemper, Dirksen et al., 2004).

(continued on page 421)

Interventions	Rationales

3. Monitor laboratory values:
  a. Serum calcium, ionized calcium
  b. CBC with differential
  c. Serum albumin, transferrin, prealbumin
  d. Blood urea nitrogen (BUN)
  e. Creatinine
  f. Electrolytes and magnesium
  g. Liver function tests
	3. Selected laboratory studies are done to monitor nutritional status and to detect early changes in renal function. Potassium and magnesium losses can occur with hydration and diuretic treatment. Hydration depends on extent of dehydration, renal excretory capacity, and cardiovascular condition (Kee, 2005; Haughney, 2004).

4. Monitor for malignant effusions (excessive accumulation of fluid in the pleural space, peritoneal cavity [ascites], or pericardial space):
  a. Pleural effusion:
    • Cough (dry)
    • Variable dyspnea
    • Pleuritic pain
    • Diminished and delayed chest movement on the involved side
    • Bulging of intercostal spaces (in a large effusion)
    • Decreased breath sounds auscultated over the effusion
    • Decreased vocal and tactile fremitus
    • Increased respiratory rate and depth
  b. Ascites:
    • Abdominal distention
    • Increased abdominal girth
    • Shortness of breath
    • Fatigue
    • Fluid wave
    • Generalized edema
    • Reduced bladder capacity
    • Ankle edema
    • Indigestion
    • Early satiety
    • Decreased serum albumin and protein values
    • Abnormal clotting factors and electrolyte values
  c. Pericardial effusion:
    • Dyspnea, dry cough, chest pain
    • Weakness and dizziness
    • Upright, forward-leaning posture
    • Muffled heart/breath sounds
    • Friction rub
    • Orthopnea
    • Neck vein distention
    • Increased central venous pressure
	4. Effusions cause pain and discomfort and inhibit function.
	
	  a. Collections of fluid (either transudates or exudates) in the pleural cavity, pleural effusions are common with cancer. Fluid pressure dynamics are affected by direct pressure by the tumor or lymphatic or venous obstruction of severe hypoproteinemia (Wagner, Johnson, & Kidd, 2006).
	
	  b. Accumulation of serous fluid in the peritoneal cavity is caused by obstruction in portal circulation. Tumors also can involve lymphatic channels that interfere with drainage of the peritoneal cavity; humoral factors may cause capillary leakage (Wagner, Johnson, & Kidd, 2006).
	
	  c. Tumors of the lung and breast, leukemia, lymphomas, melanomas, and sarcomas metastasize to the pericardium and promote pericardial effusions. These effusions interfere with cardiac function, reducing cardiac volume during diastole and decreasing cardiac output and venous return.

5. Monitor abdominal girth and weight daily.	5. These measurements help detect fluid retention and ascites.

6. Monitor for signs of narcotic toxicity:
  a. Increased sedation
  b. Drowsiness
  c. Depressed respiratory rate
	6. Many health care professionals are overly concerned about narcotic toxicity and may needlessly withhold narcotics from a terminally ill client. A client in severe pain can tolerate very high doses of narcotics without developing excessive sedation and respiratory depression.

7. As necessary, intervene for narcotic toxicity:
  a. Monitor sedation level frequently. Expect peak effects from narcotics 5–10 minutes after intravenous (IV) injection, 30 minutes after intramuscular (IM) injection, and 90 minutes after subcutaneous (SC) injection.
  b. Withhold narcotic dose if sedation level increases; assess results.
	7. Narcotic toxicity can occur if excretion is impaired (e.g., in liver dysfunction). Sedation usually precedes respiratory depression; withholding drugs when sedation occurs usually heads off respiratory depression. Narcotic antagonists reduce opioid effects by competing for the same receptor sites.

(continued on page 422)

Interventions	Rationales
c. If respirations fall below 12 breaths per minute, monitor client carefully; if below 10, notify the physician. d. If respirations continue to fall, consult with physician for a narcotic antagonist (e.g., naloxone) (Lehne, 2004).	
8. Monitor for signs and symptoms of pathologic fracture: a. Localized pain that becomes continuous and unrelenting b. Visible bone deformity c. Crepitation on movement d. Loss of movement or use e. Localized soft tissue edema f. Skin discoloration g. Tenderness to percussion over involved spine	8. Pathologic fractures occur in about 9% of clients with metastatic disease. Metastatic cancer deposits in the proximal femur may weaken the bone and cause a pathological hip fracture. Bones most susceptible to tumor invasion are those with the greatest bone marrow activity and blood flow—the vertebrae, pelvis, ribs, skull, and sternum. The most common sites for long bone metastasis are the femur and humerus (Lindqvist, Widmarkt, & Rasmussen, 2006).
9. Maintain alignment and immobilize the site if fracture is suspected.	9. Immobilization helps reduce soft tissue damage from dislocations.
10. If a stabilization device is necessary, refer to the Casts care plan for specific interventions.	10. Devices may be necessary to stabilize bones.
11. Monitor for signs and symptoms of spinal cord compression (Bader & Littlejohns, 2004). a. Early signs: • Neck or back pain—gradual onset relieved by sitting, intensified by lying or movements • Motor weakness • Sensory loss b. Late signs: • Motor loss • Urinary retention, overflow, incontinence • Constipation, incontinence, difficulty expelling stool • Poor sphincter control	11. Spinal cord compression results from tumor invasion into the epidural space or from bony erosion and altered vertebral alignment secondary to fracture. Symptoms vary, depending on the extent and location of compression. Treatments include radiation therapy and corticosteroids for compression resulting from an extradural mass, and a decompression laminectomy for compression owing to bony erosion.
12. Maintain bed rest.	12. Immobility reduces the risk of injury to the spinal cord.
13. Monitor respiratory, bowel, and bladder function.	13. The level of the cord compression influences respiratory (cervical), bowel (lumbar), and bladder (lumbar) functioning.
14. Monitor for signs and symptoms of superior vena cava syndrome (SVCS) (Wilson, 2007). a. Early signs: • Facial, trunk, upper extremity edema • Pronounced venous pattern on trunk • Neck vein distention • Cough b. Late signs: • Hoarseness • Stridor • Engorged conjunctiva • Headache • Dizziness • Visual disturbances • Change in mental status • Respiratory distress • Decreased cardiac output • Flushed edematous face • Difficulty swallowing • Tachypnea • Orthopnea	14. SVCS occurs when the superior vena cava becomes occluded by a tumor or thrombus. Commonly associated with lung cancer, breast cancer, and lymphomas, SVCS causes impaired venous return from the head and upper extremities, resulting in upper body edema and prominent collateral circulation (Wilson, 2007).

◥ Related Physician-Prescribed Interventions

Medications. Dependent on symptomatology, chemotherapy, analgesics, antiemetics
Intravenous Therapy. Replacement (fluid, electrolytes); transfusions; albumin
Laboratory Studies. Dependent on history, clinical symptomatology; serum protein; complete blood count; carcinogenic antigens; blood chemistry; electrolytes
Diagnostic Studies. Varies according to site and clinical symptomatology
Therapies. Refer to Cancer: Initial Diagnosis

Documentation

Flow records
   Daily weights
   Vital signs
   Auscultation findings (lung, heart)
   Abdominal girth
   Intake and output
Progress notes
   New complaints

Nursing Diagnoses

Acute and/or Chronic Pain Related to Direct Tumor Involvement and/or Associated With Cancer Therapy (Surgery, Radiation, Chemotherapy)

NOC Comfort Level, Pain: Disruptive Effects, Pain Control, Depression Self-Control

Goals

The client will report relief after pain measures and an increase in activity.

Indicators

• Participate in pain management decisions.
• Relate that others validate that their pain exists.
• Practice one non-invasive pain relief measure.

NIC Pain Management, Medication Management, Exercise Promotion, Mood Management, Coping Enhancement

Interventions	Rationales
1. Assist in identifying the source of pain: a. Obstruction b. Effusions c. Invasive lines d. Immobility e. Skeletal source f. Muscular source	1. Do not assume that all pain is related to tissue destruction. Pain of different origins requires different interventions for relief.
2. Convey that you acknowledge and accept his or her pain.	2. A client who believes that he or she must convince skeptical caregivers of the seriousness of his or her pain experiences increased anxiety, which can increase pain.

(continued on page 424)

Interventions	Rationales

3. Review pharmacologic options.
  a. NSAIDs
	3.
	  a. NSAIDs can be useful for metastatic bone pain from compression of tendons, muscles, pleura, and peritoneum; soft tissue pain; and non-obstructive visceral pain (Lehne, 2004; Deglin & Vallerand, 2007). NSAIDs are also effective against mild pain.

b. Steroids	b. Indirectly or directly, steroids reduce swelling, inflammation, and compression resulting from tumor growth. They also are an appetite stimulant and antiemetic (Lehne, 2004; Deglin & Vallerand, 2007).
c. Opioids	c. Opioids interfere with pain perception in the brain; they are useful for moderate to severe pain (Lehne, 2004; Deglin & Vallerand, 2007).

d. Adjuvant analgesics
    • Tricyclic antidepressants
    • Anticonvulsants
    • NMDA-receptor antagonist
    • Psychostimulants
	d. These medications enhance the action of pain-modulating symptoms, especially in the treatment of neuropathic pain (Lehne, 2004; Deglin & Vallerand, 2007).
	    • They have been found useful in relieving pain from infiltration as a result of treatment-related injury (e.g., postmastectomy pain syndrome).
	    • They have been found useful in relieving neuropathic pain.
	    • Ketamine has been found to reduce neuropathic pain.
	    • These agents counteract the sedation seen with opioid analgesics.

4. Provide selected interventions with type of medication:
  a. NSAIDs
    • Provide medicine with food or milk.
    • Monitor for GI bleeding and ulcers (e.g., Hemoccult, c/o pain, nausea).
    • Monitor liver and renal function laboratory test results.
  b. Steroids
  Refer to Corticosteroid care plan.
  c. Opioids
    • Start with low dose and increase until adequate analgesic is achieved.
    • Aggressively manage nausea and vomiting with antiemetics. Use round-the-clock medications for 1–2 weeks.
    • Provide laxatives for constipation (e.g., Metamucil, senna, lactulose, docusate).
For dry mouth, rinse often, suck on sugarless candies, and drink liquids frequently.
	4.
	  a. Prostaglandins cause loss of protective epithelial lining in the GI tract and kidneys. Elimination of drug is primarily through hepatic metabolism. The goal is to balance the incidence of side effects with effective pain management.
	
	  c. The chemoreceptor trigger zone (CTZ) is an area of the brain which receives inputs from blood-borne drugs or hormones, and communicates with the vomit center, to initiate vomiting. The CTZ is close to the area postrema, which is on the floor of the fourth ventricle and is outside of the blood–brain barrier. The neurotransmitters implicated in the control of nausea and vomiting include acetylcholine, dopamine, and 5-hydroxytryptamine (5-HT). There are also opioid receptors present, which may be the mechanism by which opiates cause nausea and vomiting (Lehne, 2004; Deglin & Vallerand, 2007). Opioids reduce peristalsis and decrease saliva production.

5. Treat breakthrough pain with immediate-release formulations.	5. Pain can vary through the day and night.

6. Differentiate pain from other symptoms (Valente, 2004; Haughney, 2004):
  a. Delirium
  b. Increased agitation
  c. Restlessness
	6. A terminally ill person may moan and grimace in response to pain as well as delirium.

(continued on page 425)

Interventions	Rationales
7. If increased pain is suspected, titrate the pain medication to a level where pain is acceptable or resolved without compromising respiratory and neurologic functioning (Valente, 2004; Haughney, 2004; Lehne, 2004).	7. If the symptoms decrease, then pain is probably the cause (Lehne, 2004).

8. Provide accurate information:
  a. Explain the cause of the pain, if known.
  b. Explain how long the pain should last.
  c. Reassure that narcotic addiction is not likely to develop from the pain relief regimen. Physical dependency may occur.
	8. A client who understands and is prepared for pain by detailed explanations tends to experience less stress—and, consequently, less pain—than a client who receives vague or no explanations. Physical dependency is easily resolved by slowly reducing the amount of pain medication when the client is free of pain (Lehne, 2004; Lindqvist, Widmarkt, & Rasmussen, 2006).

9. Provide privacy for the client during acute pain episodes.	9. Privacy reduces embarrassment and anxiety and enables more effective coping.

10. Recognize and treat pain promptly with prescribed analgesics.
  a. Determine the preferred route of administration; consult with the physician.
 	
  b. Assess vital signs, especially respiratory rate, before and after administration.
  c. Consult with a pharmacist for possible adverse interactions with other medications the client is taking, such as muscle relaxants and tranquilizers.
  d. Consult with the physician for a regular narcotic administration schedule.
 	
  e. If necessary, use the PRN approach to pain medication; administer before treatment procedures or activity, and instruct the client to request pain medications, as needed, before pain becomes severe.
  f. About ½ hour after administration, assess pain relief and client satisfaction with the pain relief plan.
	10.
	
	  a. If frequent injections are necessary, the intravenous route is preferred because it is not painful and absorption is guaranteed.
	  b. Narcotics depress the brain's respiratory center.
	
	  c. Some medications potentiate the effects of narcotics.
	
	  d. The scheduled approach may reduce the total 24-h drug dose as compared to the PRN approach and may reduce the client's anxiety associated with having to ask for and wait for PRN medications.
	  e. The PRN approach is effective for breakthrough pain or to manage additional pain from treatments and procedures.
	
	  f. Response to analgesics can vary with stress levels, fatigue, and pain intensity.

11. Consult with the physician for co-analgesic medications, as necessary:
  a. Bone pain—aspirin or ibuprofen
  b. Increased intracranial pressure—dexamethasone
  c. Postherpetic neuralgia—amitriptyline
  d. Nerve pressure—prednisone
  e. Gastric distention—metoclopramide
  f. Muscle spasm—diazepam
  g. Lymphodermia—diuretics
  h. Infection—antibiotics
  i. Neuropathic pain—Tegretol and amitriptyline
	11. In addition to narcotics, other medications can help relieve pain and discomfort.

12. Explain and assist with noninvasive pain relief measures:
  a. Splinting
  b. Positioning
  c. Distraction
  d. Massage
  e. Relaxation techniques
  f. Music therapy
	12. Certain measures can relieve pain by preventing painful stimuli from reaching higher brain centers. They also may improve the client's sense of control over pain.

(continued on page 426)

Interventions	Rationales

13. Consult with the physician for other invasive pain relief measures, if needed:
  a. Radiation
  b. Nerve block
  c. Surgery
  d. Advanced analgesic technologies (client-controlled analgesia and morphine drips)
	13. Radiation can reduce the tumor size to decrease compression on structures and reduce obstructions. Nerve blocks cause an interruption in nerve function through injection of a local anesthetic (temporary) or a neurodestructive agent (permanent). Surgery can decrease tumor bulk to reduce pressure and obstruction.

14. Emphasize the need to report unsatisfactory pain relief.	14. Prompt reporting enables rapid adjustment to control pain.

Documentation

Medication administration record
Type, dose, time, route of all medications
Progress notes
Unsatisfactory relief from pain
Noninvasive relief measures

Grieving Related to Terminal Illness, Impending Death, Functional Losses, and Withdrawal of or From Others

NOC Coping, Family Coping, Grief Resolution, Psychosocial Adjustment: Life Change

Goals

The client will acknowledge that death is expected.

Indicators

• Verbalize losses and changes.
• Verbalize feelings associated with losses and changes.

Family members will maintain an effective closure relationship as evidenced by:

• Spending time with the client
• Maintaining loving, open communication with the client
• Participating in care

NIC Family Support, Grief Work Facilitation, Coping Enhancement, Anticipatory Guidance, Emotional Support

Interventions	Rationales
1. Provide opportunities for client and family members to express feelings, discuss the loss openly, and explore the personal meaning of the loss. Explain that grief is a common and healthy reaction.	1. The knowledge that no further treatment is warranted and that death is imminent may give rise to feelings of powerlessness, anger, profound sadness, and other grief responses. Open, honest discussions can help client and family members accept and cope with the situation and their responses to it.
2. Encourage use of positive coping strategies that have proved successful in the past.	2. Positive coping strategies aid acceptance and problem-solving.
3. Encourage client to express positive self-attributes.	3. Focusing on positive attributes increases self-acceptance and acceptance of imminent death.

(continued on page 427)

Interventions	Rationales
4. Help client acknowledge and accept impending death; answer all questions honestly.	4. Grief work, the adaptive process of mourning, cannot begin until the impending death is acknowledged.

5. Promote grief work with each response:
a. Denial:
  • Encourage acceptance of the situation; do not reinforce denial by giving false reassurance.
  • Promote hope through assurances of care, comfort, and support.
  • Explain the use of denial by one family member to other members. Often, the family members cannot imagine the loved one's death and are torn between the notion that death may be a blessing or a tragedy (Valente, 2004).
  • Do not push a client to move past denial until he or she is emotionally ready.
b. Isolation:
  • Convey acceptance by encouraging expressions of grief.
  • Promote open, honest communication to encourage sharing.
  • Reinforce the client's self-worth by providing for privacy, when desired.
  • Encourage socialization as feasible (e.g., support groups, church activities).
c. Depression:
  • Reinforce client's self-esteem.
  • Employ empathetic sharing and acknowledge grief.
  • Identify degree of depression and develop appropriate strategies.
d. Anger:
  • Explain to other family members that anger represents an attempt to control the environment and stems from frustration at the inability to control the disease.
  • Encourage verbalization of anger.
e. Guilt:
  • Acknowledge the client's expressed self-image.
  • Encourage identification of the relationship's positive aspects.
  • Avoid arguing and participating in the client's system of "I should have . . ." and "I shouldn't have. . . ."
f. Fear:
  • Focus on the present and maintain a safe and secure environment.
  • Help the client explore reasons for, and meanings of, the fears.
g. Rejection:
  • Provide reassurance by explaining what is happening.
  • Explain this response to other family members.
h. Hysteria:
  • Reduce environmental stressors (e.g., limit personnel).
  • Provide a safe, private area in which to express grief.
	5. Grieving involves profound emotional responses; interventions depend on the particular response.
	
	• Anger is often perceived as negative. Anger, however, can energize behavior; facilitate expression of negative feelings, and function to help the client defend against a threat (Lewis et al., 2004).

6. Encourage client to engage in a life review by focusing on accomplishments and disappointments. Assist in attempts to resolve unresolved conflicts.	6. Life review provides an opportunity to prepare for life closure.
7. Implement measures to support the family and promote cohesiveness (Valente, 2004). a. Seek family perceptions of what is happening. b. Help them acknowledge losses and impending death.	7. Family cohesiveness is important to client support.

(continued on page 428)

Interventions	Rationales
c. Explain the grief process. d. Explain expected behaviors during terminal stages (denial, anger, depression, and withdrawal). e. Allow participation in care to promote comfort. f. Encourage discussing the relationship's significance. g. Promote adequate rest and nutrition. h. Assist with funeral home arrangements, if needed. i. Refer to a bereavement support group. j. Identify resources for helping family and children cope with cancer (booklets, social service, hospice). Family members experience significant burdens and guilt when they decide to place a loved one in an extended care facility or hospice. Often, they have exhausted all other options before placement and feel this may be the most difficult decision they have made, a decision accompanied by feelings of loss, pain, regret, and fear of the future (Valente, 2004).	
8. Promote hope by assurances of attentive care, relief of discomfort, and support.	8. Terminally ill clients most appreciate the following nursing care measures: assisting with grooming, supporting independent functioning, providing pain medications when needed, and enhancing physical comfort.

Documentation

Progress notes
Present emotional status
Interventions
Response to nursing interventions

Powerlessness Related to Change From Curative Status to Palliative Status

NOC Depression Self-Control, Health Beliefs: Perceived Control, Participation in Health Care Decisions

Goal

The client will participate in decisions regarding care and activities.

Indicators

• Identify factors that can be controlled.
• Share feelings.

NIC Mood Management, Teaching: Individual, Decision-Making Support, Self-Responsibility Facilitation, Health System Guidance, Spiritual Support

Interventions	Rationales

1.
  a. Determine client's usual response to problems.
 	
  b. Decrease ambiguity by identifying choices and options.
	1.
	  a. It is important to determine whether the client usually seeks to change own behaviors to control problems or expects others or external factors to control problems.
	  b. Understanding anticipated trajectory of disease and treatment plan promotes a sense of control, both for the client and family members, as it takes the unknown factors out of the equation (Stajduhar, Martin, & Barwich, 2008).

(continued on page 429)

Interventions	Rationales
2. Help client identify personal strengths and assets.	2. Discouraging client from focusing only on limitations can promote self-esteem.
3. Assist in identifying energy patterns and scheduling activities to accommodate these patterns.	3. A review of the client's daily schedule helps in planning appropriate rest periods.
4. Help client prioritize activities and schedule them during usual periods of high energy.	4. Scheduling can help client participate in activities that promote feelings of self-worth and dignity.

5. Help client identify components of the situation that can be controlled or maintained:
  a. Comfort
  b. Care schedule
  c. Family interaction and communication
  d. Home care decisions
  e. Death with dignity
  f. Funeral arrangements
	5. Loss of power in one area may be counterbalanced by the introduction of other sources of power or control.

6. Promote effective problem-solving by breaking activities down into parts:
  a. Things to be resolved now
  b. Things that require time to resolve
  c. Things that cannot be changed (e.g., impending death)
	6. A sense of control may be established by breaking the situation down into components that can be controlled.

7. As appropriate, provide client with opportunities to make decisions about certain aspects of the care plan.	7. Allowing client to make decisions reinforces respect for his or her right of self-determination.
8. Promote communication of feelings and concerns among family members and significant others.	8. Open communication can help to enlist the support of others (Stajduhar, Martin, & Barwich, 2008).

9. If family support is not available, do the following:
  a. Identify possible community resources for home support.
  b. Explain long-term care placement.
  c. Refer to social services or to clergy, if appropriate.
  d. Provide social support using volunteer and professional services.
	9. Although end-stage cancer cannot be cured and death will occur, clients and support persons need a sense of hope. Client should believe that he or she will be comfortable, that care needs will be met, that he or she can maintain relationships with others, and that he or she will die with dignity.

Documentation

Progress notes
  Participation in self-care decisions
  Emotional status
  Interactions

Hopelessness Related to Overwhelming Functional Losses or Impending Death

NOC Decision-Making, Depression Self-Control, Hope, Quality of Life

Goal

The client will die with dignity and peace.

Indicators

• Express confidence that he or she will receive the needed care and be comfortable.
• Share his or her suffering openly.

NIC Hope Instillation, Values Clarification, Decision-Making Support, Spiritual Support, Support System Enhancement

Interventions	Rationales
1. Discuss the medical situation honestly.	1. Promoting hope for a cure sets up the client and support persons for false hope and despair.
2. Redirect client to identify alternate sources of hope: a. Relationships b. Faith c. Things to accomplish	2. Recognizing positive aspects of one's life may facilitate coping with an aspect of one's life that is uncontrollable. Authentic relationships, self-representation, and feelings of belonging have been identified as a client's emotional needs in the living and dying phase.
3. Help client to identify realistic hope in his or her situation: a. Client will be comfortable. b. Client will receive needed care. c. Client will maintain significant relationships. d. Client will die with dignity.	3. Others can promote hope. Their support can help the client gain confidence and autonomy.
4. Encourage client to appreciate the fullness of each moment, each day.	4. Redirecting thoughts can produce growth and strength even in a time of conflict.
5. Promote a positive psychosocial environment through measures such as: a. Providing favorite foods b. Encouraging personalization of the room c. Keeping the room clean and comfortable	5. These techniques show that the client is respected and valued.
6. Help client to identify purpose in his or her life such as: a. Model for others b. Love c. Advice	6. The dying client can provide others with a gift—an example of how to live with imminent death and how to control one's death.
7. Provide client with a sense of confidence and assurance that he or she can deal with cancer. Explain that the nurse can be relied on to guide the client along the way.	7. A guide provides support and direction and introduces the client and family members to the available support groups and information to lessen the anxiety (NCI, 2008; ACS, 2007).

Documentation

Progress notes
  Dialogues
  Emotional, spiritual status

High Risk for Spiritual Distress Related to Fear of Death, Overwhelming Grief, Belief System Crisis

NOC Hope, Spiritual Health

Goal

The client will express desire to perform religious or spiritual practice.

Indicators

• Express feelings regarding beliefs.
• Discuss the meaning and purpose of illness and death.

NIC Spiritual Growth Facilitation, Hope Instillation, Active Listening, Presence, Emotional Support, Spiritual Support

Interventions	Rationales
1. Communicate willingness to listen to the client's feelings regarding spiritual distress.	1. Client may view anger at God and a religious leader as a "forbidden" topic and may be reluctant to initiate discussions of spiritual conflicts.
2. Suggest contact with another spiritual support person, such as the hospital chaplain, if client is reluctant to share feelings with his or her usual spiritual advisor.	2. Other contacts may help client move toward a new spiritual understanding.
3. Explore if client desires to engage in a religious practice or ritual and accommodate his or her request to the extent possible.	3. The client may value prayer and spiritual rituals highly.
4. Offer to pray with him or her or to read from a religious text.	4. This can help to meet client's spiritual needs.

Documentation

Progress notes
   Dialogues
   Interventions
   Spiritual status
   Referrals

High Risk for Ineffective Therapeutic Regimen Management Related to Insufficient Knowledge of Home Care, Pain Management, Signs and Symptoms of Complications, and Community Resources Available

NOC Compliance Behavior, Knowledge: Treatment Regimen, Participation in Health Care Decisions, Treatment Behavior: Illness or Injury

Goals

The goals for this diagnosis represent those associated with discharge planning. Refer to the discharge criteria.

NIC Anticipatory Guidance, Learning Facilitation, Risk Identification, Health Education, Teaching: Procedure/Treatment, Health System Guidance

Interventions	Rationales

1. Discuss home-care needs:
  a. Treatments:
    • Pressure ulcer care
    • Feeding tubes
    • Wound care
    • Tube care
    • Injections
    • Tracheostomy care
    • Ostomy care
    • Denver shunt management
	1. Each client has specific individual care needs. Understanding can maximize treatment effectiveness.

(continued on page 432)

Interventions	Rationales
b. Equipment: • Supplemental oxygen • Suction equipment • IV equipment • Assistive devices (e.g., walker, wheelchair) c. Care needs: • Positioning • Feeding and bathing techniques • Transfer techniques • Injury prevention strategies	
2. Teach home care measures and evaluate ability: a. Provide written teaching materials for treatments and equipment, when feasible. b. Demonstrate procedures, equipment, and care measures. c. Have the caregiver return demonstration under supervision until skill is evident. d. Provide for practice to increase caregiver's skill. e. Encourage verbalization of questions and concerns. f. Provide positive reinforcement.	2. Specific instructions can reduce fear related to lack of knowledge and help the nurse determine what follow-up teaching is needed.
3. If renal insufficiency is present, use opioids with short half-lives, such as oxycodone, fentanyl, or hydromorphone.	3. Renal insufficiency allows opioid metabolites, especially morphine, to accumulate and causes opioid toxicity.
4. Monitor for signs/symptoms of opioid toxicity: • Hallucinations • Myoclonus (muscle spasms) • Hyperirritability	4. Excess metabolites cause opioid toxicity, which requires lowering the dose or changing the type of opioid.
5. Consider changing type of opioid if it is ineffective or has adverse effects.	5. Changing opioids may be required until there is a balance between pain relief and side effects (Lehne, 2004; Deglin & Vallerand, 2007).
6. Consider sedation with clients who have advanced disease when intractable pain continues (Lehne, 2004; Deglin & Vallerand, 2007).	6. The primary goal is no longer prolongation of life but achieving optimal comfort for people with a do not resuscitate (DNR) status.
7. Consult with client and family for sedation use. Advise that sedation can be reduced and can be resumed anytime (Lehne, 2004; Deglin & Vallerand, 2007; Valente, 2004).	7. Consultation is needed to provide clear explanations and to acquire informed consent (Lehne, 2004; Deglin & Vallerand, 2007; Valente, 2004).
8. Clearly communicate the client's and family's decisions to the staff in the plan of care.	8. Controversies regarding the use of sedation at end of life are distinguishable from euthanasia (Valente, 2004).
9. Explain how and where to obtain needed equipment and supplies.	9. Knowledge of access postdischarge can reduce some apprehension and facilitate care.
10. Teach signs and symptoms that must be reported to a health care professional: a. Change in mental status, visual changes, or muscle coordination b. Muscle cramps, numbness c. Increasing dyspnea, edema, abdominal distention	10. Early reporting may enable prompt interventions to reduce or eliminate certain complications. a. Neurologic changes may indicate cerebral metastasis, which can be sudden or insidious. Cancers of the lung, breast, testicles, thyroid, kidney, prostate, melanoma, and leukemia are associated with cerebral metastasis. b. Muscle cramps and numbness may point to calcium imbalance. c. These symptoms may indicate malignant effusions (pleural, ascites, pericardial).

(continued on page 433)

Interventions	Rationales
d. Increasing sedation, decreasing respirations	d. Sedation and respiratory depression may indicate narcotic toxicity.
e. Skeletal pain, loss of movement	e. Pain and limited movement may indicate pathologic fracture.
f. Neck or back pain, motor deficits, sensory deficits (e.g., paresthesias)	f. These signs and symptoms may point to cord compression.
g. Change in bowel or bladder function	g. Bladder or bowel changes may result from cord compression or ascites.
h. Facial edema, dyspnea, distended neck veins	h. These effects may indicate superior vena cava syndrome (SVCS), which is associated with lung cancer, breast cancer, and lymphoma.
11. If skeletal pain, loss of movement, or neck or back pain occurs, teach client to maintain bed rest and to immobilize the area until a health care professional can examine it.	11. Immobilization helps to prevent further tissue damage.
12. Discuss possible cancer- and death-related stressors with the family, such as financial burdens, role responsibility changes, and dependency.	12. Terminal illness entails a wide range of stressors. Preparing the family for possible problems enables planning to prevent or minimize them.
13. Provide information about, or initiate referrals to, community resources (e.g., hospice, counselors, home health agencies, American Cancer Society, and National Cancer Institute) (NCI, 2008; ACS, 2007).	13. Assistance may be needed with home management and with minimizing the potential destructive effects on the client and family.

Documentation

Discharge summary record
Client teaching
Outcome achievement or status
Referrals, if indicated

Leukemia

Leukemia is a blood-related cancer, specifically of bone marrow cells, that may be chronic or acute and aggressive. It accounts for 3% of all cancer diagnoses (Rogers, 2005). Cells arising from stem cells lose the ability to differentiate into red blood cells, white blood cells, and platelets. One type of abnormal white cell prevails, preventing normal cell differentiation and development (Rogers, 2005).

Leukemia is classified according to the cell type involved, either myelogenous or lymphocytic. The leukemia is called biphenotypic if it has characteristics of both cell types (Rogers, 2005). Myelogenous indicates changes in marrow cells that generally differentiate into red cells, some white cells, and platelets. Lymphocytic indicates changes in marrow cells that differentiate into lymphocytes (The Leukemia & Lymphoma Society, 2007). Acute leukemia progresses rapidly. It is characterized by immature cells crowding out normal cells in the bone marrow. Acute myelogenous leukemia (AML) accounts for most of adult diagnoses, acute lymphocytic leukemia (ALL) is more common in pediatric clients. Chronic leukemia progresses more slowly and usually affects those over 20 years old. There is some development of normal cells; therefore, symptoms may not be detected until later stages of the disease (National Cancer Institute, 2003; Rogers, 2005).

Acute myelogenous leukemia involves a malignant clone that arises in myeloid, monocyte, erythroid, or megakaryocyte cells; stem cells usually commit to the development of neutrophils (Rogers, 2005). Acute lymphocytic leukemia involves abnormal lymphoblast clones in the marrow, thymus, and lymph nodes;

with the over-development of immature lymphocytes (Rogers, 2005). Chronic lymphocytic leukemia (CLL) involves proliferation of long-lived incompetent lymphocytes. Chronic myelogenous leukemia (CML) involves proliferation of mature granulocytes in the bone marrow (Wujcik, 2000; Rogers, 2005).

Hairy cell leukemia is a rare form of chronic leukemia (National Cancer Institute, 2003). It is called "hairy cell" because the leukemic lymphocytes have thin projections on their surface that resemble hairs when examined under a microscope (The Leukemia & Lymphoma Society, 2007). It is caused by an abnormal change in B lymphocytes.

The exact cause of leukemia is unknown, but the key event is damage to the DNA of the hematopoietic stem cells. Some presumed causes are chemicals or occupational hazards (e.g., pesticides), medications (e.g., actinomycin), smoking, ionizing radiation, genetic factors, environmental factors, and viruses (e.g., Epstein-Barr) (Rogers, 2005).

 Time Frame
Initial diagnosis

■■■■■ DIAGNOSTIC CLUSTER*

Collaborative Problems

PC: Bone Marrow Depression
PC: Leukostasis
PC: CNS Involvement
PC: Massive Splenomegaly

Nursing Diagnoses	Refer to
High Risk for Infection related to increased susceptibility secondary to leukemic process and side effects of chemotherapy	
High Risk for Ineffective Therapeutic Regimen Management related to insufficient knowledge of disease process, treatment, signs and symptoms of complications, reduction of risk factors, and community resources	
High Risk for Impaired Social Interactions related to fear of rejection or actual rejection of others after diagnosis	Cancer (Initial Diagnosis)
Powerlessness related to inability to control situation	Cancer (Initial Diagnosis)
High Risk for Ineffective Sexual Patterns related to fear secondary to potential for infection and injury	Cancer (Initial Diagnosis)

Related Care Plans

Chemotherapy
Cancer (Initial Diagnosis)

*This medical condition was not included in the validation study.

Discharge Criteria

Before discharge, the client or family will

1. Describe the home care regimen, including restrictions.
2. Identify the signs and symptoms of complications that must be reported to a health care professional.

3. Describe the necessary follow-up care.

4. Verbalize an awareness of available community resources.

5. Identify function of bone marrow, including cell lines.

Collaborative Problems

Potential Complication: Bone Marrow Depression

Potential Complication: Leukostasis

Potential Complication: CNS Involvement

Potential Complication: Massive Splenomegaly

Nursing Goal

The nurse will detect early signs and symptoms of (a) bone marrow depression, (b) leukostasis, (c) CNS involvement, and (d) massive splenomegaly, and collaboratively intervene to stabilize client.

Indicators

- Alert, oriented (c)
- Neutrophils 60%–70% (a, b, d)
- Red blood cells (a, b, d)
  - Male: 4.6–5.9 million/mm^3
  - Female: 4.2–5.4 million/mm^3
- Platelets 150,000–400,000/mm^3 (a, b, d)
- No petechiae or purpura (a, b, d)
- No gum or nasal bleeding (a, b, d)
- Regular menses (a, b, d)
- No headache (c)
- Clear vision (c)
- Intact coordination, facial symmetry, and muscle strength (c)
- No splenomegaly (d)
- Identify risk factors that can be reduced
- Relate early signs and symptoms of infection

Interventions	Rationales

1. Monitor for bone marrow depression:
  a. Decreased neutrophils
  b. Decreased red blood cells
  c. Decreased platelets
	1. Each day bone marrow produces and releases into the circulation red cells, platelets, and granulocytes to maintain hemostasis and oxygen requirements. In addition, bone marrow participates in the defense against foreign invasion with antibody synthesis, initiating phagocytosis and antigen processing (Wujcik, 2000). Leukemia cells proliferate and infiltrate the bone marrow, decreasing red blood cells, platelets, and granulocytes.

2. Monitor for disseminated intravascular coagulation (DIC):
  a. Easy bruising
  b. Epistaxis
  c. Menorrhagia
  d. Gingival bleeding
  e. Central nervous system (CNS) hemorrhage
  f. Thrombosis (chronic DIC)
	2. DIC may occur with any acute leukemia but more often with acute promyelocytic. The cause is extensive triggering of the coagulation system. Excessive circulating thromboses may be the triggering cause in leukemia. At some point, the extensive hypercoagulation consumes available clotting factors, resulting in the body's inability to form stable clots (Gobel, 2000; Wujcik, 2000).

3. Report WBC counts over 50,000 to the physician; prepare to administer high doses of cytotoxic drugs.	3. Individuals with many circulating blasts are at risk for leukostasis. Leukostasis occurs when vessel walls rupture as the result of excessive numbers of blast cells (Wujcik, 2000).

(continued on page 436)

Interventions	Rationales

4. Monitor for CNS leukemia:
  a. Altered level of consciousness/confusion (National Library of Medicine, 2006)
  b. Headaches
  c. Blurred vision
  d. Change in coordination, facial symmetry, or muscle strength
  e. Seizures (National Library of Medicine, 2006)
  f. Vomiting (National Library of Medicine, 2006)
	4. CNS involvement can result from infiltration of leukemic cells into the cerebrospinal fluid, which increases intra-cerebral pressure and compresses cerebral tissue (National Library of Medicine, 2006).

5. Complete a neurologic assessment before administering high-dose cytosine arabinoside (HDCA).	5. Cerebellar toxicity is a CNS toxic effect of high-dose cytosine arabinoside (Wujcik, 2000).

6. Monitor for massive splenomegaly:
  • Enlarged spleen
  • Thrombocytopenia (decreased platelets)
  • Petechiae (pinpoint purplish-red spots)
  • Purpura (purple areas of bruising)
	6. Leukemia cells proliferate and infiltrate the spleen. Replacement of bone marrow by leukemia cells results in decreased platelet production (Porth, 2002).

7. Teach client to assess for signs of bleeding every day to every shift as necessary (Gobel, 2000):
 	
  a. Integumentary system:
    • Petechiae
    • Ecchymoses
    • Hematomas
    • Oozing from venipuncture sites
    • Cyanotic patches on arms/legs
  b. Eyes and ears:
    • Visual disturbances
    • Periorbital edema
    • Subconjunctival hemorrhage
    • Ear pain
  c. Nose, mouth, and throat:
    • Petechiae
    • Epistaxis
    • Tender or bleeding gums
  d. Cardiopulmonary system:
    • Crackles and wheezes
    • Stridor and dyspnea
    • Tachypnea and cyanosis
    • Hemoptysis
  e. Gastrointestinal system:
    • Pain
    • Bleeding around rectum
    • Occult blood in stools
  f. Genitourinary system:
    • Bleeding
    • Increased menses
    • Decreased urine output
  g. Musculoskeletal system:
    • Painful joints
  h. Central nervous system:
    • Mental status changes
    • Vertigo
    • Seizures
    • Restlessness
	7. Regular total body assessment is necessary to detect early signs of bleeding, which is the second leading cause of death in leukemia.
	As platelet count decreases, the risk of bleeding increases, as follows (Gobel, 2000):
	  a. >100,000: no risk
	
	  b. 100,000–50,000: minimal risk
	
	  c. 50,000–20,000: moderate risk
	
	  d. <20,000: severe risk

(continued on page 437)

Interventions	Rationales
8. Transfuse blood components as ordered.	8. Potential transplant candidates should receive leuco-depleted blood products. Most clients need a specific blood component (e.g., platelets, plasma) (Gobel, 2000).
9. Minimize invasive procedures; avoid the following: a. Rectal temperatures b. Suppositories c. IM and SC injections d. Vaginal douches e. Bladder catheterization	9. Invasive procedures can cause tissue trauma and may be sources of infection (Gobel, 2000).
10. Apply pressure to puncture sites for 3–5 minutes.	10. This prevents prolonged bleeding from puncture sites, which can cause damage to underlying structures such as nerves.

Related Physician-Prescribed Interventions

Medications. Prednisone, antineoplastics, stool softeners, anthracycline, antiemetics, cyclophosphamide, analgesics, methotrexate, teniposide, 6-mercaptopurine, cytarabine, hypoxanthine, idarubicin, interferon-alfa, vitamin D_3, all-transretinoic acid

Intravenous Therapy. Granulocyte transfusion, platelet transfusion, blood transfusion, electrolyte support, medication administration, stem cell transplant. Use of a central line is preferred for most antineoplastic treatment.

Laboratory Studies. Reverse-transcriptase, polymerase chain reaction, complete blood count with differential, urinalysis, liver enzyme levels, BUN levels, chemistry, prothrombin time, blood cultures, partial thromboplastin time, uric acid level, polymerase chain reaction, serum markers (see Cancer: Initial Diagnosis)

Diagnostic Studies. Bone marrow aspiration, tomography scan, chest x-ray film, liver–spleen scan, lumbar puncture, flow cytometric typing, electron microscopy, intracranial radiation, cytochemistry, immunophenotype

Therapies. Nutritional supplements, splenectomy, bone marrow transplant

Documentation

Flow records
    Intake and output
    Vital signs
    Weight
    Physical assessment
    Neurologic checks
Progress notes
    Abnormal assessment findings
    Interventions
    Response to interventions

Nursing Diagnoses

High Risk for Infection Related to Increased Susceptibility Secondary to Leukemic Process and Side Effects of Chemotherapy

NOC Immune Hypersensitivity Response

Goal

The client will report risk factors and precautions needed.

NIC Allergy Management, Latex Precautions, Environmental Risk Protection

Interventions	Rationales

1. Institute measures to prevent exposure to known or potential sources of infection:
  a. Maintain protective isolation in accordance with institutional policy.
  b. Maintain meticulous handwashing.
  c. Provide scrupulous hygiene.
  d. Restrict visitors with colds, flu, or infections.
  e. Provide good perianal hygiene twice daily and after each bowel movement (e.g., sitz baths).
  f. Restrict fresh flowers and plants.
  g. Restrict fresh fruits and vegetables.
  h. Use mouth care protocol.
  i. Care for neutropenic clients first.
	1. These precautions minimize client's exposure to bacterial, viral, and fungal pathogens, both exogenous and endogenous.

2. Notify physician of any changes in vital signs.	2. Subtle changes in vital signs, particularly fever, may be only early signs of sepsis.
3. Obtain cultures of sputum, urine, diarrhea, blood, and abnormal body secretions, as ordered.	3. Cultures can confirm infection and identify the causative organism.
4. Explain reasons for precautions and restrictions.	4. Client's understanding may improve compliance and reduce risk factors.
5. Reassure client and family that the increased susceptibility to infection is only temporary.	5. Granulocytopenia can persist for 6–12 weeks. Understanding the temporary nature of granulocytopenia may help to prevent client and family from becoming discouraged.
6. Minimize invasive procedures (e.g., rectal and vaginal examinations, indwelling [Foley] catheter insertion, IM injections).	6. Certain procedures cause tissue trauma, increasing the susceptibility of infection.
7. Optimal nutrition supports protein synthesis and phagocytosis.	7. Explain the importance of good nutrition and vitamin and mineral supplementation.

Documentation

Flow records
  Vital signs
  Intake and output
  Assessments
  WBC/granulocyte count
Progress notes
  Abnormal findings or complaints
Discharge summary record
  Client teaching

High Risk for Ineffective Therapeutic Regimen Management Related to Insufficient Knowledge of Disease Process, Treatment, Signs and Symptoms of Complications, Reduction of Risk Factors, and Community Resources

NOC Compliance Behavior, Knowledge: Treatment Regimen, Participation in Health Care Decisions, Treatment Behavior: Illness or Injury

Goals

The goals for this diagnosis represent those associated with discharge planning. Refer to the discharge criteria.

NIC Anticipatory Guidance, Risk Identification, Learning Facilitation, Health Education

Interventions	Rationales
1. Explain leukemia to client and family, including the following aspects: a. Pathophysiology b. Function of bone marrow and its specific components c. Potential complications (e.g., infection, anemia, bleeding)	1. Providing specific information about leukemia may improve compliance by helping client and family understand the need for treatments and precautions (Wujcik, 2000).
2. Explain that anemia causes fatigue; stress the need for energy conservation (Rogers, 2005). (Refer to the nursing diagnosis Fatigue in the Inflammatory Joint Disease care plan for specific strategies.)	2. Anemia results from inadequate red blood cell production secondary to increased WBC production. Energy conservation reduces fatigue (Wujcik, 2000).
3. Teach the importance of optimal nutrition.	3. Adequate intake of protein, carbohydrates, vitamins, and minerals is required for tissue rebuilding and increased resistance to infection. Gastric irritation can occur with treatment (Rogers, 2005).
4. Provide written information about and applications for registration to the Leukemia & Lymphoma Society and local leukemia foundations.	4. These resources can provide emotional support and possibly financial assistance.
5. Teach client the importance of good oral care and to inspect oral mucous membranes daily.	5. Inadequate defense mechanisms (e.g., abnormal WBC count, bone marrow suppression) increase the risk for infection.
6. Teach client the importance of good perianal hygiene and avoiding constipation and rectal trauma (e.g., enemas, thermometers).	6. Rectal abscesses can occur from trauma and constipation, increasing the susceptibility to infection.
7. Teach to avoid all immunizations.	7. An immunosuppressed client must avoid immunization because he or she lacks the ability to build antibodies and can contract the disease from the immunization.
8. Consult with pharmacist or physician before using over-the-counter (OTC) drugs.	8. Many OTC medications inhibit platelet functioning.
9. Teach measures to avoid bacteria in the diet: a. Avoid raw fruits and vegetables. b. Avoid fried foods in restaurants.	9. These foods are a potential source of bacteria pathogens.
10. Teach client to report the following signs of: a. Infection (Rogers, 2005): • Fever • Excess cough and sputum production • Burning with urination b. Anemia: • Dyspnea • Increasing weakness c. Bleeding: • Nosebleeds • Blood in stools • Cloudy urine • Bruises	10. These signs and symptoms may indicate need for additional treatment (e.g., NSAIDs, aspirin).
11. Provide soft toothbrushes or sponges for oral hygiene. Explain the following to client and family: a. Rationales for precautions b. Signs and symptoms they must report to a health care professional	11. This can help prevent damage to oral mucosa, which is susceptible to bleeding and flossing. The client's and family's understanding can encourage compliance and reduce anxiety. Include function of platelets (Gobel, 2000).

(continued on page 440)

Interventions	Rationales
c. The need to avoid medications that interfere with platelet function; provide a list.	
12. Teach client to avoid: a. Forceful coughing, sneezing, or nose blowing b. Constipation and bowel straining	12. a. Epistaxis can be life-threatening in a client with decreased platelets (Gobel, 2000). b. Rectal bleeding can result from straining (Gobel, 2000).
13. Teach the importance of informing all health care providers about diagnosis: a. Dentist and hygienist b. Phlebotomist	13. Precautions may be needed to prevent bleeding.
14. Encourage client to continue usual social activities, as tolerated.	14. Long-term survivors report personal relationships to be the most important indicator for a positive quality of life (Zebrack, 2000).
15. Provide opportunities to discuss how the experience of leukemia has affected client's and family members' lives (Rogers, 2005).	15. Some clients living with leukemia report a high ability to cope with stressors (Zebrack, 2000).
16. Consider referrals to counselors and therapists, as needed.	16. Individuals facing a life-threatening condition may need assistance with adaption.
17. Explain the potential for hair loss (Rogers, 2005).	17. Hair will probably grow back when therapy is completed (Rogers, 2005).
18. Instruct client that skin may become dry and sensitive to sun exposure (Rogers, 2005).	18. Client should wear sunscreen and appropriate attire when outdoors (Rogers, 2005).

Documentation

Discharge summary record
    Client teaching
    Outcome achievement or status
    Referrals, if indicated

Alcohol Withdrawal Syndrome

Approximately 27% of persons between the ages of 18 and 64 meet the diagnostic criteria for alcohol dependency (McKinley, 2005). It is estimated that one in every five hospitalized persons is an alcohol abuser (McKinley, 2005). Clinically, only one of every ten alcoholics is diagnosed, and clinicians do not ask about alcohol use unless it is obvious. It is critical to identify people who abuse alcohol to prevent potentially fatal withdrawal symptoms. Surgical clients are at high risk for alcohol withdrawal syndrome because of the pre-procedural and postoperative fasting. Most signs and symptoms are caused by the rapid removal of the depressant effects of alcohol on the central nervous system. The focus of medical and nursing care is to prevent, not to observe for, the complications of alcohol withdrawal (Gordon, 2006). Prevention includes aggressive management of early withdrawal and close monitoring of the client's response.

 Time Frame
Secondary diagnosis

■■■■■■ DIAGNOSTIC CLUSTER*

Collaborative Problems	Refer to
PC: Delirium Tremens	
PC: Autonomic Hyperactivity	
PC: Seizures	
PC: Alcohol Hallucinosis	
PC: Hypovolemia	Thermal Injuries
PC: Hypoglycemia	Diabetes Mellitus

Nursing Diagnoses	Refer to
Imbalanced Nutrition. Less Than Body Requirements related to inadequate intake of balanced diet and water-soluble vitamins (thiamin, folic acid, and pyridoxine)	
High Risk for Deficient Fluid Volume related to abnormal fluid loss secondary to vomiting, diarrhea, dehydration, and diaphoresis	
High Risk for Violence related to (examples) impulsive behavior, disorientation, tremors, or impaired judgment	
Anxiety related to loss of control, memory losses, and fear of withdrawal	
Ineffective Coping: Anger, Dependence, or Denial related to inability to constructively manage stressor without alcohol (Refer to Pancreatitis care plan)	Pancreatitis
High Risk for Ineffective Therapeutic Regimen Management related to insufficient knowledge of condition, treatments available, high-risk situations, and community resources	

*This clinical situation was not included in the validation study.

Discharge Criteria

The client will

1. Recognize that alcoholism is a disease.
2. Acknowledge the negative effects of alcoholism in their lives.
3. Identify community resources available for treatment of alcoholism.

Collaborative Problems

Potential Complication: Delirium Tremens

Potential Complication: Autonomic Hyperactivity

Potential Complication: Seizures

Potential Complication: Alcohol Hallucinosis

Potential Complication: Hypovolemia

Potential Complication: Hypoglycemia

Nursing Goal

The nurse will detect early signs and symptoms of (a) delirium tremens, (b) autonomic hyperactivity, (c) seizures, (d) alcohol hallucinosis, (e) hypovolemia, and (f) hypoglycemia, and will collaboratively intervene to stabilize the client.

Indicators

- No seizure activity (a, b, c)
- Calm, oriented (a, b, d)
- Temperature 98–99.5°F (d)
- Pulse 60–100 beats/min (a, b, d)
- BP >90/60, <140/90 mmHg (a, b, d)
- No reports of hallucinations (a, d)

Interventions	Rationales
1. Carefully attempt to determine if the client abuses alcohol. Consult with the family regarding perception of alcohol consumption. Explain why accurate information is necessary.	1. It is critical to identify high-risk clients so that potentially fatal withdrawal symptoms can be prevented.
2. Obtain history of drinking patterns from the client or significant others (Kappas-Larson & Lathrop, 1993): a. When did the client have his or her last drink? b. How much was consumed on that day? c. On how many days of the last 30 did the client consume alcohol? d. What was the average intake? e. What was the most consumed?	2. Alcoholics tend to underestimate alcohol consumed; therefore, multiply the amount a man tells you by two to three drinks and for a woman by four to five drinks (Smith-DiJulio, 2001).
3. Determine the client's attitude toward drinking by asking the CAGE questions: a. Have you ever thought you should *C*ut down your drinking? b. Have you ever been *A*nnoyed by criticism of your drinking? c. Have you ever felt *G*uilty about your drinking? d. Do you drink in the morning (i.e., "*E*ye-opener") (Ewing, 1984)?	3. These questions can be used to identify possible defensiveness and similar attitudes about drinking.

(continued on page 443)

Interventions	Rationales

4. Obtain history of previous withdrawals, as applicable:
  a. Delirium tremens:
    • Time of onset
    • Manifestation
  b. Seizures:
    • Time of onset
    • Type
	4. Withdrawal occurs between 6 to and 96 h after cessation of drinking. Withdrawal can occur in individuals who are considered "social drinkers" (6 ounces of alcohol daily for 3 to 4 weeks). Withdrawal patterns may resemble those of previous episodes. Seizure patterns, unlike previous episodes, may indicate another underlying pathology (Babel, 1997).

5. Obtain complete history of prescription and nonprescription drugs taken.	5. Benzodiazepine or barbiturate withdrawal may mimic alcohol withdrawal and will complicate the picture. Substance abusers tend to cross-abuse substances (Babel, 1997).

6. Monitor all persons suspected of, or identified as, high risk for alcohol withdrawal syndrome for early signs and symptoms (The Clinical Institute Withdrawal Assessment of Alcohol Scale, McKinley, 2005):
  a. Do you feel sick to your stomach?
  b. Do you feel nervous? (Observe for restlessness, sweating.)
  c. Do you feel any pins-and-needles sensations? Any itching?
  d. Is the light too bright? Are sounds too loud? Are you afraid?
  e. Observe for tremors when the client's arms are extended and the fingers spread wide.
	6. Identification of early signs and symptoms of central nervous system impairment can prompt early interventions and prevent mortality (McKinley, 2005).

7. Consult with primary care provider regarding the client's risk and the initiation of benzodiazepine therapy, with dosage determined by assessment findings.	7. Benzodiazepine requirements in alcohol withdrawal are highly variable and client-specific. Fixed schedules may oversedate or undersedate (Babel, 1997).

8. Observe for desired effects of benzodiazepine therapy:
  a. Relief from withdrawal symptoms
  b. Client sleeping peacefully, but can be roused
	8. Benzodiazepine is the drug of choice in controlling withdrawal symptoms. Neuroleptics cause hypotension and lower seizure threshold. Barbiturates may effectively control symptoms of withdrawal but have no advantages over benzodiazepines (Babel, 1997).

9. Monitor for alcohol withdrawal syndrome:
  a. Hyperactivity (nausea, vomiting, shakiness, sweating)
  b. Neuropsychiatric responses (agitation, anxiety, audio disturbances, clouding of sensorium, visual and tactile disturbances)
	9. "These signs and symptoms occur within 24 hours after the last drink. They peak in 24–36 hours and end in 48 hours" (McKinley, 2005, p.42).

10. Monitor for withdrawal delirium or delirium tremens:
  a. Severe autonomic hyperactivity (hypertension, tachycardia, tachypnea, tremors)
  b. Neuropsychiatric signs and symptoms (hallucinations, confusion, disorientation, impaired attention)
	10. These signs and symptoms occur 48–72 h after the last drink. If untreated, death can occur from respiratory and cardiovascular collapse (McKinley, 2005).

11. Monitor for and intervene promptly in cases of status epilepticus: a. Follow the institution's emergency protocol.	11. Status epilepticus is life-threatening if not controlled immediately with IV diazepam.

12. Monitor and restore fluid and electrolyte balances:
  a. Urine output
  b. Serum potassium
  c. Serum sodium
  d. Serum magnesium
	12. Fluid and electrolyte losses from vomiting, profuse perspiration, and decreased antidiuretic hormone (from alcohol ingestion) cause dehydration. Increased neuromuscular activity can deplete magnesium and IV glucose administration can cause intracellular shift of magnesium (Porth, 2006).

13. Monitor for hypoglycemia: a. Blood glucose	13. Alcohol depletes liver glycogen stores and impairs gluconeogenesis. Alcoholics are also malnourished (Porth, 2006).

(continued on page 444)

Interventions	Rationales
14. Monitor vital signs every 30 minutes initially: a. Temperature, pulse, and respiration b. Blood pressure (BP)	14. Clients in withdrawal will have elevated heart rate, respirations, and fever. Those experiencing delirium tremens can be expected to have a low-grade fever. A rectal temperature greater than 99.9°F, however, is a clue to possible infection. Hypotension may be associated with pneumonia and a clue to infection (Porth, 2006).
15. Monitor laboratory values: a. White blood cell count (WBC) b. Liver function studies c. Serum glucose d. Occult blood e. Albumin, prealbumin f. Serum alcohol level g. Electrolytes	15. Laboratory values may indicate alcohol-related conditions. Alcohol abuse causes a range of immunopathologic events. In alcoholic liver disease, albumin is lowered because of decreased synthesis by liver and malnutrition (Porth, 2006).
16. Observe for side effects or overmedication of benzodiazepine therapy: a. Oversedation b. Slurred speech c. Ataxia d. Nystagmus	16. All medications have a therapeutic window and are not without their side effects.
17. Maintain the client IV, running continuously.	17. Necessary for fluid replacement, dextrose, thiamin bolus, benzodiazepine, and magnesium sulfate administrations. Chlordiazepoxide and diazepam should not be given intramuscularly because of unpredictable absorption (Babel, 1997).
18. Control fever nonpharmacologically through cooling blankets, ice, and the like.	18. The client may also have alcohol-related conditions, such as varices, ulcers, gastritis, and cirrhosis, that contraindicate the use of acetaminophen or ASA.

◤ Related Physician-Prescribed Interventions

Medications. Benzodiazepines, Dilantin, thiamin, multivitamins, folic acid, magnesium

Intravenous Therapy. Fluid replacement, dextrose 1 g/kg

Laboratory Studies. Complete blood cell count (CBC), serum prealbumin, liver function studies, serum potassium, serum glucose, serum sodium, serum alcohol level, serum magnesium, occult blood (stool), serum albumin, uric acid, carbohydrate deficient transferrin, mean corpuscular volume

Diagnostic Studies. Electroencephalogram, if first occurrence of seizure or pattern changes, EKG

Therapies. Well-balanced diet with multivitamin supplement

Documentation

Nursing history
Flow records
    Daily weight
    Vital signs
    Laboratory values
    Alcohol withdrawal symptoms
Progress notes
    Change in status
    Interventions
    Response to interventions

Nursing Diagnoses

Imbalanced Nutrition: Less Than Body Requirements Related to Inadequate Intake of Balanced Diet and Water-Soluble Vitamins (Thiamin, Folic Acid, and Pyridoxine)

NOC Nutritional Status

Goal

The client will relate what constitutes a well-balanced diet.

Indicators

• Describe the reasons for nutritional problems.
• Gain weight (specify amount).
• Relate need for vitamin supplements.

NIC Nutrition Management, Nutritional Monitoring

Interventions	Rationales
1. Discuss the importance of a well-balanced diet; the rationale for thiamin replacement; development and symptoms of Wernicke-Korsakoff syndrome (ophthalmoplegia, ptosis, palsy, disconjugate gaze, and altered consciousness). Effects of alcohol and thiamin depletion (Dudek, 2005).	1. Helping the client to understand the benefits of a well-balanced diet can improve compliance.
2. Provide three to four meals a day with multivitamins.	2. They will help restore proper nutritional status.
3. Maintain good oral hygiene (brush teeth and rinse mouth) before and after ingestion of food.	3. Accumulation of food particles in the mouth can contribute to foul odors and tastes that diminish appetite.

Documentation

Flow record
Weight
Intake (type and supplements)

High Risk for Deficient Fluid Volume Related to Abnormal Fluid Loss Secondary to Vomiting, Diarrhea, Dehydration, and Diaphoresis

NOC Electrolyte & Acid–Base Balance, Fluid Balance, Hydration

Goal

The client will have moist mucous membranes and pale yellow urine with a specific gravity within normal limits.

Indicators

• Describe how alcohol causes dehydration.
• Maintain weight.

NIC Fluid/Electrolyte Management, Fluid Monitoring

Interventions	Rationales
1. Monitor for early signs and symptoms of fluid volume deficit: a. Dry mucous membranes b. Amber urine	1. Decreased circulating volume causes drying tissues and concentrated urine. Early detection enables prompt fluid replacement therapy to correct deficits.
2. Do not administer antiemetic medication.	2. Antiemetics lower seizure threshold.
3. Maintain client IV running continuously.	3. This will replace fluid loss.
4. Monitor intake and output, making sure that intake compensates for output.	4. Dehydration may increase glomerular filtration rate, making output inadequate to clear wastes properly.
5. Weigh daily.	5. Accurate daily weights can detect fluid loss.

Documentation

Flow records
    Vital signs
    Intake and output
    Daily weights
    Medications
    Vomiting episodes

High Risk for Violence Related to (Examples) Impulsive Behavior, Disorientation, Tremors, or Impaired Judgment

NOC Abuse Cessation, Abusive Behavior Self-Restraint, Aggression Self-Control, Impulse Self-Control

Goal

The client will have fewer violent responses.

Indicators

• Demonstrate control of behavior with assistance from others.
• Relate causative factors.

NIC Abuse Protection Support, Anger Control Assistance, Environmental Management: Violence Prevention, Impulse Control Training, Crisis Intervention, Seclusion, Physical Restraint

Interventions	Rationales
1. Promote interactions that increase the client's sense of trust and value of self.	1. In agitated state, the client may not be able to verbally express feelings but may act out these feelings in an aggressive manner.
2. Establish an environment that decreases stimuli: a. Decrease noise level b. Soft lighting	2. The client is already in an agitated/mentally compromised state; environmental stimuli will unnecessarily aggravate this state and send the client "over the edge."

(continued on page 447)

Interventions	Rationales
c. Personal possessions d. Single/semiprivate room e. Control number of people entering the client's room	
3. Assess situations that have contributed to past violent episodes and attempt to modify the circumstances to prevent similar occurrences.	3. There can be a pattern to violence. Detecting and changing the pattern can eliminate the violence.
4. Assist the client in maintaining control over his or her behavior.	4. Losing control is a very frightening experience, more so than the violence.
5. If violence is imminent, systematically approach the client with a group of four to five individuals. a. One nurse speaks to the client and is in charge. b. One nurse for each limb.	5. This decreases the nurse's risk of danger, and the presence of four to five staff members reassures the client that the nursing staff will not let her or him lose control.
6. Use least resistive method of restraint for the shortest duration possible: a. Follow agency policy when using restraint.	6. This is in keeping with ethical and legal guidelines for restraint.
7. Make verbal contact with the client as soon as possible after the aggressive incident.	7. This maintains the client's sense of worth despite the aggressive behavior.
8. Initiate debriefing strategies among the nursing staff involved in the incident.	8. This allows the nursing staff members to center themselves after critical and often unpleasant incidents.

Documentation

Progress notes
  Aggressive incident
  Actions taken
  Evaluation/outcome
Flow record
Restraint

Anxiety Related to Loss of Control, Memory Losses, and Fear of Withdrawal

NOC Anxiety Self-Control, Coping, Impulse Self-Control

Goal

The client will report increased emotional comfort.

Indicators

• Relate cause of confusion and anxiety.
• Communicate feelings regarding present situation.

NIC Coping Enhancement, Emotional Support, Substance Use Treatment

Interventions	Rationales
1. Furnish a structured and supportive environment.	1. Structure is needed to control alcohol abuse. Support is needed to assist in the difficult task of withdrawing.

(continued on page 448)

Interventions	Rationales
2. Heighten the client's awareness of unsatisfactory protective behaviors.	2. Alcohol abuse is an ineffective method of promoting self-care.
3. Empathically assist the client to investigate thoughts and feelings so as to understand the source of pain.	3. Pain can be the outcome of childhood experiences when significant persons did not meet the child's unique needs and experiences (Nighorn, 1988).
4. Encourage the client to write down his or her thoughts, feelings, and behaviors.	4. This increases the client's awareness of the interrelationship between thoughts, feelings, and behaviors.
5. Provide alternative ways to tolerate or handle painful emotions.	5. The alcoholic has difficulty tolerating painful emotions as a result of ego dysfunction and self-care deficits. They abuse alcohol to calm intense affects.
6. Encourage productive thinking patterns through the following: a. Positive self-talk b. Examining faulty assumptions about self/others c. Imagery	6. Faulty or negative thinking is prevalent among alcoholics and stems from belief systems that started in their childhoods (Smith-DiJulio, 2001).
7. Reinforce positive coping behavior.	7. Reinforcement provides the feedback needed when new behaviors are tried.
8. Provide self-esteem–building exercises.	8. Self-esteem dysfunctions are critically involved with alcoholism (Nighorn, 1988).
9. Encourage the client to build social support networks through peer support groups and mobilization of friendship networks.	9. Chemicals lead addicts to develop a skewed sense of themselves and their relationships to the world. Peers can point out unrealistic views of self and world and also provide the needed emotional growth that was stunted by alcohol.
10. Access community programs (e.g., individual counseling, AA).	10. Sobriety is a lifelong process of one-day-at-a-time.

Documentation

Flow record
  Levels of anxiety and behavior response
Progress notes
  Unusual responses or situations

High Risk for Ineffective Therapeutic Regimen Management Related to Insufficient Knowledge of Condition, Treatments Available, High-Risk Situations, and Community Resources

NOC Compliance Behavior, Knowledge: Treatment Regimen, Participation in Health Care Decisions, Treatment Behavior: Illness or Injury

Goals

The goals for this diagnosis represent those associated with discharge planning. Refer to the discharge criteria.

NIC Substance Use Prevention, Substance Use Treatment, Behavior Modification, Support System Enhancement, Health System Guidance

Interventions	Rationales

1. Educate the client regarding the disease of alcoholism and its effects on self, family, job, and finances:
a. Loss of control:
  • Drink more than planned
  • Rules about use
  • Break/dismiss rules
b. Social problems:
  • Change in friends
  • Sexual acting out when drinking
  • Friends complaining of alcohol use
c. Legal problems:
  • Driving infractions
  • Assault
  • Solicitation
  • Burglary
  • Drug trafficking
d. Family problems:
  • Family conflict
  • Sexual problems with spouse
  • Acting out of other family members
e. Employment difficulties:
  • Coworker disputes
  • Tardiness
  • Absenteeism
  • Inconsistent performance
  • Labile, moody behavior
	1. Acknowledging alcoholism's effects on one's life can motivate a client to change behavior. It may be especially useful to do this after the person experiences the discomforts of withdrawal.

2. Teach the client to recognize and respond to the various alcohol-related medical conditions.	2. Continued alcohol abuse will lead to varying alcohol-related medical conditions as described in the collaborative problems.
3. Refer the client to community skill-building activities: a. Assertiveness training b. Stress management c. ADLs d. Anger management	3. The disease of addiction prevents individuals from learning adaptive social and other coping skills.
4. Improve family functioning through referral to community programs. a. Communication skills b. Boundaries and roles c. Education d. Al-Anon	4. Family functioning and individuals have suffered from the disease of alcoholism.

Documentation

Progress notes
  Teaching
  Response to teaching

Immobility or Unconsciousness

This care plan addresses the needs of clients who are immobile and either unconscious or conscious. In addition to the following diagnostic cluster, refer to the specific coexisting medical disease or condition (e.g., renal failure and cancer).

■■■■■ DIAGNOSTIC CLUSTER

Collaborative Problems	Refer to
▲ PC: Pneumonia, Atelectasis	Cerebrovascular Accident (Stroke)
▲ PC: Fluid/Electrolyte Imbalance	General Surgery
▲ PC: Negative Nitrogen Balance	Chronic Renal Failure
△ PC: Sepsis	Urolithiasis
▲ PC: Thrombophlebitis	General Surgery
△ Renal Calculi	Chronic Renal Failure
△ PC: Urinary Tract Infection	Chronic Renal Failure
✳ PC: Osteoporosis	Corticosteroid Therapy

Nursing Diagnoses	Refer to
△ Disuse Syndrome related to effects of immobility on body systems	
▲ (Specify) Self-Care Deficit related to immobility	
△ Powerlessness related to feelings of loss of control and the restrictions placed on life style	
▲ High Risk for Ineffective Airway Clearance related to stasis of secretions secondary to inadequate cough and decreased mobility	COPD
▲ Total Incontinence related to unconscious state	Neurogenic Bladder
△ High Risk for Impaired Oral Mucous Membrane related to immobility to perform own mouth care and pooling of secretions	Pneumonia

▲ This diagnosis was reported to be monitored for or managed frequently (75%–100%).
△ This diagnosis was reported to be monitored for or managed often (50%–74%).
✳ This diagnosis was not included in the validation study.

Nursing Diagnoses

Disuse Syndrome Related to Effects of Immobility on Body Systems

NOC Endurance, Immobility Consequences: Physiological, Immobility Consequences: Psycho-Cognitive, Mobility

Goal

The client will not experience complications of immobility.

Indicators

- Demonstrate intact skin and tissue integrity.
- Demonstrate maximum pulmonary function.
- Demonstrate maximum peripheral blood flow.
- Demonstrate full range of motion.
- Demonstrate adequate bowel, bladder, and renal functions.
- Explain rationale for treatments.

• Make decisions regarding care, when possible.
• Share feelings regarding immobile state.

NIC Activity Therapy, Energy Management, Mutual Goal Settings, Exercise Therapy, Fall Prevention, Pressure Ulcer Prevention, Body Mechanics Promotion, Skin Surveillance, Positioning, Coping Enhancement, Decision-Making Support

Interventions	Rationales
1. Explain the effects of immobility on body systems and the reason for the interventions, as indicated.	1. Understanding may help to elicit cooperation in reducing immobility.
2. Take steps to promote optimal respiratory function. a. Vary bed position, unless contraindicated, to change the horizontal and vertical positions of the thorax gradually. b. Assist with repositioning, turning from side to side every hour, if possible. c. Encourage deep breathing and controlled coughing exercises five times an hour. d. Teach to use a blow bottle or incentive spirometer every hour when awake. (A client with severe neuromuscular impairment may have to be awakened during the night as well.) e. For a child, try using colored water in the blow bottle; also have the client blow up balloons, blow soap bubbles, blow cotton balls with a straw, and other "fun" breathing exercises. f. Auscultate lung fields every 8 hours or less if altered breath sounds occur. g. Encourage small, frequent feedings.	2. Immobility contributes to stasis of secretions and possible pneumonia or atelectasis. These measures help increase lung expansion and the ability to expel secretions (Hickey, 2003).
3. Encourage increased oral fluid intake, as indicated.	3. Optimal hydration liquefies secretions for easier expectoration and prevents stasis of secretions that provide a medium for microorganism growth.
4. Explain the effects of daily activity on elimination. Assist with ambulation when possible.	4. Activity influences bowel elimination by improving muscle tone and stimulating appetite and peristalsis.

5. Promote factors that contribute to optimal elimination.
a. Balanced diet:
  • Review a list of foods high in bulk (e.g., fresh fruits with skins, bran, nuts and seeds, whole-grain breads and cereals, cooked fruits and vegetables, and fruit juices).
  • Discuss dietary preferences.
  • Encourage intake of approximately 800 g of fruits and vegetables (about four pieces of fresh fruit and a large salad) for normal daily bowel movement.
b. Adequate fluid intake:
  • Encourage intake of at least 8–10 glasses (about 2000 mL) daily, unless contraindicated.
  • Discuss fluid preferences.
  • Set up a regular schedule for fluid intake.
c. Regular time for defecation:
  • Identify normal defecation pattern before onset of constipation.
  • Review daily routine.
  • Include time for defecation as part of the regular daily routine.
	5.
	a. A well-balanced diet high in fiber content stimulates peristalsis.
	
	b. Sufficient fluid intake is necessary to maintain bowel patterns and promote proper stool consistency.
	
	c. Taking advantage of circadian rhythms may aid in establishing a regular defecation schedule.

(continued on page 452)

Interventions	Rationales

• Discuss a suitable time based on responsibilities, availability of facilities, etc.
• Suggest that the client attempt defecation about an hour after a meal and remain in the bathroom a suitable length of time.
d. Simulation of the home environment:
   • Have the client use the bathroom instead of a bedpan, if possible; offer a bedpan or a bedside commode if the client cannot use the bathroom.
   • Assist the client into position on the toilet, commode, or bedpan, if necessary.
   • Provide privacy (e.g., close the door, draw curtains around the bed, turn on a television or radio to mask sounds, and make a room deodorizer available).
   • Provide for comfort (e.g., provide reading materials as a diversion) and safety (e.g., make a call bell readily available).
e. Proper positioning:
   • Assist the client to a normal semisquatting position on toilet or commode, if possible.
   • Assist the client onto a bedpan, if necessary, elevating the head of the bed to high Fowler's position or to the elevation permitted.
   • Stress the need to avoid straining during defecation efforts.
	d. Privacy and a sense of normalcy promotes elimination.
	
	e. Proper positioning uses the abdominal muscles and the force of gravity to aid defecation.

6. Institute measures to prevent pressure ulcers. (Refer to the Pressure Ulcers care plan for specific interventions.)	6. The immobile client is at risk for pressure ulcers—localized areas of cellular necrosis that tend to occur when soft tissue is compressed between a bony prominence and a firm surface for a prolonged period. Avoiding prolonged pressure can prevent pressure ulcer formation (Maklebust & Sieggreen, 2001).
7. Promote optimum circulation when the client is sitting. a. Limit sitting time for a client at high risk for ulcer development. b. Instruct client to lift self every 10 minutes using the chair arms, if possible, or assist the client with this maneuver.	7. Capillary flow is increased if pressure is relieved and redistributed. Prolonged compromised capillary flow leads to tissue hypoxia and necrosis (Maklebust & Sieggreen, 2001).
8. With each position change, inspect areas at risk for developing ulcers: a. Ears b. Elbows c. Occiput d. Trochanter e. Heels f. Ischia g. Sacrum h. Scapula i. Scrotum	8. Certain areas over bony prominences are more prone to cellular compression (Maklebust & Sieggreen, 2001).
9. Observe for erythema and blanching, palpate for warmth and tissue sponginess, and massage vulnerable areas lightly with each position change.	9. Erythema and blanching are early signs of tissue hypoxia. Deep massage can injure capillaries, but light massage stimulates local circulation (Maklebust & Sieggreen, 2001).
10. Teach the client to do the following: a. Elevate legs above the level of the heart. (*Note:* This may be contraindicated if severe cardiac or respiratory disease is present.)	10. a,b. Immobility reduces venous return and increases intravascular pressure that contribute to venous stasis and thrombophlebitis (Porth, 2005).

(continued on page 453)

Interventions	Rationales
b. Avoid standing or sitting with legs dependent for long periods. c. Consider using Ace bandages or below-knee elastic stockings. d. Avoid using pillows behind the knees or a gatch on the bed elevated at the knees. e. Avoid leg crossing. f. Change positions, move extremities, or wiggle fingers and toes every hour. g. Avoid garters and tight elastic stockings above the knees. h. Perform leg exercises every hour when advisable.	c. Elastic stockings reduce venous pooling by exerting even pressure over the leg; they increase flow to deeper veins by reducing the caliber of the superficial vein (Porth, 2005). d–g. External venous compression impedes venous flow (Porth, 2005). h. Leg exercises promote the muscle pumping effect on the deep veins (Porth, 2005).
11. Measure the baseline circumference of calves and thighs daily if the client is at risk for deep venous thrombosis (DVT) or if it is suspected.	11. Thrombophlebitis causes edema, which enlarges the legs (Porth, 2005).
12. Institute measures to increase limb mobility. a. Perform range-of-motion (ROM) exercises as frequently as the client's condition warrants. b. Support limbs with pillows to prevent or reduce swelling. c. Encourage the client to perform exercise regimens for specific joints as prescribed by the physician or physical therapist.	12. Joints without range-of-motion exercise develop contractures in 3–7 days, because flexor muscles are stronger than extensor muscles.
13. Take steps to maintain proper body alignment. a. Use a footboard. b. Avoid prolonged periods of sitting or lying in the same position. c. Change position of the shoulder joints every 2–4 h. d. Use a small pillow or no pillow when the client is in the Fowler's position. e. Support the hand and wrist in natural alignment. f. If the client is supine or prone, place a rolled towel or small pillow under the lumbar curvature or under the end of the rib cage. g. Place a trochanter roll or sandbags alongside hips and upper thighs. h. If the client is in the lateral position, place pillow(s) to support the leg from groin to foot and a pillow to flex the shoulder and elbow slightly; if needed, support the lower foot in dorsal flexion with a sandbag. i. Use hand–wrist splints.	13. Prolonged immobility and impaired neurosensory function can cause permanent contractures (Hickey, 2003). a. This measure prevents foot drop. b. This measure prevents hip flexion contractures. c. This measure can help to prevent shoulder contractures. d. This measure prevents flexion contracture of the neck. e. This measure can help to prevent dependent edema and flexion contracture of the wrist. f. This measure prevents flexion or hyperflexion of the lumbar curvature. g. This prevents external rotation of the femurs and hips. h. These measures prevent internal rotation and adduction of the femur and shoulder and prevent foot drop. i. Splints prevent flexion or extension contractures of fingers and abduction of the thumbs.
14. Monitor for and take steps to reduce bone demineralization: a. Monitor for signs and symptoms of hypercalcemia (e.g., elevated serum calcium level, nausea and vomiting, polydipsia, polyuria, lethargy). b. Provide weight-bearing activities whenever possible; use a tilt table if indicated.	14. Lack of motion and weight-bearing results in bone destruction that releases calcium into the bloodstream and results in hypercalcemia (Porth, 2005).
15. Take measures to prevent urinary stasis and calculi formation.	15. Peristaltic contractions of the ureters are insufficient in a reclining position and result in urine stasis in the renal pelvis.

(continued on page 454)

Interventions	Rationales

a. Provide daily intake of fluid of 2000 mL or greater (unless contraindicated).
b. Maintain urine pH below 6.0 (acidic) with acid ash foods (e.g., cereals, meats, poultry, fish, cranberry juice, apple juice).
c. Teach the client to avoid these foods:
  • Milk, milk products, and cheese
  • Bran cereals
  • Cranberries, plums, raspberries, gooseberries, olives
  • Asparagus, rhubarb, spinach, kale, Swiss chard, turnip greens, mustard greens, broccoli, beet greens
  • Legumes, whole grain rice
  • Sardines, shrimp, oysters
  • Chocolate
  • Peanut butter
	a. Stones form more readily in concentrated urine.
	b. These measures reduce the formation of calcium calculi.
	c. These foods are high in calcium and oxalate and can contribute to stone formation.

16. Maintain vigorous hydration, unless contraindicated:
  a. Adult: 2000 mL/day
  b. Adolescent: 3000 to 4000 mL/day
	16. Optimal hydration reduces the blood coagulability, liquefies secretions, inhibits stone formation, and promotes glomerular filtration of body wastes.

Documentation

Flow records
    Exercise
    Turning
    Assessment results (circulatory, respiratory, skin)
Discharge summary record
    Client teaching

Self-Care Deficit (Specify) Related to Immobility

NOC See Bathing/Hygiene, Feeding, Dressing, Toileting, and or Instrumental Self-Care Deficit

Goal

The client will perform self-care activities (specify feeding, toileting, dressing, grooming, or bathing).

Indicators

• Demonstrate use of adaptive devices (specify), if necessary.
• Demonstrate optimal hygiene after care is provided.

NIC See Feeding, Bathing, Dressing, Toileting, and/or Instrumental Self-Care Deficit

Interventions	Rationales

1. Promote the client's maximum involvement in feeding activities.
  a. Ascertain from the client or family members what foods the client likes and dislikes.
  b. Have the client eat all meals in the same setting—pleasant surroundings that are not too distracting.
  c. Provide good oral hygiene before and after meals.
  d. Encourage the client to wear dentures and eyeglasses, as necessary.
	1. Eating has physiologic, psychologic, social, and cultural implications. Providing control over meals promotes overall well-being.

(continued on page 455)

Interventions	Rationales
e. Place the client in the most normal eating position suited to the physical disability (best is sitting in a chair at a table). f. Provide social contact during meals. g. Encourage eating of "finger foods" (e.g., bread, bacon, fruit, and hot dogs) to promote independence. h. To enhance independence, provide necessary adaptive devices (e.g., plate guard to avoid pushing food off plate, suction device under plate or bowl for stabilization, padded handles on utensils for a more secure grip, wrist or hand splints with clamp to hold eating utensils, special drinking cup, and rocker knife for cutting). i. Assist with setup, if needed (e.g., opening containers, napkins, and condiment packages; cutting meat; and buttering bread). j. Arrange food so the client has adequate space for eating.	
2. Promote the client's maximum involvement in bathing activities: a. Bathing time and routine should be consistent to encourage greatest independence. b. Encourage the client to wear prescribed corrective lenses or hearing aid. c. Keep the bathroom temperature warm; ascertain the client's preferred water temperature. d. Provide for privacy during the bathing routine. e. Provide for adaptive equipment, as needed (e.g., bath board for transferring to tub chair or stool, washing mitts with pocket for soap, adapted toothbrushes, shaver holders, and handheld shower spray). f. Place bathing equipment in the location most suitable to the client. g. Keep a call bell within reach if the client is to bathe alone.	2. Inability for self-care produces feelings of dependency and poor self-concept. With increased ability for self-care, self-esteem increases.
3. Promote the client's maximum involvement in toileting activities: a. Observe the client's ability to obtain equipment or to get to the toilet unassisted. b. Provide only the amount of supervision and assistance necessary. c. Provide necessary adaptive devices to enhance independence and safety (e.g., commode chairs, spill-proof urinals, fracture bedpans, raised toilet seats, and support side rails for toilets). d. Avoid use of bedpans and urinals whenever possible; provide a normal atmosphere of elimination in the bathroom; use the same toilet to promote familiarity.	3. These measures can reduce the embarrassment associated with assistance with toileting.
4. Promote or provide assistance with grooming and dressing: a. Deodorant application daily b. Cosmetics of choice c. Hair care (shampoo and styling) d. Facial hair e. Nail and foot care	4. Optimal personal grooming promotes psychological well-being.

Documentation

Progress notes
Involvement in self-care

Powerlessness Related to Feelings of Loss of Control and the Restrictions Placed on Life Style

NOC Depression Self-Control, Health Beliefs, Health Beliefs: Perceived Control, Participation in Health Care Decisions

Goal

The client will verbalize the ability to influence selected situations.

Indicators

- Identify what factors can be controlled.
- Make decisions regarding his or her care.

NIC Mood Management, Teaching: Individual, Decision-Making Support, Self-Responsibility Facilitation, Health System Guidance, Spiritual Support

Interventions	Rationales
1. Encourage the client to share his or her feelings and fears regarding restricted movement.	1. Open dialogue promotes sharing and well-being.
2. Determine the client's usual response to problems.	2. To plan effective care, the nurse must determine whether the client usually seeks to change his or her own behaviors to control problems or expects others or external factors to control problems.
3. Encourage the client to wear desired personal adornments (e.g., baseball cap, colorful socks) and clothes rather than pajamas.	3. Street clothes allow the client to express her or his individuality, which promotes self-esteem and reduces feelings of powerlessness.
4. Plan strategies to reduce the monotony of immobility: a. Vary daily routine, when possible. b. Have the client participate in daily planning, when possible. c. Try to make the routine as normal as possible (e.g., have the client dress in street clothes during the day, if feasible). d. Encourage visitors. e. Alter physical environment when possible (e.g., update bulletin boards, change pictures on the walls, rearrange furniture). f. Maintain a pleasant, cheerful environment. Position the client near a window, if possible. If appropriate, provide a goldfish bowl for visual variety. g. Provide various reading materials (or "books on tape" if impairment hinders reading ability), a television, and radio. h. Discourage excessive television watching. i. Plan some "special" activity daily to give the client something to look forward to each day. j. Consider enlisting a volunteer to read to the client or help with activities, if necessary. k. Encourage the client to devise his or her own strategies to combat boredom.	4. These measures may help to reduce the monotony of immobility and compensate for psychologic effects of immobility (e.g., decreased attention span, decreased motivation).
5. Provide opportunities for the client to make decisions regarding surroundings, activities, routines, and short- and long-term goals, as appropriate.	5. Mobility enables the client to actualize decisions (e.g., when to eat, where to go, what to do). Loss of mobility can affect autonomy and control.
6. Encourage family members to request the client's opinions when making family decisions.	6. The family can provide opportunities for the client to maintain role responsibilities; this can help to minimize feelings of powerlessness.

Documentation

Progress notes
   Interactions
    Response

Sexual Assault

There is an estimate of more than 200,000 cases of sexual assault reported in the United States yearly (Rainn, 2005) and that only 4 in 10 cases are reported. *Rape is a crime using sexual means to humiliate, dominate, and degrade the victim* (Symes, 2000). *Sexual assault is forced and violent oral, vaginal, or anal penetration of a person without his or her consent.* This care plan focuses on nursing for a client who has been sexually assaulted and is hospitalized for injuries.

 Time Frame
Coexisting with (trauma requiring hospitalization)

DIAGNOSTIC CLUSTER*

Collaborative Problems

PC: Sexually Transmitted Infection (STI)
PC: Unwanted Pregnancy
PC: Compartment Syndrome

Nursing Diagnoses

Rape Trauma Syndrome

Collaborative Problems associated with physical injuries sometimes caused by sexual assault include fractures, head injuries, abdominal injuries, and burns. Refer to the collaborative problem index for specific problems.

*This situation was not included in the validation study.

Discharge Criteria

The client will

1. Share feelings.
2. Describe rationales and treatment procedures.
3. Identify what needs to be done now and take steps toward the goals.
4. Relate the intent to seek professional help after discharge.
5. Identify members of support system and use them appropriately.

Collaborative Problems

Potential Complication: Sexually Transmitted Infection
Potential Complication: Unwanted Pregnancy

Nursing Goal

The nurse collaboratively intervenes to prevent (a) STIs and (b) unwanted pregnancy.

Indicators

- Continued negative results on pregnancy test (b)
- Continued negative results on chlamydia test (a)
- Continued negative results on gonorrhea test
- Continued negative results on microscopic examination of vaginal fluids (*Trichomonas vaginalis*)
- Continued negative results on rapid plasma reagin test (RPR)
- Continued negative HIV test

Interventions	Rationales
1. Explain the risks of STIs and pregnancy.	1. Both are possible results of sexual assault.
2. Screen individual cultures (cervical, urethral, rectal, oral) and blood specimens (syphilis, HIV).	2. Selected medications can eliminate pathogens that cause STIs.
3. Provide treatment 1 prophylaxis for: a. Chlamydia: Zithromax 1 g b. Gonorrhea: Rocephin 250 mg IM (with 1% lidocaine as dilutant) c. Trichomonas: Flagyl 2 g in two divided doses over 24 h	3. The U.S. Centers for Disease Control recommends screening of all sexual assault victims (Feldhaus, 2002).
4. Explain risks of HIV transmission and prophylaxis (if within 48 h of assault) (Moe & Grau, 2001). Consult with infectious disease specialist or institution protocol for prophylaxis.	4. The seriousness of HIV infection has prompted HIV postexposure prophylaxis for sexually assaulted persons (Moe & Ledray, 2001; Centers for Disease Control, 2008).
5. Explain side effects of medications, need for adherance, and specific instruction regarding food and other drug interactions.	5. Adherance can be improved with specific teaching.
6. Determine if the client is at risk for pregnancy: a. No contraceptive use b. No surgical sterilization c. History of infertility d. Premenopausal or postmenopausal	6. At-risk clients should be identified (Feldhaus, 2002).
7. Explain how emergency contraceptive pills (ECPs) prevents implantation of fertilized egg.	7. ECP delays ovulation and interferes with tubal transport of egg or sperm (Arcangelo & Peterson, 2005).
8. If desired, and within 72 h of assault, provide ECP medication. Explain when to take the second dose.	8. ECP can cause nausea and vomiting from high estrogen content.
9. Provide antiemetic medication, if needed.	

◣ Related Physician-Prescribed Interventions

Medications (refer to collaborative problems for specific medications). STD prophylaxis, ECP, HIV prophylaxis, antiemetics, analgesics, sedatives

Laboratory Studies. Vaginal, urine, urethra, rectal cultures; HIV testing; RPR test; serum/urine drug screens

Diagnostic Studies. Microscopic examination of vaginal fluid smear (wet mount)

Documentation

Progress notes
    Present emotional status
    Interventions
    Responses in nursing interventions, police and counselor interviews, examination for evidence
    Subjective, objective, and general reactions
    Availability of significant others for support
    Medications given and collection of specimens

Nursing Diagnoses

Rape Trauma Syndrome

NOC   Abuse Protection, Abuse Recovery Status, Coping

Goals

Refer to discharge criteria.

Interventions	Rationales

1. Provide interventions to decrease anxiety.
  a. Limit people to whom the client–victim must describe assault.
  b. Do not leave client alone.
  c. Maintain a nonjudgmental attitude.
  d. Show concern for the client.
  e. Ensure confidentiality.
  f. Encourage talking.
  g. Allow the client self-blame.
  h. Encourage problem-solving.
  i. Enlist support system.
  j. Create a plan to increase sense of safety.
	1.
	  a. Repeatedly relating the incident increases shame and anxiety.
	  b. Isolation can increase anxiety.
	  c. This will lessen shame.
	  d. Empathy will validate worth.
	  e. This will encourage sharing.
	  f. This helps the client to sort his or her feelings.
	  g. This validates the client's humanity.
	  h. It increases the client's sense of control.
	  i. Support system provides some stability and safety.
	  j. This will reduce fear and anxiety.

2. Assess for psychologic responses:
  a. Subjective:
    • Phobias, nightmares, and flashbacks
    • Disbelief
    • Denial and emotional shock
    • Anger, fear, and anxiety
    • Depression and guilt
    • Expressions of numbness, shame, and self-blame
    • Suicidal ideation
    • With older adults, fear of losing independence
    • Concerns about going mad, losing control, and having intrusive thoughts
    • Difficulty with decision-making
  b. Objective:
    • Crying
    • Silence, calm, composed
    • Trembling hands
    • Excessive bathing (seen particularly with child or adolescent)
    • Avoiding interaction with others (staff and family)
    • Wearing excessive clothing (two or three pairs of pants or panties)
    • Pacing and excessive talking
    • Mood swings and inappropriate laughing
    • Self-abusive behaviors (head banging or scratching)
    • Increased startle response
	2. Careful recording of psychologic responses assists in recording progress in therapy, planning treatment, or identifying those at greatest risk. Behavior can differ from individual to individual. Feelings can be fast and furious or slow, trance-like, mixed, or clear.
	    Victims may experience a wide range of feelings; either expressed or controlled. Previous coping skills often dissipate.

(continued on page 460)

Interventions	Rationales
3. Assist the client to identify major concerns (psychologic, medical, and legal) and his or her perception of needed help.	3. Sexual assault is always associated with coercion and threatened or actual violence. It is by this means the assailant takes control from the victim. Involving the victim in decision-making begins reestablishing a sense of control (Smith-DiJulio, 2001).
4. Whenever possible, provide crisis counseling within one hour of rape trauma event: a. Ask permission to contact the rape crisis counselor. b. Be flexible and individualize approach according to the client's needs.	4. Victim empowerment is the primary antidote to the trauma of sexual assault (Smith-DiJulio, 2001).
5. Promote a trusting relationship by providing emotional support with unconditional positive regard and acceptance: a. Stay with the client during acute stage, or arrange for other support. b. Brief the client on police and hospital procedures during acute stage. c. Assist during medical examination and explain all procedures in advance. d. Help the client to meet personal needs (bathing after examination and after evidence has been acquired). e. Listen attentively to the client's requests. f. Maintain unhurried attitude toward the client and her or his family. g. Avoid rescue feelings toward the client. h. Maintain nonjudgmental attitude. i. Support the client's beliefs and value system; avoid labeling. j. Reassure the client that the symptoms are normal responses that will lessen and improve with time.	5. Providing immediate and ongoing empathy and support prepares victims for referral to more in-depth psychologic counseling. Main issues in the acute stage are being in control, fearing being left alone, and having someone to listen (Smith-DiJulio, 2001). a–i. Helping and other deep interpersonal transactions demand a certain intensity of presence. Being with a client is attending in its deepest sense. Victims are vulnerable to any statement that can be construed as blaming. Their normal defenses are weakened. When asked too many questions, clients can feel "grilled." This interferes with the rapport between helper and client. Statements are gentler forms of probes than questions (e.g., "I can see fear in your eyes; tell me about it" versus "Are you afraid?"). j. The victim needs to understand that a wide range of behavior and emotional responses is normal.
6. Explain the care and examination she or he will experience: a. Maintaining eye contact, conduct the examinations in an unhurried manner. b. Explain every detail before action. c. During pelvic examination, explain the position and the instruments.	6. Because the victim's right to deny or consent has been violently violated, it is important to seek permission for subsequent care (Heinrich, 1987). It is important to tell the client as much as is practical or possible about what is happening and why. Even in life-threatening situations, any sense of control given to the victim is helpful. a. Unhurried and confident actions, eye contact, and affirming the victim is safe help to calm and assure that he or she is alive and worthy. b. Cognitive dysfunction impairs short-term memory (see Anxiety). c. The victim of rape needs to understand the common reactions to this experience. The evidentiary examination is especially distressing, because it can be reminiscent of the assault (Ledray, 2001).
7. Explain the legal issues and police investigation (Heinrich, 1987): a. Explain the need to collect specimens for future possible court use. b. Explain that the choice to report the rape is the victim's.	7. According to Backman (1990), reporting the crime to authorities is clearly associated with improved emotional outcomes for victims. This is an important step in helping the victim recognize the reality of the crime.

(continued on page 461)

Interventions	Rationales

c. If police interview is permitted:
- Negotiate with the victim and police for an advantageous time.
- Explain to the victim what kind of questions will be asked.
- Remain with the victim during the interview; do not ask questions or offer answers.
- If the officer is insensitive, intimidating, offensive in manner, or asks improper questions, discuss this with the officer in private. If the behavior continues, use proper channels and make a complaint.

---

8. Fulfill medical and legal responsibilities by documentation ([AALNC], 2001; Heinrich, 1987):
   a. History of rape (date, time, and place)
   b. Nature of injuries, use of force, weapons used, threats of violence or retribution, and restraints used
   c. Nature of assault (fondling, oral, anal, vaginal penetration, ejaculation, use of condom)
   d. Postassault activities (douching, bathing, showering, gargling, urinating, defecating, changing clothes, eating or drinking)
   e. Present state (use of drugs or alcohol)
   f. Medical history, tetanus immunization status, gynecologic history (last menstrual period), and last voluntary intercourse
   g. Emotional state and mental status
   h. Examination findings, smears/cultures taken, blood tests, evidence collected, and photographs (if appropriate)
   i. Document to whom, when, and what evidence is delivered
   j. Label all evidence with name, identification number, date, time collected, collector's name, and source

8. Strict adherence to procedures and policies can enhance the future legal case. When possible, a sexual assault nurse examiner (SANE) should manage the victim's care.

---

9. If the attack was a drug-facilitated sexual assault (DFSA):
   a. Assess for possible involuntary drug ingestion:
   - Reports exist that a victim appeared intoxicated within 15 minutes after drinking a beverage.
   - Victim remembers very little after drinking the beverage.
   - Victim awakens hours later undressed or partially dressed, or with vaginal or rectal soreness.
   - Victim reports nausea and vomiting upon awakening.
   b. If suspicious of DFSA (and within 72 h of ingestion), collect blood and urine specimens while maintaining proper chain of custody.
   c. Document if the victim has taken or used drugs recreationally or by prescription.

9.
   a. These signs and symptoms increase the probability of DFSA (Ledray, 2001).

   b. If the samples are to be used as evidence, proper handling must be strictly followed (Ledray, 2001).

   c. If this is not known ahead of time, the victim's credibility can be questioned (Ledray, 2001).

---

10. Provide interventions to assist with regaining control (Smith-DiJulio, 2001):
    a. Listen, listen, listen.

    b. How can I help you?

    c. Encourage verbalizing thoughts and feelings.

    d. Empower survivors by involving them in decision-making and in their treatment plan. Explore their identified needs.

10.
   a. Probably the best response is simply for the nurse to listen without judgment and ask more than once what to do to support the client's recovery (Carosella, 1995).
   b. Many traumatized people repeat their stories over and over. This is part of the healing and diminishes with time.
   c. Victims should not be forced to talk until they are ready. Having the name and number of a person to call helps when the client is ready.

(continued on page 462)

Interventions	Rationales
11. Reassure that feelings and reactions are normal responses and accept where the client is in the recovery process:	11. Expert nursing care can minimize a victims' emotional trauma, prevent further victimization, and promote recovery. Whatever help the nurse offers, honest empathy and non-judgmental listening are crucial.

a. Crying or silence
  • Sit quietly with the client.
  • Offer to listen when she or he is ready to talk.
  • Affirm and validate his or her feelings.
  • Reassure of normalcy:
   "You have a lot to be sad about."
   "I am here for you when you're ready to talk."
	a. Emotional care must aim to convey respect and understanding; communicate empathy, reassurance, and support; encourage ventilation of feelings; preserve dignity; empower the victim; provide anticipatory guidance; and ensure adequate follow-up.

b. Anger
  • Understand that anger can be displaced onto care-givers or significant others.
  • Redirect and acknowledge its validity:
   "You're very angry." "You have every right to be."
   "You were assaulted." "Who wouldn't be angry?"
  • Allow the anger.
  • Try not to personalize or be offended. It's not you the client is angry with.
  • Later, when the client is calmer, help to restore his or her dignity by calmly exploring the basis for his or her feelings.
	b. Intense anger may cause feelings of being out of control or out of touch.

c. Self-blame, self-abuse, feeling repulsive
  • Avoid using "should," "ought to," "must," "never." These words can be interpreted as blaming.
  • Assure the victim that "rape exists because there are rapists, not because there are victims" (Carosella, 1995).
  • Reassure: "You made the right decisions. You survived."
  • Provide comfort measures.
  • Provide scented soaps, bubble bath, etc.
	c.
	  • Victims of rape feel vulnerable and repulsive to others. Feeling comfortable can increase the client's sense of security.
	  • Comfort creates a sense of healing and eases feelings of dirtiness.

d. Flashbacks, dreams, night terrors.
  • Don't leave the client alone.
  • Reassure the client that he or she is safe.
  • If possible do not leave the client alone; phone support people.
  • Identify if there were triggers prompting the reaction.
  • Encourage rest and avoiding stress.
  • Problem-solve ways to feel safer. Determine where the client will be discharged to.
	d. Dreams are an attempt to make sense of what happened. The most positive way to view dreams is as an attempt to reclaim power. Identifying triggers helps to link them to a past experience, rather than only the present. This differentiation begins to make the present feel safe.
	  • Incidence of flashbacks increases with fatigue or stress.
	  • Feeling empowered means you can do something to avert or minimize future trauma.
	  • We need order to feel safe: "Everyone said what helped most was routine, routine, routine."

12. Explore available support systems. Involve significant others. a. Share with family and friends the victim's immediate needs for love and support. b. Encourage the family to express feelings and to ask questions. c. Reassure the victim that his or her reactions are normal. d. Refer to counseling services. e. Respect the victim's right to restrict unwanted visitors. f. Discuss fears of rejection. g. Explore sexual, intimate concerns. h. Encourage the survivor to recognize positive responses or support from others. i. Expect many of the same reactions as the victim/survivor.	12. a. Isolation can lead to withdrawal. d. Postponing professional help lengthens the time reactions persist and lengthens recovery.
13. Participate in community activities to raise awareness of relationship of alcohol use and sexual assault.	13. Alcohol reduces inhibitions, affects judgment, and limits one's ability to make decisions (French, Beynon, & Delaforce, 2007).

Surgical Procedures

Generic Care Plan for the Surgical Client

This care plan (Level I) presents nursing diagnoses and collaborative problems that commonly apply to clients (and their significant others) experiencing all types of surgery. Nursing diagnoses and collaborative problems specific to a surgical procedure are presented in the care plan (Level II) for that procedure.

 Time Frame
Preoperative and postoperative periods

■■■■■■ DIAGNOSTIC CLUSTER

Preoperative

Nursing Diagnosis

Anxiety/Fear related to surgical experience, loss of control, unpredictable outcome, and insufficient knowledge of preoperative routines, postoperative exercises and activities, and postoperative changes and sensations

Postoperative

Collaborative Problems

PC: Hemorrhage
PC: Hypovolemia/Shock
PC: Evisceration/Dehiscence
PC: Paralytic Ileus
PC: Infection (Peritonitis, Incision)
PC: Urinary Retention
PC: Thrombophlebitis

Nursing Diagnoses

Risk for Ineffective Respiratory Function related to immobility secondary to postanesthesia state and pain

Risk for Infection related to a site for organism invasion secondary to surgery

Acute Pain related to surgical interruption of body structures, flatus, and immobility

Risk for Imbalanced Nutrition: Less Than Body Requirements related to increased protein and vitamin requirements for wound healing and decreased intake secondary to pain, nausea, vomiting, and diet restrictions

Risk for Constipation related to decreased peristalsis secondary to immobility and the effects of anesthesia and narcotics

Activity Intolerance related to pain and weakness secondary to anesthesia, tissue hypoxia, and insufficient fluid and nutrient intake

Risk for Ineffective Therapeutic Regimen Management related to insufficient knowledge of care of operative site, restrictions (diet, activity), medications, signs and symptoms of complications, and follow-up care

Discharge Criteria

Before discharge, the client and/or family will

1. Describe any at-home activity restrictions.
2. Describe at-home wound and pain management.
3. Discuss fluid and nutritional requirements for proper wound healing.
4. List the signs and symptoms that must be reported to a health care professional.
5. Describe necessary follow-up care.

Preoperative: Nursing Diagnosis

Anxiety/Fear Related to Surgical Experience, Loss of Control, Unpredictable Outcome, and Insufficient Knowledge of Preoperative Routines, Postoperative Exercises and Activities, and Postoperative Changes and Sensations

NOC Anxiety Reduction, Coping, Impulse Control

Goal

The client will communicate feelings regarding the surgical experience, including the limitations and restrictions, and discuss any therapeutic medical devices (e.g., braces, crutches, plasters, etc), that will apply postoperatively.

Indicators

- Verbalize, if asked, what to expect regarding routines, environment, and sensations.
- Demonstrate postoperative exercises, splinting, and respiratory regimen.

NIC Anxiety Reduction, Impulse Control Training, Anticipatory Guidance

Interventions	Rationales
1. Provide reassurance and comfort: stay with the client, encourage her or him to share her or his feelings and concerns, listen attentively, and convey a sense of empathy and understanding.	1. Providing emotional support and encouraging the client to share her or his feelings allows her or him to clarify fears, and allows the nurse to give realistic feedback and reassurance.
2. Correct any misconceptions and inaccurate information that the client has about the procedure. Supply written literature, where possible, that the client and family can read for future reference and at their own leisure (Black, J., 2005).	2. Modifiable contributing factors to anxiety include incomplete and inaccurate information. Providing accurate information and correcting misconceptions may help to eliminate fears and reduce anxiety.
3. Determine if the client desires spiritual support (e.g., visit from clergy or other spiritual leader, religious article, or ritual). Arrange for this support, if necessary.	3. Many clients need spiritual support to cope with their fears and anxieties.
4. Allow and encourage family members and significant others to share their fears and concerns. Enlist their support for the client, but only if it is meaningful and productive.	4. Effective support from family members, other relatives, and friends can help the client to cope with surgery and recovery.
5. Notify the physician if the client exhibits severe or panic anxiety.	5. Immediate notification enables prompt assessment and possible pharmacologic intervention.
6. Notify the physician if the client needs any further explanations about the procedure; beforehand, the physician should explain the following: a. Nature of the surgery b. Reason for and expected outcome of the procedure c. Any risks involved d. Type of anesthetic to be used e. Expected length of recovery and any postoperative restrictions and instructions	6. The physician is responsible for explaining the surgery to the client and family; the nurse, for determining their level of understanding and then notifying the physician of the need to provide more information, if necessary.
7. Involve family members or significant others in client teaching, whenever possible.	7. Knowledgeable family members or significant others can serve as "coaches" to remind the client of postoperative instructions and restrictions.

(continued on page 466)

Interventions	Rationales
8. Provide instruction (bedside or group) on general information pertaining to the need for active participation, preoperative routines, environment, personnel, and postoperative exercises.	8. Preoperative teaching provides the client with information; this can help to reduce anxiety and fear associated with the unknown, and to enhance the client's sense of control over the situation.
9. Present information or reinforce learning using written materials (e.g., books, pamphlets, instruction sheets) or audiovisual aids (e.g., videotapes, slides, posters).	9. Simultaneous stimulation of multiple senses augments the learning process. Written materials can be retained and used as a reference after discharge. These materials may be especially useful for care-givers who did not participate in client teaching sessions.
10. Explain the importance and purpose of all preoperative procedures: a. Bowel prep b. Nothing-by-mouth (NPO) status c. Preoperative sedatives d. Laboratory studies	10. This information can help to relieve anxiety and fear associated with lack of knowledge of necessary preoperative activities and routines. a. Enemas and/or laxatives are sometimes given to empty the bowel of fecal material; this can help to reduce risk of postoperative bowel obstruction as peristalsis resumes. b. Eliminating oral fluids preoperatively reduces the risk of aspiration postoperatively. c. Preoperative sedatives reduce anxiety and promote relaxation, increasing the effectiveness of anesthesia and decreasing secretions in response to intubation. d. Tests and studies establish baseline values and help to detect any abnormalities before surgery.
11. Discuss expected intraoperative procedures and sensations: a. Appearance of operating room and equipment b. Presence of surgical staff c. Administration of anesthesia d. Appearance of postanesthesia recovery room e. Recovery from anesthesia	11. The client's understanding of expected procedures and sensations can help to ameliorate fears.
12. Explain all expected postoperative routines and sensations: a. Parenteral fluid administration b. Vital sign monitoring c. Dressing checks and changes d. Nasogastric (NG) tube insertion and care e. Indwelling (Foley) catheter insertion and care f. Other devices, such as intravenous (IV) lines, pumps, and drains g. Symptoms including nausea, vomiting, and pain h. The availability of analgesics and antiemetics, if needed	12. Explaining what the client can expect, why the procedures are done, and why certain sensations may occur, can help to reduce fears associated with the unknown and unexpected. a. Parenteral fluids replace fluids lost from NPO state and blood loss. b. Careful monitoring is needed to determine the client's status and track any changes. c. Until the wound edges heal, wound must be protected from contaminants. d. An NG tube promotes drainage, reduces abdominal distention, and prevents tension on the suture line. e. A Foley catheter drains the bladder until muscle tone returns as anesthesia is excreted. g. Nausea and vomiting are common side effects of preoperative medications and anesthesia; other contributing factors include certain types of surgery, obesity, electrolyte imbalance, rapid position changes, and psychological and environmental factors. h. Pain commonly occurs as medications lose their effectiveness.

(continued on page 467)

Interventions	Rationales
13. As applicable, teach the client (using return demonstration to ensure understanding and ability) how to do the following: a. Turn, cough, and deep-breathe. b. Support the incision site while coughing, split incision with pillow (Wagner, Johnson, & Kidd, 2006). c. Change position in bed every 1–2 hours. d. Sit up, get out of bed, and ambulate as soon as possible after surgery (prolonged sitting should be avoided).	13. The client's understanding of postoperative care measures can help to reduce anxiety associated with the unknown and promote compliance. Teaching the client about postoperative routines before surgery ensures that his or her understanding is not impaired postoperatively by the continuing effects of sedation.
14. Explain the importance of progressive activities postoperatively, including early ambulation and self-care as soon as the client is able.	14. Activity improves circulation and helps to prevent pooling of respiratory secretions. Self-care promotes self-esteem and can help to enhance recovery.
15. Explain important hospital policies to family members or significant others (e.g., visiting hours, number of visitors allowed at one time, location of waiting rooms, and how the physician will contact them after surgery).	15. Providing family members and significant others with this information can help to reduce their anxiety and allow them to better support the client.
16. Evaluate the client's and family's or significant others' abilities to achieve preset, mutually planned learning goals.	16. This assessment identifies the need for any additional teaching and support.

Documentation

Flow records
    Progress notes
    Unusual interactions
Multidisciplinary client education record
    Preoperative, postoperative, and general treatment regime teaching care plan/critical pathway

Postoperative: Collaborative Problems

Potential Complication: Hemorrhage
Potential Complication: Hypovolemia/Shock
Potential Complication: Evisceration/Dehiscence
Potential Complication: Paralytic Ileus
Potential Complication: Infection (Peritonitis, Incision)
Potential Complication: Urinary Retention
Potential Complication: Thrombophlebitis

Nursing Goal

The nurse will monitor for early signs and symptoms of (a) hemorrhage, (b) hypovolemia/shock, (c) evisceration/dehiscence, (d) paralytic ileus, (e) infection, (f) urinary retention, and (g) thrombophlebitis, and will intervene collaboratively to stabilize the client.

Indicators

• Calm, alert, oriented (a, b)
• Respirations 16–20 breaths/min (a, b)
• Respirations relaxed and rhythmic (a, b)
• Breath sound present all lobes (a, b)
• No rales or wheezing (a, b)

- Pulse 60–100 beats/min (a, b)
- BP > 90/60, <140/90 mmHg (a, b)
- Capillary refill <3 sec (a, b)
- Peripheral pulses full, equal (a, b)
- Skin warm and dry (a, b)
- Temperature 98.5–99°F (a, b, e)
- Urine output >5 mL/kg/h (a, b)
- Usual skin color (a, b)
- Surgical wound intact (c, e)
- Minimal serosanguineous drainage (e)
- Bowel sounds present (b, d)
- No nausea and vomiting (b, d)
- No abdominal distention (b, d)
- Decreasing abdominal tenderness (c, e)
- Decreasing wound tenderness (c, e)
- No bladder distension (f)
- No difficulty voiding (f)
- Negative Homans sign (no pain with dorsiflexion of foot) (g)
- No calf tenderness, warmth, or edema (g)
- White blood cells 4000–10,000/mm³ (e)
- Hemoglobin (a)
  - Male 14–18 g/dL
  - Female 12–16 g/dL
- Hematocrit (a)
  - Male 42%–52%
  - Female 37%–47%
- Oxygen saturation (SaO$_2$) >94% (a, b)

Interventions	Rationales
1. Monitor for signs and symptoms of hemorrhage/shock and promptly report changes to the surgeon: a. Increased pulse rate with normal or slightly decreased blood pressure b. Urine output <5 mL/kg/h c. Restlessness, agitation, decreased mentation d. Increased capillary refill >3 seconds e. Decreased oxygen saturation <94% (pulse oximetry) f. Increased respiratory rate g. Diminished peripheral pulses h. Cool, pale, or cyanotic skin i. Thirst	1. The compensatory response to decreased circulatory volume aims to increase blood oxygen through increased heart and respiratory rates and decreased peripheral circulation (manifested by diminished peripheral pulses and cool skin). Decreased oxygen to the brain results in altered mentation.
2. Monitor fluid status; evaluate the following: a. Intake (parenteral and oral) b. Output and other losses (urine, drainage, and vomiting)	2. Fluid loss during surgery and as a result of NPO status can disrupt fluid balance in a high-risk client. Stress can cause sodium and water retention.
3. Teach the client to splint the surgical wound with a pillow when coughing, sneezing, or vomiting.	3. Splinting reduces stress on the suture line by equalizing pressure across the wound.
4. Monitor the surgical site for bleeding, dehiscence, and evisceration.	4. Careful monitoring enables early detection of complications.
5. If dehiscence or evisceration occurs, contact the surgeon immediately and do the following: a. Place the client in low Fowler's position.	5. Rapid interventions can reduce severity of complications. a. Low Fowler's position uses gravity to minimize further tissue protrusion.

(continued on page 469)

Interventions	Rationales
b. Instruct the client to lie still and quiet. c. Cover any protruding viscera with a wet sterile dressing.	b. Lying still and quiet also minimizes tissue protrusion. c. A wet sterile dressing helps to maintain tissue viability.
6. Do not initiate fluids until bowel sounds are present; then, begin with small amounts. Monitor the client's response to resumption of fluids and foods and note the nature and amount of any emesis. 7. Monitor for signs of paralytic ileus: a. Absent bowel sounds b. Nausea, vomiting c. Abdominal distention	6,7. Intraoperative manipulation of abdominal organs and the depressive effects of narcotics and anesthetics on peristalsis can cause paralytic ileus, usually between the third and fifth postoperative day. Pain typically is localized, sharp, and intermittent.
8. Monitor for signs and symptoms of infection/sepsis (refer also to the nursing diagnosis High Risk for Infection): a. Increased temperature b. Chills c. Malaise d. Elevated white blood cell (WBC) count e. Increasing abdominal tenderness f. Wound tenderness, redness, or edema g. Hypotension h. Tachycardia i. Decreased level of consciousness (dependent on client age and severity of sepsis)	8. Microorganisms can be introduced into the body during surgery or through the incision. Circulating pathogens trigger the body's defense mechanisms: WBCs are released to destroy some pathogens, and the hypothalamus raises the body temperature to kill others. Wound redness, tenderness, and edema result from lymphocyte migration to the area.
9. Monitor for signs of urinary retention: a. Bladder distention and unrelieved associated pain (Wagner, Johnson, & Kidd, 2006) b. Urine overflows (30–60 mL, or urine every 15–30 minutes)	9. Anesthesia relaxes the muscles, affecting the bladder. As muscle tone returns, spasms of the bladder sphincter prevent urine outflow, causing bladder distention. When urine retention increases the intravesical pressure, the sphincter releases urine and control of flow is regained.
10. Instruct the client to report bladder discomfort or inability to void.	10. Bladder discomfort and failure to void may be early signs of urinary retention.
11. If the client does not void within 8–10 hours after surgery or complains of bladder discomfort, do the following: a. Warm the bedpan. b. Encourage the client to get out of bed to use the bathroom, if possible. c. Instruct a male client to stand when urinating, if possible. d. Run water in the sink as the client attempts to void. e. Pour warm water over the client's perineum.	11. These measures may help to promote relaxation of the urinary sphincter and facilitate voiding.
12. If the client still cannot void, follow the protocols for straight catheterization, as ordered.	12. Straight catheterization is preferable to indwelling catheterization, because it carries less risk of urinary tract infection from ascending pathogens.
13. Monitor for signs and symptoms of thrombophlebitis: a. Positive Homans sign (pain on dorsiflexion of the foot, due to insufficient circulation) b. Calf tenderness, unusual warmth, or redness c. Lowenberg sign (calf pain in response to lower pressure than expected upon inflation of a compressive device) (Begelman, 2002)	13. Vasoconstriction due to hypothermia decreases peripheral circulation. Anesthesia and immobility reduce vasomotor tone, resulting in decreased venous return with peripheral blood pooling. In combination, these factors increase the risk of venous thromboembolism (VTE) (Ahonen, 2007). Laparoscopic surgery leads to pneumoperitoneum, and reverse Trendelenburg position causes venous pooling in the legs. The resulting venous distention can cause endothelial damage, also promoting VTE (Ahonen, 2007).

(continued on page 470)

Interventions	Rationales
14. Apply antiembolic hose, as ordered.	14. An antiembolic hose applies even compression, enhances venous return, and reduces venous pooling.
15. Remind the client to move and flex legs every hour.	15. This increases circulation.
16. Encourage the client to perform leg exercises. Discourage placing pillows under the knees, using a knee gatch, crossing the legs, and prolonged sitting. Use elastic compression hose/compression boots, as appropriate.	16. These measures help to increase venous return and prevent venous stasis.

 Related Physician-Prescribed Interventions

Medications.
Preoperative: Sedatives, narcotic analgesics, anticholinergics
Postoperative: Narcotic analgesics, antiemetics
Intravenous Therapy. Fluid and electrolyte replacement
Laboratory Studies. Complete blood count, urinalysis, chemistry profile (especially magnesium, potassium, and calcium)
Diagnostic Studies. Chest x-ray film, electrocardiography, computed tomography, ultrasound
Therapies. Indwelling catheterization, incentive spirometry, wound care, liquid diet (progressed to full diet) as tolerated, preoperative NPO status, antiembolic hose, and pulse oximetry

Documentation

Flow records
    Vital signs (pulses, respirations, blood pressure, and temperature)
    Circulation (color, peripheral pulses)
    Intake (oral, parenteral)
    Output (urinary, tubes, specific gravity)
    Bowel function (bowel sounds, defecation, distention)
    Wound (color, drainage)
Progress notes
    Unusual complaints or assessment findings
    Interventions
Multidisciplinary client education record
    Postoperative teaching

Postoperative: Nursing Diagnoses

Risk for Ineffective Respiratory Function Related to Immobility Secondary to Postanesthesia State and Pain

 Aspiration Control, Respiratory Status

Goal

The client will exhibit clear lung fields.

Indicators

• Breath sounds present in all lobes
• Clear breath sounds in all lobes (no wheezes or congestion)
• Relaxed rhythmic respirations

NIC Airway Management, Cough Enhancement, Respiratory Monitoring, Positioning

Interventions	Rationales
1. Auscultate lung fields for diminished and abnormal breath sounds.	1. Presence of rales indicates retained secretions. Diminished breath sounds may indicate atelectasis.
2. Take measures to prevent aspiration. Position the client on his or her side, with pillows supporting the back and knees slightly flexed.	2. In the postoperative period, decreased sensorium and hypoventilation contribute to increased risk of aspiration.
3. Reinforce preoperative client teaching about the importance of turning, coughing, deep breathing, and of leg exercises every 1–2 hours.	3. Postoperative pain may discourage compliance; reinforcing the importance of these measures may improve compliance.
4. Promote the following as soon as the client returns to the unit: a. Deep breaths b. Coughing (except if contraindicated) c. Frequent turning d. Early ambulation e. Incentive spirometry every hour (10 breaths each time, or as ordered) (Wagner, Johnson, & Kidd, 2006).	4. Exercises and movement promote lung expansion and mobilization of secretions. Incentive spirometry promotes deep breathing by providing a visual indicator of the effectiveness of the breathing effort. Coughing assists in dislodging mucus plugs. Coughing is contraindicated in clients who have had a head injury, intracranial surgery, eye surgery, or plastic surgery, because it increases intracranial and intraocular pressure and tension on delicate tissues (plastic surgery).
5. Encourage adequate oral fluid intake, as indicated.	5. Adequate hydration liquefies secretions, which enables easier expectoration and prevents stasis of secretions that provide a medium for microorganism growth. It also helps to decrease blood viscosity, which lowers the risk of clot formation.

Documentation

Flow record
  Temperature
  Respiratory rate and rhythm
  Breath sounds
  Respiratory treatments and client responses
Progress notes
  Unsatisfactory response to respiratory treatments
Multidisciplinary client education record

Risk for Infection Related to a Site for Organism Invasion Secondary to Surgery

NOC Infection Status, Wound Healing: Primary Infection, Immune Status

Goal

The client will demonstrate healing of wound.

Indicators

• No abnormal drainage
• Intact, approximated wound edges

NIC Infection Control, Wound Care, Incision Site Care, Health Education

Interventions	Rationales

1. Monitor for signs and symptoms of wound infection:
   a. Increased swelling and redness
   b. Wound separation
   c. Increased or purulent drainage
   d. Prolonged subnormal temperature or significantly elevated temperature
	1. Tissue responds to pathogen infiltration with increased blood and lymph flow (manifested by edema, redness, and increased drainage) and reduced epithelialization (marked by wound separation). Circulating pathogens trigger the hypothalamus to elevate the body temperature; certain pathogens cannot survive at higher temperatures.

2. Monitor wound healing by noting the following:
   a. Evidence of intact, approximated wound edges (primary intention)
   b. Evidence of granulation tissue (secondary and tertiary intention)
	2. A surgical wound with edges approximated by sutures usually heals by primary intention. Granulation tissue is not visible and scar formation is minimal. In contrast, a surgical wound with a drain or an abscess heals by secondary intention or granulation and has more distinct scar formation. A restructured wound heals by third intention and results in a wider and deeper scar.

3. Teach the client about factors that can delay wound healing:
   a. Dehydrated wound tissue
 	
   b. Wound infection
 	
   c. Inadequate nutrition and hydration
 	
   d. Compromised blood supply
 	
   e. Increased stress or excessive activity
	3.
	   a. Studies report that epithelial migration is impeded under dry crust; movement is three times faster over moist tissue.
	   b. The exudate in infected wounds impairs epithelialization and wound closure.
	   c. To repair tissue, the body needs increased protein and carbohydrate intake and adequate hydration for vascular transport of oxygen and wastes.
	   d. Blood supply to injured tissue must be adequate to transport leukocytes and remove wastes.
	   e. Increased stress and activity result in higher levels of chalone, a mitotic inhibitor that depresses epidermal regeneration.

4. Take steps to prevent infection:
   a. Wash hands before and after dressing changes.
   b. Wear gloves until the wound is sealed.
   c. Thoroughly clean the area around drainage tubes.
   d. Keep tubing away from incision.
   e. Discard unused irrigation solutions after 24 hours.
   f. If drains are in place, ensure their patency and that they are secured properly, to prevent them from pulling against the incision (Baird, Keen, & Swearingen, 2005).
	4. These measures help to prevent the introduction of microorganisms into the wound; they also reduce the risk of transmitting infection to others.

5. Explain when a dressing is indicated for a wound healing by primary intention, and for one healing by secondary intention.	5. A wound healing by primary intention requires a dressing to protect it from contamination until the edges seal (usually by 24 hours). A wound healing by secondary intention requires a dressing to maintain adequate hydration; the dressing is not needed after wound edges seal.

6. Minimize skin irritation by the following means:
   a. Using a collection pouch, if indicated
   b. Changing saturated dressings often
	6. Preventing skin irritation eliminates a potential source of microorganism entry.

7. Protect wound and surrounding skin from drainage by these methods:
   a. Using a collection pouch if indicated
   b. Applying a skin barrier
	7. Protecting skin can help to minimize excoriation by acid drainage. A semipermeable skin barrier provides a moist environment for healing and prevents bacteria entry.

8. Teach and assist the client in the following:
   a. Supporting the surgical site when moving
   b. Splinting the area when coughing, sneezing, or vomiting
   c. Reducing flatus accumulation
	8. A wound typically requires 3 weeks for strong scar formation. Stress on the suture line before this occurs can cause disruption.

9. Consult with an enterostomal or clinical nurse specialist for specific skin care measures.	9. Management of a complex wound or impaired healing requires expert nursing consultation.

Documentation

Progress notes
    Signs and symptoms of infection
Flow records
    Temperature
    Status of wound and wound management plan (Black, 2005)

Acute Pain Related to Surgical Interruption of Body Structures, Flatus, and Immobility

NOC Comfort Level, Pain Control

Goal

A client will report progressive reduction of pain and an increase in activity.

Indicators

- Relate factors that increase pain.
- Report effective interventions.

NIC Pain Management, Medication Management, Emotional Support, Teaching: Individual, Hot/Cold Application, Simple Massage

Interventions	Rationales
1. Collaborate with the client to determine effective pain relief interventions.	1. A client experiencing pain may feel a loss of control over his body and his or her life. Collaboration can help minimize this feeling.
2. Express your acceptance of the client's pain. Acknowledge the pain's presence, listen attentively to the client's complaints, and convey that you are assessing the pain because you want to understand it better, not because you are trying to determine if it really exists.	2. A client who feels the need to convince health care providers that she or he actually is experiencing pain is likely to have increased anxiety that can lead to greater pain.
3. Reduce the client's fear and clear up any misinformation by doing the following: a. Teaching what to expect; describing the sensation as precisely as possible, including how long it should last b. Explaining pain relief methods such as distraction, heat application, and progressive relaxation	3. A client who is prepared for a painful procedure with a detailed explanation of the sensations that he or she will feel, usually experiences less stress and pain than a client who receives vague or no explanations.
4. Explain the differences between involuntary physiologic responses and voluntary behavioral responses regarding drug use. a. Involuntary physiologic responses: • Drug tolerance is a physiologic phenomenon in which, after repeated doses, the prescribed dose begins to lose its effectiveness. • Physical dependence is a physiologic state that results from repeated administration of a drug. Withdrawal is experienced if the drug is abruptly discontinued. Tapering down the drug dosage helps to manage withdrawal symptoms. b. Voluntary behavioral responses: • Drug abuse is the use of a drug in any manner that deviates from culturally acceptable medical and social uses (Lehne, 2004). Addiction is a behavioral pattern of drug use characterized by overwhelming involvement with use of the drug and securing its supply, and the high tendency to relapse after withdrawal (Lehne, 2004).	4. Many clients and families are misinformed regarding the nature and risks of drug addiction and, consequently, may be reluctant to request pain medication.

(continued on page 474)

Interventions	Rationales
5. Provide the client with privacy during his or her pain episodes (e.g., close curtains and room door, ask others to leave the room).	5. Privacy allows the client to express pain in her or his own manner, which can help to reduce anxiety and ease pain (Lehne, 2004).

6. Provide optimal pain relief with prescribed analgesics:
  a. Determine the preferred administration route—by mouth, intramuscular, intravenous, or rectal. Consult with the physician or advanced practice nurse.
 	
  b. Assess vital signs—especially respiratory rate—before and after administering any narcotic agent.
  c. Consult with a pharmacist regarding possible adverse interactions between the prescribed drug and other medications the client is taking (e.g., muscle relaxants, tranquilizers).
  d. Take a preventive approach to pain medication; that is, administer medication before an activity (e.g., ambulation) to enhance participation (but be sure to evaluate the hazards of sedation); instruct the client to request pain medication as needed before pain becomes severe.
 	
  e. After administering the pain medication, return in ½ hour to evaluate its effectiveness.
	6.
	
	  a. The proper administration route optimizes the efficacy of pain medications. The oral route is preferred in most cases; for some drugs, the liquid dosage form may be given to a client who has difficulty swallowing. If frequent injections are necessary, the intravenous (IV) route is preferred to minimize pain and maximize absorption; however, IV administration may produce more profound side effects than other routes.
	  b. Narcotics can depress the respiratory center of the brain.
	  c. Some medications potentiate the effects of narcotics; identifying such medications before administration can prevent excessive sedation (Lehne, 2004).
	
	  d. The preventive approach may reduce the total 24-hour dose as compared with the PRN approach; it also provides a more constant blood drug level, reduces the client's craving for the drug, and eliminates the anxiety associated with having to ask for and wait for PRN relief.
	  e. Each client responds differently to pain medication; careful monitoring is needed to assess individual response. For example, too often every surgical client is expected to respond to 50 mg of meperidine (Demerol) every 3–4 hours regardless of body size, type of surgery, or previous experiences (Lehne, 2004; Lewis et al., 2004).

7. Explain and assist with noninvasive and nonpharmacologic pain relief measures:
  a. Splinting the incision site
  b. Proper positioning
  c. Distraction
  d. Breathing exercises
  e. Massage
  f. Heat and cold application
  g. Relaxation techniques
	7. These measures can help to reduce pain by substituting another stimulus to prevent painful stimuli from reaching higher brain centers. In addition, relaxation reduces muscle tension and may help enhance the client's sense of control over pain.

8. Assist the client in coping with the aftermath of the pain experience:
  a. If indicated, inform the client that the painful procedure is completed and that the pain should soon subside.
  b. Encourage the client to discuss the experience.
  c. Clarify any misconceptions the client still may have.
  d. Praise the client for her or his endurance and behavior.
	8. These measures can help reduce anxiety, and help the client to regain the sense of control altered by the painful experience.

9. Teach the client to expel flatus by the following measures:
  a. Walking as soon as possible after surgery
  b. Changing positions regularly, as possible (e.g., lying prone, assuming the knee–chest position)
	9. Postoperatively, sluggish peristalsis results in accumulation of nonabsorbable gas. Pain occurs when unaffected bowel segments contract in an attempt to expel this accumulated gas. Activity speeds the return of peristalsis and the expulsion of flatus; proper positioning helps cause the gas to rise and be expelled.

Documentation

Medication administration record
    Type, route, and dosage schedule of all prescribed medications
Progress notes
    Unsatisfactory relief from pain-relief measures
Multidisciplinary client education record

Risk for Imbalanced Nutrition: Less Than Body Requirements Related to Increased Protein and Vitamin Requirements for Wound Healing and Decreased Intake Secondary to Pain, Nausea, Vomiting, and Diet Restrictions

NOC Nutritional Status, Teaching: Nutrition

Goal

The client will resume ingestion of the daily nutritional requirements.

Indicators

* Selections from the four basic food groups, taking into account cultural preferences and allergies (Lewis et al., 2004).
* 2000–3000 mL of fluids
* Adequate fiber, vitamins, and minerals

NIC Nutrition Management, Nutritional Monitoring

Interventions	Rationales

1. Explain the need for an optimal daily nutritional intake including:
  a. Increased protein and carbohydrate intake
  b. Increased intake of vitamins A, B, B_{12}, C, D, E, and niacin
  c. Adequate intake of minerals (zinc, magnesium, calcium, copper)
	1. Understanding the importance of optimal nutrition may encourage the client to comply with the dietary regimen.

2. Take measures to reduce pain:
  a. Plan care so that painful or unpleasant procedures are not scheduled before mealtimes.
  b. Administer pain medication as ordered.
  c. Position the client for optimal comfort.
	2. Pain causes fatigue, which can reduce appetite.

3. Explain to the client the possible causes of his or her nausea and vomiting:
  a. Side effect of preoperative medications and anesthesia
  b. Surgical procedure
  c. Obesity
  d. Electrolyte imbalance
  e. Gastric distention
  f. Too-rapid or strenuous movement
Reassure the client that these symptoms are normal.
	3. The client's understanding of the source and normalcy of nausea and vomiting can reduce anxiety, which may help to reduce symptoms.

4. Take steps to reduce nausea and vomiting:
  a. Restrict fluids before meals and large amounts of fluids at any time; instead, encourage the client to ingest small amounts of ice chips or sip cool, clear liquids (e.g., dilute tea, Jell-O water, flat ginger ale, or cola) frequently, unless vomiting persists.
	4.
	  a. Gastric distention from fluid ingestion can trigger the vagal visceral afferent pathways that stimulate the medulla oblongata (vomiting center) (Wagner, Johnson, & Kidd, 2006).

(continued on page 476)

Interventions	Rationales
b. Teach the client to move slowly.	b. Rapid movements stimulate the vomiting center by triggering vestibulocerebellar afferents.
c. Reduce or eliminate unpleasant sights and odors.	c. Noxious odors and sights can stimulate the vomiting center.
d. Provide good mouth care after the client vomits.	d. Good oral care reduces the noxious taste.
e. Teach deep breathing techniques.	e. Deep breaths can help to excrete anesthetic agents.
f. Instruct the client to avoid lying down flat for at least two hours after eating. (A client who must rest should sit or recline with her or his head at least four inches higher than the feet.)	f. Pressure on the stomach can trigger vagal visceral afferent stimulation of the vomiting center in the brain.
g. Ensure patency of any nasogastric (NG) tube.	g. A malfunctioning NG tube can cause gastric distention.
h. Teach the client to practice relaxation exercises during episodes of nausea.	h. Concentrating on relaxation activities may help to block stimulation of the vomiting center.
5. Maintain good oral hygiene at all times.	5. A clean, refreshed mouth can stimulate the appetite.
6. Administer an antiemetic agent before meals, if indicated.	6. Antiemetics prevent nausea and vomiting.

Documentation

Flow record
  Intake and output (amount, type, time; Wagner, Johnson, & Kidd, 2006)
  Vomiting (amount, description)
Multidisciplinary client education record

Risk for Constipation Related to Decreased Peristalsis Secondary to Immobility and the Effects of Anesthesia and Narcotics

NOC Bowel Elimination, Hydration, Symptom Control

Goal

The client will resume effective preoperative bowel function.

Indicators

* No bowel distention
* Bowel sounds in all quadrants

NIC Bowel Management, Fluid Management, Constipation/Impaction Management

Interventions	Rationales
1. Assess bowel sounds to determine when to introduce liquids. Advance diet as ordered.	1. Bowel sounds indicate the return of peristalsis.
2. Explain the effects of daily activity on elimination. Assist with ambulation when possible.	2. Activity influences bowel elimination by improving abdominal muscle tone and stimulating appetite and peristalsis.
3. Promote factors that contribute to optimal elimination. a. Balanced diet: • Review a list of foods high in bulk (e.g., fresh fruits with skins, bran, nuts and seeds, whole grain breads and cereals, cooked fruits and vegetables, and fruit juices). • Discuss dietary preferences. • Encourage intake of approximately 800 g of fruits and vegetables (about four pieces of fresh fruit and a large salad) for normal daily bowel movement.	3. a. A well-balanced diet high in fiber content stimulates peristalsis.

(continued on page 477)

Interventions	Rationales
b. Adequate fluid intake: • Encourage intake of at least 8–10 glasses (about 2000 mL) daily, unless contraindicated. • Discuss fluid preferences. • Set up a regular schedule for fluid intake.	b. Sufficient fluid intake is necessary to maintain bowel patterns and promote proper stool consistency.
c. Regular time for defecation: • Identify the normal defecation pattern before the onset of constipation. • Review daily routine. • Include time for defecation as part of the regular daily routine. • Discuss a suitable time based on responsibilities, availability of facilities, and so on. • Suggest that the client attempt defecation about 1 hour following a meal and remain in the bathroom for a suitable length of time.	c. Taking advantage of circadian rhythms may aid in establishing a regular defecation schedule.
d. Simulation of the home environment: • Have the client use the bathroom instead of a bedpan, if possible; offer a bedpan or a bedside commode if the client cannot use the bathroom. • Assist the client into position on the toilet, commode, or bedpan, if necessary. • Provide privacy (e.g., close door, draw curtains around the bed, switch on a TV or radio to mask sounds, make room deodorizer available). • Provide for comfort (e.g., provide reading materials as a diversion) and safety (e.g., make a call bell readily available).	d. Privacy and a sense of normalcy can promote relaxation, which can enhance defecation.
e. Proper positioning: • Assist the client to a normal semi-squatting position on the toilet or commode, if possible. • Assist onto a bedpan, if necessary, elevating the head of the bed to high Fowler's position or to the elevation permitted. • Stress the need to avoid straining during defecation efforts.	e. Proper positioning uses the abdominal muscles and the force of gravity to aid in defecation. Straining can activate a Valsalva response, which may lead to reduced cardiac output; in some incidences it can lead to bradycardia and fainting (Baird, Keen, & Swearingen, 2005; Wagner, Johnson, & Kidd, 2006)
4. Notify the physician if bowel sounds do not return within 6–10 hours, or if elimination does not return within 2–3 days postoperatively.	4. Absence of bowel sounds may indicate paralytic ileus; absence of bowel movements may indicate obstruction.

Documentation

Flow record
    Bowel movements
    Bowel sounds

Activity Intolerance Related to Pain and Weakness Secondary to Anesthesia, Tissue Hypoxia, and Insufficient Fluid and Nutrient Intake

NOC Activity Tolerance

Goal

The client will increase tolerance to activities of daily living (ADLs).

Indicators

• Progressive ambulation
• Ability to perform ADLs

NIC Activity Tolerance, Energy Management, Exercise Promotion, Sleep Enhancement, Mutual Goal Setting

Interventions	Rationales
1. Encourage progress in the client's activity level during each shift, as indicated: a. Allow the client's legs to dangle first; support the client from the side. b. Place the bed in high position and raise the head of the bed. c. Increase the client's time out of bed by 15 minutes each time. Allow the client to set a comfortable rate of ambulation and agree on a distance goal for each shift. d. Encourage the client to increase activity when pain is at a minimum or after pain relief measures take effect.	1. A gradual increase in activity allows the client's cardiopulmonary system to return to its preoperative state without excessive strain. a. Dangling the legs helps to minimize orthostatic hypotension. b. Raising the head of the bed helps to reduce stress on suture lines. c. Gradual increases toward mutually established, realistic goals can promote compliance and prevent overexertion.
2. Increase client's self-care activities from partial to complete self-care, as indicated.	2. The client's participation in self-care improves physiologic functioning, reduces fatigue from inactivity, and improves her or his sense of self-esteem and well-being.
3. If the client is not progressing at the expected or desired rate, do the following: a. Take vital signs prior to the activity. b. Repeat vital sign assessment after the activity. c. Repeat again after the client has rested for 3 minutes. d. Assess for abnormal responses to increased activity: • Decreased pulse rate • Decreased or unchanged systolic blood pressure • Excessively increased or decreased respiratory rate • Failure of pulse to return to near the resting rate within 3 minutes after discontinuing the activity • Complaints of confusion or vertigo • Uncoordinated movements	3. Activity tolerance depends on the client's ability to adapt to the physiologic requirements of increased activity. The expected immediate physiologic responses to activity are increased blood pressure and increased respiratory rate and depth. After 3 minutes, the pulse rate should decrease to within 10 beats/minute of the client's usual resting rate. Abnormal findings represent the body's inability to meet the increased oxygen demands imposed by activity.
4. Plan regular rest periods according to the client's daily schedule.	4. Regular rest periods allow the body to conserve and restore energy.
5. Remark on and encourage the client's progress. Keep a record of progress, particularly for a client who is progressing slowly.	5. Encouragement and realization of progress can give the client an incentive for continued advancement.

Documentation

Flow record
  Vital signs
  Ambulation (time, amount)
Progress notes
  Abnormal or unexpected response to increased activity

Risk for Ineffective Therapeutic Regimen Management Related to Insufficient Knowledge of Care of Operative Site, Restrictions (Diet, Activity), Medications, Signs and Symptoms of Complications, and Follow-up Care

NOC Compliance Behavior, Knowledge: Treatment Regimen, Participation: Health Care Decisions, Treatment Behavior: Illness or Injury

Goals

The goals for this diagnosis represent those associated with discharge planning. Refer to the discharge criteria.

NIC Anticipatory Guidance, Learning Facilitation, Risk Management, Health Education, Teaching: Procedures/Treatments, Health System Guidance

Interventions	Rationales
1. As appropriate, explain and demonstrate care of an uncomplicated surgical wound: a. Washing with soap and water b. Dressing changes using clean technique	1. Uncomplicated wounds have sealed edges after 24 hours and therefore do not require aseptic technique or a dressing; however, a dressing may be applied if the wound is at risk for injury.
2. As appropriate, explain and demonstrate care of a complicated surgical wound: a. Aseptic technique b. Hand-washing before and after dressing changes c. Avoiding touching the inner surface of the soiled dressing, and discard it in a sealed plastic bag d. Use sterile hemostats, if indicated e. Wound assessment—condition and drainage f. Wound cleaning g. Drainage tubes, if indicated h. Dressing reapplication	2. Aseptic technique is necessary to prevent wound contamination during dressing changes. Hand-washing helps to prevent contamination of the wound and the spread of infection. Proper handling and disposal of contaminated dressings helps to prevent infection transmission. Daily assessment is necessary to evaluate healing and detect complications.
3. Reinforce activity restrictions, as indicated (e.g., bending, lifting).	3. Avoiding certain activities decreases the risk of wound dehiscence before scar formation (usually after 3 weeks).
4. Explain the importance of the following: a. Avoiding ill persons and crowds b. Drinking 8–10 glasses of fluid daily c. Maintaining a balanced diet	4. Wound healing requires optimal nutrition, hydration, and rest, as well as avoiding potential sources of infection.
5. Review with the client and family the purpose, dosage, administration, and side effects of all prescribed medications.	5. Complete understanding can help to prevent drug administration errors.
6. Teach the client and family to watch for and report signs and symptoms of possible complications: a. Persistent temperature elevation b. Difficulty breathing, chest pain c. Change in sputum characteristics d. Increasing weakness, fatigue, pain, or abdominal distention e. Wound changes (e.g., separation, unusual or increased drainage, increased redness or swelling) f. Voiding difficulties, burning on urination, urinary frequency, or cloudy, foul-smelling urine g. Pain, swelling, and warmth in calf h. Other signs and symptoms of complications specific to the surgical procedure performed	6. Early detection and reporting danger signs and symptoms enables prompt intervention to minimize the severity of complications.
7. Whenever possible, provide written instructions.	7. Written instructions provide an information resource for use at home.
8. Evaluate the client's and family's understanding of the information provided.	8. Knowledge gaps may indicate a need for a referral for assistance at home.

Documentation

Flow records
  Discharge instructions documenting the method used to ensure that the client and family understand
    instructions (verbalization, return demonstration)
  Follow-up instructions arranging appointment with surgeons/physicians, as ordered, prior to the
    client leaving the hospital
Discharge summary record
  Status at discharge (pain, activity, wound healing)
  Achievement of goals (individual or family)
Multidisciplinary client education record

Abdominal Aortic Aneurysm Resection

This procedure involves surgical resection of an aneurysm with a replacement graft of the aorta or endovascular stenting. Aneurysms are localized or diffuse dilations in an arterial wall that are 50% larger than normally anticipated (Anderson, 2001; Nehler, 2001). Aneurysms can result from arteriosclerosis, arterial trauma, congenital weakness, previous infections, cystic medial necrosis, genetic predisposition, or heredity (Anderson, 2001; Beese-Bjurstrom, 2004).

There are four types of aortic aneurysms: ascending aorta, aortic arch, descending thoracic aorta, and abdominal aortic. Open repair of three types, excluding abdominal, requires cardiopulmonary bypass and hypothermia during surgery and is the only option available in emergent cases (e.g., active dissection or rupture). Non-emergent repair can be done by a less invasive procedure called percutaneous endovascular stent grafting, resulting in shorter hospital stays as well as lower morbidity and mortality rates (Beese-Bjurstrom, 2004; Mukherjee, 2003; Dillon, 2007).

 Time Frame
Preoperative and postoperative periods

■■■■■■ DIAGNOSTIC CLUSTER

Preoperative

Collaborative Problems

▲ PC: Rupture of Aneurysm

Postoperative Period

Collaborative Problems

▲ PC: Distal Vessel Thrombosis or Emboli
▲ PC: Renal Failure
△ PC: Mesenteric Ischemia/Thrombosis
△ PC: Spinal Cord Ischemia

(continued on page 481)

Nursing Diagnoses	Refer to
▲ High Risk for Ineffective Therapeutic Regimen Management related to insufficient knowledge of home care, activity restrictions, signs and symptoms of complications, and follow-up care	
▲ High Risk for Infection related to location of surgical incision	Arterial Bypass Graft
High Risk for Sexual Dysfunction (male) related to possible loss of ejaculate and erections secondary to surgery or atherosclerosis	Colostomy

Related Care Plan
General Surgery Generic care plan (Appendix II)

▲ This diagnosis was reported to be monitored for or managed frequently (75%–100%).
△ This diagnosis was reported to be monitored for or managed often (50%–74%).

Discharge Criteria

Before discharge, the client or family will

1. State wound care measures to perform at home.
2. Verbalize precautions regarding activities.
3. State signs and symptoms that must be reported to a health care professional.

Preoperative: Collaborative Problems

Potential Complication: Ruptured Aneurysm

Nursing Goal

The nurse will detect early signs and symptoms of (a) rupture of aneurysm, (b) distal vessel thrombosis/emboli, (c) renal failure, (d) mesenteric ischemia/thrombosis, and (e) spinal cord ischemia, and will collaboratively intervene to stabilize the client.

Indicators

- Calm, oriented (a, d)
- All pulses palpable and strong (a, b, e)
- No abdominal pelvic chest pain (a, b)
- Non-tender abdomen (a, b, d)
- Capillary refill <3 seconds (b)
- No numbness of extremities (b, e)
- Urine output >5 mL/kg/h (c, e)
- Blood urea nitrogen 5–25 mg/dL (c)
- Serum creatinine
  - Male 0.6–1.5 gm/dL
  - Female 0.6–1.1 gm/dL
- White blood count 4300–10,800/mm3 (d)
- Hematocrit (d)
  - Male 42%–52%
  - Female 37%–47%
- Sensory/motor intact (e)

- Bowel sounds present 5–30 times/min (d)
- Flatus present (d)
- Soft-formed bowel movements (d)

Interventions	Rationales
1. Monitor all pulses (carotid, brachial, radial, ulnar, femoral, popliteal, dorsalis pedis, and posterior tibial) and blood pressure.	1. A carotid bruit must be evaluated preoperatively to rule out risk of stroke during the operation. Assessing upper extremity pulses establishes a baseline for follow-up after arterial lines are in place and arterial punctures are made for blood gas analysis. Assessing lower extremity pulses establishes a baseline for postoperative assessment. A potential complication of aneurysm repair is thrombosis or embolus of distal vessels. Also, clients with abdominal aneurysm have a higher incidence of popliteal aneurysm than the general population.
2. Monitor for signs and symptoms of aneurysm rupture:	2. The larger the aneurysm, the greater the risk of rupture. Risk of rupture increases significantly when aneurysm size >5 cm (Anderson, 2001).
a. Acute abdominal pain with intense back, chest, or pelvic pain; pain sometimes described as "tearing" (Beese-Bjurstrom, 2004)	a. Pain results from massive tissue hypoxia and profuse bleeding into the abdominal cavity.
b. Tender, pulsating abdomen	b. Abdominal pulsations and tenderness result from rhythmic pulsations of the artery and tissue hypoxia, respectively.
c. Restlessness	c. Restlessness is a response to tissue hypoxia.
d. Shock	d. Shock may result from massive blood loss and tissue hypoxia.
3. Initiate emergency measures, as necessary: • Oxygen • Intravenous line • Antihypertensive medications	3. Surgery for ruptured aneurysm carries a mortality rate of 78%–94%; without immediate surgery, however, mortality rate is near 100% (Beese-Bjurstrom, 2004).

Documentation

Flow records
   Vital signs
Progress notes
   Unusual events
   Interventions

Postoperative: Collaborative Problems

Potential Complication: Distal Vessel Thrombosis or Emboli

Potential Complication: Renal Failure

Potential Complication: Mesenteric Ischemia/Thrombosis

Potential Complication: Spinal Cord Ischemia

Potential Complication: Aortoenteric Fistula

Potential Complication: Endoleak

Nursing Goal

The nurse will identify and report vascular complications.

Interventions	Rationales

1. Monitor for signs of thrombosis in distal vessels:
   a. Diminished distal pulses, increased capillary refill time (>3 seconds)
   b. Pallor or darkened patches of skin
	1. Prolonged hypotension may result in thrombosis because of decreased blood flow.

2. Instruct the client to report numbness or tingling in the extremities.	2. Thrombosis of an artery supplying the leg results in a cool, pale, numb, tingling, or painful extremity.
3. If the client complains of pain, assess its location and characteristics.	3. It is important to differentiate pain of surgical manipulation from ischemic pain. Microembolization from the aneurysm to the distal skin causes skin infarctions manifested by point discomfort at the infarct and a dark pink-purple discoloration.

4. Monitor for signs of renal failure (may be due to cross-clamping, hypotension, emboli, or contrast medium) (Anderson, 2001; Hall, 2003)
   a. Decreased urine output (<5 mL/kg/h)
   b. Elevated blood urea nitrogen (BUN), creatinine
   c. Occult blood in urine
	4. During abdominal aorta surgery, the renal arteries are at risk for thrombosis if they are involved in the aneurysm, are clamped for the operation, or are hypoperfused anytime during periods of hypotension. Impaired renal function can result. The endovascular technique reduces risks for subclinical renal damage and colonic ischemia (Solomon, Yee, & Soulen, 2000).

5. Monitor for signs and symptoms of mesenteric thrombosis:
 	
   a. Decreased bowel sounds
 	
   b. Constipation or diarrhea (may be bloody) (Beese-Bjurstrom, 2004)
   c. Increasing abdominal pain or girth (Beese-Bjurstrom, 2004)
   d. Elevated WBCs (20,000 to 30,000/mm^3)
	5. The mesenteric artery, like the renal artery, is at risk for thrombosis.
	   a. Bowel sounds usually are not heard before the third postoperative day.
	   b. A liquid bowel movement before the third postoperative day may point to bowel ischemia; may be bloody.
	   c. Postoperative pain normally decreases each day.
	
	   d. Elevated WBC count indicates possible bowel necrosis.

6. Monitor for signs and symptoms of spinal cord ischemia:
 	
   a. Urinary retention or incontinence
	6. The spinal arteries are at risk for thrombosis for the same reasons as the renal arteries.
	   a. Inadequate perfusion above the second lumbar vertebra (L2) can result in bladder dysfunction.

7. Carefully monitor intake, output, and hydration and renal status (e.g., central venous pressure/hemodynamic monitoring every hour for the first 24 hours postoperatively) (Anderson, 2001).	7. Hypovolemia can cause thrombosis of graft and decrease renal perfusion. Cross-clamping during surgery will disrupt blood flow to the renal arteries.
8. Monitor blood pressure and report elevations from baseline.	8. Hypertension can result from vasoconstrictor and can potentiate graft rupture.

9. Monitor for retroperitoneal bleeding (Anderson, 2001):
   a. Decreased hematocrit
   b. Hypotension
   c. Tachycardia
   d. Back pain
   e. Grey Turner sign
	9. Retroperitoneal bleeding can occur after endovascular surgery.

10. Monitor for intraabdominal bleeding:
   a. Increased abdominal girth
   b. Decreased hematocrit
   c. Hypotension
   d. Tachycardia
	10. Intraabdominal bleeding can occur during the first 24 hours postoperatively.

(continued on page 484)

Interventions	Rationales
11. Palpate or Doppler peripheral pulses every hour for the first 24 hours.	11. Early detection of graft failure can prevent limb loss.

12. Monitor for ileus:
  a. Absence of bowel sounds
  b. Absence of flatus
  c. Abdominal distention
	12. Manual manipulation and displacement of the bowel during surgery will cause bruising and resultant decreased peristalsis.

13. Monitor patency of gastrostomy or nasogastric tube.	13. Nasogastric suctioning is used for 4–5 days postoperatively to decompress the bowel until peristalsis returns.
14. Monitor for signs of infection.	14. Wound and endovascular graft infections can occur.

 Related Physician-Prescribed Interventions

Medications. Dependent on underlying etiology, antihypertensive (e.g., nitroprusside), beta blockers
Intravenous Therapy. Fluid and electrolyte replacement
Laboratory Studies. Refer to the General Surgery care plan, Appendix II.
Diagnostic Studies. Plain radiograph, CT scan, angiogram, MRI, B-mode ultrasound, computed tomographic angiography
Therapies. Oxygen, endovascular stent-graft; also refer to the General Surgery care plan.

Documentation

Flow records
Vital signs
  Circulation (distal, pulses, color)
  Bowel sounds, presence of occult blood
  Lower extremities (sensation, motor function)
  Urine (output, occult blood)
Progress notes
  Characteristics of pain
  Unrelieved pain
  Interventions
  Response to interventions

Postoperative: Nursing Diagnoses

High Risk for Ineffective Therapeutic Regimen Management Related to Insufficient Knowledge of Home Care, Activity Restrictions, Signs and Symptoms of Complications, and Follow-up Care

NOC Compliance Behavior, Knowledge: Treatment Regimen, Participation: Health Care Decisions, Treatment Behavior: Illness or Injury

Goals

The goals for this diagnosis represent those associated with discharge planning. Refer to the discharge criteria.

NIC Anticipatory Guidance, Risk Identification, Health Education, Learning Facilitation

Interventions	Rationales
1. For wound care measures and rationale, refer to the General Surgery care plan.	
2. If an aorto-bifemoral graft was performed, reinforce the need for a slouched position when sitting.	2. A slouched position helps to prevent graft kinking and possible occlusion.
3. Reinforce activity restrictions (e.g., car riding, stair climbing, lifting).	3. About 5–6 weeks after abdominal surgery for a client in good nutritional status, the collagen matrix of the wound becomes strong enough to withstand stress from activity. The surgeon may prefer to limit activity for a longer period, because certain activities place tension on the surgical site (Nichols, 1991). The period of activity restriction is significantly less with endovascular repair, as incisions are smaller.
4. If the client smokes, reinforce the health benefits of quitting and refer the client to a smoking cessation program, if available.	4. Tobacco acts as a potent vasoconstrictor that increases stress on the graft.
5. Instruct the client to report any changes in color, temperature, or sensation in the legs.	5. These signs and symptoms may indicate thrombosis or embolism that requires immediate evaluation.
6. Instruct the client to report any GI bleeding immediately.	6. Duodenal bleeding may be a sign of erosion of the aortic graft into the duodenum.
7. Instruct the client to inform all health care providers about the presence of a prosthetic graft before any invasive procedures.	7. Puncture or exposure of a prosthetic graft risks graft infection that may compromise the client's life.
8. Stress the importance of managing hypertension, if indicated.	8. Hypertension can cause false aneurysms at the anastomosis site.

Documentation

Discharge summary record
    Client and family teaching
    Response to teaching

Amputation

Amputation is the surgical severing and removal of a limb. Amputations are caused by accidents (23%), disease (74%), and congenital disorders (3%). The most common reason for amputation is peripheral vascular disease, especially for those over 50 years old (Society for Vascular Surgery, 2007). Lower extremity amputation is about 15–20 times greater in people with diabetes (Calvert, Penner, Younger, & Wing, 2007). Lower-limb constitutes 80%–85% of all amputations, with nearly two-thirds related to diabetes (Philbin, DeLuccia, Nitsch, & Maurus, 2007).

    There are six categories of lower extremity amputations: hip disarticulation, above knee, knee disarticulation, below knee, Syme (ankle and foot; Williamson, 1998), and transmetatarsal (forefoot; Calvert et al., 2007). Transmetatarsal amputation preserves most of the limb, allowing maximum function and less energy expenditure during mobilization (Calvert et al., 2007).

 Time Frame
Preoperative and postoperative periods

▪▫▪▪▪▪ DIAGNOSTIC CLUSTER

Preoperative Period

Nursing Diagnoses

▲ Anxiety related to insufficient knowledge of postoperative routines, postoperative sensations, and crutch-walking techniques

Related Care Plan

▲ General Surgery Generic care plan

Postoperative Period

Collaborative Problems

▲ PC: Edema of Stump
▲ PC: Wound Hematoma
▲ PC: Hemorrhage
✴ PC: Delayed Wound Healing

Nursing Diagnoses

△ High Risk for Disturbed Body Image related to perceived negative effects of amputation and response of others to appearance

▲ High Risk for Impaired Physical Mobility related to limited movement secondary to amputation and pain

▲ Grieving related to loss of limb and its effects on life style

▲ Acute/Chronic Pain related to phantom limb sensations secondary to peripheral nerve stimulation and abnormal impulses to central nervous system

▲ High Risk for Injury related to altered gait and hazards of assistive devices

△ High Risk for Ineffective Therapeutic Regimen Management related to insufficient knowledge of activity of daily living (ADL) adaptations, stump care, prosthesis care, gait training, and follow-up care

▲ This diagnosis was reported to be monitored for or managed frequently (75%–100%).
△ This diagnosis was reported to be monitored for or managed often (50%–74%).

Discharge Criteria

Before discharge, the client and family will

1. Describe daily stump care.
2. Explain phantom sensations and interventions to reduce them.
3. Describe measures to protect the stump from injury.
4. Demonstrate prosthesis application and care, if indicated.
5. Demonstrate ability to transfer from bed to chair safely.
6. Demonstrate ability to get to the bathroom safely.
7. Demonstrate ability to ascend and descend stairs safely.
8. Demonstrate exercises taught in physical therapy.

Preoperative: Nursing Diagnosis

Anxiety Related to Insufficient Knowledge of Postoperative Routines, Postoperative Sensations, and Crutch-walking Techniques

NOC Anxiety Control, Coping, Impulse Control

Goal

The client will identify his or her expectations of the postoperative period.

Indicators

• Ask questions.
• Express concerns.

NIC Anxiety Reduction, Impulse Control Training, Anticipatory Guidance

Interventions	Rationales

1. Explore the client's feelings about the impending surgery.
  a. Allow the client to direct discussion.
  b. Do not assume or project how the client feels.
	1. Some clients may perceive amputation as a devastating event, while others will view the surgery as an opportunity to eliminate pain and improve quality of life.

2. Help to establish realistic expectations.	2. Successful prosthetic rehabilitation requires cooperation, coordination, tremendous physical energy and fitness, and a well-fitting, comfortable prosthesis (Piasecki, 2001; Yetzer, 1996; Chin, Sawamura, & Shiba, 2006).
3. Consult with other team members (e.g., physical therapy, prosthetist, or discharge coordinator) to see the client preoperatively.	3. Preoperative instructions on postoperative activity help the client to focus on rehabilitation instead of on the surgery; this may help to reduce anxiety.

4. Discuss postoperative expectations, including the following:
 	
  a. Appearance of the stump
  b. Positioning
 	
  c. Ambulation
 	
  d. Phantom pain
	4. These explanations help to reduce fears associated with unknown situations and to decrease anxiety.
	  a. See rationales 8 and 9.
	  b. The stump will be elevated for 24 hours after surgery to prevent edema. The client will be assisted into the prone position three to four times a day to prevent hip contractures (Piasecki, 2001).
	  c. Dangling and transfer to a chair may occur on the first postoperative day. As soon as the client is strong enough, he or she may start using crutches or a walker (Piasecki, 2001).
	  d. Research suggests that 85% of amputees have phantom limb pain ranging from daily to weekly to yearly (Mortimer, Steedman, McMillan, Martin, & Ravey, 2002; Richardson, Glenn, & Horgan, 2006).

5. Instruct the client on the following postoperatively:
  a. Active and active-resistive exercises
  b. Transfer maneuvers
  c. Use of crutches or walker
	5. Training initiated preoperatively can increase mobility postoperatively (Piasecki, 2001).

6. Consult with the physician regarding whether there will be immediate prosthetic fitting or conventional delayed prosthetic fitting, as applicable.	6. Postoperative care varies with each approach (Piasecki, 2001; Yetzer, 1996).

(continued on page 488)

Interventions	Rationales
7. If immediate postsurgical prosthetic fitting is planned, explain that a rigid dressing and cast will be applied at the time of surgery.	7. A socket on the distal end of the cast provides an attachment for a pylon prosthetic unit (Piasecki, 2001).
8. If conventional delayed prosthesis fitting is planned, explain why the stump is covered with a dressing and an elastic bandage.	8. This method shrinks and shapes the stump. A temporary or intermediate prosthesis will be fitted in 3–6 weeks (Piasecki, 2001).
9. Explain that fitting for a permanent prosthesis will occur approximately three months after surgery.	9. With or without immediate postsurgical fitting, the stump needs this time for complete healing and shrinkage (Piasecki, 2001).
10. Explain that immediately following surgery, the client will perceive the amputated limb as if it were still intact and of the same shape and size as before surgery.	10. Immediately after surgery, most amputees feel the phantom limb as it was before surgery.
11. Remind the client and family to verify the amount of prosthetic coverage with the applicable health insurance company (Himiak, 2007).	11. Insurance coverage varies among companies. Some insurers cover only a fraction of the cost, others will pay for only one prosthesis in a lifetime (Himiak, 2007).

Documentation

Progress notes
    Assessment of learning readiness and ability
    Client teaching
    Response to teaching

Postoperative: Collaborative Problems

Potential Complication: Edema of Stump

Potential Complication: Wound Hematoma

Potential Complication: Hemorrhage

Potential Complication: Infection

Potential Complication: Delayed Wound Healing

Nursing Goal

The nurse will detect early signs and symptoms of (a) edema of stump, (b) wound hematoma, (c) hemorrhage, (d) infection, and (e) delayed wound healing, and will collaboratively intervene to stabilize the client.

Indicators

- Diminishing edema (a)
- No evidence of bleeding (c)
- Approximated suture line (a, b, d)
- No point tenderness (b)
- Temperature 98–99.5°F (d)
- Pulse 60–100 beats/min (c)
- BP >90/60, <140/90 mmHg (c)
- Hematocrit (c)
  - Male 42%–52%
  - Female 37%–47%
- White blood cells 4300–10,800 mm³ (d)

Interventions	Rationales
1. Elevate the stump for the first 24 hours only.	1. Elevation for the first 24 hours will reduce edema and promote venous return. Elevation of the limb after 24 hours can cause flexion contractions (Williamson, 1998).
2. Monitor the incision for the following: a. Edema along suture line b. Areas of compression (if Ace wraps are used) c. Areas of pressure (if a cast is used) d. Bleeding e. Signs of delayed healing (Calvert, Penner, Younger, & Wing, 2007)	2. Traumatized tissue responds with lymphedema. Excessive edema must be detected to prevent tension on the suture line that can cause bleeding. Tissue compression from edema can compromise circulation (Williamson, 1998). Delayed wound healing is the most common complication, especially among diabetics (Calvert, Penner, Younger, & Wing, 2007).
3. Monitor for signs of hematoma: a. Unapproximated suture line b. Ruddy color changes of skin along suture line c. Oozing dark blood from suture line d. Point tenderness on palpation	3. Amputation flaps may be pulled over large areas of "space," creating pockets that may contain old blood. Hematoma may compromise flap healing and delay rehabilitation (Ray, 2000).
4. Evaluate the fit of elastic bandages and reapply every 4–6 hours using figure-of-eight turns.	4. Proper bandaging provides wound protection, controls tissue edema, molds the limb for prosthetic fitting, and remains secure with movement (Williamson, 1998).

 Related Physician-Prescribed Interventions

Medications. Analgesics, antibiotics, and antidepressants
Laboratory Studies. Dependent on underlying condition and symptomatology
Diagnostic Studies. Dependent on symptomatology
Therapies. Physical therapy, occupational therapy, prosthesis

Documentation

Flow records
    Appearance of suture line
    Appearance of skin around suture line
    Drainage
Progress notes
    Abnormal findings

Postoperative: Nursing Diagnoses

High Risk for Disturbed Body Image Related to Perceived Negative Effects of Amputation and Response of Others to Appearance

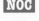 **NOC** Body Image, Child Development: (specify age), Grief Resolution, Psychosocial Adjustment: Life Change, Self-Esteem

Goal

The client will communicate feelings about his or her changed appearance.

Indicators

• Express an interest in dress and grooming.
• Discuss feelings with family.

 NIC Self-Esteem Enhancement, Counseling, Presence, Active Listening, Body Image Enhancement, Grief Work Facilitation, Support Group, Referral

Interventions	Rationales
1. Contact the client frequently and treat him or her with warm, positive regard.	1. Frequent contact by the care-giver indicates acceptance and may facilitate trust. The client may be hesitant to approach staff because of negative self-concept; the nurse must reach out (Dudas, 1997).
2. Encourage the client to verbalize feelings about appearance and perceptions of life style impacts. 3. Validate the client's perceptions and assure him or her that they are normal and appropriate.	2,3. Expressing feelings and perceptions increases the client's self-awareness and helps the nurse to plan effective interventions to address the client's needs. Validating the client's perceptions provides reassurance and can decrease anxiety (Dudas, 1997).
4. Assist the client in identifying personal attributes and strengths. 5. Facilitate adjustment through active listening.	4,5. These can help the client to focus on the positive characteristics that contribute to the whole concept of self, rather than only on the change in body image. The nurse should reinforce these positive aspects and encourage the client to reincorporate them into his or her new self-concept (Dudas, 1997). Body image is strongly related to depression, perception of poor quality of life, low self-esteem, increased general anxiety, lowers levels of satisfaction with prosthetic, participation in activity, and social isolation (Gallagher, Horgan, Franchignoni, Giordano, & MacLachlan, 2007; Yazicioglu et al., 2007).
6. Encourage optimal hygiene, grooming, and other self-care activities.	6. Participation in self-care and planning promotes positive coping with the change.
7. Encourage the client to perform as many activities as possible unassisted.	7. Nonparticipation in self-care and overprotection by care-givers tends to promote feelings of helplessness and dependence.

8. When appropriate, do the following:
  a. Share your perceptions of the loss and the client's response to it.
  b. Explain the nature of the loss.
  c. Discuss the anticipated changes in life style.
	8. Open, honest discussions—expressing that changes will occur but that they are manageable—promote feelings of control.

9. Prepare the client's family and significant others for physical and emotional changes.	9. Support can be given more freely and more realistically if others are prepared (Dudas, 1997).
10. Discuss with the client's support system the importance of communicating his or her value and importance.	10. This will enhance self-esteem and promote adjustment.
11. Facilitate the use of prosthesis as soon as possible.	11. Restoration of mobility has a positive effect on self-concept (Williamson, 1992).
12. Refer a client at high risk for unsuccessful adjustment to counseling, as appropriate.	12. Professional counseling is indicated for a client with poor ego strengths and inadequate coping resources.

Documentation

Progress notes
  Present emotional status
  Dialogues

High Risk for Impaired Physical Mobility Related to Limited Movement Secondary to Pain

NOC Ambulation: Walking, Joint Movement: Active, Mobility Level

Goal

The client will report increased use of affected limb.

Indicators

- Demonstrate safe use of adaptive devices.
- Use safety measures to prevent injury.

NIC Exercise Therapy: Joint Mobility, Exercise Promotion: Strength Training, Exercise Therapy: Ambulation, Positioning, Teaching: Prescribed Activity/Exercise, Teaching: Assistive Device, Teaching: Strategy

Interventions	Rationales
1. Elevate the limb for the first 24 hours only.	1. Elevation will reduce edema. Continued elevation after 24 hours can cause flexion contractures (Williamson, 1992).
2. Initiate transfer to chair and ambulation as soon as indicated.	2. These activities are usually initiated 12–24 hours after surgery (Williamson, 1992).
3. Consult with a physical therapist to begin exercises.	3. Exercises are indicated for muscle strengthening and to prevent abduction and flexion contractures (Williamson, 1992).
4. Assist the client into a prone position three to four times a day for at least 15 minutes. 5. Encourage the client to sleep in this position.	4,5. Abdominal lying places the pelvic joints in an extended position that extends the extensor muscles and prevents contractures (Williamson, 1992).
6. Teach the client to perform active ROM exercises on unaffected limbs at least four times a day. (*Note:* Perform passive ROM only if the client cannot do active ROM.)	6. Active ROM increases muscle mass, tone, and strength, and improves cardiac and respiratory functioning.
7. Teach the client to avoid prolonged sitting.	7. Prolonged sitting can cause hip flexion contractures.
8. Discuss the increased energy requirements needed to use a prosthesis.	8. Walking with a prosthesis requires more effort because of its weight and the loss of the usual muscle coordination. Clients who are successful see more advantages than disadvantages with prosthetic use (Williamson, 1992).
9. Explore with the client activities that are important to resume her or his life style (e.g., bowling or swimming). Engaging in sports as part of rehabilitation also helps with psychosocial problems (Yazicioglu et al., 2007).	9. Successful adaption to prosthesis use is dependent on the client's belief that one's behavior will improve one's situation (Bandura, 1992). Psychosocial factors influence prosthetic rehabilitation (Gallagher et al., 2007).
10. If appropriate, arrange for someone who has successfully adapted to a prosthesis to visit the client.	10. Successful coping is promoted by witnessing others successfully coping (Bandura, 1992).
11. Remark on the client's progress, no matter how small. Convey that the client can successfully manage adaptation to the prosthesis.	11. Other people's belief that they can successfully cope increases one's own confidence (Bandura, 1992).

Documentation

Flow records
    Exercises
Progress notes
    Range of motion

Nursing Diagnosis

Grieving Related to Loss of a Limb and Its Effects on Life Style

> **NOC** Coping, Family Coping, Grief Resolution, Psychosocial Adjustment: Life Change
>
> Goal
>
> The client will describe the meaning of the loss.
>
> Indicators
>
> * Express grief.
> * Report an intent to discuss feelings with family members or significant others.
>
> **NIC** Anticipatory Guidance, Risk Management, Health Education, Learning Facilitation

Interventions	Rationales
1. Provide opportunities for the client and family members to ventilate feelings, discuss the loss openly, and explore the personal meaning of the loss. Explain that grief is a common and healthy reaction.	1. Amputation may give rise to feelings of powerlessness, anger, profound sadness, and other grief responses. Open, honest discussions can help the client and family members to accept and cope with the situation and their responses to it (Butler, Turkal, & Seidl, 1992; Williamson, 1998).
2. Encourage the use of positive coping strategies that have proved successful in the past.	2. Positive coping strategies aid in acceptance and problem-solving (Piasecki, 2001).
3. Encourage the client to express positive self-attributes.	3. Focusing on positive attributes increases self-acceptance and acceptance of the loss (Piasecki, 2001).
4. Assess the family's or significant others' responses to the situation by focusing on the following: a. Their perception of the short- and long-term effects of disability b. Past and present family dynamics	4. Successful adjustment depends on the client's and support clients' realistic perceptions of the situation (Piasecki, 2001).
5. Help family members and significant others to cope. a. Explore to share their guilt with significant others. b. Identify behaviors that facilitate adaptation. c. Encourage them to maintain usual roles and behaviors. d. Encourage including the client in family decision-making. e. Discuss the reality of everyday emotions such as anger, guilt, and jealousy; relate the hazards of denying these feelings. f. Explain the dangers of trying to minimize grief and interfering with the normal grieving process.	5. A positive response by client's family or significant others is one of the most important factors in the client's own acceptance of the loss (Butler, Turkal, & Seidl, 1992).

6. Promote grief work with each response.
a. Denial:
  • Encourage acceptance of the situation; do not reinforce denial by giving false reassurance.
  • Promote hope through assurances of care, comfort, and support.
  • Explain the use of denial by one family member to other members.
  • Do not push a client to move past denial until he or she is emotionally ready.
b. Isolation:
	6. Grieving involves profound emotional responses; interventions depend on the particular response.

(continued on page 493)

Interventions	Rationales

• Convey acceptance by encouraging expressions of grief.
• Promote open and honest communication to encourage sharing.
• Reinforce the client's self-worth by providing for privacy, when desired.
• Encourage socialization, as feasible (e.g., support groups or church activities).
c. Depression:
  • Reinforce the client's self-esteem.
  • Employ empathetic sharing and acknowledge grief.
  • Identify the degree of depression and develop appropriate strategies.
d. Anger:
  • Explain to other family members that anger represents an attempt to control the environment, stemming from frustration at the inability to control the disease.
  • Encourage verbalization of anger.
e. Guilt:
  • Acknowledge the client's expressed self-image.
  • Encourage to share their guilt with significant others.
  • Avoid arguing and participating in the client's system of "I should have . . ." and "I shouldn't have . . ."
f. Fear:
  • Focus on the present and maintain a safe and secure environment.
  • Help the client to explore reasons for and meanings of the fears.
g. Rejection:
  • Provide reassurance by explaining what is happening.
  • Explain this response to other family members.
h. Hysteria:
  • Reduce environmental stressors (e.g., limit personnel).
  • Provide a safe, private area in which to express grief.	

7. Refer the client to amputee support group. Have an amputee visitor see client.	7. This allows the client and his or her family the opportunity to ventilate and ask questions.

Documentation

Progress notes
  Present emotional status
  Interventions
  Response to interventions

*This diagnosis is not currently on the NANDA list but has been included for clarity or usefulness.

Acute/Chronic Pain Related to Phantom Limb Sensations Secondary to Peripheral Nerve Stimulation and Abnormal Impulses to Central Nervous System

NOC Comfort Level, Pain: Disruptive Effects, Pain Control, Depression Control

Goal

The client will report decreased phantom pain.

Indicators

- State the reasons for phantom sensation.
- Demonstrate techniques for managing phantom sensation.

NIC Pain Management, Medication Management, Exercise Promotion, Mood Management, Coping Enhancement

Interventions	Rationales
1. Explain that the sensations are normal and encourage the client to report them. Sensations are physiologic, not psychologic in origin. Clients prefer personal education regarding phantom sensations rather than reading about it (Mortimer, Steedman, McMillan et al., 2002).	1. The client may be hesitant to discuss phantom sensations for fear of appearing abnormal. Nearly 100% of clients with amputations report phantom pain sensation of varying degree during their first six months (Mortimer et al., 2002). Education reduces anxiety and opens lines of communication (Mortimer et al., 2002).
2. Explain that phantom sensations and/or pain are common phenomena. Phantom sensations are non-painful sensations that may manifest as sensations of position of the amputated limb (proprioception or kinesthetic); of movement (kinetic); of feelings within the missing limb (exteroceptive) such as paresthesia, tickling, itching, warmth or cold, something touching the phantom limb, or numbness; or sensations as if an object, such as a ring, watch, or shoe, is still on the limb (superadded). Phantom pain is any sensation so intense it manifests as pain (Bosmans et al., 2007; Richardson, Glenn, & Hogan, 2006). Phantom sensations occur in 29%–78% of clients with amputations; phantom pain occurs in 49%–83% (Bosmans, Suurmeijer, Hulsink et al., 2007).	2. Phantom sensations are caused by stimulation of the nerve proximal to the amputation that previously extended to the limb. The client perceives the stimulation as originating from the absent limb. On the other hand, there is no agreement yet on the exact cause of phantom limb pain. Stimulus of peripheral nerves proximal to the amputation is thought to be a cause. Another explanation is that severed nerves may send impulses that are perceived by the brain as abnormal (Davis, 1993; Katz, 1996).
3. Explain that stress, anxiety, fatigue, depression, excitement, and weather changes may intensify phantom limb pain (Wilkens, McGrath, Finley, & Katz, 2004).	3. Psychological stressors do not cause phantom limb pain, but can trigger or increase it (Katz, 1996).
4. Explain measures that have been effective in alleviating phantom limb pain. a. Applying heat to stump b. Applying pressure to stump (e.g., elastic bandages) c. Distraction, diversion techniques, and relaxation exercises d. Massage therapy (after two weeks postoperatively)	4. Stimulation causing a second sensation may serve to override the phantom sensation (Williamson, 1992).
5. Avoid administering narcotics or analgesics for phantom pain. Check with the physician about administration of other medications.	5. Narcotics are ineffective for phantom limb pain, but are effective for surgical stump pain (Katz, 1996).
6. Advise the client to consult with pain specialists if phantom limb pain is unmanageable.	6. Phantom limb pain may cause disability and loss of employment, depending on its intensity (Bosmans et al., 2007). Phantom pain influences physical and social well-being and quality of life. The most important determinant is the sense of independence (Bosmans et al., 2007).
7. Advise the client that phantom pain may begin right after surgery or not until 2–3 months later.	7. This explanation will help to reduce fears associated with unknown situations.

Documentation

Progress notes
    Reports of pain
    Interventions
    Response to interventions

High Risk for Injury Related to Altered Gait and Hazards of Assistive Devices

NOC Risk Control, Safety Status: Falls Occurrence

Goal

The client will not injure self.

Indicators

• Relate the potential safety problems associated with use of a prosthesis or an assistive device.
• Ask for assistance, as needed.

NIC Fall Prevention, Environmental Management: Safety, Health Education, Surveillance: Safety, Risk Identification

Interventions	Rationales
1. Reinforce exercise and activities prescribed by the physical therapist.	1. Exercises increase muscle strength needed for transfers and ambulation.
2. Provide an assistive device (such as walker or cane) to compensate for altered gait, as necessary.	2. The client may need an assistive device for walking or to reduce the risk of falling.
3. Teach the client to eliminate environmental hazards from the home, such as the following: a. Throw rugs b. Clutter c. Dim lighting d. Uneven or slippery floors	3. Removing hazards can reduce risks of slipping and falling.
4. Encourage the client to request assistance, as needed, when in an unfamiliar environment or situation.	4. Assistance may help to prevent injury.
5. Encourage the client to report altered gait to the physician or prosthetist.	5. Altered gait may be due to a poorly fitted prosthesis or other reasons; it requires further evaluation.

Documentation

Progress notes
    Assessment of learning readiness/ability
    Ability to perform ADLs
Discharge summary record
    Client teaching
    Response to teaching

High Risk for Ineffective Therapeutic Regimen Management Related to Insufficient Knowledge of Activity of Daily Living (ADL) Adaptations, Stump Care, Prosthesis Care, Gait Training, and Follow-up Care

NOC Compliance Behavior, Knowledge: Treatment Regimen, Participation: Health Care Decisions, Treatment Behavior: Illness or Injury

Goals

The goals for this diagnosis represent those associated with discharge planning. Refer to the discharge criteria.

NIC Anticipatory Guidance, Risk Identification, Health Education, Learning Facilitation

Interventions	Rationales
1. Teach foot care for the remaining foot including the following: 　a. Daily foot bath 　b. Thorough drying 　c. Daily inspection for corns, calluses, blisters, and signs of infection 　d. Professional nail cutting 　e. Wearing clean socks daily 　f. Wearing sturdy slippers or shoes	1. Daily care is necessary to deflect or prevent injury, especially if a circulatory disorder was a contributing factor to amputation (Yetzer, Kauffman, & Sopp, 1994).
2. Instruct the client to place a chair or other large object next to the bed at home to prevent him or her from getting out of bed at night and attempting to stand on the stump when not fully awake.	2. Phantom sensations include a kinesthetic awareness of the absent limb. A half-asleep client arising during the night may fall and damage the healing stump (Davis, 1993).
3. Instruct the client to avoid tobacco; refer to a smoking cessation program, if necessary.	3. Nicotine in tobacco constricts arterial vessels, which decreases blood flow to the healing stump. If amputation was related to atherosclerosis, tobacco use may threaten the stump's survival (Rudolph, 1992).
4. Explain the risks for infection and the need to report: 　a. Fever 　b. Increased pain 　c. Increased swelling 　d. Skin necrosis	4. Hematomas of the wound contribute to infection. Coexisting diabetes mellitus reduces resistance to bacteria and causes diminished circulation. Tissue necrosis also can result from decreased circulation, chronic swelling, and infection.
5. Teach the client to prepare the stump for a prosthesis, as appropriate: 　a. Regularly examine the stump for expected changes (e.g., muscle and scar atrophy) and unexpected changes (e.g., skin breakdown, redness, tenderness, increased warmth or coolness, numbness or tingling). 　b. When the incision is closed, perform daily stump care, including the following: 　　• Washing with soap and water 　　• Drying thoroughly 　　• Avoiding creams and ointments 　c. Wrap the stump with Ace bandages using figure-of-eight turns.	5. Knowing how to avoid skin trauma promotes healthy, comfortable function (Chin et al., 2006). 　a. Shrinkage occurs as scar tissue retracts. Increasing redness or tenderness may indicate infection. 　b. Daily cleansing helps to prevent infection. Creams and ointments may soften the skin to the point at which it is easily broken down. 　c. Elastic compression reduces edema in the stump. Edema interferes with wound healing and prolongs the rehabilitation time. Wrapping using figure-of-eight turns also helps to shape the stump for better fit into the prosthesis. Ace bandages wrapped horizontally can impede circulation.
6. Reinforce the need to continue exercises at home. (For more information, see the nursing diagnosis High Risk for Impaired Physical Mobility in this care plan).	6. Active ROM exercises increase muscle mass, tone, and strength; pressure joint mobility; and improve cardiac and respiratory function.
7. Evaluate the client's ability to manage the home, shop, prepare food, and do other ADLs. If indicated, initiate referrals to community and social service agencies (e.g., amputee support group).	7. Referrals may be indicated to provide additional assistance after discharge.
8. Refer the client to a rehabilitative facility.	8. The sooner the client engages in rehabilitation, the more successful the prosthetic ambulation.

Documentation

Discharge summary record
　Client and family teaching
　Response to teaching
　Referrals, if indicated

Arterial Bypass Grafting in the Lower Extremity

This open surgical procedure involves grafting an autogenous vein or an artificial graft to bypass an arterial occlusion and restore continuous blood flow (Hirsch et al., 2006; Morgan, 2005). Depending on the extent of the occlusion, the bypass graft can reach from the top of the femoral artery to the proximal popliteal artery, to the tibioperoneal trunk, or to small arteries in the ankle (Folcarelli & Carleton, 1997). Eighty percent (80%) of acute arterial occlusions originate in the heart, affecting the lower extremities much more than the upper extremities. The other 20% of occlusions are related to arterial embolization of plaque or thrombus (Mitchell, Mohler, & Carpenter, 2007).

Revascularization may also be accomplished using endovascular techniques which are less traumatic and with lower morbidities and mortalities, but it may be less durable then open procedures. Endovascular procedures include: catheter-directed therapy with thrombolytic agents, thrombectomies, balloon angioplasties, stent placement (Aronow, 2005; Morgan, 2005; Sieggreen, 2007), arthrectomy and endovascular radiation (Zaetta, Mohler, & Baum, 2007).

 Time Frame
Preoperative and postoperative periods

■■■■■ DIAGNOSTIC CLUSTER

Collaborative Problems

▲ PC: Thrombosis of Graft
△ PC: Compartment Syndrome
△ PC: Lymphocele
▲ PC: Disruption of Anastomosis

Nursing Diagnoses

▲ High Risk for Infection related to location of surgical incision

△ High Risk for Impaired Skin Integrity related to immobility and vulnerability of heels

▲ Acute Pain related to increased tissue perfusion to previous ischemic tissue

△ High Risk for Ineffective Therapeutic Regimen Management related to insufficient knowledge of wound care, signs and symptoms of complications, activity restrictions, and follow-up care

Related Care Plans

▲ General Surgery Generic care plan
▲ Abdominal Aortic Aneurysm Resection

▲ This diagnosis was reported to be monitored for or managed frequently (75%–100%).
△ This diagnosis was reported to be monitored for or managed often (50%–74%).

Discharge Criteria

Before discharge, the client and/or family will

1. Demonstrate proper wound care.
2. Demonstrate correct pulse palpation technique.
3. State the signs and symptoms that must be reported to a health care professional.

Collaborative Problems

Potential Complication: Thrombosis of Graft
Potential Complication: Compartment Syndrome

Potential Complication: Lymphocele
Potential Complication: Disruption of Anastomosis or Puncture Site
Potential Complication: Renal Failure Related to Myoglobinemia Associated with Reperfusion

Nursing Goal

The nurse will detect early signs and symptoms of (a) thrombosis of graft, (b) compartment syndrome, (c) lymphocele, and (d) disruption of anastomosis, and will collaboratively intervene to stabilize the client.

Indicators

- Capillary refill <3 seconds (a, b, d)
- Peripheral pulses: full, present (a)
- Warm, not mottled limbs (a, b)
- Intact sensation (a, b)
- Minimal limb edema (b)
- No pain with passive stretching (a, b)
- Intact muscle tension (a, b)
- Increasing wound drainage (c)
- Increasing local swelling (b, c)
- No bounding pulsation over graft (d)
- Can move toes (b)

Interventions	Rationales
1. Keep the bed's side rails up within the boundaries of restraint regulations. Bed rest, as ordered (Morgan, 2005).	1. Every practical measure should be taken to prevent graft trauma from injury.
2. Keep the limb warm but *do not* use electric heating pads or hot water bottles.	2. Peripheral nerve ischemia causes diminished sensation. High temperatures of heating devices may damage tissue without the client feeling discomfort.
3. Instruct the client to sit in a "slouched" position and not to cross legs. If leg elevation is ordered, elevate the entire leg and pelvis to heart level.	3. Sharp flexion and pressure on the graft must be avoided to prevent graft damage (Edwards, Abullarade, & Turnbull, 1996).
4. Monitor graft patency, palpate a graft patency, palpate a graft near the skin surface, and assess distal pulses for changes from the baseline (e.g., Doppler pressure).	4. Graft patency is essential to arterial circulation.
5. Monitor circulatory status, color, temperature, sensation, and motor function in the affected leg every hour and as ordered/needed (Morgan, 2005).	5. A sudden change in temperature, drop in pressure, or absence of pulses indicates graft thrombosis. Changes in sensation or motor function can indicate compartment syndrome (Edwards, Abullarade, & Turnbull, 1996).
6. Immediately report changes in color, temperature, sensation, pulses, or pressure to the physician (e.g., pain in toes or foot).	6. Sudden decrease in arterial flow, indicating thrombosed graft, is an emergency requiring immediate surgical exploration of the graft (Edwards, Abullarade, & Turnbull, 1996).

(continued on page 499)

Interventions	Rationales

7. Monitor for signs and symptoms of compartment syndrome:
   a. Edema of revascularized limb
   b. Complaints of pain with passive stretching of the muscle
   c. Decreased sensation, motor function, or paresthesias of the distal limb
   d. Increased tension and firmness of muscle
	7. After a period of ischemia comes a period of increased capillary wall permeability. Restoration of arterial flow causes plasma and extracellular fluid to flow into the tissues, producing massive swelling in the calf muscles. The edema compresses the blood vessels and nerves within the non-expanding fascia (Sieggreen, 2007). The nerves become anoxic, causing paresthesias and motor deficits (Tumbarello, 2000). Urgent fasciotomy is required to relieve pressure and preserve the limb (Sieggreen, 2007).

8. Immediately report changes in status to the physician.	8. Postoperative edema is expected in the new revascularized limb. Careful assessment alerts the nurse to edema severe enough to cause compartment syndrome. Treatment must be initiated within 8 hours to preserve function of the extremity (Edwards, Abullarade, & Turnbull, 1996).

9. Monitor for signs and symptoms of lymphocele:
   a. Discomfort accompanied by local swelling
   b. Large amounts of clear or pink-tinged drainage
	9. A major lymphatic channel courses through the inner thigh area. If the lymphatic chain is lacerated during the operation, drainage may occur. The large amount of accumulated fluid seeks the path of least resistance and usually drains through the incision.

10. Support the affected leg and
   a. Discontinue elevation and ice.
   b. Loosen dressings.
	10. Support can reduce muscle spasms.

11. Apply compression dressings only if ordered by physician.	11. Although compression may possibly halt the flow of lymph long enough for the lymphatic vessel to seal, this usually is not the case; surgical intervention may be required to repair the draining lymphatic chain. Compression should be used only on the physician's order; overly vigorous compression may damage the new graft.

12. Monitor for disruption of anastomosis:
   a. Decrease in perfusion of distal extremity
   b. Bounding aneurysmal pulsation over the anastomosis site. If bleeding occurs, apply firm, constant pressure over the site and notify the physician.
	12. Hemorrhage from anastomotic disruption is an emergency requiring immediate surgical intervention.

 Related Physician-Prescribed Interventions

Medications. Vasodilators, anticoagulant therapy, mannitol, analgesics antiplatelet therapy, cholesterol-reducing medications, antihypertensive

Intravenous Therapy. Fluid/electrolyte replacement

Laboratory Studies. Prothrombin time, platelet count, serum creatinine phosphokinase, urine creatinine clearance, triglycerides, complete blood cell count, partial prothrombin time

Diagnostic Studies. Doppler ultrasonography, angiography, ankle-brachial index, magnetic resonance angiography (MRA), computed tomographic angiography

Therapies. Hyperbaric oxygen therapy; also refer to the General Surgery care plan

Documentation

Flow records
   Vital signs
   Distal pulses
   Circulatory status

Progress notes
  Presence and description of pain
  Unusual events, actions, responses
  Wound drainage and appearance

Nursing Diagnoses

High Risk for Infection Related to Location of Surgical Incision

NOC Infection Status, Wound Healing: Primary Intention, Immune Status

Goal

The client will exhibit wound healing free of infection.

Indicators

- State early signs of infection.
- Demonstrate wound care.

NIC Infection Control, Wound Care, Incision Site Care, Health Education

Interventions	Rationales
1. If the wound does not have a polyurethane film dressing from the operating room, cover it with a dry, sterile gauze dressing. Be certain that no skin surfaces come in contact with each other.	1. Minimizing moisture in the groin wound decreases the risk of infection (Maklebust & Sieggreen, 2001).
2. If the client has a pendulous abdomen, instruct him or her regarding body positioning so that the abdomen does not cover the groin wound.	2. Keeping the wound free of skin overlays decreases moisture, which is a medium for microorganism growth (Maklebust & Sieggreen, 2001).
3. If the tissue becomes macerated, change the gauze dressings more frequently. Expose the groin to air for 15-minute periods during the day. Consider obtaining an order to leave incision open to air.	3. Air will help to dry the wound.
4. Teach the client the importance of avoiding wound maceration and graft infection.	4. Graft failure can result from a wound infection.
5. Refer to Generic Surgical care plan for additional interventions.	

Documentation

Flow records
  Interventions
  Response to interventions

High Risk for Impaired Skin Integrity Related to Immobility and Vulnerability of Heels

NOC Tissue Integrity: Skin and Mucous Membrane

Goal

The client will maintain intact skin over heels intact.

Indicators

• Describe measures to protect the heels.
• Relate why the heels are at risk.

NIC Pressure Management, Pressure Ulcer Care, Skin Surveillance, Positioning

Interventions	Rationales
1. Observe for signs and symptoms of tissue ischemia (e.g., blanching or redness). Palpate for changes in tissue consistency beneath the skin.	1. Pressure ulcer formation may begin deep in the tissue. A client with peripheral vascular disease secondary to atherosclerosis is at high risk for pressure ulcer formation because of the ischemia already present in the tissue (Maklebust & Sieggreen, 2001).
2. Explain why the heels are especially vulnerable to skin breakdown from excessive pressure.	2. A compromised arterial supply may be just enough to maintain viability of a leg but inadequate to heal an ulcer in the leg (Sieggreen, 2007).
3. Take measures to alleviate pressure on the heels (e.g., elevate the heels from the bed and avoid heel protectors).	3. Skin pressure triggers ulcer formation. Elevation reduces direct pressure; heel protectors are a direct pressure device (Maklebust & Sieggreen, 2001).
4. Protect the feet by reducing weight on them with the use of foot cradles and vascular boots (Aronow, 2005).	4. See #1 & 3.

Documentation

Flow records
   Skin condition
   Interventions

Acute Pain Related to Increased Tissue Perfusion to Previous Ischemic Tissue

NOC Comfort Level, Pain Control

Goal

The client will report pain relief after interventions.

Indicators

• State the reason for the pain.
• Relate signs and symptoms of ischemia.

NIC Pain Management, Medication Management, Emotional Support, Teaching: Individual, Heat/Cold Application, Simple Massage

Interventions	Rationales
1. Explain the source of pain and reassure the client that the sensation is temporary and will decrease each day.	1. Pain results from the reperfusion of previously ischemic sensory nerve endings. Pain lessens as reperfusion progresses.
2. Assess carefully to differentiate between the pain of reperfusion and the pain of ischemia (reperfused tissue is warm and	2. Ischemic pain may indicate graft failure and warrants immediate evaluation. Monitor the "Six P's" of acute ischemia

(continued on page 502)

Interventions	Rationales
edematous; ischemic tissue is cool). Notify the physician immediately if you suspect ischemia.	related to arterial occlusion: pain, poikilothermia (coolness), pulselessness, pallor, paresthesia, and paralysis (begins with generic motor deficits) (Sieggreen, 2007).
3. Refer to the nursing diagnosis Acute Pain in the General Surgery care plan (Appendix II) for more information.	

Documentation

Progress notes
    Unrelieved pain
    Interventions
    Response to interventions

High Risk for Ineffective Therapeutic Regimen Management Related to Insufficient Knowledge of Wound Care, Signs and Symptoms of Complications, Activity Restrictions, and Follow-up Care

NOC Compliance Behavior, Knowledge: Treatment Regimen, Participation: Health Care Decisions, Treatment Behavior: Illness or Injury

Goals

The goals for this diagnosis represent those associated with discharge planning. Refer to the discharge criteria.

NIC Anticipatory Guidance, Risk Management, Health Education, Learning Facilitation

Interventions	Rationales
1. Teach the client and family the proper wound care techniques. (Refer to the nursing diagnosis High Risk for Ineffective Therapeutic Regimen Management in the General Surgery care plan, Appendix II, for specific measures.)	1. Proper wound care can prevent infection that delays healing (Edwards, Abullarade, & Turnbull, 1996).
2. Reinforce teaching regarding activity restrictions and mobility (Edwards, Abullarade, & Turnbull, 1996). a. Increase activity as prescribed. b. Avoid long periods (>20 minutes) of standing or sitting with legs bent at the groin and knee. c. Ambulate as advised; plan a walking or exercise program (Sieggreen, 2006).	2. The client's understanding may encourage compliance with the therapeutic regimen. a. Activity should be increased gradually to promote circulation and reduce loss of strength. b. Dependent positioning of the legs increases postoperative swelling. Positions of hip–knee flexion impede venous return. c. Early ambulation is recommended to restore muscle activity and enhance venous blood return.
3. Teach the client and family or support persons how to assess graft patency. a. Assess pulses and capillary refill. b. Palpate the graft for pulsations, if near the surface.	3. Monitoring circulatory status must be continued at home.
4. Teach the client and family or significant others to recognize signs and symptoms of problems and report them immediately.	4. Reporting these signs of compromised circulation, infection, or possible graft failure promptly enables intervention to prevent serious complications. Diminished circulation

(continued on page 503)

Interventions	Rationales
a. Absence of pulses b. Change in temperature of the leg or foot c. Paresthesias and other changes in sensation d. Pain e. Wound or sore in the affected leg f. Changes in the incision site (e.g., redness, drainage)	impedes healing; infection can cause graft failure (Edwards, Abullarade & Turnbull, 1996; Hirsch et al., 2006).
5. Reinforce teaching regarding foot care and prevention of injury to the leg. Refer to Peripheral Arterial care plan for specific teaching.	5. Continued care and precautions are necessary at home.
6. Discuss the options if impotence results (e.g., referral to a urologist or counselor).	6. Operative disruption of internal iliac blood supply or sympathetic fibers may cause impotence.
7. Teach the client and family about the vascular disease process and prevention of further arterial occlusions (Sieggreen, 2007).	7. Addressing risk factors and encouraging regular follow-up with the physician may prevent the client from experiencing a similar event (Bick, 2003; Hirsch et al., 2006; Sieggreen, 2007).

Documentation

Discharge summary record
    Client and family teaching
    Response to teaching

Breast Surgery (Lumpectomy, Mastectomy)

The treatment for breast cancer is removal of the tumor followed by radiation, chemotherapy, hormonal therapy, or combinations of these. The types of surgery differ in the amount of breast tissue removed, dissection of lymph nodes, and removal of pectoral muscles. *Lumpectomy* is the removal of the cancerous tissue and a small amount of adjacent tissue with overlying skin left in place. Axillary nodes may be dissected through a separate incision. Research shows that a lumpectomy followed by radiation therapy is equally as effective as a mastectomy for certain cancer presentations (BreastCancer.org, 2007). *Total mastectomy* is the removal of the entire breast but no other tissue or lymph nodes. *Modified radical mastectomy* is the removal of the entire breast and some of the axillary lymph nodes. *Radical mastectomy* is the removal of the entire breast, skin, pectoral muscles, and all axillary lymph nodes. If the breast is removed, breast reconstruction with implants and nipple–areolar construction or autologous transplants are planned (Chapman & Goodman, 2000; Susan B. Koman for the Cure, 2007a, 2007b).

 Time Frame
Preoperative and postoperative periods

■■■■■ **DIAGNOSTIC CLUSTER**

Preoperative Period

Nursing Diagnoses

▲ Anxiety/Fear related to perceived effects of mastectomy (immediate: pain, edema; postdischarge: relationships, work) and prognosis

(continued on page 504)

Postoperative Period

Collaborative Problems

▲ PC: Neurovascular Compromise
Refer to General Surgery care plan for additional collaborative problems.

Nursing Diagnoses	Refer to
▲ High Risk for Impaired Physical Mobility (arm, shoulder) related to lymphedema, nerve/muscle damage, and pain	
▲ High Risk for Injury related to compromised lymph drainage, motor, and sensory function in affected arm	
▲ High Risk for Disturbed Self-Concept related to perceived negative effects of loss on functioning	Cancer: Initial Diagnosis
▲ Grieving related to loss of breast and change in appearance	Cancer (Initial Diagnosis)
▲ High Risk for Ineffective Therapeutic Regimen Management related to insufficient knowledge of wound care, exercises, breast prosthesis, signs and symptoms of complications, hand/arm precautions, community resources, and follow-up care	

Related Care Plan

General Surgery Generic care plan

▲ This diagnosis was reported to be monitored for or managed frequently (75%–100%).

Discharge Criteria

Before discharge, the client and family will

1. Demonstrate hand and arm exercises.
2. Describe hand and arm precautions.
3. Demonstrate breast self-examination.
4. State care measures to perform at home.
5. Discuss strategies for performing ADLs.
6. State necessary precautions.
7. State the signs and symptoms that must be reported to a health care professional.
8. Verbalize an intent to share feelings and concerns with significant others.
9. Identify available community resources and self-help groups.

Preoperative: Nursing Diagnosis

Anxiety/Fear Related to Perceived Mastectomy and Prognosis

Goal

The client will share concerns regarding the surgery and its outcome.

Indicators

• Describe actions that can help to reduce postoperative edema and immobility.
• State the intent to share feelings with family, significant other, or friends.

Interventions	Rationales
1. Encourage the client to verbalize her concerns and fears. Stay with the client and family as much as possible and convey empathy and concern.	1. Both lumpectomy and mastectomy clients report anxiety and depression. The anxiety of lumpectomy clients is attributed to feelings of uncertainty regarding prognosis and possible reoccurrence. Mastectomy clients reported anxiety regarding the impact of surgery on relationships and appearance (Hoskins et al., 1996).
2. Initiate dialogue regarding concerns about the cancer diagnosis.	2. Many women have heard "horror stories" about mastectomy. Many of these stories involve older types of surgery that often did involve widespread tissue destruction. However, the goal of today's most drastic surgery is more targeted and precise, aiming at maximal preservation of breast tissue (BreastCancer.org, 2007).
3. If the client is agreeable, arrange for a visitor from Reach to Recovery.	3. Women have cited family support as essential in helping them to cope (Hoskins et al., 1996). Computer access allows women to search libraries and websites, as well as join discussion groups while on her own schedule and at her own pace. Identify support groups and information hotlines (Hoskins & Haber, 2000).
4. Explain expected events simply, such as the following: a. Preoperative and postoperative routines b. Possible development of lymphedema and sensory changes after surgery c. Postoperative positioning and exercises d. Presence of drainage tubes	4. Explaining what to expect can help to reduce fear of the unknown and anxiety over unexpected events. Simple explanations will not overwhelm an already stressful situation.
5. Explain that a temporary soft prosthesis can be worn immediately.	5. A temporary prosthesis enhances the appearance and reduces the sense of imbalance that can result from breast removal. Understanding that a prosthesis can be worn immediately after recovery can help to allay anxiety associated with appearance.
6. Allow the client's partner to share his or her concerns in private.	6. Research has shown that satisfaction with marital support and support from other adults positively affects the woman's adjustment (Hoskins et al., 1996). Partners may feel unsure of how to show support and affection (Susan B. Koman for the Cure, 2007d).
7. Assure the client and partner that their concerns and fears are normal and expected.	7. Validation can help to reduce fear associated with such feelings as rejection, repulsion, abandonment, and loss of attractiveness. Open communication between partners is very important (Susan B. Koman for the Cure, 2007d).
8. Discuss with the client and significant other that the greatest period of distress is 2–3 months postsurgery and that counseling may be helpful.	8. Research has shown that the initial emotional appraisal of threat gradually changes over time to a cognitive appraisal that leads to uncertainty and increased anxiety (Hoskins et al., 1996).
9. Discuss with the client and significant other possible responses of others (e.g., minimization or avoidance).	9. Research reports lumpectomy clients receive less psychologic support from friends, family, and coworkers who minimize the seriousness of that surgery versus mastectomy (Hughes, 1993).

(continued on page 506)

Interventions	Rationales
10. Encourage the client to discuss options with the physician regarding breast reconstruction or tissue expansion. It is a good idea to discuss one's consideration of reconstructive surgery with both the surgeon and plastic surgeon before the mastectomy. This provides an opportunity to plan the best individualized treatment (American Cancer Society, 2007; Johns Hopkins Breast Cancer Center, 2007).	10. Breast reconstruction can be done at the time of mastectomy or any time thereafter, depending on the treatment plan (American Cancer Society, 2007; Johns Hopkins Breast Cancer Center, 2007).

Documentation

Progress notes
　Dialogues
　Interventions
Response to interventions

Postoperative: Collaborative Problems

Potential Complication: Neurovascular Compromise

Nursing Goal

The nurse will detect early signs and symptoms of neurovascular compromise and collaboratively intervene to stabilize client.

Indicators

- Radial pulses full, bounding
- No numbness or tingling of hand
- Capillary refill <3 seconds
- Warm, not mottled extremity
- Intact finger flexion and extension

 Fall Prevention, Environmental Management: Safety, Health Education, Surveillance: Safety, Risk Identification

Interventions	Rationales
1. Monitor for signs and symptoms of neurovascular compromise by comparing findings between limbs. a. Diminished or absent radial pulse b. Numbness or tingling in hand c. Capillary refill time >3 seconds d. Pallor, blanching, or cyanosis, and coolness of extremity e. Inability to flex or extend fingers	1. Removal of lymph nodes causes edema, leading to entrapment of peripheral nerves at the cervical outlet or wrist; edema is marked by decreased sensation, movement, and circulation. The degree of lymphedema is dependent on the amount of collateral lymphatic avenues removed (Chapman & Goodman, 2000).

 Related Physician-Prescribed Interventions

Medications. Refer to the Cancer: Initial Diagnosis and General Surgery care plans.
Diagnostic Studies. Mammogram; thermography; ultrasound; computed tomography (CT) scan; xeroradiography; breast node biopsies (fine-needle core, wire localization); positron emission tomography (PET); scintimammography, magnetic resonance imaging (MRI), and galactography (Nettina, 2006)
Therapies. Back brace, physical therapy, temporary soft prosthesis, radiation, breast reconstruction, prosthesis, implants

Documentation

Flow records
  Radial pulse assessment
  Affected arm: color, sensation, capillary refill time, movement

Postoperative: Nursing Diagnoses

High Risk for Impaired Physical Mobility (Arm, Shoulder) Related to Lymphedema, Nerve/Muscle Damage, and Pain

NOC Ambulation: Walking, Joint Movement: Active, Mobility Level

Goal

The client will demonstrate progressive mobility to the extent possible within limitations imposed by the surgery.

NIC Exercise Therapy: Joint Mobility, Exercise Promotion: Strength Training, Exercise Therapy: Ambulation, Positioning, Teaching: Prescribed Activity/Exercise, Teaching: Procedure/Treatment

Interventions	Rationales
1. Explain the need to increase mobility to the maximum extent tolerated, and specify the hazards of immobility.	1. Explanations can help to elicit cooperation despite discomfort or fear of falling.
2. Provide appropriate pain relief. (Refer to the General Surgery care plan in Appendix II for specific interventions.)	2. Pain reduces the ability and motivation to perform ROM and other exercises, and to walk.
3. Explain the reasons for poor balance; accompany client while she walks.	3. A large compression bandage and impaired arm movement can interfere with balance and increase the risk of falling.
4. Instruct client to elevate the affected arm on a pillow when sitting or reclining.	4. Elevation facilitates lymphatic drainage and prevents pooling.
5. Provide the client with written instructions for the following exercises to be performed three times a day (5–10 times each) (Chapman & Goodman, 2000): a. Postoperatively days 1–5: Rotate wrist in circular fashion, touch fingers to shoulder, and extend arm fully (Nettina, 2006). b. After drains are removed (Nettina, 2006): • Stand and hold a chair with other arm and bend over slightly. Swing your affected arm in small circles and gradually increase in size. Make 10 circles; then rest and repeat in the opposite direction. • Swing arm forward and back as far as you can without pulling on the incision. • Bend over slightly and swing arms across the chest in each direction. • Sit in a chair with both arms at your sides. Shrug both shoulders, then relax. • While sitting or standing, pull shoulders back, then bring shoulder blades together. c. After sutures are removed: • Lie in bed with arm extended, raise arm over your head, and extend backward.	5. a. These exercises increase circulation and help with preventing edema. b. These exercises promote muscle movement without stretching (Chapman & Goodman, 2000). c. These exercises will stretch and regain ROM in shoulders if done in all directions every day (Chapman & Goodman, 2000).

(continued on page 508)

Interventions	Rationales
• Lie in bed, grasp a cane or short pole with both hands across your lap. Extend arms straight up and over your head and return. • Repeat, rotating the cane clockwise then counterclockwise while raised over your head. • Stand and extend arm straight over your head and down. • Extend your elbow out from your side at a 90-degree angle; hold it for 10 seconds, then relax. • Extend your arm straight out from your side even with your shoulder; extend arm straight up toward the ceiling. • Stand sideways to the wall. Extend arm out so fingers touch the wall. Creep up the wall a little more each day. Repeat while facing wall. d. After 6 weeks: • Water aerobics • Overall fitness program	d. A regular exercise program three times a week will strengthen the arm and shoulder and help client to regain previous function (Chapman & Goodman, 2000).
6. Initiate passive ROM exercises on the affected arm as prescribed.	6. These exercises increase circulation and help to maintain function.
7. As activities are increased, encourage client to use the affected arm as much as possible.	7. Frequent arm movement prevents lymphedema and contractures.

Documentation

Progress notes
    Level of function
    Exercises (type, frequency)

High Risk for Injury Related to Compromised Lymph Drainage, Motor, and Sensory Function in Affected Arm

NOC Risk Control, Safety Status: Falls Occurrence

Goal

The client will report no injuries to the affected arm.

Indicators

• Relate the factors that contribute to lymphedema.
• Describe activities that are hazardous to the affected arm.

NIC Fall Prevention, Environmental Management: Safety, Health Education, Surveillance: Safety, Risk Identification

Interventions	Rationales
1. Monitor for signs and symptoms of sensorimotor impairment: a. Impaired joint movement b. Muscle weakness c. Numbness or tingling	1. These signs can indicate entrapment of nerves at the cervical outlet or wrist from lymphedema or damage to the thoracodorsal nerve.

(continued on page 509)

Interventions	Rationales
2. Monitor regular measurements of arm circumference for changes.	2. Regular measurements can detect increasing lymphedema.
3. Consult with the physician for additional interventions as needed, such as diuretics, elastic wraps, and intermittent pneumatic compression. Remind the client to wear a compression sleeve and drink plenty of fluids when flying in an airplane (Susan B. Koman for the Cure, 2007c).	3. If lymphedema increases, more aggressive therapy may be indicated.
4. Teach the client to avoid the following: a. Vaccines, blood samples, injections, and blood pressure measurements on affected arm b. Constrictive jewelry and clothing c. Carrying a shoulder bag or heavy object with the affected arm d. Brassieres with thin shoulder straps (use wide–strap or no-strap brassieres instead) e. Lifting objects weighing more than 5–10 pounds f. Strenuous exercise for 3–6 weeks after any breast surgery (Johns Hopkins Breast Cancer Center, 2007). g. Leaning on arm	4. a,b. Constriction of the arm can exacerbate lymphedema. c. Shoulder bags and heavy objects increase pressure at the shoulder joint and increase blood flow to the affected arm. d. Thin straps also produce constriction on the shoulder. e,f,g. Anything that increases blood flow to the affected area contributes to lymphedema (Chapman & Goodman, 2000).
5. Teach the client precautions to prevent trauma to the affected arm and hand: a. Using long-gloved potholders b. Avoiding cuts, scratches, and bruises c. Avoiding injections and venipunctures of any kind d. Using a thimble when sewing e. Avoiding strong detergents or other chemical agents f. Wearing heavy gardening gloves and avoiding gardening in thorny plants g. Using electric razor under arms h. Protect from sunburn and avoid excessive heat (e.g., saunas, hot tubs, or tanning beds) i. Keep skin clean and well moisturized j. Do not cut cuticles k. Promptly treat infections of hand and arm (National Cancer Institute, 2007; Susan B. Koman for the Cure, 2007c)	5. Trauma to tissue with compromised lymphatic drainage exacerbates lymphedema (Chapman & Goodman, 2000).
6. Teach the client to cleanse arm or hand wounds promptly, and to observe carefully for early signs of infection (e.g., redness, increased warmth). Stress the need to report any signs promptly.	6. Compromised lymph drainage weakens the body's defense against infection; this necessitates increased emphasis on infection prevention. Studies show that prophylactic antibiotics significantly reduce the incidence of surgical site infection, lowering potential morbidity (Cunningham, Bunn, & Handscomb, 2006).
7. Teach the client to keep the wrist higher than the elbow and the elbow higher than the heart whenever possible.	7. This will reduce edema.
8. Teach methods of reducing lymphedema (Susan B. Koman for the Cure, 2007c)	8. Complete decongestive physiotherapy exercise (e.g., opening & closing the hand), manual lymphatic drainage (a specific type of massage), and physical therapy have been shown to reduce swelling and lymphedema-related infection (Susan B. Koman for the Cure, 2007c).

Documentation

Discharge summary record
  Client teaching
  Outcome achievement or status

High Risk for Ineffective Therapeutic Regimen Management Related to Insufficient Knowledge of Wound Care, Exercises, Breast Prosthesis, Signs and Symptoms of Complications, Hand/Arm Precautions, Community Resources, and Follow-up Care

NOC Compliance Behavior, Knowledge: Treatment Regimen, Participation: Health Care Decisions, Treatment Behavior: Illness or Injury

Goals

The goals for this diagnosis represent those associated with discharge planning. Refer to the discharge criteria.

NIC Anticipatory Guidance, Risk Identification, Health Education, Learning Facilitation

Interventions	Rationales
1. Teach the client breast self-examination techniques; instruct her to examine both breasts periodically.	1. Periodic, careful breast self-examination can detect problems early; this improves the likelihood of successful treatment (Nettina, 2006).
2. Teach the client wound care measures (refer to the General Surgery care plan in Appendix II for details) and to avoid using strong deodorants and shaving of axilla for two weeks after surgery (Chapman and Goodman, 2000).	2. Proper wound care is essential to reduce risk of infection. Irritation of the axilla should be avoided to decrease risk of infection (Chapman and Goodman, 2000).
3. Provide information about breast prostheses. Emphasize the importance of a properly fitted prosthesis.	3. A prosthesis of optimal contour, size, and weight provides normal appearance, promotes good posture, and helps to prevent back and shoulder strain.
4. Explain the benefits of strengthening and aerobic exercises.	4. Strengthening exercises increase lymph flow with muscle-pumping action. Aerobic activity elevates the heart and respiratory rates; this stimulates the lymphatic transport (Chapman & Goodman, 2000).
5. Encourage the client to maintain ideal body weight.	5. Adipose tissue compresses and reduces lymphatic transport (Chapman & Goodman, 2000).
6. Refer to a specialist in lymphedema, if needed.	6. Early interventions at the first sign of lymphedema can reduce long-term complications.
7. Explain the use of a compression sleeve, if ordered.	7. Compression increases lymphatic return and reduces edema.
8. Explain to expect fatigue in the months after surgery (Badger, Braden, & Michel, 2001).	8. Fatigue has been found to be the most frequently reported side effect (Badger, Braden, & Michel, 2001).
9. Encourage the client to seek professional counseling for assistance with coping and depression.	9. Depression is common and affects the client's quality of life significantly (Badger, Braden, & Michel, 2001).
10. Provide written instructions for exercises to perform at home and reemphasize their importance.	10. Research has shown that, after breast surgery, women experience significant attention deficits, regardless of the extent of surgery (Cimprich, 1992).

(continued on page 511)

Interventions	Rationales
11. Instruct the client to inspect her arm and hand daily, and to report promptly any signs and symptoms of complications, including these: a. Increasing edema or weakness b. Numbness or tingling c. Impaired hand or arm movement d. Warmth, redness, or rashes e. Pain	11. These signs and symptoms point to increasing lymphedema, which can lead to impaired sensorimotor function or infection.
12. Discuss available community resources (e.g., Reach for Recovery, ENCORE). Encourage contact and initiate referrals, if appropriate. Home health care may be helpful due to short length of hospitalization after surgery (Nettina, 2006).	12. Personal sources of information have been found to be more important than written materials.
13. As appropriate, explore the client's feelings concerning radiation therapy or chemotherapy, if planned.	13. Both radiation and chemotherapy have side effects that necessitate client teaching to enhance self-care and coping.

Documentation

Discharge summary record
    Client and family teaching
    Outcome achievement or status
    Referrals, if indicated

Carotid Endarterectomy

The surgical removal of atherosclerotic plaque or thrombus from the inside of the carotid artery, carotid endarterectomy is indicated to prevent cerebrovascular accident in clients who have a 60%–90% occlusion of the carotid artery, whether symptomatic or asymptomatic (American Heart Association [AHA], 2004; Greelish, Mohler, & Fairman, 2006c; National Institute of Neurological Disorders and Stroke [NINDS], 2004). Symptomatic occlusion indicates the occurrence of a transient ischemic attack (TIA) or cerebral vascular accident (Greelish, Mohler, & Fairman, 2006b). The procedure may be performed under general or local anesthesia; local anesthesia significantly reduces morbidity and mortality. If bilateral carotid endarterectomies are required, staging the procedures is suggested (Greelish et al., 2006c).

 Time Frame
Preoperative and postoperative periods

■■■■■ DIAGNOSTIC CLUSTER

Preoperative Period

Nursing Diagnosis

▲ Anxiety related to anticipated surgery and unfamiliarity with preoperative and postoperative routines and postoperative sensations

(continued on page 512)

Postoperative Period

Collaborative Problems

Circulatory
▲ PC: Thrombosis
▲ PC: Hypotension
▲ PC: Hypertension
▲ PC: Hemorrhage
▲ PC: Cerebral Infarction
Neurological
▲ PC: Cerebral Infarction
Cranial Nerve Impairment
▲ PC: Facial
▲ PC: Hypoglossal
▲ PC: Glossopharyngeal
△ PC: Vagal
△ PC: Local Nerve Impairment
▲ PC: Respiratory/Airway Obstruction

Nursing Diagnoses

▲ High Risk for Injury related to syncope secondary to vascular insufficiency

△ High Risk for Ineffective Therapeutic Regimen Management related to insufficient knowledge of home care, signs and symptoms of complications, risk factors, activity restrictions, and follow-up care

Related Care Plan

General Surgery Generic care plan

▲ This diagnosis was reported to be monitored for or managed frequently (75%–100%).
△ This diagnosis was reported to be monitored for or managed often (50%–74%).

Discharge Criteria

Before discharge, the client and family will

1. Describe wound care techniques.
2. State activity restrictions for home care.
3. Demonstrate range-of-motion (ROM) exercises.
4. State the signs and symptoms that must be reported to a health care professional.
5. Identify risk factors and describe their relationship to arterial disease.

Preoperative: Nursing Diagnosis

Anxiety Related to Anticipated Surgery and Unfamiliarity With Preoperative and Postoperative Routines and Postoperative Sensations

NOC Anxiety Level, Coping, Impulse Control

Goal

The client will relate postoperative expectations.

NIC Health Education, Health System Guidance, Learning Facilitation, Learning Readiness Enhancement, Risk Identification, Self-Modification Assistance

Interventions	Rationale
1. Discuss with the client the possible effect of surgery on facial nerve function (i.e., numbness and asymmetry) (Greelish et al., 2006c).	1. Alerting the client to what to expect can reduce anxiety associated with fear of the unknown.
2. Refer to the nursing diagnosis Anxiety in the General Surgery care plan, Appendix II, for specific interventions and rationales for preoperative anxiety.	

Documentation

Progress notes
  Assessment results
  Client teaching
  Response to teaching

Postoperative: Collaborative Problems

Potential Complications: Circulatory Problems, Thrombosis, Hypotension, Hypertension, Hemorrhage, Cerebral Infarction

Potential Complications: Neurologic Problems, Cerebral Infarction, Cranial Nerve Impairment, Local Nerve Impairment

Potential Complication: Respiratory/Airway Obstruction

Nursing Goals

The nurse will detect early signs and symptoms of (a) vascular problems, (b) neurologic deficits, and (c) respiratory obstruction, and will collaboratively intervene to stabilize the client.

Indicators

- Respirations—quiet, regular, unlabored (a, b, c)
- Respirations 16–20 breaths/min (a, b, c)
- BP >90/60, <140/90 mmHg (a, b)
- Pulse 60–100 beats/min (a, b, c)
- Temperature 98–99.5°F (a)
- Alert, oriented (b)
- Pupils, equal, reactive to light (b)
- Intact motor function (b)
- Clear speech (b)
- Swallowing reflex intact (b)
- Facial symmetry (b)
- Full ROM upper/lower limbs (b)
- Urine output >5 mL/kg/h (a, b, c)
- Oxygen saturation (SaO_2) 94–100 mmHg (a, b, c)
- Carbon dioxide ($PaCo_2$) 35–45 mmHg (a, b, c)
- pH 7.35–7.45 (a, b, c)
- Hemoglobin
  - Male 13–15 gm/dL (a, b, c)
  - Female 12–10 gm/dL (a, b, c)
- Hematocrit
  - Male 42%–50% (a, b, c)
  - Female 40%–48% (a, b, c)
- Mean arterial pressure 60–160 mmHg (a, b, c)
- White blood count 4000–10,800 mm^3 (a, b, c)

Interventions	Rationales
1. Monitor for the following: a. Respiratory obstruction (check trachea for deviation from midline; listen for respiratory stridor) b. Peri-incisional swelling or bleeding	1. Edema or hematoma at the surgical site can cause mechanical obstruction.
2. Monitor for changes in neurologic function (Greelish et al., 2006c): a. Level of consciousness b. Pupillary response c. Motor/sensory function of all four extremities (check hand grasps and ability to move legs)	2. Stroke is a possible, and most common, complication of carotid endarterectomy. Manifestations of cerebral infarction include neuromuscular impairment of the contralateral body side (Greelish et al., 2006c).
3. Monitor for cranial nerve dysfunction (Greelish et al., 2006c): a. Hypoglossal nerve: • Difficulty with speech • Dysphagia • Upper airway obstruction b. Facial nerve: • Upward protrusion of lower lip c. Accessory nerves: • Sagging shoulder • Difficulty raising arm or shoulder d. Vagus nerve: • Loss of gag reflex • Hoarseness • Asymmetrical movements of vocal cords	3. The surgical procedure can temporarily or permanently disrupt cranial nerve functions (Greelish et al., 2006c; National Library of Medicine, 2004). Most cranial nerve injuries resolve over a few months, permanent injuries are rare (Greelish et al., 2006c). a. The hypoglossal nerve controls intrinsic and extrinsic muscles for tongue movement. b. The facial nerve controls facial motor function and taste. c. The accessory nerve controls the trapezius and sternocleidomastoid muscles. d. The vagus nerve regulates movements of swallowing and sensation to the pharynx and larynx. Laryngeal nerve (branches of vagus nerve) damage may cause unilateral vocal cord paralysis (Greelish et al., 2006c). Stimulation of the glossopharyngeal nerve may cause hypotension and bradycardia. Dissection of trigeminal nerve may lead to sensory loss in affected area
4. Monitor for hypertension.	4. Hypertension can be anticipated in certain clients exhibiting predisposing factors, such as preoperative hypertension or postoperative hypoxia and excessive fluid replacement.
5. As necessary, consult with the physician for IV pharmacologic management to prevent hypertensive episodes.	5. Hypertension can increase the risk of hemorrhage or disruption of arterial reconstruction.
6. Monitor for hypotension and bradycardia.	6. The removal of atherosclerotic plaque may cause increased pressure waves on the carotid sinus, leading to hypotension. Bradycardia may result from pressure on the carotid sinus during the operation or from postoperative edema. Postoperative cardiac complications are the leading cause of morbidity following carotid endarterectomy (Hickey, 1996; Greelish et al., 2006c).

 Related Physician-Prescribed Interventions

Medications: Antiplatelet therapy, statins
Diagnostic Studies: Ultrasound, arteriography, magnetic resonance angiography, computed tomography angiography
Intravenous Therapies: Refer to the General Surgery care plan, Appendix II

Documentation

Flow records
    Vital signs
    Patency of the temporal artery on the operative side
    Level of consciousness
    Pupillary response
    Motor function (hand grasp, leg movement)
    Cranial nerve function
    Wound assessment

Postoperative: Nursing Diagnoses

High Risk for Injury Related to Syncope Secondary to Vascular Insufficiency

NOC Risk Control, Safety Status: Falls Occurrence

Goals

The client will no longer report syncopic episodes.

Indicators

1. Relate methods of preventing sudden decreases in cerebral blood flow caused by orthostatic hypotension.
2. Demonstrate maneuvers to change position to avoid orthostatic hypotension.
3. Relate a decrease in episodes of dizziness or vertigo.

NIC Fall Prevention, Environmental Management: Safety, Health Education, Surveillance: Safety, Risk Identification

Interventions	Rationales
1. Remain with the client during initial postoperative activity. 2. Instruct the client to call for assistance when getting out of bed.	1,2. Syncope necessitates assistance to prevent injury.
3. Teach the client to move slowly and step-by-step from the supine to the upright position to avoid orthostatic hypotension: a. Raise the head. b. Lower one leg at a time over the side of the bed. c. Sit for a few minutes before standing. d. Stand for a few minutes before walking.	3. Slow movements minimize sudden decrease in cerebral blood flow by reducing the vascular rush to the large muscles.
4. Explain the relationship of dehydration, alcohol intake, and prolonged bed rest to orthostatic hypotension.	4. Dehydration and the vasodilating effects of alcohol decrease circulating blood volume. Prolonged bed rest increases venous pooling that contributes to orthostatic hypotension upon arising. The client's understanding of these effects may encourage compliance with preventive measures.
5. Monitor use of antihypertensive medications.	5. Orthostatic hypotension can occur with certain antihypertensives.

Documentation

Progress notes
    Complaints of vertigo

Discharge summary record
Client teaching

High Risk for Ineffective Therapeutic Regimen Management Related to Insufficient Knowledge of Home Care, Signs and Symptoms of Complications, Risk Factors, Activity Restrictions, and Follow-up Care

NOC Compliance Behavior, Knowledge: Treatment Regimen, Participation: Health Care Decisions, Treatment Behavior: Illness or Injury

Goals

The goals for this diagnosis represent those associated with discharge planning. Refer to the discharge criteria.

NIC Anticipatory Guidance, Risk Management, Health Education, Learning Facilitation

Interventions	Rationales
1. Teach the client and family to watch for and report the following: a. Swelling of, or drainage from, the incision b. Numbness or weakness of opposite arm or leg c. Changes in speech or swallowing d. Changes in vision	1. These signs are indicative of progressive nerve or tissue compression.
2. Discuss the relationship of arterial disease and certain risk factors (American Heart Association, 2004). a. Smoking b. Hyperlipidemia c. Obesity	2. a. Nicotine is a potent vasoconstrictor that reduces blood flow b. Lipoprotein abnormalities have been related to an increase in vascular diseases c. Obesity is usually associated with increased dietary intake of fats and cholesterol
3. Explore ways in which the client can reduce or eliminate applicable risk factors. (Refer to the Atherosclerosis care plan for more information.) 4. Explain the need for regular ROM exercises of head and neck.	3,4. The client's awareness that he or she can modify risk factors may encourage compliance with the treatment regimen.
5. Refer the client to appropriate resources for assistance with risk factor modification: a. Dietitian for diet and weight loss counseling b. Smoking cessation program c. Exercise program (if approved by the physician)	5. The client may need assistance for sustained management of risk factors after discharge.

Documentation

Discharge summary record
Client teaching
Outcome achievement or status
Referrals, if indicated

Cataract Extraction

Cataract extraction involves the removal of the cloudy lens (opacified lens), from the eye and replacing it with a clear plastic lens (Allen, 2006). The extraction of the cataracts can be done by using several different methods, such as the intracapsular and the extracapsular procedures. The intracapsular procedure is not done routinely today as it required the client to be hospitalized and bedridden for a week. This long hospitalization was needed because it included the removal of the lens, the entire lens capsule, and its attachments from the eye. Moreover, the lens was not replaced and thick glasses were needed after surgery (Ottawa Eye Institute, 2006; Lewis et al., 2004). The extracapsular method, however, is a day surgery procedure where the entire cataract (anterior capsule, lens cortex, and nucleus) is removed through a small hole made in the lens capsule and all its attachments are left intact (Ottawa Eye Institute, 2006; Lewis et al., 2004).

Cataract removal is done with instruments or, more frequently, using the Kelman phacoemulsification procedure that uses ultrasound waves to disintegrate the lens, which is then suctioned out through a smaller 3 mm incision (Ottawa Eye Institute, 2006). Regardless of the procedure, extraction allows insertion of an intraocular lens implant.

Time Frame
Preoperative and postoperative periods

DIAGNOSTIC CLUSTER

Preoperative Period

Nursing Diagnosis

▲ Fear related to upcoming surgery and potential failure to improve vision

Postoperative Period

Collaborative Problems

▲ PC: Hemorrhage
✳ PC: Increased Intraocular Pressure (IOP)
▲ PC: Endophthalmitis
✳ PC: Bullous Keratopathy
✳ PC: Retinal Detachment, Retinal Hole or Tear
✳ PC: Iritis
✳ PC: Glaucoma
✳ PC: Macular Edema
✳ PC: Secondary Cataract

Nursing Diagnoses

△ Acute Pain related to increased intraocular pressure

▲ Risk for Infection related to increased susceptibility: surgical interruption of body surface

▲ Risk for Injury related to visual limitations and presence in unfamiliar environment

▲ High Risk for Ineffective Therapeutic Regimen Management related to insufficient knowledge of activities permitted, medications, complications, and follow-up care

▲ This diagnosis was reported to be monitored for or managed frequently (75%–100%).
△ This diagnosis was reported to be monitored for or managed often (50%–74%).
✳ This diagnosis was not included in the validation study.

Discharge Criteria

Before discharge, the client and family will

1. Discuss management of ADLs and activity restrictions, and encourage return demonstration by both client and family (Lewis et al., 2004).

2. Verbalize understanding of medication regimen.

3. Demonstrate application of eye drops, if necessary (Lewis et al., 2004).

4. Confirm follow-up appointments (Lewis et al., 2004).

5. State the signs and symptoms of any postoperative complications that must be reported to a health care professional.

Preoperative: Nursing Diagnosis

Fear Related to Upcoming Surgery and Potential Failure to Attain Improved Vision

NOC Anxiety Control, Fear Control

Goal

The client will express any fears and concerns regarding the upcoming surgery.

Indicators

- Verbalize an understanding of perioperative routines and care measures.
- Ask questions regarding the surgery.

NIC Anxiety Reduction, Coping Enhancement, Presence, Counseling, Relaxation Therapy

Interventions	Rationales
1. Encourage the client to express views and feelings about the procedure; listen attentively.	1. Verbalizing feelings and concerns helps the nurse to identify sources of anxiety.
2. Reassure the client that anxiety and fear are normal and expected responses to upcoming cataract surgery.	2. Validation and reassurance may help to reduce anxiety.
3. Address any misconceptions the client expresses and provide accurate information, such as: a. Surgery removes the cataract, not the eye. b. A cataract is not a film over the eye, but a clouded lens in the eye. c. Most cataract surgeries are performed under local anesthesia. d. Thirty percent of cataract-extraction clients develop clouding of the back of the capsular bag postsurgery (known as a secondary cataract), usually within a few months or a few years. This is due to cells moving onto this part of the capsule. If this happens, it is easily treated with a YAG (yttrium-aluminum-garnet) laser capsulotomy (Allen, 2006).	3. Misconceptions can contribute to anxiety and fear.
4. Present information using a variety of instructional methods and media: a. Print pamphlets b. Eye model c. Audiovisual programs	4. Simultaneous stimulation of multiple senses enhances the teaching–learning process. Written materials also provide a reference source after discharge.
5. Explain required preadmission activities. a. Adherence to dietary instructions provided by anesthesia services b. Adjustments in medication regimen as ordered by the surgeon, anesthesiologist, or client's physician c. Use of antibiotic eye drops the day before surgery	5. Depending on the client's general health status, presence of concurrent medical problems, time of surgery, and physician's preferences, adjustments may be needed in diet (nothing by mouth for a specified period) and medications (e.g., withholding diuretics, decreasing insulin dose).

(continued on page 519)

Interventions	Rationales

6. Discuss expected preoperative care measures:
  a. Dilating drops and mobility restrictions (Allen, 2006)
  b. Intravenous (IV) access
  c. Bladder emptying
  d. Preoperative sedation prior to transport
 	
7. Provide information about activities, sights, and sounds associated with the intraoperative period.
  a. Presence and purpose of various personnel
  b. Noises of equipment
  c. Importance of lying still during the procedure
  d. Importance of communicating the need to move or cough before doing so during surgery
	6,7. Because cataract surgery is performed under local anesthesia and the client is awake, information about what to expect can help to reduce anxiety associated with fear of the unknown. It also enables the client to participate better in care measures.

8. Reinforce the physician's explanations of options for visual rehabilitation after surgery, as appropriate.
  a. Intraocular lenses (IOL): These miniature plastic lenses are usually implanted during the surgery, but can be implanted later. They provide the best visual correction, compared with other methods. One disadvantage is that they can dislocate occasionally.
  b. Contact lenses: These create less than 5% image distortion and provide more focused central and peripheral vision than aphakic spectacles. Disadvantages include increased care and maintenance, high replacement costs, and intolerance in some clients.
  c. Aphakic spectacles: Hardly ever used in the United States because they cause distortion. They increase an object's image size by 25%–30% and cause objects to look barreled.
	8. Explaining options enables the client to make informed decisions.

Documentation

Progress notes
Medication documentation of preoperative drops (Lewis et al., 2004)
  Client teaching
  Client understanding of the procedures, which includes preoperative, intraoperative, and postoperative teaching and responses (Lewis et al., 2004; Allen, 2006)

Postoperative: Collaborative Problems

Potential Complication: Hemorrhage (Suprachoroidal)
Potential Complication: Increased Intraocular Pressure (IOP)
Potential Complication: Endophthalmitis
Potential Complication: Bullous Keratopathy
Potential Complication: Iritis
Potential Complication: Retinal Tear, Hole, or Detachment
Potential Complication: Glaucoma
Potential Complication: Macular Edema

Nursing Goal

The nurse will detect early signs and symptoms of (a) hemorrhage, (b) increased intraocular pressure, (c) endophthalmitis, (d) bullous keratopathy (e) retinal tear, hole, or detachment, (f) iritis, (g) glaucoma, (h) macular edema, (i) secondary cataract, and will collaboratively intervene to stabilize the client.

Indicators

- No complaints of eye pain (c, d, e, f, h)
- No complaints of orbital pain (c, e, f, h)
- No sudden change in vision (b, c, e, f, g, h, i)
- No complaints of eyebrow pain (b, g, h, i)
- No complaints of nausea (b, e, h, g, i)
- No complaints of halos around lights (b, g, h, i)
- No vomiting (b, e, h, g, i)
- No frontal headache (b, g, h, i)
- No red eye (a, b, c, e, f, h)
- No photophobia (b, e, f, h)

Interventions	Rationales
1. Monitor for signs and symptoms of hemorrhage: a. Pain in or around eyes b. Sudden onset of eye pain c. Changes in vision	1. Ocular tissue is very vulnerable to bleeding because of its high vascularity and fragile vessels. Blood in the anterior chamber (hyphemia) or in the vitreous chamber of the eye alters vision.
2. Monitor for signs and symptoms of increased intraocular pressure: a. Eyebrow pain b. Nausea c. Halos around lights	2. IOP may increase in response to surgery or medications such as steroid eye drops.
3. Remind the client to follow postoperative home eye care that should be explained preoperatively (e.g., keeping eye shield on at night and wearing eyeglasses during the day and sunglasses when outside.	3. Eye shields or glasses are aimed at avoiding accidental bumping, scratching, or trauma.
4. Teach the client to monitor for sign/symptoms of infection, IOP, and bleeding. Refer to Risk for Infection.	4. Because of the short hospitalization, the client and family will be instructed to monitor for postoperative complications.
5. Monitor for signs and symptoms of endophthalmitis: a. Severe eye pain b. Orbital pain c. Change in vision (blurry) d. A red eye	5. Endophthalmitis is a serious condition involving inflammation (swelling) within the eyeball. It is most often caused by infection with bacteria or other microorganisms. It can also occur as a rare complication of cataract extraction or other eye surgery (Lehmann, 2000; Lewis et al., 2004; Ottawa Eye Institute, 2006).
6. Monitor for signs and symptoms of bullous keratopathy: a. Change in vision b. Photophobia c. Moderate to severe pain d. Orbital pain	6. Bullous keratopathy is caused by edema of the cornea, resulting from failure of the corneal endothelium to maintain the normally dehydrated state of the cornea. Most frequently it is due to Fuchs corneal endothelial dystrophy or corneal endothelial trauma. Corneal endothelial trauma can occur during intraocular surgery (e.g., cataract removal) or after placement of a poorly designed or malpositioned intraocular lens implant (Lehmann, 2000; Lewis et al., 2004; Ottawa Eye Institute, 2006).
7. Monitor for signs and symptoms of retinal tear, hole, or detachment: a. Eye pain b. Orbital pain c. Change in vision d. Nausea e. Vomiting	7. Retinal detachment is separation of the neural retinal layer from the underlying retinal pigment epithelium layer. Retinal detachments are often associated with a tear or hole in the retina through which eye fluids may leak. This causes separation of the retina from the underlying tissues. Retinal detachment often occurs on its own without an underlying cause. However, it may also be caused by

(continued on page 521)

Interventions	Rationales
f. Photophobia g. Flashing lights and numerous floaters	trauma, diabetes, or an inflammatory disorder. Sometimes it may be caused by a related condition called posterior vitreous detachment (Lehmann, 2000; Lewis et al., 2004; Ottawa Eye Institute, 2006).
8. Monitor for signs and symptoms of iritis: a. Eye pain b. Orbital pain c. Change in vision d. Photophobia	8. Iritis is the most common type of uveitis, which is inflammation of the concentric middle layer of the eye (uvea). The cause of iritis, which involves inflammation of the iris and other structures at the front of the eye, cannot always be determined. It often occurs in otherwise healthy people. Known causes of iritis include injury to the eye (which could be a result of eye surgery), infection of the eye with the herpes virus, autoimmune disorders such as inflammatory bowel disease or rheumatoid arthritis, and gout (Lehmann, 2000; Lewis et al., 2004; Ottawa Eye Institute, 2006).
9. Monitor for signs and symptoms of glaucoma and secondary glaucoma: a. Orbital pain b. Nausea c. Vomiting d. Frontal headache e. Change in vision	9. A cataract is a clouding of the lens in the eye that affects vision. Secondary cataracts can form after surgery for other eye problems, such as glaucoma; this is due to cells moving onto this part of the capsule. Cataracts also can develop in people who have other health problems, such as diabetes, and are sometimes linked to steroid use. Cataracts can also result, sometimes years later, from trauma which can develop after eye injury (Lehmann, 2000; Lewis et al., 2004; Ottawa Eye Institute, 2006).
10. Monitor for signs and symptoms of macular edema. a. Eye pain b. Orbital pain c. Eyebrow pain d. Nausea e. Vomiting f. Halos around lights g. Frontal headache h. Photophobia. i. Changes in vision	10. Most of the eye's interior is filled with vitreous, a gel-like substance that fills about 80% of the eye and helps it maintain a round shape. The vitreous contains millions of fine fibers that are attached to the surface of the retina. Sometimes, when the vitreous pulls away from the retina, there is microscopic damage to the retina's surface. When this happens, the retina begins a healing process to the damaged area and forms a scar tissue, or an epiretinal membrane, on the surface of the retina. This scar tissue is firmly attached to the retinal surface. Macular edema can be triggered by certain eye diseases and disorders, such as a detached retina and inflammation of the eye (uveitis). Also, people with diabetes sometimes develop an eye disease called diabetic retinopathy, which can cause a macular edema. A macular edema can also be caused by trauma from either surgery or an eye injury (Lehmann, 2000; Lewis et al., 2004; Ottawa Eye Institute, 2006).

 Related Physician-Prescribed Interventions

Medications. Antiemetics, analgesics, cycloplegics, antibodies (topical), antibiotic eye drops
Intravenous Therapy. Refer to the General Surgery care plan.
Laboratory Studies. Refer to the General Surgery care plan.
Diagnostic Studies. Snellen eye chart, ophthalmoscopic examination, gonioscopy, B-scan ultrasonography, visual fields, potential acuity meter, brightness acuity testing, tonometry, slit-lamp examination
Therapies. Eye care

Documentation

Flow records
 Vital signs
 Eye assessment (suture lines, edema, pupils, vision)

Postoperative: Nursing Diagnoses

Acute Pain Related to Increased Intraocular Pressure

NOC Comfort Level, Pain Control

Goal

The client will relate progressive pain reduction and pain relief after interventions.

Indicators

* Relate what increases pain.
* Relate what decreases pain.

NIC Pain Management, Medication Management, Emotional Support, Teaching: Individual, Hot/Cold Application, Simple Massage

Interventions	Rationales
1. Assist the client in identifying effective pain-relief measures.	1. The client has the most intimate knowledge of his or her pain and the effectiveness of relief measures.
2. Explain that pain may not occur until several hours after surgery.	2. Pain may not occur until the local anesthetic wears off; understanding this can help to reduce the client's anxiety associated with the unexpected.
3. Support pain-relief measures with prescribed analgesics.	3. Pharmacologic therapy, such as mild analgesic, may be needed to provide adequate pain relief.

Documentation

Progress notes
    Complaints of pain
    Interventions
    Response to interventions

Risk for Infection Related to Increased Susceptibility to Surgical Interruption of Body Surfaces

NOC Infection Status, Wound Healing: Primary Intention, Immune Status

Goal

The client will exhibit healing of surgical site with no symptoms of infection.

Indicators

* Describe methods to protect eye.
* Demonstrate aseptic technique needed for medication administration.

NIC Infection Control, Wound Care, Incision Site Care, Health Education

Interventions	Rationales

1. Promote wound healing.
  a. Encourage a well-balanced diet and adequate fluid intake.
  b. Instruct the client to keep a patch over the affected eye until the first eye drops are started 4–6 hours after surgery.
	1. Optimal nutrition and hydration improve overall good health; this promotes healing of any surgical wound. Wearing an eye patch promotes healing by decreasing the irritative force of the eyelid against the suture line.

(continued on page 523)

Interventions	Rationales

2. Use aseptic technique to instill eye drops:
  a. Wash hands before beginning.
  b. Hold dropper slightly away from eye so as not to touch the eyelashes.
  c. When instilling, avoid contact between the eye, the drop, and the dropper. Teach the technique to the client and family members.
	2. Aseptic technique minimizes the introduction of micro-organisms and reduces the risk of infection.

3. Assess for signs and symptoms of infection:
  a. Reddened, edematous eyelids
  b. Conjunctival injection (prominent blood vessels)
  c. Drainage on eyelids and lashes
  d. Purulent material in anterior chamber (between the cornea and iris)
  e. Elevated temperature
  f. Decreased visual acuity
  g. Abnormal laboratory values (e.g., elevated WBC count, abnormal culture, and sensitivity results)
	3. Early detection of infection enables prompt treatment.

4. Notify the physician of any suspicious-looking drainage from the eye.	4. Abnormal drainage requires medical evaluation and possible initiation of pharmacologic treatment.

Documentation

Flow records
  Vital signs
  Condition of eye and suture line
Progress notes
  Abnormal findings

Risk for Injury Related to Visual Limitations and Presence in an Unfamiliar Environment

NOC Risk Control, Safety Status. Falls Occurrence

Goal

The client will not experience injury or tissue trauma while on unit.

Indicators

- Identify risks factors present.
- Describe safety measures needed.

NIC Fall Prevention, Environmental Management: Safety, Health Education, Surveillance: Safety, Risk Identification

Interventions	Rationales
1. Orient client to the environment upon arrival on the surgical unit.	1. The client's familiarity with the environment may help to prevent accidents.
2. Place ambulation aids where the client can see and reach them easily. Instruct the client to request assistance before ambulating. Monitor the client's use of ambulation aids.	2. These measures can help to minimize the risk of falls.
3. Teach the client the importance of hand-washing before eye care.	3. Hand-washing is the most effective method of preventing infection.

Documentation

Progress notes
  Visual acuity (preoperative)
Discharge summary record
  Client teaching and return demonstration of understanding

High Risk for Ineffective Therapeutic Regimen Management Related to Insufficient Knowledge of Activities, Permitted Medications, Complications, and Follow-up Care

NOC Compliance Behavior, Knowledge: Treatment Regimen, Participation: Health Care Decisions, Treatment Behavior: Illness or Injury

Goals

The goals for this diagnosis represent those associated with discharge planning. Refer to the discharge criteria.

NIC Health Education, Risk Management, Learning Facilitation, Anticipatory Guidance, Eye Care

Interventions	Rationales
1. Discuss activities permitted after surgery: a. Reading b. Watching television c. Driving d. Cooking e. Light housekeeping f. Shower or tub bathing	1. Beginning your discussions by outlining permitted activities rather than restrictions focuses the client on the positive rather than the negative aspects of recovery.
2. Reinforce activity restrictions specified by the physician. These may include avoiding the following activities: a. Lifting anything weighing over 20 lbs b. Showering c. Straining during bowel movements d. Certain head positions (Lewis et al., 2004) e. Valsalva maneuver (Lewis et al., 2004)	2. Restrictions are needed to reduce eye movements and prevent increased intraocular pressure. Specific restrictions depend on various factors, including the nature and extent of surgery, the physician's preference, and the client's age and overall health status. The client's understanding of the reasons for these restrictions can encourage compliance with them.
3. Reinforce the importance of avoiding rubbing or bumping the eye, keeping the protective patch or shield in place throughout the first postoperative day, and instilling the prescribed eye drops (Lewis et al., 2004). Glasses should also be worn during the day (and the eye shield at night).	3. Rubbing or bumping the eye may interrupt suture line integrity and provide an entry point for microorganisms. Keeping the eye protected reduces the risk of injury.
4. Explain the following information for each prescribed medication: a. Name, purpose, and action b. Dosage schedule (amount, times) c. Administration technique d. Special instructions or precautions	4. Providing accurate information before discharge can promote compliance with the medication regimen and helps prevent errors in administration.
5. Instruct the client and family to report the following signs and symptoms: a. Persistent vision loss b. Eye pain not relieved by analgesics c. Vision abnormalities (e.g., light flashes or spots) d. Redness, increased drainage, or elevated temperature	5. Early reporting of these signs and symptoms enables prompt intervention to prevent or minimize infection, increased intraocular pressure, hemorrhage, retinal detachment, or other complications.

(continued on page 525)

Interventions	Rationales
6. Instruct the client on ocular hygiene measures (e.g., removing crusty drainage by wiping the closed eyelid with a cotton ball moistened with ocular irrigating solution).	6. Secretions may adhere to the eyelids and eyelashes; removal promotes comfort and reduces the risk of infection by eliminating a source of microorganisms.
7. Stress the importance of adequate follow-up care with the schedule to be determined by the surgeon. The client should know the date and time of his or her first scheduled appointment before discharge.	7. Follow-up allows evaluation of healing and enables early detection of complications.
8. Provide written instructions on discharge.	8. Written instructions provide the client and family with a source of information that they can consult as needed.

Documentation

Discharge summary record
    Client and family teaching
    Outcome achievement or status

Colostomy

A colostomy is an opening between the colon and the abdominal wall. The proximal end of the colon is sutured to the skin. Indications for colostomy include diverticulitis, trauma, and cancer (tumors) of the mid-transverse colon. This procedure bypasses the rectum by diverting feces into an external appliance.

There are different names for colostomies, which is dependent on where the stoma is created. There is the *Ascending colostomy* which has an opening created from the ascending colon, and is found on the right abdomen. Because the stoma is created from the first section of the colon, stool is more liquid and contains digestive enzymes that irritate the skin. This type of colostomy is the least common.

The *transverse colostomy* may have one or two openings in the upper abdomen, middle, or right side, which are created from the transverse colon. If there are two openings in the stoma, (called a double–barrel colostomy) one is used to pass stool and the other, mucus. The stool has passed through the ascending colon, so it tends to be liquid to semi-formed. This method is mostly used for temporary colostomies.

In a *Descending or Sigmoid colostomy*, the descending or sigmoid colon is used to create the stoma, typically on the left lower abdomen. This is the most common type of colostomy surgery and generally produces stool that is semi-formed to well-formed because it has passed through the ascending and transverse colon (Lewis et al., 2004).

 Time Frame
Preoperative and postoperative periods

■■■■■ DIAGNOSTIC CLUSTER

Preoperative Period

Nursing Diagnosis

▲ Anxiety related to lack of knowledge of colostomy care and perceived negative effects on life style

(continued on page 526)

Postoperative Period

Collaborative Problems

▲ PC: Peristomal Ulceration/Herniation
▲ PC: Stomal Necrosis, Retraction, Prolapse, Stenosis, Obstruction
✳ PC: Intra-abdominal sepsis
✳ PC: Large Bowel Obstruction
✳ PC: Perforation of Genitourinary Tract

Nursing Diagnoses

▲ High Risk for Disturbed Self-Concept related to effects of ostomy on body image and life style

△ High Risk for Ineffective Sexuality Patterns related to perceived negative impact of ostomy on sexual functioning and attractiveness

High Risk for Sexual Dysfunction related to physiological impotence secondary to damage to sympathetic nerves (male) or inadequate vaginal lubrication (female)

△ High Risk for Loneliness related to anxiety over possible odor and leakage from appliance

▲ High Risk for Ineffective Therapeutic Regimen Management related to insufficient knowledge of stoma pouching procedure, colostomy irrigation, peristomal skin care, perineal wound care, and incorporation of ostomy care into activities of daily living (ADLs)

△ Grieving related to implications of cancer diagnosis (*refer to:* Cancer: Initial Diagnosis)

Related Care Plan

General Surgery Generic care plan

▲ This diagnosis was reported to be monitored for or managed frequently (75%–100%).
△ This diagnosis was reported to be monitored for or managed often (50%–74%).
✳ This diagnosis was not included in the validation study.

Discharge Criteria

Before discharge, the client and family will

1. Discuss and give return demonstration in relation to ostomy care at home, including stoma, pouching, irrigation, and skin care.
2. Discuss strategies for incorporating ostomy management into ADLs.
3. Verbalize precautions for food intake and use of medications.
4. State signs and symptoms that must be reported to a health care professional.
5. Verbalize an intent to share with significant others' feelings and concerns related to ostomy.
6. Identify available community resources and self-help groups:
   a. Visiting nurse
   b. United Ostomy Association
   c. Recovery of Male Potency: Help for Impotent Male
   d. American Cancer Foundation
   e. Community supplier of ostomy equipment
   f. Financial reimbursement for ostomy equipment

Preoperative: Nursing Diagnosis

Anxiety Related to Lack of Knowledge of Colostomy Care and Perceived Negative Effects on Life Style

NOC   Anxiety Level, Coping, Impulse Control

Goal

The client will verbalize decreased anxiety related to fear of the unknown.

Indicators

- State reason for colostomy.
- Describe anatomic changes following colostomy surgery.
- Identify the type of colostomy done, and why it was selected.

NIC   Anxiety Reduction, Impulse Control Training, Anticipatory Guidance

Interventions	Rationales
1. Identify and dispel any misinformation or misconception the client has regarding ostomy (Richbourg, Thorpe, & Rapp, 2007).	1. Replacing misinformation with facts can reduce anxiety.
2. Explain the normal anatomical structure and function of the gastrointestinal (GI) tract.	2. Knowledge boosts confidence; confidence enhances control and reduces anxiety.
3. Explain the effects of the client's particular disorder on affected organs.	3. Understanding the disorder can help the client accept the need for colostomy.
4. Use an anatomical diagram or model to show the resulting altered route of elimination.	4. Understanding how body waste is eliminated after the rectum and anus are removed can help to allay anxiety related to altered body function.
5. Describe the stoma's appearance and anticipated location. Explain the following about the stoma: a. It will be of the same color and moistness as oral mucous membrane. b. It will not hurt when touched because it has no sensory endings. c. It may bleed slightly when wiped; this is normal and not of concern. d. It will become smaller as the surgical area heals; the color will remain the same. e. It may change in size depending on illness, hormone levels, and weight gain or loss (Black, 2000).	5. Explaining expected events and sensations can help to reduce anxiety associated with the unknown and unexpected. Accurate descriptions of the stoma's appearance help to ease shock at the first sight of it after ostomy surgery.
6. Discuss the function of the stoma pouch. Explain that it serves as an external receptacle for storage of feces, much as the colon acts as an internal storage receptacle.	6. Understanding the purpose and need for a pouch encourages the client to accept it and participate in ostomy management.
7. Encourage the client to handle the stoma pouching equipment.	7. Many clients are relieved to see the actual size and material of a stoma pouch. Often, uninformed clients have visions of large bags and complicated, difficult-to-manage equipment that can produce anxiety.
8. Plan a consult with an ostomy nurse specialist.	8. This specialist can provide specific explanations.

Documentation

Progress notes
> Present emotional status
> Client teaching

Postoperative: Collaborative Problems

Potential Complication: Peristomal Ulceration/Herniation

Potential Complication: Stomal Necrosis, Prolapse, Retraction, Stenosis, Obstruction

Potential Complication: Intra-abdominal Sepsis

Potential Complication: Large Bowel Obstruction

Potential Complication: Perforation of Genitourinary Tract

Nursing Goal

The nurse will detect early signs and symptoms of (a) peristomal ulceration/herniation, (b) stomal complications, (c) intra-abdominal sepsis, (d) large bowel obstruction, and (e) perforation of genitourinary tract, and will collaboratively intervene to stabilize the client.

Indicators

- Intact bowel sounds in all quadrants (d)
- Intact peristomal muscle tone (a, b)
- Free-flowing ostomy fluid (a, b)
- No evidence of bleeding (a, b)
- No evidence of infection (c)
- No complaints of nausea/vomiting/hiccups (c, d)
- Non-distended abdomen (d)
- Perineal wound intact (if sutured) (c)
- Temperature 98–99.5°F; no chills (c)
- BP >90/60, <140/90 mmHg (c)
- Pulse 60–100 beats/min (c)
- Respirations 16–20 breaths/min
- White blood cells 4000–10,800/mm³ (c, e)
- Hemoglobin (e, j)
  - Males 13–19 gm/dL
  - Females 12–16 gm/dL
- Hematocrit (e)
  - Males 42%–50%
  - Females 40%–48%
- Urine output >5 mL/kg/h (e, j)

Interventions	Rationales
1. Monitor the peristomal area for the following: a. Decreased peristomal muscle tone b. Bulging beyond the normal skin surface and musculature c. Persistent ulceration	1. Early detection of ulcerations and herniation can prevent serious tissue damage (Colwell & Beitz, 2007).
2. Monitor the following: a. Color, size, and shape of the stoma; and mucocutaneous separation	2. a. These changes can indicate inflammation, retraction, prolapse, or edema.

(continued on page 529)

Interventions	Rationales
b. Color, amount, and consistency of ostomy effluent	b. These changes can indicate bleeding or infection. Decreased output can indicate obstruction.
c. Complaints of cramping abdominal pain, nausea and vomiting, and abdominal distention	c. These complaints may indicate obstruction.
d. Fit of ostomy appliance and appliance belt	d. An improperly fitting appliance or belt can cause mechanical trauma to the stoma (Colwell & Beitz, 2007).
3. If mucocutaneous separation occurs: • Fill separated area with absorptive powder or granules. • Cover with paste. • Reapply a new pouch.	3. Special techniques are needed to prevent fecal contamination.
4. Monitor perineal wound: a. Signs and symptoms of infection b. Bleeding c. Drainage	4. If perineal wound is closed, a drain will have to be put in place.
5. If the wound is open, follow wound care protocol.	5. If risk of infection is high, the wound will not be sutured closed and will need packing and irrigation.
6. Monitor for intra-abdominal sepsis: a. Complaints of nausea, hiccups b. Spiking fevers, chills c. Tachycardia d. Elevated WBC	6. Leakage of GI fluid into the peritoneal cavity (e.g., a leak at the anastomotic site) can cause serious infections (e.g., staphylococcal).
7. Prepare for drainage procedure and/or surgical intervention.	7. Surgical intervention may be needed to drain abscess.
8. Monitor for large bowel obstruction; notify the physician, if detected. a. Decreased bowel sounds b. Nausea, vomiting c. Abdominal distension	8. Intraoperative manipulation of the abdominal organs and the depressive effects of anesthesia and narcotics can cause decreased peristalsis.
9. For additional collaborative problems (hemorrhage, hypovolemia, infection, urinary retention, thrombophlebitis), refer to General Surgery care plan.	

 ### Related Physician-Prescribed Interventions

Refer also to the General Surgery care plan.

Medications. Antibiotics (e.g., kanamycin, erythromycin, neomycin); chemotherapy; immunotherapy; laxatives (preoperative)

Laboratory Studies. Carcinoembryonic antigen (CEA)

Diagnostic Studies. Flat plate of abdomen, computed tomography (CT) scan of abdomen

Therapies. Radiation therapy (preoperative, intraoperative, postoperative)

Documentation

Flow records
   Intake and output
   Bowel sounds
   Wound status
Progress notes
   Stoma condition
Changes in physiologic status

Postoperative: Nursing Diagnoses

High Risk for Disturbed Self-Concept Related to Effects of Ostomy on Body Image and Life Style

NOC Anxiety Reduction, Coping, Impulse Control

Goal

The client will communicate feelings about the ostomy, addressing the changes in their body and function, and acknowledge the reason for the surgery (Haugen, Bliss, & Savik, 2006).

Indicators

- Acknowledge changes in body structure and function.
- Participate in stoma care.

NIC Hope Instillation, Mood Management, Values Clarification, Counseling, Referral, Support Group, Coping Enhancement

Interventions	Rationales
1. Contact the client frequently and treat him or her with warm, positive regard.	1. Frequent contact by caregiver indicates acceptance and may facilitate trust. The client may be hesitant to approach staff because of a negative self-concept (Colwell & Beitz, 2007).
2. Incorporate emotional support into technical ostomy self-care sessions.	2. This allows resolution of emotional issues during acquisition of technical skills. Richbourg, Thorpe, and Rapp (2007) have identified four stages of psychologic adjustment that ostomy clients may experience: a. *Narration.* Each client recounts his or her illness experience and reveals understanding of how and why he or she finds self in this situation. b. *Visualization and verbalization.* The client looks at and expresses feelings about his or her stoma. c. *Participation.* The client progresses from observer to assistant, then to independent performer of the mechanical aspects of ostomy care. d. *Exploration.* The client begins to explore methods of incorporating the ostomy into his or her life style. Use of this adjustment framework helps to establish guidelines for planning the client's experiences in an organized manner.
3. Have client look at and touch the stoma.	3. The nurse should not make assumptions about a client's reactions to ostomy surgery. The client may require help in accepting the reality of the altered body appearance and function, or in dealing with an overwhelming situation (Richbourg, Thorpe, & Rapp, 2007).
4. Encourage the client to verbalize feelings (both positive and negative) about the stoma and perceptions of its anticipated effects on his or her life style. Direct the client to the appropriate professional to help overcome negative feelings and perceptions (Richbourg, Thorpe, & Rapp, 2007; Junkin & Beitz, 2005).	4. Sharing gives the nurse an opportunity to identify and dispel misconceptions and allay anxiety and self-doubt.
5. Validate the client's perceptions and reassure that such responses are normal and appropriate.	5. Validating the client's perceptions promotes self-awareness and provides reassurance.

(continued on page 531)

Interventions	Rationales
6. Have the client practice using a pouch clamp on an empty pouch.	6. Beginning client teaching with a necessary skill that is separate from the body may be less threatening and may ease the fear of failure when performing on his or her own body.
7. Assist the client with pouch emptying, as necessary.	7. Discreetness in doing ostomy care procedures is important: clients will watch health care professionals for signs of revulsion. The nurse's attitude and support are of primary importance (Junkin & Beitz, 2005).
8. Have the client participate in pouch removal and pouch application. Provide feedback on progress; reinforce positive behavior and proper techniques.	8. Effective, thorough teaching helps the client learn to master procedures.
9. Have the client demonstrate the stoma pouching procedure independently in the presence of support persons.	9. Return demonstration lets nurse evaluate the need for any further teaching.
10. Involve support persons in learning ostomy care principles. Assess the client's interactions with support persons.	10. Other people's response to the ostomy is one of the most important factors influencing a client's acceptance of it.
11. Encourage the client to discuss plans for incorporating ostomy care into his or her life style.	11. Evidence that the client will pursue his or her goals and life style reflects positive adjustment (Junkin & Beitz, 2005).
12. Encourage the client to verbalize positive self-attributes.	12. Identifying personal strengths promotes self-acceptance and positive self-concept.
13. Suggest that the client meet with a person from the United Ostomy Associations of America (UOAA) who can share similar experiences.	13. In addition to the clinical expertise of the professional nurse, the ostomy client may choose to take advantage of a UOAA visitor's actual experience with an ostomy (Junkin & Beitz, 2005).
14. Identify a client at risk for unsuccessful adjustment; look for these characteristics (Richbourg, Thorpe, & Rapp, 2007; Junkin & Beitz, 2005): a. Poor ego strength b. Ineffective problem-solving ability c. Difficulty in learning new skills d. Lack of motivation e. External focus of control f. Poor health g. Unsatisfactory preoperative sex life h. Lack of positive support systems i. Unstable economic status j. Rejection of counseling	14. Successful adjustment to ostomy is influenced by factors such as the following: a. Previous coping success b. Achievement of pre-surgery developmental tasks, which includes the education and acceptance of the ostomy requirement and placement (Haugen, Bliss, & Savik, 2006). c. Extent to which the disability interferes with goal-directed activity d. Sense of control e. Realistic perception of the event by the client and support persons
15. Refer an at-risk client for professional counseling (Colwell & Beitz, 2007).	15. In such a client, follow-up therapy is indicated to assist with effective adjustment (Haugen, Bliss, & Savik, 2006; Junkin & Beitz, 2005).

Documentation

Progress notes
    Present emotional status
    Interventions
    Response to interventions

High Risk for Ineffective Sexuality Patterns Related to Perceived Negative Impact of Ostomy on Sexual Functioning and Attractiveness

NOC Body Image, Self-Esteem, Role Performance, Sexual Identity: Acceptance

Goal

The client will discuss own feelings and partner's concerns regarding the effect of ostomy surgery on sexual functioning.

Indicators

- Verbalize the intent to discuss concerns with partner before discharge.
- Relate resources available after discharge.
- Patient to address their own, as well as partner's, thoughts and ideas regarding the effect on their lives of ostomy surgery on sexual functioning.

NIC Behavior Management: Sexual, Counseling, Sexual Counseling, Emotional Support, Active Listening, Teaching: Sexuality

Interventions	Rationales
1. Reaffirm the need for frank discussion between sexual partners and the need of time for the partner to become accustomed to changes in the client's body.	1. The client may worry about his or her partner's acceptance; the partner may be afraid of hurting the client and needs to know that the stoma is not harmed by sexual activity.
2. Role-play ways for the client and partner to discuss concerns about sex.	2. Role-playing helps a person to gain insight by placing him or her in the position of another. It also may promote more spontaneous sharing of fears and concerns.
3. Discuss the possibility that the client may project his or her own feelings onto the partner. Encourage frequent validation of feelings between partners.	3. The client may have erroneous assumptions about the partner (e.g., may erroneously assume that the partner is "turned off" by the ostomy).
4. Reaffirm the need for closeness and expressions of caring; involve the client and partner in touching, stroking, massage, and the like.	4. Sexual pleasure and gratification are not limited to intercourse. Other expressions of caring may prove more meaningful.
5. Explore any fears the client may express regarding mutilation, unacceptability, and other concerns that might limit his or her involvement in relationships (Junkin & Beitz, 2005).	5. These fears might limit involvement in relationships.
6. Discuss the possible availability of a penile prosthesis if the client is physiologically unable to maintain or sustain an erection sufficient for intercourse. Explain that penile implants provide the erection needed for intercourse and do not alter sensations or the ability to ejaculate (Haugen, Bliss, & Savik, 2006; Junkin & Beitz, 2005).	6. Realizing that a prosthesis may be available may reassure the client and reduce anxiety about performance; this actually could help to improve function.
7. Refer the client to a certified sex or mental health counselor, if desired.	7. Certain sexual problems require continuing therapy and the advanced knowledge of therapists.

Documentation

Progress notes
    Assessment data
    Interventions
    Response to interventions
    Referrals, if indicated

High Risk for Sexual Dysfunction Related to Physiologic Impotence Secondary to Damage to Sympathetic Nerve (Male) or Inadequate Vaginal Lubrication (Female)

NOC Body Image, Self-Esteem, Role Performance, Sexual Identity: Acceptance

Goal

The client will describe possible physiologic effects of surgery on sexual functioning.

Indicators

- Relate alternative methods of sexual expression.
- Relate intent to seek counseling, if needed.

NIC Behavior Management: Sexual, Counseling, Sexual Counseling, Emotional Support, Active Listening, Teaching: Sexuality

Interventions	Rationales

1. Explain the effects of the surgery on sexual function.
  a. In men, abdominoperineal resection often damages sympathetic nerves in the presacral area that controls emission. This may result in retrograde ejaculation into the bladder and a "dry" orgasm. During abdominoperineal surgery, the parasympathetic nerves that control blood flow to the penis can be damaged, possibly resulting in erectile dysfunction.
  b. In women, there is little objective evidence of sexual dysfunction following abdominoperineal resection. The most common female sexual complaint is dyspareunia, which may result in "female impotence" (Junkin & Beitz, 2005).
	1. Explanations of the possible effects on sexual function can help reduce fear of the unknown.

2. In men:
  a. Suggest that sexual activity need not always culminate in vaginal intercourse, and that orgasm can be reached through non-coital manual or oral stimulation. Remind the client that sexual expression is not limited to intercourse, but includes closeness, communication, touching, and giving pleasure to another (Junkin & Beitz, 2005).
  b. Explain the function of a penile prosthesis. Both semirigid and inflatable penile prostheses have high rates of success.
  c. Suggest counseling with a certified sex therapist.
	2.
	  a. Alternative methods of sexual expression and gratification promote positive sexual function.
	
	  b. Penile implants provide the erection needed for intercourse and do not alter sensations or the ability to ejaculate.
	  c. Certain sexual problems require continuing therapy and the advanced knowledge of therapists.

3. In women:
  a. Suggest using a water-based vaginal lubricant for intercourse.
  b. Teach the client to perform Kegel exercises, and instruct her to do them regularly.
 	
  c. Suggest that she sit astride her partner during intercourse.
	3.
	  a. Water-based lubricants can help to prevent dyspareunia related to inadequate vaginal lubrication.
	  b. Kegel exercises promote control of the pubococcygeal muscles around the vaginal entrance; this can ease dyspareunia.
	  c. A woman on top can control the depth and rate of penetration; this can enhance vaginal lubrication and relaxation.

Documentation

Progress notes
  Interventions
  Response to interventions

High Risk for Loneliness Related to Anxiety about Possible Odor and Leakage from Appliance

NOC Loneliness, Social Involvement

Goal

The client will state the intent to reestablish preoperative socialization pattern.

Indicators

• Discuss methods to control odor and appliance leakage.
• Participate in self-help groups with similar experiences.

NIC Socialization Enhancement, Spiritual Support, Behavior Modification: Social Skills, Presence, Anticipatory Guidance

Interventions	Rationales
1. Select an appropriate odor-proof pouching system and explain to the client how it works.	1. Fear of accidents and odor can be reduced through effective management. Some pouches have charcoal filters to reduce odor from flatus.
2. Stress the need for good personal hygiene. 3. Teach the client care of a stoma appliance.	2,3. Proper hygiene and appliance care removes odoriferous retained fecal material.

4. Discuss methods for reducing odor.
  a. Avoid odor-producing foods, such as onions, fish, eggs, cheese, and asparagus (Hyland, 2002).
  b. Use internal chlorophyll tablets or a liquid appliance deodorant (Hyland, 2002).
  c. Empty or change the ostomy pouch regularly, when the pouch is one-third to one-half full (Hyland, 2002).
	4. Minimizing odor improves self-confidence and can permit more effective socialization. Bacterial proliferation in retained effluent increases odor with time. A full pouch also puts excessive pressure on seals, which increases risk of leakage.

5. Encourage the client to reestablish his or her pre-operative socialization pattern. Help the client through such measures as progressively increasing his or her socializing time in the hospital, role-playing possible situations that the client feels may cause anxiety, and encouraging him or her to visualize and anticipate solutions to "worst-case scenarios" for social situations.	5. Encouraging and facilitating socialization help to prevent isolation. Role playing can help the client to identify and learn to cope with potential anxiety-causing situations in a nonthreatening environment.
6. Suggest that the client meet with a person from the UOA who can share similar experiences.	6. Others in a similar situation can provide a realistic appraisal and may provide information to answer the client's unasked questions.

Documentation

Progress notes
  Dialogues
Discharge summary record
  Client teaching
Outcome achievement or status

High Risk for Ineffective Therapeutic Regimen Management Related to Insufficient Knowledge of Stoma Poaching Procedure, Colostomy Irrigation, Peristomal Skin Care, Perineal Wound Care, and Incorporation of Ostomy Care into Activities of Daily Living (ADLs)

NOC Compliance Behavior, Knowledge: Treatment Regimen, Participation: Health Care Decisions, Treatment Behavior: Illness or Injury

Goals

The goals for this diagnosis represent those associated with discharge planning. Refer to the discharge criteria.

NIC Anticipatory Guidance, Ostomy Care, Learning Facilitation, Risk Management, Health Education

Interventions	Rationales
1. Consistently use the same sequence in client teaching.	1. Consistency reinforces learning and may enhance the client's sense of control over the situation.
2. Teach the client basic stoma pouching principles, including the following: a. Keep the peristomal skin clean and dry. b. Use a well-fitting appliance. c. Change the pouch when the least amount of drainage is anticipated (usually on arising). d. Empty the pouch when it is one-third to one-half full and change it routinely before leakage occurs (Pontieri-Lewis, 2006). e. Change the pouch if the skin under the appliance itches or feels like burning. f. Observe the condition of the stoma and peristomal skin during pouch changes.	2. Proper pouching techniques can prevent leakage and skin problems. a. This ensures that the appliance adheres to the skin. b. Proper fit protects the surrounding skin surface from contact with drainage. c. This prevents copious drainage from interfering with pouch changes. d. A pouch filled more than halfway exerts greater pressure on the seal; this increases the risk of leakage. e. Burning or itching may indicate that ostomy effluent has undermined the skin barrier; prompt intervention is necessary to prevent skin breakdown. f. Regular observation enables early detection of skin problems.
3. Teach the client the procedure for preparing a stoma pouch (Collett, 2002): a. Select the appropriate stoma pouching system. b. Measure the stoma carefully. c. Use the appliance manufacturer's stoma measuring card, if possible. If the card does not accommodate the stoma's size or shape, teach the client to make a customized stoma pattern: (1) place a clear plastic wrap over the stoma; (2) trace the stoma with a marking pen; and (3) cut a hole in the plastic wrap to accommodate the stoma. d. Cut an opening in the center of the skin barrier slightly larger (approximately ⅛ inch) than the stoma (Pontieri-Lewis, 2006; Hyland, 2002). e. Secure an appropriate odor-proof pouch onto the skin barrier wafer (if using a two-piece appliance system).	3. Preparing a new pouch beforehand ensures that it is ready to apply as soon as the used pouch is removed; this helps to minimize drainage on the skin surface.
4. Teach the procedure for changing a disposable stoma pouch: a. Remove the old pouch by gently pushing the skin away from the paper tape and skin barrier wafer. b. Fold the old pouch over on itself and discard it in a plastic bag. c. Cleanse the peristomal skin with a wash cloth and warm tap water. d. Blot or pat the skin dry. e. Apply the new pouch to the abdomen, carefully centering the hole in the skin barrier wafer over the stoma. Press on the wafer for a few minutes. f. Secure the pouch by "picture framing" the wafer with four strips of hypo-allergenic paper tape (if the wafer does not already have a tape attached).	4. Correct pouch removal and attachment techniques minimize irritation and injury of the peristomal skin and ensure a tight, reliable seal between the pouch and skin.

(continued on page 536)

Interventions	Rationales

5. Teach the procedure for emptying a stoma pouch.
  a. Put some toilet paper in the toilet bowl and sit on the toilet seat.
  b. Remove the clamp from the tail of the pouch and carefully empty the pouch contents into the toilet.
  c. Clean the inside and outside of the pouch tail with toilet paper and squeeze ostomy appliance deodorant into the end of the pouch.
	5. Correct techniques can reduce spillage, soiling, and odor. Placing toilet paper in the bowl prevents water from splashing as the pouch contents are emptied.

6. Teach client the ostomy irrigation procedure.
 	
  a. Assemble all equipment:
    • Water container and water
    • Irrigating sleeves and stoma
    • Items for cleaning the skin and stoma
    • Way to dispose of old pouch
    • Clean pouch and closure
    • Skin care items
  b. Cleanse the stoma and surrounding skin with water and let dry. Observe their condition and color.
  c. Apply the irrigating sleeve and belt securely. If using a karaya washer, dampen and apply this first. You may lubricate the inside of the irrigation sleeve with oil to help the stool slide through the sleeve.
  d. Fill the irrigating container with about one quart of tepid water.
  e. Suspend the irrigating container so that the bottom of the container is even with the top of the shoulder.
 	
  f. Remove all air from the tubing.
 	
  g. Gently insert the irrigating cone into the stoma, holding it parallel to the floor. Start the water slowly. If water does not flow easily, try or check the following:
    • Slightly adjust the body position or the angle of the cone.
    • Check for kinks in the tubing from the irrigating container.
    • Check the height of the irrigating container.
    • Relax and take some deep breaths.
  h. Instill water into the bowel; the amount of fluid instillation varies. *Do not force water into the bowel.* If cramping occurs, if the flow of water stops, or if water is forcefully returning around the irrigating cone or catheter, stop the flow.
  i. If bloating or constipation develops, irrigate again on the same day with about ½ quart more water than previously, or use a mild laxative.
  j. Most of the stool should be released in about 15 minutes. When most of the stool is expelled, rinse the sleeve with water, dry the bottom edge, roll the sleeve up, and close the end.
  k. Allow 30–45 minutes more for the bowels to finish emptying.
  l. Remove the irrigation sleeve and apply a clean closed-end pouch or a stoma cover.
	6. The purpose of colostomy irrigation is to establish a regular bowel evacuation pattern; this makes a colostomy pouch unnecessary.
	  a. Assembling all equipment beforehand prevents delays during the procedure.
	
	  b. Thorough cleansing removes drainage from the skin.
	
	  c. Preapplication makes cleaning easier.
	
	  d. Hot water traumatizes the bowel; cold water causes cramping.
	  e. At a lower height, the water may not flow easily. Higher height would give too much force to the water, causing cramping or incomplete emptying.
	  f. Removing air from the tubing helps to prevent gas pains during irrigation.
	  g. Gentle and slow movements help reduce tissue trauma. Relaxation decreases muscle tension and resistance.
	
	  h. Forcing water can cause tissue damage.
	
	  i. Increasing the amount of water may promote evacuation.
	
	  j. The clamped irrigation sleeve acts as a temporary pouch until all stool is expelled.
	
	  k. Complete emptying helps to prevent later leakage.
	
	  l. Just a stoma cover is appropriate if the client can achieve total control by irrigation. Manufacturers are currently

(continued on page 537)

Interventions	Rationales
	testing stoma occluding devices that can be inserted and removed intermittently to allow fecal elimination; this would serve as an alternative to an external colostomy pouch.
m. Rinse the irrigation sleeve and hang it up to dry.	m. Thorough rinsing and drying decreases odor.

7. Teach strategies for prevention and management of potential peristomal skin problems:
  a. Shave peristomal skin with an electric razor rather than a blade; avoid using shaving cream, soap, and detergents except when showering.
  b. Evaluate all skin products for possible allergic reaction; patch-test all suspect products elsewhere on the abdomen.
  c. Do not change brands of skin barriers and adhesives casually; assess for allergic reaction before using a new brand.
  d. Avoid irritation from contact with ostomy effluent.
  e. Avoid prolonged skin pressure, especially if fair-skinned or with thin, atrophic skin due to long-term corticosteroid therapy.
  f. Use corticosteroid creams sparingly and briefly; they can cause dryness and irritation.
  g. If bacterial or fungal infection is suspected, use a specific antibacterial or antifungal cream or powder.
  h. Use a liquid film barrier; avoid a tincture of benzoin compound that can dry the skin.
  i. Avoid aluminum paste and greasy ointments that can mask skin problems and also interfere with pouch adherence.
  j. Protect the skin with barriers.
  k. Expect the stoma to shrink slightly over time. This necessitates re-measuring the stoma to ensure proper appliance fit.
	7. A client with a stoma is at increased risk for peristomal skin breakdown. Factors that influence skin integrity include composition, quantity, and consistency of the ostomy effluent; allergies; mechanical trauma; the underlying disease and its treatment (including medications); surgical construction and location of the stoma; the quality of ostomy and peristomal skin care; availability of proper supplies; nutritional status; overall health status; hygiene; and activity level.

8. Teach the procedure for perineal wound care:
  a. Take sitz baths or irrigate the area with warm water to cleanse the wound thoroughly.
  b. Wear a peripad to protect the wound and contain the drainage until the wound heals.
  c. Watch for and report signs and symptoms of infection or abscess (e.g., pain or purulent drainage).
  d. If the rectum is missing (e.g., due to ostomy), thermometers, suppositories, or other devices cannot be inserted.
	8. Removal of the rectum results in a large perineal wound that may be left open to heal by secondary intention. Some clients with a colostomy do not have the rectum and anus removed but have a rectal stump sutured across the top. This becomes a nonfunctioning internal pouch (Hartmann pouch). In this situation, the client continues to expel mucus through the anus, produced by the remaining rectal mucosa.

9. Address nutrition and diet management:
  a. Teach how the ostomy affects absorption and use of nutrients, and discuss dietary implications.
  b. Assess food tolerances by adding new foods one at a time and in small amounts.
  c. Teach the client to eat regularly and slowly, to chew food well, and to avoid high-fiber foods that can promote stomal blockage.
  d. Discuss dietary modifications that can help to decrease odor and flatus.
  e. List dietary modifications to prevent or manage diarrhea and constipation, as indicated.
	9. Proper nutritional intake and dietary management are important factors in ostomy management.

(continued on page 538)

Interventions	Rationales
f. Instruct the client to monitor weight and report any loss or gain of more than 10 pounds. g. Explain the importance of adequate fluid intake (water and juices) to prevent or manage fluid and electrolyte problems related to altered elimination.	

10. Explain the effects of certain medications on ostomy function:
  a. Antibiotics may induce diarrhea.
  b. Narcotics and aluminum- or calcium-containing antacids can promote constipation.
  c. Internal or external deodorizers can control fecal odor. Internal deodorizers may have a mild laxative effect.
  d. Suppositories cannot be used after the rectum and anus are removed.
Instruct the client to notify a physician or pharmacist if a drug problem is suspected.
	10. Counseling the client about the possible harmful effects of home remedies and of indiscriminate self-medication may help to prevent minor or serious problems.

11. Promote measures to help the client incorporate ostomy care into ADLs (Collett, 2002; Hyland, 2002; Pontieri-Lewis, 2006).
  a. *Working/traveling:* Keep extra supplies at work. When traveling, carry supplies rather than pack them in a suitcase and risk losing them; keep in mind that pectin-based wafers melt in high environmental temperatures. Take a list of ostomy supplies when traveling.
  b. *Exercise:* The only limits involve contact sports, during which trauma to the stoma may occur. Normal exercise is beneficial and may help to stimulate bowel evacuation and, in some cases, can eliminate the need for irrigation. Successful use of exercise to regulate the bowel depends on the presurgical bowel pattern and regularity of elimination. Other contributing factors include the consistency of the fecal contents, motivation, diet, ability to exercise, and practice.
  c. Bathing/showering/swimming: These activities may be done while wearing an ostomy appliance. "Picture-frame" the skin barrier with paper tape to seal the edges and keep the barrier edge from getting wet. Showering may be done without an appliance and, in fact, is recommended on days of appliance changes.
  d. *Wardrobe:* Ostomy appliances are invisible under clothing. Any clothing worn preoperatively may be worn postoperatively. Dress comfortably.
  e. More wardrobe tips:
    • Wear two pairs of underpants. The inside pair should be a low-rise or bikini-height cotton knit worn *under* the ostomy appliance to absorb perspiration and keep the pouch away from the skin. The outside pair can be cotton or nylon, should be waist high, and worn *over* the ostomy appliance.
    • The ostomy pouch can be tucked between the two pairs of underwear like a kangaroo pouch. Special pouch covers are expensive, soil rapidly, and are not necessary.
    • Avoid too-tight clothing that can restrict the appliance and cause leakage. A boxer-type bathing suit is preferable for men. For women, a patterned bathing suit with shirring can camouflage the appliance well.
	11. Successful incorporation of ostomy management into ADLs allows the client to resume his or her pre-colostomy life style and pursue goals and interests before surgery. If the ostomate had a strong supportive relationship before surgery, there usually are no problems after surgery (Haugen, Bliss, & Savik, 2006; Colwell & Beitz, 2007).

(continued on page 539)

Interventions	Rationales

f. Diet:
- Chew all food well.
- Noise from passing flatus will decrease postoperatively with progression to a regular diet.
- Eat on a regular schedule to help decrease the noise from an empty gut.
- Avoid mushrooms, Chinese vegetables, popcorn, and other foods that may cause blockage. (*Note:* Pillsbury microwave popcorn is specially made to be tolerated because adequate chewing can finely grind the kernels.)
- Keep in mind that fish, eggs, and onions cause odor in the stool.
- Drink at least several 8-oz glasses of water a day to prevent dehydration in an ileostomate and constipation in a colostomate. Concentrated urine or decreased urinary output is a good indicator of dehydration.

g. Odor control:
- Explain that odor is caused from bacteria in the stool.
- Because most ostomy appliances are made to be odor-proof, do not poke a hole in the ostomy appliance to allow flatus to escape; constant odor will result.
- Control offensive odors with good hygiene and ostomy pouch deodorants. (Super Banish appliance deodorant works best because it contains silver nitrate, which kills the bacteria.) Hydrogen peroxide and mouthwashes such as Binaca can be placed in the ostomy pouch as inexpensive appliance deodorants.
- Do not use aspirin tablets as a deodorant in the ostomy pouch; aspirin tablets coming in contact with the stoma may cause stomal irritation and bleeding.
- Avoid foods that increase flatus (beer, beans, cabbage, onions, and fish).
- Avoid foods that increase odor (onions, cabbage, eggs, fish, and beans).
- Eating yogurt and cranberry juice may help to reduce fecal odor. Certain oral medications reduce fecal odor, but these should be used only with the advice of a physician.

h. Hygiene:
- Use a hand-held shower spray to wash the skin around the stoma and irrigate perineal wounds.
- Showers can be taken with the ostomy appliance on or off. On days when the appliance is changed, a shower can be taken when the old pouch is removed, but before the new pouch is applied.
- The new pouch should be readied before getting in the shower. On days between appliance changes, showering with the appliance on requires only that the paper tape around the wafer be covered with a liquid sealant to waterproof the tape.

i. Exercise:
- Normal activities (even strenuous sports, in most cases) can be resumed after recovery from surgery.
- Be aware that increased incidence of peristomal herniation is associated with heavy lifting.
- Also keep in mind that increased perspiration from strenuous exercise may require more frequent ostomy appliance changes due to increased melting of the appliance skin barrier.

(continued on page 540)

Interventions	Rationales

j. Travel:
  • Take all ostomy supplies along when traveling; if by air, put them in a carry-on bag (Collett, 2002).
  • Do not leave ostomy appliances in automobiles parked in the sun, because the heat will melt the skin barrier.
  • When flying, always keep appliances in carry-on luggage to avoid loss.
k. Sexual activity:
  • Remember that an ostomy does not automatically make a person undesirable. On the other hand, as in any sexual encounter, the client may have to indicate sexual interest to his or her partner who may be afraid of hurting the ostomy.
  • Wearing a stretch tube top around the midriff will cover the ostomy appliance while leaving the genitals and breasts exposed.
  • If male impotence is a problem, the man can be referred to a urologist for discussion or investigation of a penile prosthesis.	

12. Discuss community resources/self-help groups, including: a. Visiting nurse b. United Ostomy Associations, www.uoaa.org c. National Foundation for Ileitis and Colitis (800-343-3637) d. American Cancer Foundation e. Community suppliers of ostomy equipment f. Financial reimbursement for ostomy equipment	12. Personal sources of information have been found to be more important than written materials (Richbourg, Thorpe, & Rapp, 2007).

Documentation

Discharge summary record
    Client and family teaching
    Response to teaching as well as achieved outcomes or the status of each goal

Coronary Artery Bypass Grafting

Indicated for clients with coronary artery disease, coronary artery bypass grafting (CABG) increases blood flow to the heart by either anastomosis of an autograft vessel (i.e., saphenous vein or inferior epigastric artery) to an area proximal and distal to the coronary artery occlusion, or by use of an autograft vessel (i.e., internal mammary or gastroepiploic artery) grafted distal to the coronary artery occlusion. Internal mammary grafts have a 90% patency rate at 10 years compared to 40%–60% for saphenous veins.

Surgery most often involves a median sternotomy incision with cardiopulmonary bypass, or extracorporeal circulation, to circulate and oxygenate the blood while diverting it from the heart and lungs to provide a bloodless operative field for the surgeon. A more recent trend in cardiac surgery is a minimally invasive procedure known as "off-pump coronary artery bypass," in which the heart is not stopped for suturing of the bypass graft(s). Cardiopulmonary bypass is not used; the incision is smaller and may have a thoracotomy approach; complications are reduced and recovery is faster (American Heart Association, 2007; Martin & Turkelson, 2006; Shatzer, George, & Wei, 2007).

Over the last few years, advancements have allowed the robot-assisted endoscopic CABG approach to expand with substantially less complications and more rapid recovery (Pike & Gundry, 2003).

 Time Frame
Preoperative and postoperative periods (not intensive care period)

■■■■■ DIAGNOSTIC CLUSTER

Preoperative Period

Nursing Diagnosis

▲ Fear (individual/family) related to the client's health status, need for coronary artery bypass graft surgery, and unpredictable outcome

Postoperative Period

Collaborative Problems

▲ PC: Cardiovascular Insufficiency
▲ PC: Respiratory Insufficiency
▲ PC: Renal Insufficiency
✳ PC: Hyperthermia
✳ PC: Postcardiotomy Delirium

Nursing Diagnoses

△ Fear related to transfer from intensive environment of the critical care unit and potential for complications

△ Interrupted Family Processes related to disruption of family life, fear of outcome (death, disability), and stressful environment (ICU)

△ High Risk for Disturbed Self-Concept related to the symbolic meaning of the heart and changes in life style

△ High Risk for Ineffective Therapeutic Regimen Management related to insufficient knowledge of incisional care, pain management (angina, incisions), signs and symptoms of complications, condition, pharmacologic care, risk factors, restrictions, stress management techniques, and follow-up care

▲ Impaired Comfort related to surgical incisions, chest tubes, and immobility secondary to lengthy surgery (refer to General Surgery)

Related Care Plans

General Surgery Generic care plan
Thoracic Surgery

▲ This diagnosis was reported to be monitored for or managed frequently (75%–100%).
△ This diagnosis was reported to be monitored for or managed often (50%–74%).
✳ This diagnosis was not included in the validation study.

Discharge Criteria

Before discharge, the client and family will

1. Demonstrate insertion site care.
2. Relate at-home restrictions and follow-up care.
3. State signs and symptoms that must be reported to a health care professional.
4. Relate a plan to reduce risk factors, as necessary.

Preoperative: Nursing Diagnosis

Fear (Individual/Family) Related to the Client's Health Status, Need for Coronary Artery Bypass Graft Surgery, and Unpredictable Outcome

NOC Anxiety Control, Fear Control

Goals

The client or family will verbalize concerns regarding surgery.

Indicators

- Verbalize, if asked, what to expect before surgery (e.g., routines and tests).
- Verbalize, if asked, an understanding of the CABG procedure.
- Verbalize, if asked, what to expect post-CABG (e.g., monitoring and care).
- Demonstrate postoperative exercises, turning, splinting, and respiratory regimen.

NIC Anxiety Reduction, Coping Enhancement, Presence, Counseling

Interventions	Rationales
1. Reinforce previous teaching about coronary artery disease, as necessary.	1–6. Preoperative teaching provides information to help reduce the client's and family's fears of the unknown, and enhance their sense of control over the situation (Kirkeby-Garstad et al., 2006).
2. Reinforce, as necessary, the physician's explanation of CABG surgery and why it is needed. Notify the physician if additional explanation is indicated.	
3. Explain necessary preoperative tests and procedures, such as the following: a. 12-Lead electrocardiogram (ECG) b. Chest x-ray film c. Cardiac catheterization d. Urinalysis e. Blood work: electrolytes, coagulation studies, complete blood count, type and cross-match f. Nuclear studies, if indicated	
4. Provide instruction about preoperative routines beyond those of general surgery, such as the following: a. Chlorhexidine gluconate (Hibiclens or Betadine) shower the night before and the morning of surgery b. Sending belongings home with family members c. Measures in operating room holding area: skin preparation, IV and other invasive line insertions, and indwelling (Foley) catheter insertion	
5. Discuss postoperative measures, routines, and expectations, including the following (Kirkeby-Garstad et al., 2006): a. Endotracheal intubation and mechanical ventilation b. Chest tubes c. Multiple IV lines d. Sedative the evening before e. Pulmonary artery catheter f. Arterial line g. Epidural cardiac pacing h. Cardiac monitoring i. Indwelling urinary catheter j. Autotransfusion/blood replacement k. Weight increase	

(continued on page 543)

Interventions	Rationales

l. Nasogastric tube
m. Pain
n. Frequent assessment of vital signs, dressing, heart and lung sounds, peripheral pulses, skin, and capillary refill time
o. TEDs stockings
 	
6. Discuss expectations for intensive care (Kirkeby-Garstad et al., 2006):
  a. Environment, noises
  b. Length of stay
  c. Care measures
  d. Visiting policies
  e. Early ambulation (Kirkeby-Garstad et al., 2006)
  f. Cough and deep breathing exercises/incentive spirometry (Kirkeby-Garstad et al., 2006)	

7. Explain specific pain-relief measures that will be used and the comfort level goals (e.g., splinting) (Kirkeby-Garstad et al., 2006)	7. Knowledge of the pain expected and the ability to control pain can reduce fear and increase pain tolerance (Kirkeby-Garstad et al., 2006).
8. Discuss possible emotional and mental reactions post-CABG surgery.	8. The heart is a symbol of life; cardiac dysfunction and surgery typically invoke a profound emotional reaction. Anesthesia, fluid loss from surgery, and pain medications can temporarily cloud thinking.
9. Present information or reinforce learning using written materials (e.g., booklets, posters, or instruction sheets) and audiovisual aids (e.g., slides, videotapes, models, or diagrams).	9. Using various teaching materials and approaches provides multisensory stimulation that can enhance effectiveness of teaching and learning and improve retention.
10. Offer a tour of intensive care unit.	10. Individuals who have a preoperative tour of ICU report a benefit from the experience (Lynn-McHale, Wiegand, & Carlson, 1997).

Documentation

Progress notes
  Present emotional status
  Interventions
  Response to interventions
Client teaching record or discharge summary record
  Client and family teaching
  Response to teaching
  Outcome achievement or status

Postoperative: Collaborative Problems

Potential Complication: Cardiovascular Insufficiency

Potential Complication: Respiratory Insufficiency

Potential Complication: Renal Insufficiency

Potential Complication: Hyperthermia

Potential Complication: Postcardiotomy Delirium

Nursing Goal

The nurse will detect early signs and symptoms of (a) cardiovascular insufficiency, (b) respiratory insufficiency, (c) renal insufficiency, (d) hyperthermia, and (e) postcardiotomy delirium, and will collaboratively intervene to stabilize the client.

Indicators

- Oriented, calm (a, b, c, d, e)
- No change in vision (a)
- Normal sinus rhythm (EKG) (a, b)
- Heart rate 60–100 beats/min (a, b)
- BP >90/60, <140/90 mmHg (a, b)
- No complaints of syncope, palpitations (a, b)
- Mean arterial pressure 70/90 mmHg (a, b)
- Pulmonary artery wedge pressure 4–12 mmHg (a, b)
- Cardiac output/index >2.4 (a, b)
- Pulmonary artery systolic pressure 20–30 mmHg (a, b)
- Pulmonary artery diastolic pressure 10–15 mmHg (a, b)
- Temperature 98–99.5°F (d)
- Minimal change in pulse pressure (a, b)
- Respirations 16–20 breaths/min (a, b)
- Urine output >5 mL/kg/h (a, b, c)
- Capillary refill <3 seconds (a, b)
- Skin warm, no pallor, cyanosis, or grayness (a, b)
- No complaints of palpitations, syncope, chest pain (a, b)
- No neck vein distension (a, b)
- Cardiac enzymes (a)
  - Myoglobin up to 85 ng/mL
  - Creatine phosphokinase (CK)
    - Male 50–325 mU/mL
    - Female 50–250 mU/mL
  - Troponin complex (C, I, T)
  - Hemoglobin (a)
    - Males 13–18 gm/dL
    - Females 12–16 gm/dL
  - Hematocrit (a)
    - Males 42%–50%
    - Females 40%–48%
- Partial thromboplastin time (PTT) 20–45 seconds (a)
- International Normalized Ratio (INR) 1.0 (a)
- Platelets 100,000–400,000/mm³ (a)
- Prothrombin time (PT) >20 seconds (a)
- Urine specific gravity 1.005–1.025 (a, b, c)
- Blood urea nitrogen 8–20 mg/dL (a, b, c)
- Creatinine 0.6–1.2 mg/dL (c)
- Potassium 3.5–5.0 mEq/L (c)
- Magnesium 1.84–3.0 mEq/L (c)
- Sodium 135–145 mEq/L (c)
- Calcium 8.5–10.5 mg/dL (c)
- Oxygen saturation (SaO$_2$) 4–100 mmHg (a, b)
- Carbon dioxide (PaCO$_2$) 35–45 mmHg (a, b)
- pH 7.35–7.45 (a, b)
- Relaxed, regular, deep, rhythmic respirations (a, b)
- No rales, crackles, wheezing (b)
- Wound approximated, minimal drainage (d)
- Chest tube drainage <200 mL/h (d)
- Full, easy to palpate pulses (a, b)
- No evidence of petechiae (pinpoint round, reddish lesions) or ecchymoses (bruises) (a)
- No seizure activity (a, d, e)

Interventions	Rationales

1. Monitor for the following as per unit standard (Martin & Turkelson, 2006):
  a. Dysrhythmias, abnormal rate or conduction
  b. ECG changes: ST segment depression or elevation; T-wave changes; PR, QRS, or QT interval changes
  c. Peripheral pulses (pedal, tibial, popliteal, femoral, radial, brachial)
  d. Blood pressure (arterial, left atrial, pulmonary artery)
  e. Pulmonary artery diastolic pressure (PAD)
  f. Pulmonary artery wedge pressure (PAWP)
  g. Cardiac output/index
  h. Cardiac enzymes daily (e.g., creatine phosphokinase, troponin complex)
  i. Urine output
  j. Skin color, temperature
  k. Capillary refill
  l. Palpitations
  m. Syncope
  n. Cardiac emergencies (e.g., arrest or ventricular fibrillation)
	1. Myocardial ischemia results from reduction of oxygen to myocardial tissue. Ischemic muscle is electrically unstable, leading to dysrhythmias. Dysrhythmias also may result from surgical manipulation, hypothermia, and acidosis. Atrial dysrhythmias may also be due to mechanical remodeling or injury or conductive delays (Porth, 2005).

2. Monitor select electrolytes (Porth, 2005):
 	
  a. Potassium
 	
  b. Magnesium
 	
  c. Sodium
  d. Calcium
	2. Specific levels of electrolytes are necessary for both extracellular and intracellular body fluids
	  a. Inadequate intake, diuretics, vomiting, nasogastric drainage, and stress can decrease potassium. Renal insufficiency, increased intake, tissue necrosis, and adrenal cortical insufficiency can increase potassium levels.
	  b. Decreased intake, alcoholism, excess intake of calcium, and increased excretion after surgery; diabetic ketoacidosis; primary aldosteronism; and primary hyperparathyroidism cause decreased magnesium levels. Renal failure and excess intake of medications with magnesium (antacids, cathartics) increase magnesium levels.
	  c. Increased water intake causes decreased sodium levels.
	  d. Alkalosis and multiple transfusions of citrated blood products cause low calcium levels. Prolonged immobility causes increased calcium levels.

3. Monitor for signs and symptoms of hypotension and low cardiac output syndrome (Martin & Turkelson, 2006):
  a. Cardiac index <2.4
  b. Increased pulmonary arteriole wedge pressure (PAWP)
  c. Increased central venous pressure (CVP)
  d. SvO_2 <60%
  e. Development of S_3 or S_4
  f. Neck vein distention
  g. Decreased systolic BP (90 mmHg or 30 mmHg below baseline)
  h. Irregular pulse
  i. Cool, moist skin
  j. Decreased urine output (<5 mL/kg/h)
  k. Increased pulse and respirations
  l. Increased restlessness
  m. Lethargy or confusion
  n. Increased rales/crackles
  o. Weak peripheral pulses
	3. These effects can result from severe pain or greatly reduced cardiac output secondary to severe tissue hypoxia; inadequate preload and inadequate myocardial contractility; dysrhythmias; and ventricular failure. Decreased circulating volume and cardiac output can lead to kidney hypoperfusion and overall decreased tissue perfusion, triggering a compensatory response of decreased circulation to the extremities and increased heart and respiratory rates. Cerebral hypoperfusion also may result.

(continued on page 546)

Interventions	Rationales

4. Monitor for signs and symptoms of cardiac tamponade:
   a. Decreased systolic BP (90 mmHg or 30 mmHg below baseline)
   b. Muffled heart sounds
   c. Pericardial friction rub
   d. Pulsus paradoxus
   e. Kussmaul respirations
   f. Neck vein distention
   g. Narrowing pulse pressure
   h. Anginal pain
   i. Restlessness or stupor
   j. Equalizing CVP and pulmonary arterial wedge pressure (PAWP)
   k. Significant increase in or cessation of chest tube drainage
   l. Decreased electrocardiograph (ECG) voltage
	4. Cardiac tamponade is a condition in which excess fluid collects within the pericardial space and impairs cardiac filling. It occurs because of graft leakage, inadequate hemostasis, or inadequate chest tube drainage (Porth, 2005).

5. Monitor for signs and symptoms of respiratory failure:
   a. Increased respiratory rate
   b. Dyspnea
   c. Use of accessory muscles of respiration
   d. Cyanosis
   e. Increasing crackles or wheezing
   f. Increased pCO_2, decreased O_2 saturation, decreased pH
   g. Decreased SvO_2
   h. Restlessness
   i. Decreased capillary refill time >3 seconds
	5. In the immediate postoperative period, hypoventilation may result from central nervous system depression caused by narcotics and anesthesia, impaired respiratory effort resulting from pain, fatigue, and immobility, or incomplete reinflation of lungs collapsed during surgery. Pulmonary dysfunction occurs in 30%–60% of postoperative CABG clients (Martin & Turkelson, 2006).

6. Monitor for signs and symptoms of hypertension or hypervolemia (Martin & Turkelson, 2006):
   a. Systolic blood pressure >140 mmHg
   b. Diastolic blood pressure >90 mmHg
   c. Mean arterial pressure >90 mmHg
   d. Increased systemic vascular resistance
	6. Hypervolemia and hypertension can result from a response to circulating catecholamines and renin secretion following cardiopulmonary bypass, which causes sodium and water retention. Hypertension can lead to bleeding at anastomosis sites (Martin & Turkelson, 2006).

7. Monitor for signs and symptoms of hemorrhage or hypovolemia:
   a. Incisional bleeding
   b. Chest tube drainage >200 mL/h
   c. Increased heart rate, decreased blood pressure, increased respirations
   d. Weak or absent peripheral pulses
   e. Cool, moist skin
   f. Dizziness
   g. Petechiae
   h. Ecchymoses
   i. Bleeding gums
   j. Decreased hemoglobin and hematocrit
   k. Increased prothrombin time (PT), partial thromboplastin time (PTT), international normalized ratio (INR), and decreased platelet count
	7. Hemorrhage can be caused by inadequate surgical hemostasis, inadequate heparin reversal, or hypertension.

8. Monitor for signs and symptoms of myocardial infarction:
   a. Chest pain or pressure
   b. Increased heart rate
   c. Hypotension
   d. Tachypnea
	8. Cardiac pain results from cardiac tissue hypoxia secondary to narrowing or blockage of the coronary arteries, increased myocardial oxygen consumption, or collapse of the newly grafted bypass.

(continued on page 547)

Interventions	Rationales

e. Abnormal heart sounds
f. Restlessness, lethargy, or confusion
g. Elevated CVP and PAWP
h. Nausea and vomiting
i. ECG changes: ST segment elevation, abnormal Q waves
j. Increased cardiac enzymes
k. Decreased SvO$_2$
l. Neck vein distention
m. Weak peripheral pulses
n. Moist, cool skin
o. Decreased urine output (<0.5 mL/kg/h)

---

9. Monitor for signs and symptoms of renal failure (Martin & Turkelson, 2006):
   a. Elevated BUN, creatinine, and potassium
   b. Decreased urine output (<0.5 mL/kg/h)
   c. Elevated urine specific gravity (>1.030)
   d. Weight gain
   e. Elevated CVP and PAP

9. Cardiopulmonary bypass causes destruction of some red blood cells (RBCs), producing free hemoglobin that may occlude renal arteries. Hypovolemia or poor myocardial contractility may decrease circulation to the kidneys, resulting in hypoperfusion and eventual renal failure.

---

10. Monitor for signs and symptoms of cerebrovascular accident (stroke):
    a. Unequal pupil size and reaction
    b. Paralysis or paresthesias in extremities
    c. Decreased level of consciousness
    d. Dizziness
    e. Blurred vision
    f. Seizure activity
    g. Slurred speech
    h. Confusion
    i. Altered motor and sensory function (Martin & Turkelson, 2006)

10. CVA may result from embolization or hypoperfusion that obstructs or interrupts blood flow to the central nervous system.

---

11. Monitor for signs and symptoms of postcardiotomy delirium:
    a. Disorientation
    b. Confusion
    c. Hallucinations or delusions

11. This disorder may result from surgery-related microemboli, sensory overload or deprivation, altered sleep pattern, hypoxia, medications, metabolic disorders, or hypotension.

---

12. Monitor for hyperthermia:
    a. Increased temperature
    b. Increased heart rate
    c. Hypotension

12. Hyperthermia can indicate infection or postpericardiotomy syndrome (pericarditis) (Porth, 2005).

---

13. Assess readiness for early extubation (Martin & Turkelson, 2006).

13. Early extubation promotes reduced pulmonary complications (Martin & Turkelson, 2006).

---

14. Monitor for gastrointestinal (GI) complications (Martin & Turkelson, 2006)
    a. GI bleeding
    b. Decreased Hct & Hgb
    c. Reduced or absent bowel sounds
    d. Nausea & vomiting
    e. Abdominal distention
    f. Nasogastric tube output

14. GI complications occur in 0.12%–2% of clients and include: peptic ulcer disease, perforated ulcer, pancreatitis, bowel ischemia, diverticulitis, acute cholecystitis, and liver failure (Martin & Turkelson, 2006).

---

15. Monitor for sleep disturbance (Martin & Turkelson, 2006)

15. Sleep disturbances can result from poor pain control. Sleep deprivation can lead to negative outcomes (Martin & Turkelson, 2006).

Related Physician-Prescribed Interventions

Medications. Antibiotics, anticoagulants, analgesics, stool softeners, diuretics, beta-blockers, aspirin (postoperatively), antidysrhythmics, calcium-channel blockers, H_2 blockers, vasoactive medications

Intravenous Therapy. Fluid/electrolyte replacement

Laboratory Studies. Complete blood count, arterial blood gas analysis, glucose, creatinine, cardiac enzymes, amylase, electrolytes, BUN, blood chemistry profile, coagulation levels

Diagnostic Studies. Ear/pulse oximetry, chest x-ray film, ECG, cardiac echocardiogram, cardiac catheterization

Nuclear Studies. Egthallium-221

Therapies. Supplemental oxygen, pulse oximetry, hemodynamic monitoring and others, dependent on symptomatology

Documentation

Flow records
   Vital signs
   Cardiac rhythm
   Peripheral pulses
   Skin color, temperature, moisture
   Neck vein distention
   Respiratory assessment
   Neurologic assessment
   Intake (oral, IVs, blood products)
   Incisions (color, drainage, swelling)
   Output (chest tubes, nasogastric tube)
   Bowel function (bowel sounds, distention)
   Sputum (amount, tenaciousness, color)
Progress notes
   Change in physiologic status
   Interventions
   Response to interventions

Postoperative: Nursing Diagnoses

Fear Related to Transfer From Intensive Environment of the Critical Care Unit and Potential for Complications

 NOC Anxiety Control, Fear Control

Goal

The client will report a decreased level of anxiety or fear.

Indicators

• Verbalize any concerns regarding the completed surgery, possible complications, and the critical care environment.
• Verbalize the intent to share fears with one person after discharge.

NIC Anxiety Reduction, Coping Enhancement, Presence, Counseling

Interventions	Rationales

1. Take steps to reduce the client's levels of anxiety and fear.
  a. Reassure the client that you or other nurses are always close by and will respond promptly to requests.
  b. Convey a sense of empathy and understanding.
	1. Reducing anxiety, fear, and stress can decrease demands made on an already compromised heart.

(continued on page 549)

Interventions	Rationales
c. Minimize external stimuli (e.g., close the room door, dim the lights, speak in a quiet voice, decrease the volume level of equipment alarms, and position equipment so that alarms are diverted away from the client). d. Plan care measures to provide adequate periods of uninterrupted rest and sleep. e. Promote relaxation; encourage regular rest periods throughout the day. f. Explain each procedure before performing it.	
2. Encourage the client to verbalize concerns and fears. Clarify any misconceptions and provide positive feedback regarding progress.	2. This sharing allows the nurse to correct any erroneous information the client may believe, and to assure the client that concerns and fears are normal; this may help to reduce anxiety.
3. Encourage the client to identify and call on reliable support persons, and to recall coping mechanisms that have worked well in the past.	3. Support persons and coping mechanisms are important factors in anxiety reduction.
4. Consult with the physician for medications, as necessary.	4. Pharmacologic assistance may be necessary if anxiety is at an unmanageable level; severe pain may also be interfering with the client's ability to cope.
5. Prepare the client for progression through the intensive care unit (ICU) and for stepdown to the general care unit.	5. Explanations can prevent serious complications related to unexpected relocations or transfers.

Documentation

Progress notes
    Present emotional status
    Interventions
    Response to interventions

Interrupted Family Processes Related to Disruption of Family Life, Fear of Outcome (Death, Disability), and Stressful Environment (ICU)

NOC Family Coping, Family Environment: Internal, Family Normalization, Parenting

Goal

The family members or significant others will report continued adequate family functioning during the client's hospitalization.

Indicators

- Verbalize concerns regarding CABG outcome and client prognosis.
- Verbalize concerns regarding the discharge.

NIC Family Involvement Promotion, Coping Enhancement, Family Integrity Promotion, Family Therapy, Counseling, Referral

Interventions	Rationales
1. Spend time with family members or significant others and convey a sense of empathetic understanding.	1. Frequent contact and communicating a sense of caring and concern can help to reduce stress and promote learning.
2. Allow family members or significant others to express their feelings, fears, and concerns.	2. Sharing allows the nurse to identify fears and concerns, then plan interventions to address them.

(continued on page 550)

Interventions	Rationales
3. Explain the ICU environment and equipment.	3,4. This information can help to reduce anxiety associated with the unknown.
4. Explain expected postoperative care measures and progress, and provide specific information on the client's progress, as appropriate.	
5. Teach family members or significant others ways in which they can be more supportive (e.g., show them how they can touch the client; encourage them to talk with and touch the client and to maintain a sense of humor, as appropriate).	5. This information can ease fears associated with doing or saying the wrong thing and can promote normal interaction with the client.
6. Encourage frequent visits and participation in care measures.	6. Frequent visits and participation in care can promote continued family interaction and support.
7. Consult with, or provide referrals to, community and other resources (e.g., social service agency) as necessary.	7. Families with problems such as financial needs, unsuccessful coping, or unresolved conflicts may need additional resources to help maintain family functioning.

Documentation

Progress notes
    Present family functioning
    Interventions
    Response to interventions
Discharge summary record
    Referrals, if indicated

High Risk for Disturbed Self-Concept Related to the Symbolic Meaning of the Heart and Changes in Life Style

NOC Quality of Life, Depression Level, Self-Esteem, Coping

Goal

The client will demonstrate healthy coping skills.

Indicators

• Report realistic changes in life style.
• Appraise situation realistically.

NIC Hope Instillation, Mood Management, Values Clarification, Counseling, Referral, Support Group, Coping Enhancement

Interventions	Rationales
1. Encourage the client to express feelings and concerns about necessary life style changes and changes in level of functioning.	1. Sharing gives nurse the opportunity to correct misconceptions, provide realistic feedback, and reassure the client that his or her concerns are normal.
2. Stress the client's role in preventing recurrence of athero-sclerosis. Emphasize steps the client can take and encourage progress.	2. The client's knowledge of control over the situation can enhance ego strength. Stressing the positive promotes hope and reduces frustration.

(continued on page 551)

Interventions	Rationales
3. Allow the client to make choices regarding daily activities.	3. A decrease in power in one area can be counterbalanced by providing opportunities for choices and control in other areas.
4. Encourage the client to participate actively in the care regimen.	4. Participation in self-care mobilizes the client and promotes decision-making, which enhances self-concept.
5. Identify a client at risk for poor ego adjustment (Shipes, 1987): a. Poor ego strength b. Ineffective problem-solving ability c. Difficulty learning new information or skills d. Lack of motivation e. External locus of control f. Poor health g. Unsatisfactory preoperative sex life h. Lack of positive support systems i. Unstable economic status j. Rejection of counseling	5. Successful adjustment to CABG surgery is influenced by factors such as the following: a. Previous coping success b. Achievement of development tasks before surgery c. The extent to which resulting life style changes interfere with goal-directed activity d. Sense of control over the situation e. Realistic perceptions by the client and support persons
6. Refer an at-risk client for counseling.	6. Follow-up therapy is indicated to assist with effective adjustment.

High Risk for Ineffective Therapeutic Regimen Management Related to Insufficient Knowledge of Incisional Care, Pain Management (Angina, Incisions), Signs and Symptoms of Complications, Condition, Pharmacologic Care, Risk Factors, Restrictions, Stress Management Techniques, and Follow-up Care

NOC Compliance Behavior, Knowledge: Treatment Regimen, Participation: Health Care Decisions, Treatment Behavior. Illness or Injury

Goal

The goals for this diagnosis represent those associated with discharge planning. Refer to the discharge criteria.

NIC Anticipatory Guidance, Risk Identification, Health Education, Learning Facilitation

Interventions	Rationales
1. Explain and demonstrate care of uncomplicated surgical incisions. a. Wash with soap and water (bath and shower, as permitted; use lukewarm water). b. Wear loose clothing until incision areas are no longer tender.	1. Correct technique is needed to reduce the risk of infection.
2. Provide instruction for pain management. a. For incision pain (sore, sharp, stabbing): • Take pain medication as prescribed and before activities that cause discomfort. • Continue to use the splinting technique, as needed.	2. a. Adequate instruction in pain management can reduce the fear of pain by providing a sense of control. Combining analgesics and nonsteroidal anti-inflammatory agents may increase the effectiveness of pain management (Martin & Turkelson, 2006).

(continued on page 552)

Interventions	Rationales
b. For angina (tightness, squeezing, pressure, pain, or mild ache in chest; indigestion; choking sensation; pain in jaw, neck, and between shoulder blades; numbness, tingling, and aching in either arm or hand): • Stop whatever you are doing and sit down. • Take nitroglycerin, as prescribed (e.g., one tablet every 5 minutes sublingually until pain subsides or a maximum of three tablets have been taken). • If pain is unrelieved by three nitroglycerin tablets, call for immediate transportation to the emergency room.	b. Angina is a symptom of cardiac tissue hypoxia. Immediate rest reduces the tissues' oxygen requirements. Nitroglycerin causes coronary vasodilation, which increases coronary blood flow in an attempt to increase myocardial oxygen supply.
3. Provide instruction regarding the client's condition and reduction of risk factors. a. Reinforce the purpose and outcome of CABG surgery. b. Explain the risk factors that need to be eliminated or reduced (e.g., obesity, smoking, high cholesterol, sedentary life style, regular heavy alcohol intake, excessive stress, hypertension, or uncontrolled diabetes mellitus).	3. Surgery does not replace the need to reduce risk factors. a. Preoperative anxiety may have interfered with retention of preoperative teaching. b. Emphasizing those risk factors that can be reduced may decrease the client's sense of powerlessness regarding those factors that cannot be reduced, such as heredity.
4. Teach the client about safe and effective weight loss methods, if indicated. Consult a dietitian, and refer the client to appropriate community resources.	4. Weight reduction reduces peripheral resistance and cardiac output.
5. Provide instruction about smoking cessation, if indicated; refer to a community program.	5. Smoking's immediate effects include vasoconstriction and decreased blood oxygenation, elevated blood pressure, increased heart rate, and possible dysrhythmias, and increased cardiac workload. Long-term effects include an increased risk of coronary artery disease and myocardial infarction. Smoking also contributes to hypertension, peripheral vascular disease (e.g., leg ulcers), and chronically abnormal arterial blood gases (low oxygen, or PO_2, and high carbon dioxide, or PCO_2).
6. Teach about a low-fat, high-fiber, low-cholesterol diet; consult with a dietitian.	6. A low-fat, high-fiber, and low-cholesterol diet can reduce or prevent arteriosclerosis in some clients.
7. Provide instruction in a progressive activity program. a. Increase activity gradually. b. Consult with a physical therapist and cardiac rehabilitation specialist. c. Schedule frequent rest periods throughout the day for the first 6–8 weeks. Balance periods of activity with periods of rest. d. Consult with the physician before resuming work, driving, strenuous recreational activities (e.g., jogging, golfing, and other sports), and travel (airplane or automobile). e. Try to get 8–10 hours of sleep each night. f. Avoid isometric exercises (e.g., lifting anything over 10 lb). Avoid pushing anything weighing more than 10 lb (e.g., vacuum cleaner, grocery cart) for 6–8 weeks. g. Limit stair climbing to once or twice a day.	7. a. Progressive regular exercise increases cardiac stroke volume, thus increasing the heart's efficiency without greatly altering rate. b. These professionals can provide specific guidelines. c. Rest periods reduce myocardial oxygen demands. d. Caution is needed to reduce risk of myocardial hypoxia from overexertion. e. Sleep allows the body restorative time. f. Isometric exercises and straining increase cardiac workload and peripheral resistance. They also place stress on the healing sternum. g. Stair climbing increases cardiac workload.

(continued on page 553)

Interventions	Rationales
8. Provide instructions for stress management strategies (Cheng et al., 2005). a. Identify stressors. b. Avoid stressors, if possible. c. Use techniques to reduce stress response (e.g., deep breathing, progressive relaxation, guided imagery, or exercise within postoperative constraints).	8. Although the relationship of stress and atherosclerotic changes is not clear, stress may increase cardiac workload.
9. Provide instructions for sexual activity. a. Consult with the physician about when sexual activity can be resumed. b. Rest before and after engaging in sexual activity. c. Stop sexual activity if angina occurs. d. Try different positions to decrease exertion (e.g., both partners side-lying or the client on bottom). e. If prescribed, take nitroglycerin before sexual activity. f. Avoid sexual activity in very hot or cold temperatures, within 2 hours of eating or drinking, when tired, after alcohol intake, with an unfamiliar partner, and in an unfamiliar environment.	9. Although resumption of sexual activity is encouraged, the client needs specific instructions focusing on reducing cardiac workload and avoiding certain situations that increase anxiety or vasoconstriction.
10. Provide instructions regarding prescribed medications (i.e., purpose, dosage and administration techniques, and possible side effects).	10. Understanding can help to improve compliance and reduce the risk of overdose and morbidity.
11. Teach the client and family to report these signs and symptoms of complications to the physician: a. Redness, drainage, warmth, or increasing pain at incision site b. Increasing weakness, fatigue c. Elevated temperature d. Anginal pain e. Difficulty breathing f. Weight gain exceeding 3 lb in one day or 5 lb in one week g. Calf swelling, tenderness, warmth, or pain h. Dehiscence (Cheng et al., 2005)	11. Early reporting of complications enables prompt interventions to minimize their severity. a–c. These signs and symptoms may indicate infection. Wounds from graft donation sites may be more painful than the sternotomy site; endovascular harvesting reduces these risks (Cheng et al., 2005). d. Anginal pain indicates myocardial hypoxia. e,f. Difficulty breathing and abnormal weight gain may point to fluid retention. g. These signs and symptoms may indicate thrombophlebitis.
12. Provide information regarding community services (e.g., American Heart Association, "Mended Hearts Club").	12. Community resources after discharge can assist with adaptation and self-help strategies (Cheng et al., 2005), including home health and telehealth interventions (Barnason, Zimmerman, Nieveen, & Hertzog, 2006).

Documentation

Discharge summary record
    Client and family teaching
    Response to teaching
    Referrals, if indicated

For a Care Map on Cardiac Surgery, visit http://thePoint.lww.com.

Cranial Surgery

Cranial surgery involves surgical access through the skull to the intracranial structures; the approach depends on the location of the lesion or trauma. The surgical procedure can be done only by using a method referred to as "burr holes," by procedures called craniotomy (sometimes this is done while the client is awake, as with brain mapping) (American Association of Neuroscience Nurses [AANN], 2006), or by decompressive craniectomy which entails removal of bone (this is to allow the brain to swell to minimize secondary injury in traumatic brain injury cases, the bone flap in these cases is left off in the acute phase and replaced at a later date with metal plates).

Cranial surgery is indicated to remove a tumor, control hemorrhage, remove a hematoma, or to clip or coil aneurysms and arteriovenous malformations (vascular abnormalities), or as an emergent procedure to reduce increased intracranial pressure (Wright, 2007, p. 1174; AANN, 2006; Reddy, 2006; Lejeune & Howard-Fain, 2002). In cranial surgeries to remove brain tumors and repair arteriovenous malformations, the bone flap is generally replaced at the end of the surgery (Wagner, Johnson, & Kidd, 2006, p. 454; Wright, 2007, p. 1178).

 Time Frame
Preoperative and postoperative periods
Post intensive care unit

■■■■■■ DIAGNOSTIC CLUSTER

Preoperative Period

Nursing Diagnosis

△ Anxiety related to impending surgery and perceived negative effects on life style

Postoperative Period

Collaborative Problems

▲ PC: Increased Intracranial Pressure
▲ PC: Brain Hemorrhage, Hematoma, Hygroma
▲ PC: Cranial Nerve Dysfunctions
▲ PC: Fluid/Electrolyte Imbalances
△ PC: Meningitis/Encephalitis
▲ PC: Sensory/Motor Losses
▲ PC: Cerebral/Cerebellar Dysfunction
▲ PC: Hypo or Hyperthermia
△ PC: Diabetes Insipidus
△ PC: SIADH
▲ PC: Cerebrospinal Fluid (CSF) Leaks
▲ PC: Seizures
✳ PC: Cardiac Dysrhythmias

Nursing Diagnoses

▲ Acute Pain related to compression/displacement of brain tissue and increased intracranial pressure

△ High Risk for Impaired Corneal Tissue Integrity related to inadequate lubrication secondary to tissue edema

△ High Risk for Ineffective Therapeutic Regimen Management related to insufficient knowledge of wound care, signs and symptoms of complications, restrictions, and follow-up care

Related Care Plan

General Surgery Generic care plan

▲ This diagnosis was reported to be monitored for or managed frequently (75%–100%).
△ This diagnosis was reported to be monitored for or managed often (50%–74%).
✳ This diagnosis was not included in the validation study.

Discharge Criteria

Before discharge, the client or family will

1. Explain surgical site care, discussing signs and symptoms of wound infection (AANN, 2006).
2. Discuss management of activities of daily living (ADLs). This would include ensuring the client's support systems (i.e., physical therapy, occupational therapy, and social services) and potential discharge needs are assessed prior to discharge (AANN, 2006).
3. Verbalize precautions to take for medication use.
4. State the signs and symptoms that must be reported to a health care professional.
5. Ensure that the client has follow-up appointments scheduled at approximately 10–14 days postsurgery for suture or staple removal, and at 6–8 weeks to discuss progress, medications, further treatment, imaging plans, driving, and work issues, etc., as indicated (AANN, 2006, p, 28–29; Wright, 2007, p. 1180).

Preoperative: Nursing Diagnosis

Anxiety Related to Impending Surgery and Perceived Negative Effects on Life Style

NOC Anxiety Reduction, Coping, Impulse Control

Goal

The client will verbalize decreased anxiety related to impending surgery.

Indicators

- State the reason for the surgery and verbalize (as well as sign) the informed consent for it (Wright, 2007, p. 1176).
- Describe postoperative restrictions.

NIC Anxiety Reduction, Impulse Control Training, Anticipatory Guidance

Interventions	Rationales
1. Elicit from the client and family their concerns regarding a. Surgical procedure b. Prognosis c. Postoperative period d. Function (loss or return) e. Current disability	1. Studies show that these concerns were most frequently cited (Hickey, 2003).
2. Ensure that the client understands the effects of disease on the affected brain area and the need for surgery.	2. This information can help the client accept the need for surgery and ready him- or herself psychologically, which may reduce anxiety.
3. Explain the specific postoperative experiences, which may include the following: a. A large head dressing b. Swollen eyes c. Tracheostomy or endotracheal intubation d. Intracranial pressure monitoring equipment (AANN, 2006) e. Ventriculostomy drainage system (AANN, 2006) f. Nerve deficits (may be temporary or permanent) (AANN, 2006)	3. Knowing what to expect can reduce anxiety associated with the unknown.
4. Discuss the possibility of cognitive and behavioral changes related to the site of surgery. a. Frontal: • lack of spontaneity and initiative	4. Cognitive and behavioral changes have been reported in 50%–70% of clients postcraniotomy (Hickey, 2003).

(continued on page 556)

Interventions	Rationales

- child-likeness
- impulsivity
- decreased concentration and attention
- loss of recent memory
- inability to plan/organize
b. Temporal:
  - Dyssomnia
  - Aphasia
  - Test-taking deficits
  - Impairments
  - Apathy
  - Placidity
c. Parietal:
  - Cognitive deficits
  - Inattention
  - Language disorders
  - Astereognosis
  - Apraxia
  - Apathy
d. Occipital:
  - Visual agnosia
  - Alexia

5. Discuss the uncertainty of resolution of previous cognitive or behavior patterns.	5. Cognitive and behavior changes frequently diminish or disappear six weeks to six months after surgery (Hickey, 2003).
6. Assess and document cognitive functions preoperatively: a. Orientation (place, person, and time) b. Short-term memory (ask to repeat a set of words) c. Long-term memory (ask to identify name of high school) d. Affect (apathetic, hostile, or labile) e. General behavior (appropriate/inappropriate) f. Abstract reasoning (ask to relate the meaning of a proverb) g. Ability to calculate h. Attention (easily distracted or attentive) i. Full range of movements and, especially, gait (AANN, 2006)	6. Baseline data will permit clear and accurate communication of the client's condition changes postoperatively.
7. Inform the client if an alternate form of communication to speech (e.g., note pad and pencil or hand signals) will be necessary postoperatively.	7. The client may require other means of communication if large head dressings inhibit hearing, periorbital edema impairs sight, or tracheostomy or endotracheal intubation prevents speech. Preoperative teaching prepares the client for this possibility and may ease anxiety.
8. Refer to the General Surgery care plan for more interventions and rationales.	

Documentation

Progress notes (including verification of NPO status, allergies, baseline neurologic assessment and documents accurately any deficits) (Wright, 2007, p. 1177).

Present emotional status
Interventions
Response to interventions

Postoperative: Collaborative Problems (Most complications will occur in the first 6 hours following surgery; AANN, 2006)

Potential Complication: Increased Intracranial Pressure

Potential Complication: Brain Hemorrhage, Hematoma, Hygroma

Potential Complication: Cranial Nerve Dysfunction

Potential Complication: Fluid and Electrolyte Imbalances

Potential Complication: Meningitis or Encephalitis

Potential Complication: Sensory and Motor Losses

Potential Complication: Cerebral or Cerebellar Dysfunction

Potential Complication: Hypothermia or Hyperthermia

Potential Complication: Diabetes Insipidus

Potential Complication: SIADH

Potential Complication: Cerebrospinal Fluid Leakage

Potential Complication: Seizure Activity

Potential Complication: Cardiac Arrhythmias Secondary to Increased Intracranial Pressure

Nursing Goal

The nurse will detect early signs and symptoms of (a) increased ICP, (b) brain hemorrhage, hematoma, hygroma, (c) cranial nerve dysfunction, (d) fluid and electrolyte imbalances, (e) cardiac dysrhythmias, (f) meningitis, encephalitis, (g) sensory and motor losses, (h) cerebellar dysfunction, (i) hypothermia or hyperthermia, (j) diabetes insipidus, (k) SIADH, (l) cerebrospinal fluid leakage, and (m) seizure activity, and will collaboratively intervene to stabilize the client.

Indicators

- Alert, calm, oriented (a, b)
- No seizures (l)
- Appropriate speech (a, b)
- Pupils equal; reactive to light and accommodation (a, b)
- Intact extraocular movements (a, b)
- Pulse 60–100 beats/min (a, b, e)
- Respirations 16–20 breaths/min (a, b)
- Respirations regular, easy (a, b)
- BP >90/60, <140/90 mmHg (a, b) (This parameter would be dependent on the surgeon; if cerebral vasospasm is to be avoided, surgeons tend to run systolic and diastolic rates 20–30 points higher that client's normal range. This also depends on client's condition as surgeons tend, on occasion, to use the theory of Triple H therapy—hypertension, hypervolemia, and hemodilution as a postoperative measure.) (Smith, 2007, p. 403).
- Stable pulse pressure (the difference between diastolic and systolic readings not widening, as this is a late sign of Cushing's triad) (a, b)
- Normal sinus rhythm
- Temperature 98–99.5°F (e, h)
- No shivering (e, h)
- No complaints of nausea/vomiting (a, b)
- Mild or no headache (a, b)
- Intact gag reflex (c)
- Intact swallowing (c)
- Symmetrical face (c)
- Symmetrical tongue movements (c)

- Intact sensory function (c, f)
- Full range of motion (c, f)
- Intact strength (c, f)
- Stable gait (c, g, f)
- Wound approximated (b, k)
- No or minimal bleeding/drainage (b, k)
- Urine output >5 mL/kg/h (d, i, j)
- Urine specific gravity 1.005–1.025 (d, i, j)
- Urine osmolality
  - Adult 50–1200 mOsm/kg H_2O
  - Child 50–1200 mOsm/kg H_2O
  - Newborn 100–600 mOsm/kg H_2O (Kee, 2004, p. 263).
- Electrolytes
- Sodium 135–145 mEq/L (d, i, j)
- Potassium 3.5–5.0 mEq/L (d)
- White blood count 4000–10,800 mm³ (e)
- Hemoglobin (b)
  - Males 13–15 gm/dL
  - Females 12–16 gm/dL
- Hematocrit (b)
  - Males 42%–50%
  - Females 40%–48%
- ICP monitoring (a) <20 mmHg (Baird, Keen, & Swearingen, 2005, p. 99)
- Mean arterial pressure 60–160 mmHg (a) 70–105 mmHg (Baird, Keen, & Swearingen, 2005, p. 25)
- Oxygen saturation (SaO_2) 94%–100 mm/Hg (a)
- Carbon dioxide ($PaCo_2$) 35%–45 mm/Hg (a)
- pH 7.35–7.45 (a)

Interventions	Rationales
1. Maintain and monitor increased intracranial pressure (ICP) (Baird, Keen, & Swearingen, 2005, p. 99):	1,2. ICP can be monitored by an intraventricular catheter or a fiberoptic transducer-tipped catheter inserted in the brain tissue or the ventricle
a. A waves	a. A waves are transient, paroxysmal waves that may last 5–20 minutes with amplitudes from 50–100 mmHg. They indicate cerebral ischemia.
b. B waves	b. B waves have a shorter duration (30 seconds to 2 minutes) with amplitudes of up to 50 mmHg. They may precede A waves and indicate intracranial hypertension.
c. C waves	c. C waves are small oscillations (about 6 per minute) that are rhythmic to respirations and systemic arterial blood pressure.
2. Follow the institution's procedures regarding ICP monitoring (e.g., calibration, draining, maintenance).	
3. Monitor for signs and symptoms of increased intracranial pressure (ICP).	3. Cerebral tissue is compromised by deficiencies of the cerebral blood supply caused by hemorrhage, hematoma, cerebral edema, thrombus, or emboli. Monitoring intracranial pressure (ICP) serves as an indicator of cerebral perfusion (Hickey, 2003).
a. Assess the following: • Best eye opening response: spontaneously to auditory stimuli, to painful stimuli, or no response • Best motor response: obeys verbal commands, localizes pain, flexion-withdrawal, and abnormal flexion-decorticate, abnormal extension-decerebrate, or no response	a. These responses evaluate the client's ability to integrate commands with conscious and involuntary movement. Cortical function can be assessed by evaluating eye opening and motor responses. No response may indicate damage to the midbrain (Hickey, 2003).

(continued on page 559)

Interventions	Rationales
• Best verbal response: oriented to person, place, and time; confused conversation; inappropriate speech; incomprehensible sounds; or no response b. Assess for changes in vital signs:	b. These vital-sign changes may reflect increasing ICP (Hickey, 2003).
• Pulse changes: slowing rate to 60 or below or increasing rate to 100 or above	• Changes in pulse may indicate brain-stem pressure—slowed at first, then increasing to compensate for hypoxia.
• Respiratory irregularities: slowing of rate with lengthening periods of apnea	• Respiratory patterns vary with impairments at various sites. Cheyne-Stokes breathing (a gradual increase followed by a gradual decrease, then a period of apnea) points to damage in both cerebral hemispheres, midbrain, and upper pons. Ataxic breathing (irregular with random sequence of deep and shallow breaths) indicates medullar dysfunction.
• Rising blood pressure or widening pulse pressure	• Blood pressure and pulse pressure changes are late signs indicating severe hypoxia.
• Decreased oxygen saturation (pulse oximetry)	• Pulse oximetry provides ongoing assessment of cardiovascular and respiratory status.
c. Assess pupillary response:	c. Pupillary changes indicate pressure on oculomotor or optic nerves (Hickey, 2003).
• Inspect pupils with a bright pinpoint light to evaluate size, configuration, and reaction to light. Compare both eyes for similarities and differences.	• Pupil reactions are regulated by the oculomotor nerve (cranial nerve III) in the brain stem.
• Evaluate gaze to determine whether it is conjugate (paired, working together) or if eye movements are abnormal.	• Conjugate eye movements are regulated from parts of the cortex and brain stem.
• Evaluate ability of eyes to adduct and abduct.	• Cranial nerve VI, the abducens nerve, regulates abduction and adduction of the eyes. Cranial nerve IV, the trochlear nerve, also regulates eye movement.
d. Note the presence of the following: • Vomiting	d. • Vomiting results from pressure on the medulla that stimulates the brain's vomiting center.
• Headache (constant, increasing in intensity, or aggravated by movement or straining)	• Compression of neural tissue movement increases ICP and pain.
• Subtle changes (e.g., lethargy, restlessness, forced breathing, purposeless movements, and changes in mentation)	• These changes may be early indicators of ICP changes.
4. Assist with cerebrospinal fluid (CSF) drainage through ventriculostomy drain.	4. Decreasing CSF will rapidly decrease ICP.
5. Elevate the head of the bed 15–30 degrees, unless contraindicated. Avoid changing the client's position hastily.	5. Slight head elevation can aid venous drainage to reduce cerebrovascular congestion (Hickey, 2003; Baird, Keen, & Swearingen, 2005).
6. Avoid the following:	6. These situations or maneuvers can increase ICP (Hickey, 2003; Baird, Keen, & Swearingen, 2005).
a. Carotid massage	a. Carotid massage slows the heart rate and reduces systemic circulation, which is followed by a sudden increase in circulation.
b. Neck flexion or extreme rotation	b. Neck flexion or extreme rotation disrupt circulation to the brain.
c. Digital anal stimulation d. Breath holding e. Straining f. Extreme flexion of hips and knees g. If client is ventilated, use only ear-to-ear endotracheal tapes (Baird, Keen, & Swearingen, 2005)	c–e. These activities initiate Valsalva maneuver, which impairs venous return by constricting the jugular veins and increases ICP.

(continued on page 560)

Interventions	Rationales
7. Consult with the physician for stool softeners as a prophylactic measure (Baird, Keen, & Swearingen, 2005).	7. Stool softeners prevent constipation and straining, which initiates Valsalva maneuver.
8. Maintain a quiet, calm, softly lit environment. Plan activities to minimize interruptions.	8. These measures promote rest and decrease stimulation, helping decrease ICP.

9. Assess cranial nerve function by evaluating the following:
  a. Pupillary responses
  b. Corneal reflex
  c. Gag reflex
  d. Cough
  e. Swallow
  f. Facial movements
  g. Tongue movements
	9. Cranial nerve pathways may be damaged directly by ischemia, trauma, or increased pressure.

10. Assess motor and sensory functions by observing each extremity separately for strength and normalcy of movement, and responses to stimuli.	10. The frontal and parietal lobes contain the neurons responsible for motor and sensory functions and may be affected by ischemia, trauma, or increased pressure.

11. Assess cerebellar function by observing for the following:
  a. Ataxic movements
  b. Loss of equilibrium
	11. Cerebellar function may be affected by ischemia, trauma, or increased pressure.

12. Carefully monitor hydration status; evaluate fluid intake and output, electrolytes, serum osmolality, and urine specific gravity and osmolality.	12. Fluid and electrolyte imbalances are not uncommon after cranial surgery. They result when water load exceeds renal excretion (hyposmolar) from excess fluid loss or inadequate intake (hyperosmolar) (Hickey, 2003; Baird, Keen, & Swearingen, 2005).

13. Identify possible causes of hyposmolar state.
  a. Excess IV fluids
  b. Inappropriate antidiuretic hormone secretion
	13. A lowered serum osmolarity releases the antidiuretic hormone (ADH).

14. Identify possible causes of hyperosmolar state.
  a. Fever
  b. Diarrhea
  c. Osmotic diuretic
  d. High-protein tube feeding
  e. Surgically induced diabetes insipidus
  f. Hyperglycemia
	14. Fever and diarrhea increase fluid losses. High solute tube feeding draws water from tissues by osmosis (Hickey, 2003; Baird, Keen, & Swearingen, 2005).

15. Monitor intake and administer necessary IV fluids via infusion pump.	15. Strict control of infusion is imperative to prevent fluid overload or dehydration.

16. Monitor for diabetes insipidus.
  a. Excessive urinary output
  b. Excessive thirst
  c. Increased serum sodium
  d. Prolonged capillary filling
	16. Surgery around the pituitary gland and hypothalamus can cause a deficiency of ADH, resulting in diabetes insipidus. Increased ICP causes cessation of blood flow to the brain. One result is decreased secretion of ADH, causing excessive urine output (Porth, 2002; Hickey, 2003; Baird, Keen, & Swearingen, 2005).

17. Monitor for syndrome of inappropriate secretion of antidiuretic hormone (SIADH).
  a. Decreased urine output
  b. Decreased serum sodium
  c. Decreased BUN
	17. Surgery can cause direct pressure on the hypothalamic-posterior pituitary structures, stimulating secretion of ADH (Porth, 2002; Hickey, 2003; Baird, Keen, & Swearingen, 2005).

(continued on page 561)

Interventions	Rationales
18. Monitor urinary output and urine specific gravity every hour.	18. Trauma to the brain results in increased aldosterone production and sodium retention, which intensifies hypertonicity and decreases urine output.
19. Monitor temperature for elevations, and use cooling blanket, as needed.	19. Hyperthermia increases cerebral metabolic demands and leads to depletion of energy stores in the brain. Fever can result from impaired hypothalamic function, urinary tract infections, atelectasis, or wound infection (Hickey, 2003; Baird, Keen, & Swearingen, 2005).
20. If the client shivers, notify the physician for possible pharmacologic treatment.	20. Shivering will increase cranial pressure. Thorazine may be prescribed (Baird, Keen, & Swearingen, 2005; Deglin & Vallerand, 2007, p. 274).
21. Monitor the wound site for the following: a. Bleeding b. Bulging c. CSF leakage d. Infection	21. A visible bulge under the wound may indicate localized bleeding or hygroma (collection of CSF). CSF leakage through the incision must be dealt with using strict asepsis to avoid ascending infection.
22. Consult with the physician if the client experiences seizures.	22. Seizures must be controlled to avoid hypoxia and resultant increased PCO_2 and increased ICP.
23. Teach the client to avoid the following: a. Coughing b. Neck hyperextension c. Neck hyperflexion d. Neck turning	23. Head and neck alignment must be maintained to prevent jugular vein compression that can inhibit venous return and result in increased ICP. Coughing increases intrathoracic pressure, which also has these effects (Hickey, 2003; Baird, Keen, & Swearingen, 2005).
24. Avoid sequential performance of activities that increase ICP (e.g., coughing, suctioning, repositioning, and bathing).	24. Research has validated that such sequential activities can cause a cumulative increase in ICP (Hickey, 2003).
25. Limit suctioning to two suction passes at a time, each pass being <10 seconds; hyper-oxygenate the client using 100% oxygen both before and after suctioning; use negative suction pressure <120 mmHg.(Baird, Keen, & Swearingen, 2005, p. 103–104).	25. These measures help to prevent hypercapnia that can increase cerebral vasodilation, raise ICP, and prevent hypoxia and that may increase cerebral ischemia (Hickey, 2003; Baird, Keen, & Swearingen, 2005).
26. Prevent hypoxia and atelectasis.	26. Hypoxia is the most common cause of decreased level of consciousness.

 ### Related Physician-Prescribed Interventions

Medications. Antihypertensives, stool softeners, peripheral vasodilators, osmotic diuretics, anticoagulants, corticosteroids, anticonvulsants

Intravenous Therapy. Fluid and electrolyte replacement

Laboratory Studies. Complete blood count, urinalysis, blood chemistry profile, drug levels, prothrombin time, urine chemistries

Diagnostic Studies. Computed tomography (CT) scan of head, lumbar puncture, cerebral angiography, magnetic resonance imaging (MRI), positron emission tomography (PET) scan, brain scan, Doppler ultrasonography, electroencephalography, skull x-ray film

Therapies. Antiembolism stockings, speech therapy, physical therapy, enteral feedings, occupational therapy, ventriculostomy drain, pulse oximetry, CP monitor, ICP monitoring

Documentation

Flow records
   Vital signs
   Intake and output

Body systems assessment findings
Neurologic assessment findings
Progress notes
Assessment findings deviating from normal
Seizures
Complaints of vomiting, headache

Postoperative: Nursing Diagnoses

Acute Pain Related to Compression/Displacement of Brain Tissue and Increased Intracranial Pressure

NOC Comfort Level, Pain Control

Goal

The client will report progressive pain reduction after pain-relief measures.

Indicators

• Report strategies that reduce pain.
• Report position restrictions.

NIC Pain Management, Medication Management, Emotional Support, Teaching: Individual, Hot/Cold Application, Simple Massage

Interventions	Rationales
1. Ascertain the location, nature, and intensity of the pain.	1. Pressure exerted on the baroreceptors in blood vessel walls causes generalized headache. Other sources of discomfort may include dressings, IV lines, edema, and poor positioning.
2. If the pain is a headache, slightly raise the head of the bed, dim the lights, minimize noise in the room, and loosen constrictive head dressings.	2. These measures may help to reduce increased ICP and relieve headache.
3. Provide non-pharmacologic relief measures, as appropriate: a. For eye edema: eye patches b. For immobility: frequent position changes and back rubs	3. The nurse should make every attempt to minimize the use of narcotic analgesics.
4. Observe for a decrease in the level of consciousness (LOC) and respiratory rate after narcotic administration. (*Note:* The nurse must be able to arouse the client fully to ascertain actual LOC.)	4. Narcotics constrict the pupils, depress respiration and may mask eye sign changes.
5. Refer to General Surgery care plan under Pain.	

Documentation

Medication administration record
Type, dosage, and route of all medications
Progress notes
Unsatisfactory pain relief

High Risk for Impaired Corneal Tissue Integrity Related to Inadequate Lubrication Secondary to Tissue Edema

NOC Risk Control

Goal

The client will demonstrate continued corneal integrity.

Indicators

* Relate rationale for eye drops.
* Relate why eyes are at risk.

NIC Eye Care

Interventions	Rationales
1. If eyelids do not close completely, use an eye shield or tape the lids closed, per protocol.	1. Corneal abrasion or erosion can occur within 4–6 hours if the eyelids do not close and dryness occurs (Baird, Keen, & Swearingen, 2005).
2. Loosen any tight dressings over the eyes.	2. Minimize direct pressure on the eyes.
3. Instill normal saline or hydroxyethylcellulose (Artificial Tears), as necessary.	3. Moisture provides lubrication and prevents dryness (Hickey, 2003).
4. Assess for irritation and drainage.	4. Early recognition of inflammation enables prompt intervention to prevent serious damage.
5. Apply cool compresses to the eye area, if necessary.	5. This can help to reduce periocular edema by decreasing lymphatic response to injured tissue.

Documentation

Flow records
  Eye assessment findings (vision, edema)

High Risk for Ineffective Therapeutic Regimen Management Related to Insufficient Knowledge of Wound Care, Signs and Symptoms of Complications, Restrictions, and Follow-up Care

NOC Compliance Behavior, Knowledge: Treatment Regimen, Participation: Health Care Decisions, Treatment Behavior: Illness or Injury

Goals

The goals for this diagnosis represent those associated with discharge planning. Refer to the discharge criteria.

NIC Anticipatory Guidance, Risk Management, Health Education, Learning Facilitation

Interventions	Rationales
1. Explain that mild headaches will persist but gradually decrease.	1. Knowing what to expect can reduce the client's anxiety associated with headaches.
2. Explain surgical site care:	2. This knowledge enables the client and family to participate in care.

(continued on page 564)

Interventions	Rationales
a. Wear a cap after bandages are removed. b. Hair can be shampooed after suture removal, but scrubbing near the incision should be avoided. c. Pat the incision area dry.	a. This helps to protect incision site. b. Hair regrowth indicates adequate wound closure. c. Vigorous rubbing can separate the wound edges.
3. Explain the need to avoid hair dryers or hot curlers until the hair has regrown.	3. Direct heat can burn the unprotected surgical site.

4. Teach the client not to do the following:
  a. Hold breath
  b. Strain during defecation
  c. Lift heavy objects
  d. Blow nose
  e. Cough, sneeze
	4. These activities activate Valsalva maneuver, which impairs venous return by compressing the jugular veins, and can increase ICP.

5. Teach the client to exhale during certain activities (e.g., defecating, turning, or bending).	5. Exhaling causes the glottis to open, which prevents Valsalva maneuver (Hickey, 2003).

6. Teach the client and family to watch for and report the following:
  a. Drainage from surgical site, nose, or ear
 	
  b. Intensifying headaches
  c. Elevated temperature, stiff neck, photophobia, hyper-irritability
	6. Early detection enables prompt intervention to prevent serious complications (Baird, Keen, & Swearingen, 2005).
	  a. Leakage may be CSF, which represents an entry route for microorganisms.
	  b. Intensifying headaches may point to increasing ICP.
	  c. These signs may indicate infection or meningitis.

7. If motor-sensory deficits remain, refer to the index for specific nursing diagnoses (e.g., Impaired Communication, Self-Care Deficits, Caregiver Role Strain, and Disturbed Thought Processes).	
8. Discuss with the client and family their perceptions of cognitive and behavior changes.	8. Evaluation of the client's personal system is essential to plan interventions (Hickey, 2003; Baird, Keen, & Swearingen, 2005).

9. Depending on the client's and family's readiness for more information, explain the following:
  a. Specific problems that may arise:
    • Decreased concentration
    • Difficulty with multiple stimuli
    • Emotional lability
    • Easy fatigability
    • Decreased libido
    • Allusiveness
  b. Different problems can occur throughout the recovery period.
	9. Family caregivers who are more informed are better prepared to help the client to compensate (Hickey, 2003; Baird, Keen, & Swearingen, 2005).

10. Discuss need to evaluate the effects of changes on the following:
  a. Safety
  b. Self-care ability
  c. Communication
  d. Family system
	10. The negative impact of deficits can be decreased by identifying strategies to be used at home (Hickey, 2003; Baird, Keen, & Swearingen, 2005).

11. Expand community services that may be indicated:
  • Home health care
  • Respite care
  • Counseling
  • National Head Injury Foundation (800-444-6443)
  • The Brain Injury Association (www.biaUSA.org)
	11. More intensive therapy may be necessary for adaptation.

Documentation

Discharge summary record
> Client and family teaching and return demonstration (physical or verbal), to ensure understanding of education.
> Outcome achievement or status

Enucleation

Enucleation is the surgical removal of the eyeball. The primary indication for enucleation is a blind, painful eye, which may result from absolute glaucoma, infection, or trauma. Enucleation may also be indicated in ocular malignancies, or for cosmetic improvement for a blind eye. The surgical procedure includes severing the extraocular muscles close to their insertion on the globe and inserting an implant to maintain the intraorbital anatomy (Lewis et al., 2004). The ocular muscles are sutured onto a hydroxyapatite sphere that has been covered with donor sclera of fascia. Alternatively, a synthetic porous sphere is placed into the ocular cavity, and a temporary conformer is inserted after the extraocular muscles have been sutured (Merbs, Grant, & Illiff, 2004). Between 4–6 weeks after surgery, an ocular prosthesis can be created for the client to insert, which restores natural appearance and some movement.

 Time Frame
Preoperative and postoperative periods

■■■■■ DIAGNOSTIC CLUSTER

Preoperative Period

Nursing Diagnosis

▲ Fear related to upcoming surgery, uncertain cosmetic outcome of surgery

Postoperative Period

Collaborative Problem

✳ PC: Bleeding (refer to General Surgery)

Nursing Diagnoses

△ Risk for Infection related to increased susceptibility secondary to surgical interruption of body surface and use of prosthesis (ocular)

▲ Acute Pain related to surgical interruption of body surfaces

△ Grieving related to loss of eye and its effects on life style

△ High Risk for Disturbed Self-Concept related to effects of change in appearance on life style (acute)

△ High Risk for Impaired Home Maintenance Management related to inability to perform activities of daily living (ADLs) secondary to change in visual abilities and loss of depth perception

△ High Risk for Ineffective Therapeutic Regimen Management related to insufficient knowledge of activities permitted, self-care activities, medications, complications, and plans for follow-up care

▲ This diagnosis was reported to be monitored for or managed frequently (75%–100%).
△ This diagnosis was reported to be monitored for or managed often (50%–74%).
✳ This diagnosis was not included in the validation study.

Discharge Criteria

Before discharge, the client and family will

1. Demonstrate site care, including instruction on the method of inserting the conformer into the socket in case it falls out (Lewis et al., 2004).
2. Verbalize precautions to take in order to protect the remaining eye (e.g., wearing protective glasses at all times).
3. State the signs and symptoms that must be reported to a health care professional.
4. Verbalize an intent to share with significant others feelings and concerns related to surgery.
5. Identify available community resources and self-help groups.

Preoperative: Nursing Diagnosis

Fear Related to Upcoming Surgery, Uncertain Cosmetic Outcome of Surgery

Goal

The client will express concerns regarding upcoming surgery during dialogues.

Indicators

- Describe postoperative restrictions.
- Describe expected postoperative cause.

NIC   Anxiety Reduction, Coping Enhancement, Presence, Counseling, Relaxation Therapy

Interventions	Rationales
1. Promote an environment in which the client will express feelings and concerns. Listen actively, validate the client's fears, and reassure the client and family that anxiety and fear are normal and expected responses to the upcoming surgery, while supporting the client and family (Lewis et al., 2004).	1. Verbalizing feelings and concerns increases the client's self-awareness and helps the nurse to identify sources of anxiety. Validation and reassurance promote self-esteem and may help to reduce anxiety.
2. Present information using a variety of instructional methods and media, such as the following: a. Audiovisual programs b. Ball implant and conformer models c. Sample prosthesis	2. Simultaneous stimulation of multiple senses enhances the teaching–learning process. Written materials also provide a source for referral after discharge.
3. Explain required preadmission activities: a. Adherence to dietary instructions provided by anesthesia services b. Adjustments in medication regimen as ordered by the surgeon, anesthesiologist, or the client's physician	3. Depending on the client's general health status, concurrent medical problems, time of surgery, and the physician's preferences, adjustments may be needed in diet (nothing by mouth for a specified period) and medications (e.g., withholding diuretics, decreasing insulin dose).
4. Discuss expected preoperative care measures, including the following: a. Preoperative sedation b. IV fluid infusion for medications c. Bladder emptying	4. Information about what to expect can help to reduce anxiety associated with fear of the unknown. Knowledge also enables the client to participate better in care measures and enhances his or her sense of control.
5. Explain when the pressure dressing will be removed. 6. Explain general postoperative care measures, such as: a. Ice compresses b. Antibiotic/steroid eye drops/ointment	5,6. Information about what to expect can reduce fear of the unknown. Explaining postoperative care before surgery allows the client to absorb the information and ask other questions while not under the effects of sedation. It also can help to improve compliance and facilitates the discharge planning process.

Documentation

Progress notes
  Client teaching
    Client's understanding of teaching and response
Progress notes
  Dialogues

Postoperative: Collaborative Problems

Potential Complication: Bleeding

Potential Complication: Infection

Potential Complication: Persistent Swelling

Potential Complication: Wound Separation

Potential Complication: Scarring

Nursing Goal

The nurse will detect early signs and symptoms of bleeding and collaboratively intervene to stabilize the client.

Indicators

- No blood on dressing
- Urine output >30 mL/h

Interventions	Rationale
1. Monitor for bleeding through the pressure patch.	1. Surgical disruption can cause trauma and bleeding. The pressure patch usually is removed in one week.

 Related Physician-Prescribed Interventions

Medications. Antibiotics/steroid drops/ointment
Laboratory Studies. Liver function studies, refer to the General Surgery care plan, Appendix II
Diagnostic Studies (preoperative). Dependent on underlying etiology, CT scan, MRI, A scan, B scan
Therapies. Ophthalmic site care

Documentation

Flow records
  Vital signs
Progress notes
  Unusual complaints

Postoperative: Nursing Diagnoses

Risk for Infection Related to Increased Susceptibility Secondary to Surgical Interruption of Body Surface and Use of Prosthesis (Ocular)

NOC Infection Status, Wound Healing: Primary Intention, Immune Status

Goal

The client will demonstrate evidence of wound healing without infection.

Indicators

- Demonstrate aseptic technique with eye care.
- Explain precautions.

NIC Infection Control, Wound Care, Incision Site Care, Health Education

Interventions	Rationales
1. Promote wound healing: a. Encourage a well-balanced diet and adequate fluid intake. b. Instruct the client to keep the pressure dressing over the eye for 12–15 hours for hydroxyapatite implants, or 4–5 days for synthetic Porex implants.	1. Optimal nutrition and hydration improve overall good health, which promotes healing of any surgical wound. Wearing a pressure patch decreases swelling.
2. Instruct the client to use aseptic technique to care for the socket and prosthesis: a. Wash hands first. b. Gently clean the eyelids of any discharge by wiping the lashes from nose to cheek with clean gauze (Lewis et al., 2004). c. Once the prosthesis is in place, remove and clean it weekly, as ordered. d. With the prosthesis removed, inspect the cavity for signs of conjunctival infection or other problems.	2. Aseptic technique minimizes the introduction of micro-organisms and reduces risk of infection.

Documentation

Progress notes
   Client teaching
   Signs of infection

Acute Pain Related to Surgical Interruption of Body Surfaces

NOC Comfort Level, Pain Control

Goal

The client will voice progressive pain reduction and pain relief after interventions.

Indicators

- State pain-relief measures.
- Report what increases pain.

NIC Pain Management, Medication Management, Emotional Support, Teaching: Individual, Heat/Cold Application, Simple Massage

Interventions	Rationales
1. Assist the client in identifying effective pain relief measures.	1. The client has the most intimate knowledge of his or her pain and the effectiveness of relief measures.
2. Provide information to allay anxiety and fear, such as the following: a. Give reassurance that pain is not always directly related to the development of complications.	2. This information can help to reduce anxiety associated with the unexpected; anxiety and fear actually increase pain.

(continued on page 568)

Interventions	Rationales
b. Explain how and when pain reduction interventions will begin working.	
3. Use ice compresses over the enucleation site 3–4 times a day.	3. Ice compresses will decrease swelling.
4. Support pain relief measures with prescribed analgesics, as necessary.	4. For some clients, pharmacologic therapy may be needed to provide adequate pain relief.
5. Notify the physician if pain is unrelieved within ½ hour of drug administration, if pain is accompanied by nausea, or if there is drainage on the eye patch or shield.	5. These signs may indicate increased intraocular pressure or other complications.

Documentation

Progress notes
    Complaints of pain
    Interventions
    Response to interventions

*Grieving Related to Loss of Eye and Its Effects on Life Style

NOC Coping, Family Coping, Grief Resolution, Psychosocial Adjustment: Life Change

Goal

The client will express grief.

Indicators

• Report an intent to discuss feelings with significant others.
• Describe meaning of loss.

NIC Family Support, Grief Work Facilitation, Coping Enhancement, Anticipatory Guidance, Emotional Support

Interventions	Rationales
1. Provide opportunities for the client and family members to vent feelings, discuss the loss openly, and explore the personal meaning of the loss. Explain that grief is a common and healthy reaction.	1. Loss of an eye and vision may give rise to feelings of powerlessness, anger, profound sadness, and other grief responses. Open, honest discussions can help the client and family members to accept and cope with the situation and their responses to it.
2. Encourage use of positive coping strategies that have proved successful in the past.	2. Positive coping strategies can help to decrease feelings of hopelessness and aid with problem-solving.
3. Encourage the client to express positive self-attributes.	3. Focusing on positive attributes increases self-acceptance.
4. Implement measures to support the family and promote cohesiveness: a. Support the family at its level of functioning. b. Encourage members to reevaluate their feelings and to support one another.	4. Family cohesiveness is important to client support.

*This diagnosis is not currently on the NANDA list but has been included for clarity and usefulness.

Documentation

Progress notes
    Present emotional status
    Interventions
    Response to interventions

High Risk for Disturbed Self-Concept Related to Effects of Change in Appearance on Life Style (Acute)

NOC Quality of Life, Depression Self-Control, Self-Esteem, Coping

Goal

The client will demonstrate self-care.

Indicators

- Acknowledge the change in appearance.
- Communicate feelings regarding the effects of loss of an eye and changes in appearance on client's life style.
- Participate in self-care.

NIC Hope Instillation, Mood Management, Values Clarification, Counseling, Referral, Support Group, Coping Enhancement

Interventions	Rationales
1. Encourage the client to verbalize feelings about the surgery and anticipated altered appearance and self-concept.	1. Interactions seeking to improve a client's self-concept must begin with assessing how the client feels about the illness, surgery, and self at this stress-producing time.
2. Help the client to identify personal attributes and strengths.	2. This may help the client to shift focus from the change in appearance to the positive aspects that contribute to his or her self-concept.
3. Facilitate adjustment through active listening.	3. By doing so, the nurse can reinforce positive attributes and help the client to reincorporate them into his or her new self-concept.
4. Encourage regular hygiene, grooming, and other self-care activities; assist as necessary. Allow the client to make decisions about care and participate in planning, as appropriate.	4. Participation in self-care and planning helps to facilitate positive coping with the change.
5. Encourage visitors and telephone conversations.	5. Maintaining social contacts can promote positive coping.
6. Reinforce that an ocular prosthesis (usually fitted 2–6 weeks after surgery) restores cosmetic appearance.	6. This information can minimize anxiety related to fear of a radical change in appearance.
7. Discuss strategies for socialization, as necessary (e.g., continued involvement in presurgical activities, or exploration of new activities and interests).	7. Minimizing life style changes promotes adjustment and coping. Isolation can contribute to negative self-concept.

8. Assess for signs of negative adjustment to change in appearance:
  a. Refusal to discuss the loss
  b. Refusal to discuss future care, including prosthesis fitting
	8. These signs may indicate that the client is at high risk for unsuccessful adjustment.

9. Refer an at-risk client for professional counseling.	9. The client may need follow-up counseling to assist with successful adjustment.

Documentation

Progress notes
   Present emotional status
   Interventions
      Response to interventions

High Risk for Impaired Home Maintenance Management Related to Inability to Perform Activities of Daily Living (ADLs) Secondary to Change in Visual Ability and Loss of Depth Perception

NOC Family Functioning

Goal

Before discharge, the client and family will verbalize ways to adjust the home environment to accommodate the client's current abilities.

Indicators

- Review safety risks.
- Identify community resources available.

NIC Home Maintenance Assistance, Environmental Management: Safety, Environmental Management

Interventions	Rationales
1. Help the client identify problem areas such as stairs or curbs.	1. A client experiencing vision loss needs to adapt the home environment to his or her current ability. As the client adjusts to altered depth perception and other changes, home maintenance abilities will improve.

2. Assist with adaptations to address problems:
  a. Transportation needs: Call on family, friends, or public transportation.
  b. Shopping: Arrange for delivery from the market; call on community resources.
  c. Food preparation: Obtain assistance from friends and family; arrange for Meals-on-Wheels.
	2. The nurse should make every feasible attempt to promote self-care and independence.

3. Refer the client to community agencies, as necessary (e.g., Lions Club for financial aid).	3. Specialized assistance may be required.

Documentation

Progress notes
   Needs identified
   Interventions
   Response to interventions

High Risk for Ineffective Therapeutic Regimen Management to Insufficient Knowledge of Activities Permitted, Self-Care Activities, Medications, Complications, and Plans for Follow-up Care

NOC Compliance Behavior, Knowledge: Treatment Regimen, Participation: Health Care Decisions, Treatment Behavior: Illness or Injury

Goals

The goals for this diagnosis represent those associated with discharge planning. Refer to the discharge criteria.

NIC Anticipatory Guidance, Risk Identification, Health Education, Learning Facilitation

Interventions	Rationales

1. Reinforce postoperative activity restrictions, such as avoiding the following:
  a. Swimming, for 2 weeks after surgery
  b. Driving too close to other cars
	1. Activity restrictions are aimed at reducing strain on the suture line and, in the case of driving, at eliminating situations that could be hazardous due to impaired depth perception and visual field loss.

2. Reinforce required self-care activities:
  a. Wear eye protection at all times during waking hours. Suggest wearing glasses even when no vision correction is required.
  b. Cleanse eyelids and eyelashes of mucus threads as necessary.
	2.
	  a. Because only one operative eye remains, that eye must be protected to preserve vision.
	
	  b. Daily face washing reduces risk of infection.

3. Instruct the client to notify the physician of the following:
  a. Periorbital redness and edema
  b. Purulent drainage
  c. Pain
	3. These signs and symptoms can indicate infection; early detection enables prompt intervention to prevent serious infection.

4. Provide information about scheduled follow-up care. Stress the importance of keeping appointments with the surgeon and ocularist. Make sure the client has the date and time of the first scheduled appointment after discharge.	4. Follow-up care enables early detection of problems.
5. Review instructions for and clients ability to use sterile technique to reinsert conformers, if dislodged.	5. The conformer maintains the integrity of the eyelids.
6. Explain to client that the ocularist will give specific instructions on prosthetic care.	6. Specific instructions and return demonstrations will provide practical information.

Documentation

Discharge summary record
    Client teaching with return demonstration, both verbal and physical, where applicable (Merbs, Grant, & Illiff, 2004).
    Outcome achievement or status

Fractured Hip and Femur

There are many subtypes of hip fractures; however a true hip fracture involves the hip joint. Nevertheless, the following fractures are also referred to as hip fractures: femoral head fracture, femoral neck fracture, inter-trochanteric fracture, and sub-trochanteric fracture. The differences between these fractures are important, as they are treated differently. The femoral head fracture involves a fracture to the femoral head as a result of high trauma; dislocation of the hip joint is common with this fracture. The femoral neck fracture (neck of femur [NOF], subcapital, or intracapsular fracture), is a fracture adjacent to the femoral head in the neck between the head and the greater trochanter. This type of fracture has a tendency to damage the blood supply to the femoral head, which can result in avascular necrosis. Intertrochanteric fractures indicate a fracture line between the greater and lesser trochanter on the intertrochanteric line. This is the most common type of hip fracture and, if the client is healthy, the prognosis for bone healing is good. The subtrochanteric fracture involves the shaft of the femur immediately below the lesser trochanter and may extend down the shaft of the femur (Cukierman, Gatt, Hiller, & Chajek-Shaul, 2005; Tinetti, 2003).

    Surgical treatment will depend on the type of fracture. It can be a standard surgical treatment which involves fixation of the fracture in situ with screws or a sliding plate/screw, which can take up to three to six months to heal properly. A hemiarthroplasty, which involves replacing the broken part of the bone with metal implants, allows the client to move around without having to wait for complete healing (Cukierman et al., 2005; Tinetti, 2003). Elderly clients are more vulnerable to hip fractures because of osteoporosis and mobility problems. Between 38% and 60% of hip fractures require permanent institutional care.

 Time Frame
Preoperative and postoperative periods

◼◼◼◼◼ DIAGNOSTIC CLUSTER

Preoperative Period

Nursing Diagnosis	Refer to
▲ Anxiety related to recent trauma, upcoming surgery, and insufficient knowledge of preoperative routines, postoperative routines, and postoperative sensations	General Surgery

Postoperative Period

Collaborative Problems	Refer to
▲ PC: Fat Emboli	
▲ PC: Compartment Syndrome	
▲ PC: Peroneal Nerve Palsy	
▲ PC: Displacement of Hip Joint	
△ PC: Venous Stasis/Thrombosis	
△ PC: Avascular Necrosis of Femoral Head	
△ PC: Sepsis	
PC: Hemorrhage/Shock	General Surgery
PC: Pulmonary Embolism	General Surgery

Nursing Diagnoses	Refer to
▲ Acute Pain related to trauma and muscle spasms	
▲ Impaired Physical Mobility related to pain, impaired gait, and postoperative position restrictions	
▲ (Specify) Self-Care Deficit related to prescribed activity restrictions	
▲ Fear related to anticipated dependence postoperatively	
△ Acute Confusion related to the multiple stressors associated with fractured hip and surgery	
▲ High Risk for Ineffective Therapeutic Regimen Management related to insufficient knowledge of activity restrictions, assistive devices, home care, follow-up care, and supportive services	
▲ High Risk for Constipation related to immobility	Immobility or Unconsciousness
▲ High Risk for Impaired Skin Integrity related to immobility and urinary incontinence secondary to inability to reach toilet quickly enough between urge to void and need to void	

(continued on page 574)

Related Care Plan
General Surgery Generic care plan

▲ This diagnosis was reported to be monitored for or managed frequently (75%–100%).
△ This diagnosis was reported to be monitored for or managed often (50%–74%).

Discharge Criteria

Before discharge, the client and family will

1. Demonstrate care of the surgical site and use of assistive devices.
2. Relate at-home restrictions and follow-up care.
3. State the signs and symptoms that must be reported to a health care professional.
4. Demonstrate a clear understanding of medications.

Postoperative: Collaborative Problems

Potential Complication: Fat Emboli

Potential Complication: Compartment Syndrome

Potential Complication: Peroneal Nerve Palsy

Potential Complication: Hip Joint Displacement

Potential Complication: Venous Stasis/Thrombosis

Potential Complication: Avascular Necrosis of the Femoral Head

Potential Complication: Sepsis

Nursing Goal

The nurse will detect early signs and symptoms of (a) fat emboli, (b) compartment syndrome, (c) peroneal nerve palsy, (d) hip joint displacement, (e) venous stasis/thrombosis, (f) avascular necrosis of femoral head, and (g) sepsis, and will collaboratively intervene to stabilize the client.

Indicators

- Alert, calm, oriented (g)
- Temperature 98.5–99°F (a, f, g)
- Heart rate 60–100 beats/min (a, g)
- Respirations 16–20 breaths/min (a, g)
- Deep relaxed respirations (a, g)
- BP >90/60, <140/90 mmHg (a, g)
- Peripheral pulses: full, equal, strong (b)
- Sensation intact (b)
- No pain with passive dorsiflexion (calf, toes) (b)
- Mild edema (b)
- Pain relieved by analgesics (b)
- No tingling in legs (b, c)
- Can move legs (b, c, d)
- No calf or thigh redness, warmth (e)
- Negative Homans sign (e)
- Affected extremity aligned (d)
- No petechiae (upper trunk, axilla) (a)
- Urine output >5 mL/kg/h (a, g)
- White blood cells 4000–10,800 (g)
- Oxygen saturation 94%–100% (a, g)
- Capillary refill <3 seconds (b)
- Blood urea nitrogen 10–20 mg/dL (g)
- Creatinine 0.7–1.4 mg/dL (g)

Interventions	Rationales

1. Assess high-risk clients for postoperative complications:
  a. Low serum albumin
 	
  b. Co-mobilities of cardiac disease, COPD, serum creatinine >1.7, pneumonia, digestive system disorder
	1.
	  a. A decrease in serum albumin will cause fluid to shift from the vessels to the tissues, resulting in edema (Kee, 2004).
	  b. These factors increase (in decreasing order) mortality after a hip fracture.

2. Monitor for signs and symptoms of fat emboli (Baird, Keen, & Swearingen, 2005):
  a. Fever
  b. Tachycardia
  c. Dyspnea
  d. Cough
  e. Petechiae (pinpoint reddish lesions) on upper trunk and axillae (secondary to thrombocytopenia)
  f. Neurologic deterioration (confusion, delirium, and coma)
  g. Restlessness
  h. Hypertension
  i. Inspiratory crowing (stridor); and expiratory wheezes
  j. Hemoptysis (coughing up of blood)
	2. Fat emboli can occur after long bone fractures, especially in older clients. Signs and symptoms indicate an inflammatory response or obstruction (Wagner, Johnson, & Kidd, 2006; Baird, Keen, & Swearingen, 2005).

3. Monitor for signs and symptoms of compartment syndrome:
  a. Deep, throbbing pain at the fracture site
  b. Increasing pain with passive movement
  c. Decreased sensation to light touch
  d. Inability to distinguish between sharp and dull sensation in the first web space of toes, sole, and the dorsum and lateral aspects of the foot
  e. Diminished or absent pedal pulses
  f. Increased edema and indurations in extremity
  g. Increased capillary refill (>3 seconds)
	3. Edema at the fracture site can compromise muscular vascular perfusion. Stretching damaged muscle causes pain. Sensory deficit is an early sign of nerve ischemia; the specific area of change indicates the affected compartment (Wagner, Johnson, & Kidd, 2006; Baird, Keen, & Swearingen, 2005).

4. Ensure proper positioning of the client:
  a. Before surgical treatment, turn toward fracture with pillows between legs
  b. Post-surgery, turn away from fracture until able to tolerate operative side with pillow between legs.
	4. This will avoid dislocation or further displacement.

5. Monitor for signs and symptoms of peroneal nerve palsy:
  a. Decreased sensation to light touch (numbness and tingling at the top of the foot) (Baird, Keen, & Swearingen, 2005)
  b. Inability to distinguish between sharp and dull sensations
  c. Paralysis
  d. Foot drop (Baird, Keen, & Swearingen, 2005)
  e. Walking abnormalities (Baird, Keen, & Swearingen, 2005)
  f. Slapping gait (Baird, Keen, & Swearingen, 2005)
  g. Toes drag while walking (Baird, Keen, & Swearingen, 2005)
	5. Pressure of the strap from skeletal traction (Buck traction) over the fibular head can compress the peroneal nerve, resulting in paresthesias and ultimately paralysis due to nerve ischemia (Buck traction is not commonly used in acute care settings) (Wagner, Johnson, & Kidd, 2006).

6. Prevent dislocation during turning by placing a pillow between the client's legs.	6. The pillow will maintain abduction and alignment.

7. Monitor for signs and symptoms of hip joint displacement:
  a. External rotation of affected extremity
  b. Affected extremity shorter than unaffected extremity
  c. Increased pain
	7. Damaged tissue and muscles may not provide adequate support for the hip joint, resulting in displacement.

(continued on page 576)

Interventions	Rationales
8. Monitor for signs and symptoms of venous stasis thrombosis: a. Calf pain b. Inflammation with redness, and warm to touch c. Positive Homans sign	8. The incidence of DVT in individuals with hip fractures ranges from 40%–74% (Pellino et al., 1998). The rate of pulmonary embolus in clients after hip surgery is as much as 15%, with the incidence of fatality being as high as 10%. Aspirin, subcutaneous or IV heparin, and low-dose Coumadin are the most commonly used therapies (Wagner, Johnson, & Kidd, 2006; Baird, Keen, & Swearingen, 2005; Deglin & Vallerand, 2007).
9. Maintain external compression devices (graded compression elastic stockings, intermittent external pneumatic compression [IPC], impulse boots).	9. Venous return is increased; pooling is decreased. Some devices (IPC and impulse) increase rate and velocity of venous flow that promote clearance and decrease hypercoagulability (Wagner, Johnson, & Kidd, 2006; Baird, Keen, & Swearingen, 2005).
10. Institute measures to decrease risks of deep vein thrombosis (DVT) (Wagner, Johnson, & Kidd, 2006): a. Discourage smoking pre- and postoperation. b. Elevate the foot of the bed without bending the client's knee. c. Encourage rhythmic and plantar flexion of the foot each hour. d. Ambulate as soon as possible.	10. a. Nicotine causes vasoconstriction. b. Elevation promotes venous return. c. This increases blood flow in the lower extremities and through the femoral vein (Wagner, Johnson, & Kidd, 2006; Baird, Keen, & Swearingen, 2005).
11. Monitor for signs and symptoms of avascular necrosis of the femoral head: a. Redness b. Warmth	11. Hematoma formation results from tearing and rupture of blood vessels within the bone. Extensive blood loss with disruption of blood supply can result in bone death.
12. Monitor for signs and symptoms of sepsis: a. Temperature >101°F or <98.6°F b. Abnormal laboratory values: increased creatinine; decreased pH; WBC count may be normal, elevated, or decreased. The presence of more than 10% of bands indicates an inflammatory response (Wagner, Johnson, & Kidd, 2006). c. Decreased urine output d. Heart rate >90 beats/min e. Respiratory rate >20 breaths/min f. Change in mentation (elderly)	12. Sepsis results in massive vasodilation and hypovolemia, leading to tissue hypoxia with decreased renal function and cardiac output. This triggers a compensatory response of increased heart and respiratory rates in an attempt to correct hypoxia and acidosis (Wagner, Johnson, & Kidd, 2006; Baird, Keen, & Swearingen, 2005).

 Related Physician-Prescribed Interventions

Medications. Anticoagulant use (low-weight heparin, warfarin); antibiotic prophylaxis (cephalosporin IM 2 hours prior to surgery); also refer to the General Surgery care plan

Intravenous Therapy. Refer to the General Surgery care plan

Laboratory Studies. Coagulation studies; also refer to the General Surgery care plan

Diagnostic Studies. Femur x-ray film, bone scans, MRI, computed tomography (CT) scan

Therapies. Wound care, compression stocking, external pneumatic compression, assistive devices, anticoagulant therapy, physical therapy, impulse devices, pulse oximetry, Buck traction

Documentation

Flow records
   Vital signs
   Distal limb sensation, paresthesias, circulation

Intake (oral, parenteral)
Output (urine, urine specific gravity)
Wound (color, drainage, swelling, rate of health)

Postoperative: Nursing Diagnoses

Acute Pain Related to Trauma and Muscle Spasms

NOC Comfort Level, Pain Control

Goal

The client will report satisfactory relief as evidenced by the indicators listed below:

Indicators

- Increased participation in activities of recovery.
- Reduction in reported pain using 0–10 pain scale.

NIC Pain Management, Medication Management, Emotional Support, Teaching: Individual, Hot/Cold Application, Simple Massage

Interventions	Rationales
1. Position the client in proper alignment. Handle the client gently, supporting the leg with your hands or a pillow.	1. Optimal alignment reduces pressure on nerves and tissues; this reduces pain. Muscle spasms accompany movement.
2. Use a trochanter roll to support the involved extremity in the neutral position (Lewis et al., 2004).	2. The trochanter roll prevents or minimizes external rotation.
3. Preoperatively, roll only on affected side with pillow between legs (Lewis et al., 2004).	3. This prevents dislocation or further displacement.
4. Take steps to maintain the effectiveness of Buck traction (Lewis et al., 2004): a. Evaluate for appropriate use of weights. b. Ensure that weights hang freely. c. Ensure proper pulley functioning. d. Ensure that the heel does not rest on the mattress. e. Assess for paresthesias in the involved extremity.	4. Proper use of Buck traction immobilizes the involved extremity, reducing muscle spasms and minimizing further tissue destruction from bone fragments. Recent research has found that skeletal and skin traction showed no greater benefits over other treatments (Lewis et al., 2004; Wagner, Johnson, & Kidd, 2006; Baird, Keen, & Swearingen, 2005).
5. Provide an orthopedic (fracture) bedpan rather than a standard bedpan.	5. Use of an orthopedic bedpan helps to maintain proper body alignment during elimination.
6. Explain and demonstrate patient-controlled analgesia (PCA) (Lehne, 2004).	6. PCA gives the client control and decreases fear and anxiety (Deglin & Vallerand, 2007).
7. Encourage the client to use PCA before the pain becomes unbearable (Lehne, 2004).	7. A steady blood level of analgesia can prevent severe pain.
8. Consult with the physician or advanced practice nurse if the pain is not relieved.	8. Unrelieved pain indicates a change in the pain management plan.
9. Refer to the General Surgery care plan for general pain-relief interventions.	

Documentation

Flow records
Participation in self-care

Impaired Physical Mobility Related to Pain, Impaired Gait, and Postoperative Position Restrictions

NOC   Ambulation: Walking, Joint Movement: Active, Mobility Level

Goal

The client will report progressive increase in range of motion and ambulation.

Indicators

- Demonstrate the use of assistive devices.
- Demonstrate measures to increase mobility.
- Report pain to be tolerable during physical therapy.

NIC   Exercise Therapy: Joint Mobility, Exercise Promotion: Strength Training, Exercise Therapy: Ambulation, Positioning, Teaching: Prescribed Activity/Exercise, Teaching: Procedure/Treatment

Interventions	Rationales
1. Explain the rationale for bed exercises and early ambulation.	1. Aggressive pursuit of range-of-motion exercises and early ambulation can decrease deep-vein thrombosis and muscle wasting and increase strength (Lewis et al., 2004; Wagner, Johnson, & Kidd, 2006; Baird, Keen, & Swearingen, 2005).
2. Implement the institution's physical therapy (PT) plan on unit. Progress client management per the PT treatment program (e.g., gait training, transfers).	2. PT is an important intervention to help with early mobilization.
3. Stress the importance of pain management.	3. Pain must be controlled for the client to actively participate in exercise.
4. Explain the importance of aggressive postdischarge PT and at-home exercises.	4. The literature reports that less than 50% of people with hip fractures achieve this preinjury status (Ward, Renni, & Hager, 1998).
5. Encourage the use of trapeze.	5. Shoulder and arm muscles need strengthening to use this assistive device.
6. Refer to discharge instructions under Ineffective Therapeutic Regimen Management.	6.
7. Arrange for home visit (nursing, PT) to evaluate adaptations needed (e.g., raised toilet seat, throw rugs).	7. Adaptations will be needed to reduce injury and prevent dislocation.

(Specify) Self-Care Deficit Related to Prescribed Activity Restrictions

NOC   See Bathing/Hygiene, Feeding, Dressing, Toileting, and/or Instrumental Self-Care Deficit

Goal

The client will participate in self-care activities.

Indicators

- Identify when assistance is needed.
- Demonstrate optimal hygiene.

NIC   See Feeding, Bathing, Dressing, Toileting, and/or Instrumental Self-Care Deficit

Interventions	Rationales
1. Collaborate with the client to prioritize self-care tasks.	1. The client is more likely to participate in the self-care activities that he or she values. Prioritizing activities also gives the client a sense of control over the situation.
2. Encourage the client to participate in doable, high-priority self-care tasks to the fullest extent possible.	2. Achieving success at some tasks encourages the client to attempt other activities that can promote progression in self-care ability.
3. Provide physical therapy (e.g., ROM exercises, instruction in proper transfer techniques, and use of assistive devices). (*Note:* The client, particularly if elderly, may have other problems that require modifications to the standard assistive devices.)	3. This can help to increase muscle strength, endurance, and mobility.
4. Pace activities to ensure adequate rest periods.	4. Pacing activities helps to avoid fatigue and ensure sufficient energy to perform tasks.
5. Evaluate progression of ability and refer to a rehabilitation center, if necessary.	5. The client needs referral if he or she is unable to return to his or her former setting safely.
6. As necessary, consult with occupational therapy for assistance in adapting self-care activities such as dressing and cooking. 7. Instruct the client or family in ways to modify the home environment to ease access to the bathroom, kitchen, and other areas.	6,7. Assistance with tasks can help the client to perform them; this promotes independence. In turn, independence increases motivation and decreases feelings of helplessness.

Documentation

Medication administration record
   Type, dosage, route of all medications
Progress notes
   Unsatisfactory response
   Positioning

Fear Related to Anticipated Dependence Postoperatively

NOC Anxiety Control, Fear Control

Goal

The client will express a progressive reduction in fear.

Indicators

- Demonstrate a decrease in pulse and respiratory rates.
- Differentiate real from unrealistic fears.
- Identify effective coping strategies.

NIC Anxiety Reduction, Coping Enhancement, Presence, Counseling

Interventions	Rationales
1. Encourage the client to express his or her feelings regarding the impact of the fracture and surgery on self-care ability and life style.	1. Fear of adverse health effects and loss of independence has a significant impact on a client's psychosocial functioning. Encouraging the client to share these fears gives the nurse the opportunity to validate them and possibly to correct any misconceptions.

(continued on page 580)

Interventions	Rationales
2. If appropriate, tell the client that persons with active life styles before surgery have high recovery rates.	2. Several studies have supported this (Lewis et al., 2004; Wagner, Johnson, & Kidd, 2006; Baird, Keen, & Swearingen, 2005).
3. Stress the importance of complying with the treatment regimen.	3. Compliance can speed up rehabilitation and promotes a return to preoperative functioning.
4. Encourage the highest possible level of independent functioning.	4. Self-care promotes self-esteem and reduces feelings of dependency.
5. Involve family members or significant others in the care regimen to the fullest extent possible.	5. Support-systems involvement has been shown to promote a speedier recovery (Lewis et al., 2004).
6. Plan diversional activities for stress management.	6. Diversional activities can help the client to refocus on matters other than his or her condition and associated fears.

Documentation

Progress notes
    Interventions
    Response to interventions

Acute Confusion Related to the Multiple Stressors Associated With Fractured Hip and Surgery

NOC Cognitive Orientation, Safety Behavior: Personal, Distorted Thought Control, Information Processing

Goal

The client will resume presurgical orientation postoperatively.

Indicators

- Be oriented.
- Engages in meaningful presurgical dialogue.

NIC Delirium Management, Cognitive Stimulation, Calming Technique, Reality Orientation, Environmental Management: Safety

Interventions	Rationales
1. Provide education to family, significant others, and caregivers regarding the situation and methods of response while ensuring a total understanding of all aspects of care.	1. Explanations regarding causes of acute confusion can help to alleviate fears.

2. Maintain standards of empathetic, respectful care.
  a. Be an advocate when other caregivers are insensitive to the individual's needs.
  b. Function as a role model with coworkers.
  c. Provide other caregivers with up-to-date information on confusion.
  d. Expect empathetic, respectful care and monitor its administration.
	2. "Confusion" is a term frequently used by nurses to describe an array of cognitive impairments. Recognizing a client as confused is just an initial step.

(continued on page 581)

Interventions	Rationales
3. Attempt to obtain information that will provide useful and meaningful topics for conversations (likes, dislikes; interests, hobbies; work history).	3. Assessing the client's personal history can provide insights into her or his current behavior patterns and communicates interest in the client (Lewis et al., 2004).
4. Encourage significant others and caregivers to speak slowly with a low voice pitch and average volume (unless hearing deficits are present) as one adult to another, with eye contact, and as if expecting the client to understand.	4. Sensory input must be carefully planned to reduce excess stimuli that increase confusion.
5. Show respect and promote sharing: a. Pay attention to what client is saying. b. Pick out meaningful comments and encourage conversation. c. Call the client by name and introduce yourself each time contact is made; use touch, if welcomed. d. Use a name the client prefers; avoid "Pops" or "Mom," which can increase confusion and is inappropriate. e. Convey to the client that you are concerned and friendly (through smiles, an unhurried pace, humor, and praise; do not argue). f. Focus on feeling beyond the spoken word or action.	5. This demonstrates unconditional positive regard and communicates acceptance and affection to a client who has difficulty interpreting his or her environment (Lewis et al., 2004).
6. Keep the client oriented to time and place. a. Refer to the time of day and the place each morning. b. Provide the client with a clock and calendar large enough to see. c. If dementia is severe, remove all visual mirrors. d. Use night lights or dim lights at night. e. Use indirect lighting. f. Turn lights on before dark. g. Provide the client with opportunity to see daylight and dark through a window, or take client outdoors. h. Single out holidays with cards or pins (e.g., lighting, glasses, hearing aids).	6. Overstimulation, under-stimulation, or misleading stimuli can cause dysfunctional episodes because of impaired sensory interpretation (Lewis et al., 2004).
7. Encourage the family to bring in familiar objects from home (e.g., photographs with non-glare glass, afghan). 8. Discuss current events, seasonal events (snow, water activities); share your interests (travel, crafts).	7,8. Topics and objects that the client has experiences with can increase orientation.
9. Explain all activities. a. Offer simple explanations of tasks. b. Allow the client to handle equipment related to each task. c. Allow the client to participate in tasks such as washing his or her face. d. Inform the client when you are leaving and say when you will return.	9. Assessing the individual's personal history can provide insight into current behavior patterns and communicates interest in the individual (Lewis et al., 2004).
10. Do not aggravate the client's confusion. a. Do not argue with the client. b. Never agree with confused statements. c. Direct the client back to reality; do not allow him or her to ramble. d. Adhere to the set schedule; if changes are necessary, advise the client of them. e. Avoid talking to coworkers about other topics in client's presence.	10. Overstimulation, under-stimulation, or misleading stimuli can cause dysfunctional episodes because of impaired sensory interpretation (Lewis et al., 2004).

(continued on page 582)

Interventions	Rationales
f. Provide simple explanations that cannot be mis-interpreted. g. Remember to acknowledge your entrance with a greeting and your exit with a closure (e.g., "I'll be back in 10 minutes.") h. Avoid open-ended questions. i. Replace five- to six-step tasks with two- or three-step ones.	

11. Avoid use of restraints; explore other alternatives.
  a. Put the client in a room with others who can help watch him or her.
  b. Enlist the aid of family or friends to watch the client during confused periods.
  c. If the client is pulling out tubes, use mitts instead of wrist restraints; use minimal restraints to maintain client safety (Lewis et al., 2004).
	11. Research has validated that restraints increase fear, which increases confusion (Lewis et al., 2004).

Documentation

Progress notes
  Level of orientation which is reflected with accurate documentation

High Risk for Ineffective Therapeutic Regimen Management Related to Insufficient Knowledge of Activity Restrictions, Assistive Devices, Home Care, Follow-up Care, and Supportive Services

NOC Compliance Behavior, Knowledge: Treatment Regimen, Participation: Health Care Decisions, Treatment Behavior: Illness or Injury

Goals

The goals for this diagnosis represent those associated with discharge planning. Refer to the discharge criteria.

NIC Anticipatory Guidance, Risk Management, Learning Facilitation, Health Education, Teaching: Procedure/Treatment, Health System Guidance

Interventions	Rationales
1. Evaluate the client's ability to ambulate and perform ADLs.	1. The nurse must evaluate the client's self-care abilities before discharge to determine the need for referrals.
2. Evaluate mental status and presence of depression.	2. Individuals with confusion and depressive symptomatology have very high risk for prolonged disability and death (Lewis et al., 2004).
3. Consult with a specialist for management of depression, as necessary.	3. Early detection and treatment of depression can reduce hospital stay and long-term disabilities.

4. Provide instruction on postoperative exercises per PT plan; these may include the following:
  a. Quadriceps setting
  b. Gluteal strengthening
	4. Exercises facilitate use of assistive devices by maintaining or enhancing present level of muscle function in unaffected limbs.

(continued on page 583)

Interventions	Rationales
c. Dorsiplantar flexion d. Range-of-motion for upper and non-affected lower extremities	
5. Teach the client how to ambulate without weight-bearing, using crutches or a walker; request a return demonstration to evaluate ability. Consult with the physician regarding amount of weight-bearing allowed (Lewis et al., 2004).	5. The client, particularly if elderly, may have impaired balance or decreased upper body strength that necessitates the use of a walker to maintain mobility. Depending on the internal fixation device used, this need may persist for 3–7 days after surgery.
6. Teach the client and family to do the following: a. Use proper techniques to transfer to a chair: Place the chair on the affected side, abduct and support the affected leg, and pivot on the unaffected leg. b. Use pillows to maintain abduction while seated. c. For 5–10 days after surgery, sit without flexing the hip more than 60 degrees. d. For at least two months after surgery, avoid adducting the affected extremity beyond the midline. e. Use proper body mechanics within limitations. f. Use an elevated toilet seat.	6. These measures may help to reduce risk of injury. a. Proper transfer technique prevents weight-bearing on the affected side. b. Leg abduction relieves stress on the internal fixation device and fracture site. c. Hip flexion puts stress on the internal fixation device and fracture site. d. Leg adduction puts stress on the internal fixation device and fracture site. e. Proper body mechanics prevent injury to muscles and ligaments. f. Using an elevated toilet seat decreases flexion and minimizes stress on fracture site. It also facilitates independent toileting.
7. Present information or reinforce learning using written materials (e.g., booklets or instruction sheets) and audiovisual aids (e.g., slides, videotapes, models, or diagrams).	7. Using a variety of teaching materials stimulates learning and enhances retention, particularly for an elderly client who may have visual or hearing impairment.
8. Explain the importance of progressive care (i.e., from early non–weight-bearing ambulation to self-care within the client's abilities).	8. The risk of complications increases with each day of immobility, particularly in an elderly client (Lewis et al., 2004; Wagner, Johnson, & Kidd, 2006; Baird, Keen, & Swearingen, 2005).
9. Teach the client and family to watch for and report subtle signs of infection: a. Increased temperature chills b. Malaise c. Pain unrelieved with analgesia (Lewis et al., 2004).	9. Hip fracture typically affects elderly clients who have a decreased ability to compensate for physiologic and immunologic system changes that may mask pronounced signs and symptoms of infection.
10. Explain anticoagulation therapy. Refer to Anticoagulation care plan.	

Documentation

Discharge summary record
    Client and family teaching and return demonstration of understanding of education
    Outcome achievement or status
    Referrals, if indicated

For a Care Map on an Operable Fractured Femur, visit http://thePoint.lww.com.

Hysterectomy

There are various types of hysterectomies performed today, depending on the client diagnosis. The *Supracervical* hysterectomy (Subtotal hysterectomy) involves removal of the uterus while leaving the cervix intact. *Total hysterectomy* removes both the uterus and the cervix. *Radical hysterectomy* or *modified radical hysterectomy* is indicated if cancer is diagnosed). This method removes the uterus and cervix, may remove part of the vagina (if cancer is involved), ovaries (oophorectomy), fallopian tubes (salpingectomy), and lymph nodes (in order to stage the cancer and to determine how far the cancer is spread, if involved) (Harmanli et al., 2004; Paparella et al., 2004).

There are several approaches to performing a hysterectomy and again it is dependent on patient diagnosis. The *open approach* (*abdominal hysterectomy*) is where the uterus, fallopian tubes and such are removed from a 6–12 inch incision in the lower abdomen. The *vaginal approach*, where the uterus is removed through the vagina. *Laparoscopic hysterectomy* removes the uterus either vaginally or through a small incision made in the abdomen. This method offers the surgeons better visualization of affected structures than either *vaginal* or *abdominal* alone, as a 2D video monitor is used (Johnson et al., 2005).

A new method, called the *Da Vinci hysterectomy*, is said to be one of the most effective and least invasive treatments. It is performed by using the Da Vinci Surgical System, 'which enables the surgeons to perform with unmatched precision and control—using only a few small incisions' (Da Vinci Hysterectomy, 2007). The benefits of this surgery include a considerable decrease in postoperative pain, blood loss, fever complications, scarring, length of hospitalization, and faster return to normal daily living (Da Vinci Hysterectomy, 2007).

 Time Frame
Preoperative and postoperative periods

■ ■ ■ ■ ■ DIAGNOSTIC CLUSTER

Preoperative Period

Refer to General Surgery Generic Care Plan

Postoperative Period

Collaborative Problems

- ▲ PC: Ureter, Bladder, Bowel Trauma
- ▲ PC: Vaginal Bleeding
- ▲ PC: Deep Vein Thrombosis
- ▲ PC: Neurological Deficits Secondary to Epidural Therapy

Nursing Diagnoses

△ High Risk for Disturbed Self-Concept related to perceived effects on sexuality and feminine role

△ High Risk for Ineffective Therapeutic Regimen Management related to insufficient knowledge of perineal/incisional care, signs of complications, activity restrictions, loss of menses, hormone therapy, and follow-up care

▲ This diagnosis was reported to be monitored for or managed frequently (75%–100%).
△ This diagnosis was reported to be monitored for or managed often (50%–74%).

Discharge Criteria

Before discharge, the client and family will

1. State wound care procedures to follow at home, especially ensuring that the client can monitor for wound infection and separation, if the abdominal approach is used.
2. Verbalize precautions to take regarding activities, especially the lifting restrictions of no more that 5 lbs until cleared by doctor (usually after six weeks).
3. State the signs and symptoms that must be reported to a health care professional, such as fever, drainage, redness, swelling, unresolved pain, and discharge associated with itching and bad-smelling odors.
4. Verbalize an intent to share feelings and concerns with significant others.

Postoperative: Collaborative Problems

Potential Complication: Ureter, Bladder, Bowel Trauma
Potential Complication: Vaginal Bleeding
Potential Complication: Deep Vein Thrombosis
Potential Complication: Neurological Deficits Associated with Epidural Injection

Nursing Goal

The nurse will detect early signs and symptoms of (a) ureter, bladder, and bowel trauma, (b) vaginal bleeding, (c) deep vein thrombosis, (d) infection, (e) hemodynamic instability, and (f) neurologic and neuromuscular deficits associated with epidural therapy, and collaboratively intervene to stabilize the client.

Indicators

- Urine output >0.5–1.0 mL/kg/h (Baird, Keen, & Swearingen, 2005) (a)
- Clear urine (a)
- Intact bowel sounds all quadrants (a)
- Flatus present (a)
- No leg pain (c)
- No leg edema (c)
- No pain with dorsiflexion of feet (Homans sign) (c)
- Light-colored vaginal drainage (b)
- No headache (particularly, spinal headache due to epidural therapy) (e, f) (Lehne, 2004)
- Monitor signs of hypotension (due to epidural therapy) (e, f) (Lehne, 2004)
- No fever (d)
- No cardiac arrhythmias (e, f)
- No decreased level of consciousness (e, f)

Interventions	Rationales
1. Monitor for signs and symptoms of ureter, bladder, or rectal trauma: a. Urinary retention b. Prolonged diminished bowel sounds c. Bloody, cloudy urine d. Absence of flatus	1. Proximity of these structures to the surgical site may predispose them to atony because of edema or nerve trauma.
2. Monitor for signs and symptoms of deep-vein thrombosis (DVT). a. Leg or calf pain b. Leg swelling c. Referred pain in abdomen or buttocks d. Positive Homans sign	2. Gynecologic surgery increases the risk of DVT because of operative time and surgical positioning.
3. Monitor for adverse reactions to epidural therapy, if in place (Lehne, 2004): a. hemodynamic stability b. decreased level of consciousness c. decreased respiratory rate and effort d. allergic reactions	3. An opioid or a combination of opioid and local anesthetic is infused into the space just before the dura mater. The opioid diffuses across the dura mater and binds to the opioid receptors. This route requires lower doses of analgesia and, as a result, minimizes the potential side effects. Providing analgesia outside of the central nervous system (CNS), on the other hand, affects drowsiness and respiratory depression. The rationale for hourly assessment is to recognize early signs and symptoms of systemic toxicity before signs of bradycardia, heart blocks, cardiac arrest,

(continued on page 586)

Interventions	Rationales
	CNS excitation (possible convulsion), followed by CNS depressions and coma, occur. This is achieved by monitoring blood pressure, heart rate and rhythm, respiratory rate and regulation, and level of consciousness (Wagner, Johnson, & Kidd, 2006; Lehne, 2004).
4. Apply elastic stockings, as ordered.	4. Stockings provide even compression to increase venous return.
5. Perform leg exercises every hour while client is in bed. Ambulate the client early, unless she is on epidural anesthesia, then mobilize as ordered (Wagner et al., 2006; Baird, Keen, & Swearingen, 2005).	5. Leg exercises and ambulation contract leg muscles, stimulate the venous pump, and reduce stasis. Movement reduces stasis and vascular pooling in legs; pressure under knees can interfere with peripheral circulation (Harmanli et al., 2004; Paparella, Sizzi, De Benedictine et al., 2004).

6. If the surgical route is vaginal, monitor vaginal bleeding every 2–4 hours:
  a. Monitor vaginal drainage. Record amount and color.
 	
  b. If packing is used, notify the physician if packing is saturated or clots are passed.
  c. Notify the physician if perineal pad is saturated.
	6.
	
	  a. Drainage is expected. Frank vaginal bleeding, if it occurs, should be light (Porth, 2005).
	  b,c. Packing is used if hemostasis is a problem during surgery. Excess bleeding or clots can indicate abnormal bleeding.

7. If the route is abdominal, monitor for incisional and vaginal bleeding every 2 hours.	7. The female pelvis has an abundant supply of blood vessels, creating a high risk for bleeding (Harmanli et al., 2004; Paparella, Sizzi, De Benedictine et al., 2004).

 Related Physician-Prescribed Interventions

Medications. Estrogen therapy (selected cases)
Intravenous Therapy. Refer to the General Surgery care plan
Laboratory Studies. STD screening; also refer to the General Surgery care plan
Diagnostic Studies. Ultrasound or computed tomography (CT) scan
Therapies. Urinary or suprapubic catheter; pelvic ultrasound; hysterosalpingography; also refer to the General Surgery care plan

Documentation

Flow records (including hourly monitoring of epidural therapy)
  Vital signs (including adverse reactions to epidural therapy)
  Perineal drainage
  Intake and output
  Turning, ambulation

Postoperative: Nursing Diagnoses

High Risk for Disturbed Self-Concept Related to Significance of Loss

NOC Quality of Life, Depression Level, Self-Esteem, Coping

Goal

The client will acknowledge change in body structure and function.

Indicators

• Communicate feelings about the hysterectomy.
• Participate in self-care within the restricted guidelines set by surgeon.

NIC Hope Instillation, Mood Management, Values Clarification, Counseling, Referral, Support Group, Coping Enhancement

Interventions	Rationales
1. Contact the client frequently and treat her with warm, positive regard.	1. Frequent contact by the caregiver indicates acceptance and may facilitate trust. The client may be hesitant to approach staff because of a negative self-concept.
2. Incorporate emotional support into the technical care teaching sessions (e.g., wound care and bathing) (Meloni-Rosa et al., 2006; Katz, 2005; Zalon, 2004).	2. This encourages resolution of emotional issues while teaching technical skills (Meloni-Rosa et al., 2006; Katz, 2005; Zalon, 2004).
3. Encourage the client to verbalize her feelings about the surgery and its consequent impact on her life style. Validate her perceptions and reassure her that the responses are normal and appropriate.	3. Sharing concerns and ventilating feelings provides an opportunity for the nurse to correct any misinformation. Validating the client's perceptions increases self-awareness (Meloni-Rosa et al., 2006; Katz, 2005; Zalon, 2004).
4. Replace myths with facts (e.g., hysterectomy usually does not affect physiologic sexual response) (Meloni-Rosa et al., 2006; Katz, 2005; Zalon, 2004).	4. Misinformation may contribute to unfounded anxiety and fear. Providing accurate information can help to reduce these emotional stressors.
5. Discuss the surgery and its effects on functioning with family members or significant others; correct any misconceptions. Encourage client to share her feelings and perceptions with family and significant others (Meloni-Rosa et al., 2006; Katz, 2005; Zalon, 2004).	5. The support of family members or significant others is often critical to client's acceptance of changes and positive self-concept (Meloni-Rosa et al., 2006; Katz, 2005; Zalon, 2004).
6. Refer the client at high risk for unsuccessful adjustment for professional counseling.	6. Follow-up therapy to assist with effective adjustment may be indicated.

Documentation

Progress notes
    Present emotional status
    Interventions
        Response to interventions

High Risk for Ineffective Therapeutic Regimen Management Related to Insufficient Knowledge of Perineal/Incisional Care, Signs of Complications, Activity Restrictions, Loss of Menses, Hormone Therapy, and Follow-up Care

NOC Compliance Behavior, Knowledge: Treatment Regimen, Participation: Health Care Decisions, Treatment Behavior: Illness or Injury

Goals

The goals for this diagnosis represent those associated with discharge planning. Refer to the discharge criteria.

NIC Anticipatory Guidance, Health Education, Risk Management, Support Group, Learning Facilitation

Interventions	Rationales
1. Discuss expectations for recovery based on type and extent of surgery. Explain that vaginal hysterectomy generally affords more rapid recovery and causes less	1. Understanding expectations for recovery can help the client and family to plan strategies for complying with the postoperative care regimen.

(continued on page 588)

Interventions	Rationales
postoperative discomfort but has several disadvantages, including the following: a. Greater risk of postoperative infection. b. Reduced ability (as compared with abdominal hysterectomy) to deal with unexpected difficulties of surgery or complications (Meloni-Rosa et al., 2006; Katz, 2005; Zalon, 2004). Explain that abdominal hysterectomy allows better visualization during surgery and has fewer contraindications, but it involves longer recovery periods, increased use of anesthesia, and greater postoperative pain.	
2. Explain care of an uncomplicated wound (abdominal hysterectomy); teach the client to do the following: a. Wash with soap and water (bath or shower when able). b. Towel-dry thoroughly; separate skin folds to ensure complete drying. c. Consult with physician for care of a complicated wound.	2. Proper wound care helps to reduce microorganisms at the incision site and prevent infection.
3. Explain perineal care (vaginal hysterectomy); teach the client to do the following: a. Maintain good hygiene. b. Wash thoroughly with soap and water. c. Change the peripad frequently. d. After elimination, wipe from the front to back using a clean tissue for each front-to-back pass.	3. Proper perineal care reduces microorganisms around the perineum and minimizes their entry into the vagina.
4. Explain the need to increase activity, as tolerated, while maintaining restrictions such as no lifting greater than 5 lbs (Meloni-Rosa et al., 2006; Zalon, 2004).	4. Physical activity, especially early and frequent ambulation, can help to prevent or minimize abdominal cramps, a common complaint during recovery from abdominal hysterectomy.
5. Teach the client and family to watch for and report the following: a. Changes in perineal drainage (e.g., unusual drainage, bright red bleeding, foul odor) b. Urinary retention, burning, frequency c. Cloudy, foul-smelling urine d. Blood in urine e. Change in bowel function (constipation, diarrhea)	5. Because of the abundance of blood vessels in the female pelvis, hysterectomy carries a higher risk of postoperative bleeding than most other surgeries. Bleeding most often occurs within 24 hours after surgery, but high risk also occurs on the fourth, ninth, and 21st postoperative days, when the sutures dissolve. A small amount of pink, yellow, or brown serous drainage or even minor frank vaginal bleeding (no heavier than normal menstrual flow) is normal and expected (Kramer & Reiter, 1997; Meloni-Rosa et al., 2006; Zalon, 2004; Zepf, 2002).
6. Explain the effects of surgery on menstruation and ovulation. Instruct the client to report symptoms of the climacteric (cessation of menses). a. Hot flashes b. Headache c. Nervousness d. Palpitations e. Fatigue f. Depression, feelings of uselessness, and other emotional reactions	6. Removal of the uterus but keeping the ovaries theoretically should not produce menopausal symptoms; however, the client may experience them temporarily, apparently because of increased estrogen levels resulting from surgical manipulation of the ovaries. Removal of both ovaries artificially induces menopause; this causes more severe symptoms than typically experienced in a normal climacteric. To help reduce these symptoms, a portion of the ovary often is left in place unless contraindicated. Estrogen therapy relieves symptoms and may be indicated except in cases of malignancy (Meloni-Rosa et al., 2006; Zalon, 2004; Zepf, 2002).

(continued on page 589)

Interventions	Rationales
7. Explain activity restrictions; teach client to do the following: a. Expect fatigue and weakness during the recovery period. b. Delegate tasks to others (e.g., vacuuming or lifting) for at least 1 month. c. Walk in moderation; gradually increase distance and pace. d. Resume driving 2 weeks after surgery if the car is equipped with an automatic transmission. e. Avoid sitting and standing for prolonged periods. f. Avoid aerobic activity. g. Avoid horseback riding.	7. Adequate rest allows the body to repair surgical tissue trauma. Walking improves muscle strength and endurance to speed up recovery. Prolonged sitting or standing may cause pelvic congestion and thrombosis formation. Repetitive activities also cause pelvic congestion.
8. Explore the client's concerns regarding the impact of surgery on sexual feelings and function. Explain that she should be able to resume intercourse anywhere from 3 weeks (with a vaginal hysterectomy) to 16 weeks after surgery; confirm a specific time frame with the physician.	8. In most cases, hysterectomy should not affect sexual response or functioning. For 3–4 months after surgery intercourse may be painful due to abdominal soreness and temporary shrinking of the vagina. Intercourse helps to stretch the vaginal walls and eventually relieves the discomfort (Katz, 2005).
9. If a subtotal hysterectomy was performed, explain that menses will continue because a portion of the uterus and its endometrial lining remain 10. Explain that total removal of the uterus prevents pregnancy and results in loss of menses, but as long as even a portion of an ovary remains, the client may experience monthly premenstrual symptoms such as bloating and abdominal cramps (Meloni-Rosa et al., 2006; Zepf, 2002).	9,10. Explanations of what to expect from surgery can help reduce anxiety associated with the unknown and allow effective coping (Redman & Thomas, 1996; Meloni-Rosa et al., 2006; Zalon, 2004; Katz, 2005). Subtotal hysterectomies left 7% of women with menstrual bleeding (Zalon, 2004).
11. Explain the effects of estrogen deficiency on (Katz, 2005, Zalon, 2004): a. Osteoporosis b. Depression c. Decreased sexual drive d. Vaginal dryness, pain during sex e. Stress incontinence	11. Decreased levels of estrogen will influence sexual function, libido, tissue structure, and self-concept. Bone loss is increased with estrogen deficiency (Meloni-Rosa et al., 2006).
12. Advise the client to discuss with her surgeon the above effects, if they occur, or strategies to prevent them	12. Strategies to reduce or prevent these complications can be instituted after discharge.
13. Discuss follow-up care and that a postoperative check is scheduled for 4–6 weeks after discharge. Reinforce the importance of keeping scheduled appointments (Meloni-Rosa et al., 2006; Zalon, 2004).	13. Regular follow-up care is necessary to evaluate the results of surgery and estrogen therapy, if indicated, and to detect any complications (Katz, 2005; Zepf, 2002).

Documentation

Discharge summary record
  Client and family teaching
  Outcome achievement or status

Ileostomy

Ileostomy is the surgical creation of an opening between the ileum and the abdominal wall for the purpose of fecal diversion. An ileostomy is typically indicated for clients with pathologic small bowel conditions, such as ulcerative colitis, cancer complications, Crohn Disease, and familial polyposis (Lewis et al., 2004; Hyland, 2002). An ileostomy may be temporary or permanent, and may be constructed as an end stoma, a loop stoma, or a double-barrel stoma.

Ileostomies are usually sited above the groin on the right hand side of the abdomen (Hyland, 2002). Ileostomy differs from colostomy in that the feces have a more liquid consistency, digestive enzymes are present, and the flow of contents is uncontrolled, so that a collection appliance must be used continuously.

There are 3 types of Ileostomy (when the entire colon is removed): the standard or Brook ileostomy, continent ileostomy (abdominal pouch), and ileoanal reservoir (Collett, 2002; Clark, 2006). The type of ileostomy employed depends on the disease process, age, general health, and the preference of the client.

A standard ileostomy requires the client to wear an external ostomy postsurgery. Two internal pouching procedures, however, can replace this external ostomy pouch. A *Kock continent ileostomy* pouch is an internal fecal reservoir constructed of ileum and containing a nipple valve that maintains continence of stool and flatus. An *ileoanal reservoir* is an ileal pouch located in the pelvis. Various pouch configurations are possible, the most common being an S- or J-shaped pouch.

Ileostomy surgery is done in two stages. The first operation involves an abdominal colectomy, construction of an ileal pouch, mucosectomy of the rectum, ileoanal anastomosis, and creation of a diverting ileostomy. The second operation removes the temporary ileostomy to restore the continuity of the fecal stream (Lewis, Heitkemper, & Dirkson et al., 2004; Hyland, 2002; Collett, 2002).

🕐 Time Frame
Preoperative and postoperative periods

■■■■■ DIAGNOSTIC CLUSTER

Preoperative Period

Nursing Diagnoses

▲ Anxiety related to lack of knowledge of ileostomy care and perceived negative effects on life style

Postoperative Period

Collaborative Problems

▲ PC: Peristomal Ulceration/Herniation
▲ PC: Stomal Necrosis, Retraction Prolapse, Stenosis, Obstruction
▲ PC: Fluid and Electrolyte Imbalances
△ PC: Ileal Reservoir Pouchitis (Kock Pouch)
△ PC: Failed Nipple Valve (Kock Pouch)
△ PC: Ileoanal Kock Pouchitis
△ PC: Cholelithiasis
△ PC: Urinary Calculi

Nursing Diagnoses

▲ High Risk for Disturbed Self-Concept related to effects of ostomy on body image and life style

△ High Risk for Ineffective Sexuality Patterns related to perceived negative impact of ostomy on sexual functioning and attractiveness

△ High Risk for Sexual Dysfunction related to physiologic impotence secondary to damaged sympathetic nerve (male) or inadequate vaginal lubrication (female)

(continued on page 591)

△ High Risk for Loneliness related to anxiety over possible odor and leakage from appliance

△ High Risk for Ineffective Therapeutic Regimen Management related to insufficient knowledge of stoma pouching procedure, peristomal skin care, perineal wound care, and incorporation of ostomy care into activities of daily living (ADLs)

△ High Risk for Ineffective Therapeutic Regimen Management related to insufficient knowledge of care of ileoanal reservoir

High Risk for Ineffective Therapeutic Regimen Management related to insufficient knowledge of intermittent intubation of Kock continent ileostomy

Related Care Plan

General Surgery Generic care plan

▲ This diagnosis was reported to be monitored for or managed frequently (75%–100%).
△ This diagnosis was reported to be monitored for or managed often (50%–74%).

Discharge Criteria

Before discharge, the client and family will

1. Discuss and give return demonstration in relation to ostomy care at home, including stoma, pouching, irrigation, skin care
2. Discuss strategies for incorporating ostomy management into ADLs.
3. Verbalize precautions for medication use and food intake.
4. State signs and symptoms that must be reported to a health care professional.
5. Verbalize an intent to share feelings and concerns related to ostomy with significant others.
6. Identify available community resources and self-help groups:
   a. Visiting nurse
   b. United Ostomy Associations of America (UOAA)
   c. Recovery of Male Potency: Help for Impotent Male
   d. American Cancer Foundation
   e. Community supplier of ostomy equipment
   f. Financial reimbursement for ostomy equipment
7. If the client has a Kock continent ileostomy, he or she should demonstrate ability to perform intermittent self-intubation (Collett, 2002).

Preoperative: Nursing Diagnosis

Anxiety Related to Lack of Knowledge of Ileostomy Care and Perceived Negative Effects on Life Style

NOC Anxiety Control, Coping, Impulse Control

Goal

The client will verbalize decreased anxiety related to fear of the unknown.

Indicators

- State reason for ileostomy.
- Describe anatomic changes following ileostomy surgery.
- Identify his/her own type of ileostomy, and why that particular one was selected (Pontieri-Lewis, 2006).

NIC Anxiety Reduction, Coping, Impulse Control

Interventions	Rationales
1. Identify and dispel any misinformation or misconceptions the client has regarding ileostomy (Richbourg, Thorpe, & Rapp, 2007).	1. Replacing misinformation with facts can reduce anxiety.
2. Explain the normal anatomical structure and function of the gastrointestinal (GI) tract.	2. Knowledge boosts confidence; confidence enhances control and reduces anxiety.
3. Explain the effects of the client's particular disorder on affected organs.	3. Understanding the disorder can help the client accept the need for ileostomy.
4. Use an anatomic diagram or model to show the resultant altered route of elimination.	4. Understanding how body waste elimination occurs after the rectum and the anus are removed can help to allay anxiety related to altered body function.
5. Describe the stoma's appearance and anticipated location. Explain the following about the stoma: a. It will be of the same color and moistness as oral mucous membrane. b. It will not hurt when touched, because it has no sensory endings. c. It may bleed slightly when wiped; this is normal and not of concern. d. It will become smaller as the surgical area heals; the color will remain the same. e. It may change in size depending on illness, hormone levels, and weight gain or loss (Black, 2000).	5. Explaining expected events and sensations can help to reduce anxiety associated with the unknown and unexpected. Accurate descriptions of the stoma appearance help to ease shock at the first sight of it after ostomy surgery.
6. Discuss the function of the stoma pouch. Explain that it serves as an external receptacle for storage of feces, much as the colon acts as an internal storage receptacle.	6. Understanding the purpose and need for a pouch encourages the client to accept it and participate in ostomy management.
7. Encourage the client to handle the stoma pouching equipment.	7. Many clients are relieved to see the actual size and material of a stoma pouch. Often, the uninformed client's visions of large bags and complicated, difficult-to-manage equipment can produce anxiety.

Documentation

Progress notes
Present emotional status
Teaching records
   Client teaching

Postoperative: Collaborative Problems

Potential Complication: Peristomal Ulceration/Herniation

Potential Complication: Stomal Necrosis, Retraction, Prolapse, Stenosis, Obstruction

Potential Complication: Fluid and Electrolyte Imbalances

Potential Complication: Ileal Reservoir Pouchitis (Kock Pouch)

Potential Complication: Failed Nipple Valve (Kock Pouch)

Potential Complication: Ileoanal Kock Pouchitis

Potential Complication: Cholelithiasis

Potential Complication: Urinary Calculi

Nursing Goal

The nurse will detect early signs and symptoms of (a) peristomal ulceration/herniation, (b) stomal necrosis, retraction, (c) prolapse, stenosis, obstruction, (d) fluid and electrolyte imbalances, (e) ileal reservoir pouchitis (Kock pouch), (f) failed nipple valve (Kock pouch), (g) ileoanal Kock pouchitis, (h) cholelithiasis, and (i) urinary calculi, and collaboratively intervene to stabilize the client.

Indicators

- Intact peristomal muscle tone (a)
- No stomal ulceration (a)
- No complaints of abdominal cramping or pain (b, e, g)
- No abdominal or flank pain (h, i)
- No nausea or vomiting (b, d, e, g)
- No abdominal distention (b, d, h)
- Urine output >30 mL/h (d, e, g)
- Minimal or no weight loss (d, e, g)
- Clear, pale urine (d, e, g)
- Urine specific gravity 1.005–1.030 (d, e, g)
- No change in stool color (d, e, g)
- Serum sodium (d, e, g)
- Serum potassium (d, e, g)
- Serum magnesium (d, e, g)
- Serum cholesterol (d, e, g)
- No epigastric fullness (h)
- No jaundice (h)
- Temperature 98.5–99°F (e, g)

Interventions	Rationales

1. Monitor for signs of peristomal ulceration or herniation:
  a. Decreased peristomal muscle tone
  b. Bulging beyond normal skin surface and musculature
  c. Persistent ulceration
	1. Early detection of ulcerations and herniation can prevent serious tissue damage (Colwell & Beitz, 2007).

2. Monitor for stomal necrosis, prolapse, retraction, stenosis, and obstruction. Assess the following:
  a. Color, size, and shape of stoma
  b. Color, amount, and consistency of ostomy effluent
  c. Complaints of cramping, abdominal pain, nausea and vomiting, and abdominal distension
  d. Ostomy appliance and appliance belt fit
	2. Daily assessment is necessary to detect early changes in stoma condition:
	  a. These changes can indicate inflammation, retraction, prolapse, or edema.
	  b. These changes can indicate bleeding or infection. Decreased output can indicate obstruction.
	  c. These complaints may indicate obstruction.
	  d. Improperly fitting appliance or belt can cause mechanical trauma to the stoma (Colwell & Beitz, 2007).

3. Monitor for signs of fluid and electrolyte imbalance:
  a. High volume of watery ostomy output (more than five ⅓- to ½-filled pouches or >1000 mL daily)
  b. Decreased serum sodium, potassium, magnesium levels, and cardiac arrhythmias (Wagner, Johnson, & Kidd, 2006; Lewis et al., 2004).
  c. Weight loss
  d. Nausea and vomiting, anorexia, abdominal distention
	3. Fluid and electrolyte imbalances most commonly result from diarrhea. Major causes of acute diarrhea include infection, diuretic therapy, obstruction, and hot weather. Chronic diarrhea can result from ileal resection or "short gut syndrome," radiation therapy, or chemotherapy (Richbourg, Thorpe, & Rapp, 2007; Wagner, Johnson, & Kidd, 2006; Lewis et al., 2004).

4. Administer fluid and electrolyte replacement therapy, as ordered.	4. Replacement therapy may be needed to prevent serious electrolyte imbalance or fluid deficiency, and cardiac arrhythmias (ventricular ectopic, ventricular tachycardia and Torsades de pointes) (Wagner, Johnson, & Kidd, 2006; Lewis et al., 2004).

(continued on page 594)

Interventions	Rationales
5. Monitor for signs and symptoms of ileal reservoir or ileoanal pouchitis: 　a. Acute increase in effluent flow 　b. Evidence of dehydration 　c. Abdominal pain and bloating, nausea and vomiting 　d. Fever	5. Pouchitis or ileitis involves inflammation of the ileal pouch. The cause is unknown, but bacterial growth in the pouch is a suspected causative factor. Insufficiently frequent pouch emptying increases the risk; it occurs in about 10% of clients with a Kock ileostomy.
6. Connect an indwelling catheter to continuous straight drainage.	6. This measure promotes continuous urine drainage of the Kock Pouch
7. Monitor for stool leakage from a stoma with a nipple valve.	7. Nipple valve failure—pulling apart of the bowel segment forming the valve—most commonly occurs within the first 3 months after surgery.
8. Irrigate the ileoanal reservoir daily to flush out mucus.	8. Daily irrigation helps to prevent stomal obstruction.
9. Monitor for cholelithiasis (gallstones): 　a. Epigastric fullness 　b. Abdominal distention 　c. Vague pain 　d. Very dark urine 　e. Grayish or clay colored stools 　f. Jaundice 　g. Elevated cholesterol	9. Changes in absorption of bile acids postoperatively increase cholesterol levels and can cause gallstones (Colwell & Beitz, 2007; Wagner, Johnson, & Kidd, 2006).
10. If symptoms occur, collaborate with the physician or advanced practice nurse to prepare for a diagnostic evaluation (e.g., ultrasound, cholecystography).	10. Diagnostic studies will be indicated to confirm gallstones and to determine severity.
11. Monitor for urinary calculi (stones): 　a. Lower abdominal pain 　b. Flank pain 　c. Hematuria 　d. Decreased urine output 　e. Increased urine specific gravity	11. Large volumes of fluid lost through the ileostomy can cause urinary stones as a result of dehydration.

 Related Physician-Prescribed Interventions

Depending on the underlying problem. Refer also to the General Surgery care plan at the beginning of Section II.

Documentation

Flow records
　Intake and output
　Bowel sounds
　Wound status
Progress notes
Stoma condition
Changes in physiologic status

Postoperative: Nursing Diagnoses

High Risk for Disturbed Self-Concept Related to Effects of Ostomy on Body Image

NOC Quality of Life, Coping, Depression, Self-Esteem

Goal

The client will acknowledge change in body structure and function.

Indicators

- Communicate feelings about the ostomy.
- Participate in stoma care.

NIC Hope Instillation, Mood Management, Values Clarification, Counseling, Referral, Support Group, Coping Enhancement

Interventions	Rationales
1. Contact client frequently and treat him or her with warm, positive regard.	1. Frequent contact by the caregiver indicates acceptance and may facilitate trust. The client may be hesitant to approach staff because of negative self-concept (Colwell & Beitz, 2007).
2. Incorporate emotional support into technical ostomy self-care sessions.	2. This allows resolution of emotional issues during acquisition of technical skills. Richbourg, Thorpe, and Rapp (2007) have identified four stages of psychological adjustment that ostomy clients may experience: a. *Narration.* The client recounts his or her illness experience and reveals understanding of how and why he or she finds self in this situation. b. *Visualization and verbalization.* The client looks at and expresses feelings about his or her stoma. c. *Participation.* The client progresses from observer to assistant, then to independent performer of the mechanical aspects of ostomy care. d. *Exploration.* The client begins to explore methods of incorporating the ostomy into her or his life style. This adjustment framework helps to establish guidelines for planning the client's experiences in an organized manner.
3. Have the client look at and touch the stoma.	3. The nurse should not make assumptions about a client's reaction to ostomy surgery. The client may require help in accepting the reality of altered body appearance and function or in dealing with an overwhelming situation (Richbourg, Thorpe, & Rapp, 2007).
4. Encourage the client to verbalize feelings (both positive and negative) about the stoma, and perceptions of its anticipated effects on his or her life style. Direct the client to the appropriate professional, to help overcome negative feelings and perceptions, if any (Richbourg, Thorpe, & Rapp, 2007; Junkin & Beitz, 2005).	4. Sharing gives the nurse an opportunity to identify and dispel misconceptions and allay anxiety and self-doubt.
5. Validate the client's perceptions and reassure her or him that such responses are normal and appropriate.	5. Validating the client's perceptions promotes self-awareness and provides reassurance.
6. Have the client practice using a pouch clamp on an empty pouch.	6. Beginning client teaching with a necessary skill that is separate from the body may be less threatening and may ease the fear of failure when performing on his or her own body.

(continued on page 596)

Interventions	Rationales
7. Assist the client with pouch emptying, as necessary.	7. During ostomy care procedures, the client watches health care professionals for signs of revulsion. The nurse's attitude and support are of primary importance (Junkin & Beitz, 2005).
8. Have the client participate in pouch removal and pouch application. Provide feedback on progress; reinforce positive behavior and proper techniques.	8. Effective, thorough teaching helps the client learn to master procedures.
9. Have the client demonstrate the stoma pouching procedure independently in the presence of support persons.	9. Return demonstration lets the nurse evaluate the need for any further teaching.
10. Involve support persons in learning ostomy care principles. Assess the client's interactions with support persons.	10. Other people's response to the ostomy is one of the most important factors influencing the client's acceptance of it.
11. Encourage the client to discuss plans for incorporating ostomy care into his or her life style.	11. Evidence that the client will pursue his or her goals and life style reflects positive adjustment (Junkin & Beitz, 2005).
12. Encourage the client to verbalize positive self-attributes.	12. Identifying personal strengths promotes self-acceptance and positive self-concept.
13. Suggest that the client meet with a person from the UOA who can share similar experiences.	13. In addition to the professional nurse's clinical expertise, the ostomy client may choose to take advantage of a UOA visitor's actual experience with an ostomy (Junkin & Beitz, 2005).
14. Identify a client at risk for unsuccessful adjustment (Richbourg, Thorpe, & Rapp, 2007; Junkin & Beitz, 2005): a. Poor ego strength b. Ineffective problem-solving ability c. Difficulty learning new skills d. Lack of motivation e. External focus of control f. Poor health g. Unsatisfactory preoperative sex life h. Lack of positive support systems i. Unstable economic status j. Rejection of counseling	14. Successful adjustment to ostomy is influenced by factors such as the following: a. Previous coping success b. Achievement of developmental tasks presurgery, which includes the education and acceptance of the ostomy requirement and placement (Haugen, Bliss, & Savik, 2006). c. Extent to which the disability interferes with goal-directed activity d. Sense of control e. Realistic perception of the event by the client and support persons
15. Refer an at-risk client for professional counseling.	15. In such a client, follow-up therapy is indicated to assist with effective adjustment (Haugen, Bliss, & Savik, 2006; Junkin & Beitz, 2005).

Documentation

Progress notes
    Present emotional status
    Interventions
    Response to interventions

High Risk for Ineffective Sexuality Patterns Related to Perceived Negative Impact of Ostomy on Sexual Functioning and Attractiveness

NOC   Body Image, Self-Esteem, Role Performance, Sexual Identity: Acceptance

Goal

The client will discuss own feelings and partner's concerns regarding the effect of ostomy surgery on sexual functioning.

Indicators

- Verbalize the intent to discuss concerns with partner before discharge.
- Discuss own feelings and partner's concerns regarding the effect of ostomy surgery on sexual functioning.

NIC   Behavior Management: Sexual, Counseling, Emotional Support, Active Listening, Teaching: Sexuality

Interventions	Rationales
1. Reaffirm the need for frank discussion between sexual partners and the need for time for the partner to become accustomed to changes in the client's body.	1. Individuals report that their lives have suffered as a result of their surgeries (Richbourg, Thorpe, & Rapp, 2007).
2. Role-play ways for the client and partner to discuss concerns about sex.	2. Role-playing helps a client to gain insight by placing him- or herself in the position of another. It also may promote more spontaneous sharing of fears and concerns.
3. Discuss the possibility that the client may project his or her own feelings onto the partner. Encourage frequent validation of feelings between partners.	3. The client may have erroneous assumptions about the partner (e.g., he or she may erroneously assume that the partner is "turned off" by the ostomy).
4. Reaffirm the need for closeness and expressions of caring; involve the client and partner in touching, stroking, massage, and so on.	4. Sexual pleasure and gratification are not limited to intercourse. Other expressions of caring may prove more meaningful.
5. Explore any fears the client may express regarding mutilation, unacceptability, and other concerns that might limit his or her involvement in relationships (Junkin & Beitz, 2005).	5. These fears might limit involvement in relationships.
6. Discuss the possible availability of a penile prosthesis if the client is physiologically unable to maintain or sustain an erection sufficient for intercourse. Explain that a penile implant provides the erection needed for intercourse and does not alter sensations or the ability to ejaculate (Haugen, Bliss, & Savik, 2006; Junkin & Beitz, 2005).	6. Realizing that a prosthesis may be available can reassure the client and reduce anxiety about performance; this actually could help to improve function.
7. Refer the client to a certified sex or mental health counselor, if desired.	7. Certain sexual problems require continuing therapy and the advanced knowledge of therapists.

Documentation

Progress notes
    Assessment data
    Interventions
    Response to interventions
    Referrals, if indicated

High Risk for Sexual Dysfunction Related to Physiologic Impotence Secondary to Damaged Sympathetic Nerve (Male) or Inadequate Vaginal Lubrication (Female)

NOC   Body Image, Self-Esteem, Role Performance, Sexual Identity: Acceptance

Goal

The client will state alternatives to deal with physiologic impotence.

Indicators

- Explain the surgery's effects on erections.
- Report community resources available.

NIC Sexual Counseling, Emotional Support, Active Listening, Teaching: Sexuality

Interventions	Rationales

1. Explain the effects of surgery on sexual function:
  a. In men, a wide resection for Crohn disease occasionally damages the sympathetic nerves in the presacral area that control emission. This may result in retrograde ejaculation into the bladder and a "dry" orgasm. During abdominoperineal surgery, the parasympathetic nerves that control blood flow to the penis can be damaged, possibly resulting in erectile dysfunction (Maklebust, 1990; Krebs, 2000).
  b. In women, body image fears are focused on aesthetics (e.g., appearance, odor).
  c. One study reported that women pre/post-ostomy surgery related fear of stool leakage; odor; and change in body appearance, sexual love play, and intercourse (Pieper & Mikols, 1996).
 	
2. Provide the client and partner opportunities to share their fears and concerns.
	1,2. Explanations and discussions of what to expect can reduce fears regarding the unknown.

3. In men:
  a. Suggest that sexual activity need not always culminate in vaginal intercourse and that orgasm can be reached through noncoital manual or oral stimulation. Remind the client that sexual expression is not limited to intercourse, but includes closeness, communication, touching, and giving pleasure to another (Junkin & Beitz, 2005).
  b. Suggest counseling with a certified sex therapist.
	3.
	  a. Alternative methods of sexual expression and gratification promote positive sexual function.
	
	  b. Certain sexual problems require continuing therapy and the advanced knowledge of therapists.

4. In women:
  a. Suggest using a water-based vaginal lubricant for intercourse.
  b. Teach the client to perform Kegel exercises and instruct her to do them regularly.
 	
  c. Suggest that she sit astride her partner during intercourse.
	4.
	  a. Water-based lubricants can help to prevent dyspareunia related to inadequate vaginal lubrication.
	  b. Kegel exercises promote control of the pubococcygeal muscles around the vaginal entrance; this can ease dyspareunia.
	  c. A woman on top can control the depth and rate of penetration; this can enhance vaginal lubrication and relaxation.

Documentation

Progress notes
  Interventions
  Response to interventions

High Risk for Loneliness Related to Anxiety over Possible Odor and Leakage from Appliance

NOC Loneliness, Social Involvement

Goal

The client will state the intent to reestablish preoperative socialization pattern.

Indicators

- Discuss methods to control odor and appliance leakage.
- Identify foods that increase odor and gas.

NIC Socialization Enhancement, Spiritual Support, Behavior Modification: Social Skills, Presence, Anticipatory Guidance

Interventions	Rationales
1. Select an appropriate odor-proof pouching system, and explain to the client how it works.	1. Fear of accidents and odor can be reduced through effective management. Some pouches have charcoal filters to reduce odor from flatus.
2. Stress the need for good personal hygiene. 3. Teach the client care of a stoma appliance.	2,3. Proper hygiene and appliance care remove odoriferous retained fecal material.

4. Discuss methods for reducing odor:
  a. Avoid odor-producing foods such as onions, fish, eggs, cheese, asparagus (Hyland, 2002).
  b. Use internal chlorophyll tablets or a liquid appliance deodorant (Hyland, 2002).
  c. Empty or change the ostomy pouch regularly—when it is one-third to one-half full (Hyland, 2002).
	4. Minimizing odor improves self-confidence and can permit more effective socialization. Bacterial proliferation in retained effluent increases odor with time. A full pouch also puts excessive pressure on seals, which increases the risk of leakage.

5. Encourage the client to reestablish his or her preoperative socialization pattern. Help through measures such as progressively increasing the client's socializing time in the hospital, role-playing possible situations that the client feels may cause anxiety, and encouraging the client to visualize and anticipate solutions to "worst-case scenarios" for social situations.	5. Encouraging and facilitating socialization help to prevent isolation. Role-playing can help the client to identify and learn to cope with potential anxiety-causing situations in a nonthreatening environment.
6. Suggest that the client meet with a person from the UOA who can share similar experiences.	6. Others in a similar situation can provide a realistic appraisal of the situation and may provide information to answer the client's unasked questions.

Documentation

Progress notes
  Dialogues
Discharge summary record
  Client teaching
  Outcome achievement or status

High Risk for Ineffective Therapeutic Regimen Management Related to Insufficient Knowledge of Stoma Pouching Procedure, Peristomal Skin Care, Perineal Wound Care, and Incorporation of Ostomy Care into Activities of Daily Living (ADLs)

NOC Compliance Behavior, Knowledge: Treatment Regimen, Participation: Health Care Decisions, Treatment Behavior: Illness or Injury

Goals

The goals for this diagnosis represent those associated with discharge planning. Refer to the discharge criteria.

NIC Ostomy Care, Anticipatory Guidance, Risk Identification, Learning Facilitation, Health Education

Interventions	Rationales
1. Consult with a wound care/ostomy specialist.	1. Experts in intervening with ostomy clients are needed to increase client and family confidence and to provide specific information on what to expect.

2. Teach client the basic stoma pouching principles:
 	
   a. Keeping the peristomal skin clean and dry.
   b. Using a well-fitting appliance.
 	
   c. Changing the pouch when the least amount of drainage is anticipated (usually on arising).
   d. Emptying the pouch when it is one-third to one-half full, and changing routinely before a leak occurs (Pontieri-Lewis, 2006).
   e. Changing the pouch if burning or itching occurs under the appliance.
 	
   f. Observing the condition of the stoma and peristomal skin during pouch changes.
	2. Proper pouching techniques can prevent leakage and skin problems:
	   a. This ensures that the appliance adheres to the skin.
	   b. Proper fit protects the surrounding skin surface from contact with drainage.
	   c. This prevents copious drainage from interfering with pouch changes.
	   d. A pouch filled more than halfway exerts increased pressure on the seal, which increases risk of leakage.
	
	   e. Burning or itching may indicate that ostomy effluent has undermined the skin barrier; prompt intervention is necessary to prevent skin breakdown.
	   f. Regular observation enables early detection of skin problems.

3. Teach the procedure for preparing a stoma pouch:
   a. Select the appropriate stoma pouching system.
   b. Measure stoma carefully.
   c. Use the appliance manufacturer's stoma measuring card, if possible. If the card does not accommodate stoma size or shape, teach the client to make a customized stoma pattern: (1) Place clear plastic wrap from the skin barrier wafer over the stoma; (2) trace the stoma with a marking pen; and (3) cut a hole in the plastic wrap to accommodate the stoma.
   d. Cut an opening in the center of the skin barrier slightly larger (approximately ⅛ inch) than the stoma (Pontieri-Lewis, 2006; Hyland, 2002).
   e. Secure an appropriate odor-proof pouch onto the skin barrier wafer, if using a two-piece appliance system.
	3. Preparing a new pouch beforehand ensures that it is ready to apply as soon as the used pouch is removed; this helps to minimize drainage on skin surface.

4. Teach the procedure for changing a disposable stoma pouch:
   a. Remove the old pouch by gently pushing the skin away from the paper tape and skin barrier wafer.
   b. Fold the old pouch over on itself and discard in a plastic bag.
   c. Cleanse the peristomal skin with a washcloth and warm tap water.
   d. Blot or pat the skin dry.
   e. Apply the new pouch to the abdomen, carefully centering the hole in the skin barrier wafer over the stoma. Press on the wafer for a few minutes.
   f. Secure the pouch by "picture framing" the wafer with four strips of hypoallergenic paper tape (if the wafer does not already have tape attached).
	4. Correct pouch removal and attachment techniques minimize irritation and injury of peristomal skin and ensure a tight, reliable seal between pouch and skin.

5. Teach the procedure for emptying a stoma pouch:
   a. Put some toilet paper in the toilet bowl and sit on the toilet seat.
   b. Remove the clamp from the tail of the pouch, and carefully empty pouch contents into the toilet.
	5. Correct techniques can reduce spillage, soiling, and odor. Placing toilet paper in the bowl prevents water from splashing as the pouch contents are emptied.

(continued on page 601)

Interventions	Rationales
c. Clean the inside and outside of the pouch tail with toilet paper and squeeze ostomy appliance deodorant into the end of the pouch.	
6. Teach strategies for prevention and management of potential peristomal skin problems: a. Shave the peristomal skin with an electric razor rather than a blade; avoid using shaving cream, soap, and detergents, except when showering. b. Evaluate all skin products for possible allergic reaction; patch-test all suspect products elsewhere on the abdomen. c. Do not change brands of skin barriers and adhesives casually; assess for allergic reaction before using a new brand. d. Avoid irritation from contact with ostomy effluent. e. Avoid prolonged skin pressure, especially if the skin is fair or thin and atrophic as a result of long-term corticosteroid therapy. f. Use corticosteroid creams sparingly and briefly; they can cause dryness and irritation. g. If bacterial or fungal infection is suspected, use a specific antibacterial or antifungal cream or powder. h. Use a liquid film barrier; avoid tincture of benzoin compound, which can dry skin. i. Avoid aluminum paste and greasy ointments that can mask skin problems and interfere with pouch adherence. j. Protect the skin with barriers. k. Expect the stoma to shrink slightly over time. This will necessitate remeasuring the stoma to ensure proper appliance fit.	6. A client with a stoma is at increased risk for peristomal skin breakdown. Factors that influence skin integrity include: composition, quantity, and consistency of the ostomy effluent; allergies; mechanical trauma; the underlying disease and its treatment (including medications); surgical construction and location of the stoma; the quality of ostomy and periostomal skin care; availability of proper supplies; nutritional status; overall health status; hygiene; and activity level.
7. Address nutrition and diet management: a. Teach how the ostomy affects absorption and use of nutrients; discuss dietary implications. b. Assess food tolerances by adding new foods one at a time and in small amounts. c. Teach the client to eat regularly and slowly, to chew food well, and to avoid high-fiber foods that can promote stomal blockage. d. Discuss dietary modifications that can help decrease odor and flatus. e. List dietary modifications to prevent or manage diarrhea and constipation, as indicated. f. If fecal discharge is too watery, increase fibrous foods (whole grain cereals, fresh fruit skins, beans, corn). g. If fecal discharge is too dry, increase salt intake if not contraindicated. h. Instruct the client to monitor weight and report any loss or gain of more than 10 pounds. i. Explain the importance of adequate fluid intake (water, sports drinks, juices) to prevent or manage fluid and electrolyte problems related to excessive perspiration and diarrhea.	7. Proper nutrition and dietary management are important factors in ostomy management.
8. Explain the effects of certain medications on ostomy function: a. Antibiotics may induce diarrhea.	8. Counseling the client about the possible harmful effects of home remedies and indiscriminate self-medication may help to prevent minor or serious problems.

(continued on page 602)

Interventions	Rationales

b. Fecal odor may be controlled by internal or external deodorizers. Internal deodorizers may have a mild laxative effect.

c. Suppositories cannot be used if the rectum and anus are removed. Instruct the client to notify a physician or pharmacist if a drug problem is suspected.

9. Promote measures to help the client incorporate ostomy care into ADLs (Collett, 2002; Hyland, 2002; Pontieri-Lewis, 2006)·

   a. *Working/traveling:* Keep extra supplies at work. When traveling, carry supplies rather than packing them in a suitcase and risk losing them; keep in mind that pectin-based wafers melt in high environmental temperatures. Take a list of ostomy supplies when traveling.

   b. *Exercise:* The only limits involve contact sports during which trauma to the stoma may occur. Normal exercise is beneficial and may help to stimulate bowel evacuation; in some cases exercise can eliminate the need for irrigation. Successful use of exercise to regulate the bowel depends on the presurgical bowel pattern and regularity of elimination. Other contributing factors include the consistency of fecal contents, motivation, diet, ability to exercise, and practice.

   c. *Wardrobe:* Ostomy appliances are invisible under clothing. Any clothing worn preoperatively may be worn postoperatively; dress comfortably.

     • Wear two pairs of underpants. The inside pair should be low-rise or bikini-height cotton knit worn *under* the ostomy appliance to absorb perspiration and keep the pouch away from the skin. The outside pair can be cotton or nylon, should be waist-high, and worn *over* the ostomy appliance.

     • The ostomy pouch can be tucked between the two pairs of underwear like a kangaroo pouch. Special pouch covers are expensive, soil rapidly, and are not necessary.

     • Avoid too-tight clothing that can restrict the appliance and cause leakage. A boxer-type bathing suit is preferable for men. For women, a patterned bathing suit with shirring can camouflage the appliance well.

   d. *Bathing/showering/swimming:* These activities may be done while wearing an ostomy appliance. "Picture-frame" the skin barrier with paper tape to seal the edges and keep the barrier edge from getting wet. Showering may be done without an appliance and, in fact, is recommended on days of appliance changes.

   e. *Diet:*

     • Chew all food well.

     • The noise from passing flatus will decrease postoperatively with progression to a regular diet.

     • Eat on a regular schedule to help decrease the noise from an empty gut.

     • Avoid mushrooms, Chinese vegetables, popcorn, and other foods that may cause blockage. (*Note:* Pillsbury microwave popcorn is specially made to be tolerated because adequate chewing can finely grind the kernels.)

9. Successful incorporation of ostomy management into ADLs allows the client to resume preileostomy life style and pursue goals and interests.

(continued on page 603)

Interventions	Rationales

- Keep in mind that fish, cabbage, eggs, and onions cause odor in the stool.
- Drink at least several 8-oz glasses of water a day to prevent dehydration in an ileostomate and constipation in a colostomate. Concentrated urine or decreased urinary output is a good indicator of dehydration.

f. *Odor control:*
- Explain that odor is caused by bacteria in the stool.
- Because most ostomy appliances are made to be odor-proof, do not poke a hole in the ostomy appliance to allow flatus to escape; constant odor will result.
- Control offensive odors with good hygiene and ostomy pouch deodorants. Super Banish appliance deodorant works best because it contains silver nitrate, which kills the bacteria. Hydrogen peroxide and mouthwashes such as Binaca can be placed in the ostomy pouch as inexpensive appliance deodorants.
- Do not use aspirin tablets as a deodorant in the ostomy pouch; aspirin tablets in contact with the stoma may cause stomal irritation and bleeding.
- Eating yogurt and cranberry juice may help to reduce fecal odor. Certain oral medications reduce fecal odor, but these should be used only with the advice of a physician.

g. *Hygiene:*
- Use a hand-held shower spray to wash the skin around the stoma and irrigate perineal wounds.
- Showers can be taken with the ostomy appliance on or off. On days when the appliance is changed, a shower can be taken when the old pouch is removed, but before the new pouch is applied.
- The new pouch should be readied before getting in the shower. On days between appliance changes, showering with the appliance on requires only that the paper tape around the wafer be covered with a liquid sealant to waterproof the tape.

h. *Exercise:*
- Normal activities (even strenuous sports, in most cases) can be resumed after recovery from surgery.
- Be aware that increased incidence of peristomal herniation is associated with heavy lifting.
- Also keep in mind that increased perspiration from strenuous exercise may require more frequent ostomy appliance changes because of increased melting of the appliance skin barrier.

i. *Travel:*
- Take all ostomy supplies along when traveling, if by airplane, put in carry-on bag (Collett, 2002).
- Do not leave ostomy appliances in automobiles parked in the sun because the heat will melt the skin barrier.
- When flying, always keep appliances in carry-on luggage to avoid loss.

j. *Sexual activity:*
- Remember that an ostomy does not automatically make the client undesirable; as in any sexual encounter, the client may have to indicate sexual interest to his or her partner, who may be afraid of hurting the ostomy.

(continued on page 604)

Interventions	Rationales
• Wearing a stretch tube top around the midriff will cover the ostomy appliance while leaving the genitals and breasts exposed. • If male impotence is a problem, the man can be referred to a urologist for discussion or consideration of a penile prosthesis. • Keep in mind that in many cases, sexual problems following ostomy surgery are manifestations of problems that existed before surgery. If the ostomate had a strong supportive relationship before surgery, there usually are no problems after surgery.	
10. Teach the client to monitor the stoma and adjacent skin for changes: a. Color, size, and shape b. Color, amount, and consistency of effluent c. Ulceration	10. These changes can indicate inflammation, retraction, prolapse, edema, or obstruction.
11. Instruct the client to call the physician, an advanced practice nurse, or ostomy specialist if changes occur.	11. The client will be informed if the changes are expected or if an intervention is needed.
12. Discuss community resources/self-help groups: a. Visiting nurse b. United Ostomy Association c. Foundation for Ileitis and Colitis d. Recovery of Male Potency—Help for the Impotent Male e. American Cancer Foundation f. Community suppliers of ostomy equipment g. Financial reimbursement for ostomy equipment	

Documentation

Discharge summary record
  Client and family teaching
  Outcome achievement or status

High Risk for Ineffective Therapeutic Regimen Management Related to Insufficient Knowledge of Care of Ileoanal Reservoir

NOC Compliance Behavior, Knowledge: Treatment Regimen, Participation: Health Care Decisions, Treatment Behavior: Illness or Injury

Goals

The goals for this diagnosis represent those associated with discharge planning. Refer to the discharge criteria.

NIC Anticipatory Guidance, Risk Identification, Ostomy Care

Interventions	Rationales
1. Instruct client to practice Kegel exercises regularly.	1. Regular performance of Kegel exercises can strengthen sphincter muscle tone.
2. Teach the client how to intubate the anus and irrigate the ileoanal pouch.	2. Irrigation is needed to remove mucus and prevent clogging.

(continued on page 605)

Interventions	Rationales
3. Teach client to protect the perianal skin by using a liquid skin sealant prophylactically, and wearing minipads at night to absorb anal drainage.	3. These measures can help to protect against perianal skin denudation resulting from frequent stools.

Documentation

Discharge summary record
Client teaching
Outcome achievement or status

High Risk for Ineffective Therapeutic Regimen Management Related to Insufficient Knowledge of Intermittent Intubation of Kock Continent Ileostomy

NOC Compliance Behavior, Knowledge: Treatment Regimen, Participation: Health Care Decisions, Treatment Behavior: Illness or Injury

Goals

The goals for this diagnosis represent those associated with discharge planning. Refer to the discharge criteria.

NIC Ostomy Care, Risk Identification

Interventions	Rationales
1. Explain the need for continuous drainage postoperatively.	1. Continuous drainage is needed to decrease pressure on the suture line.
2. If indicated, teach the client intermittent self-intubation to drain the pouch; cover such measures as the following: a. Gradually decreasing the number of intubations to 3–4 times/day b. Irrigating if stool is thick c. Using lubricant on a large-bore catheter	2. Proper intubation technique helps to maximize pouch capacity, provides complete drainage, and prevents tissue trauma.
3. Encourage thorough chewing of food before swallowing; caution the client against eating high-fiber foods.	3. Bulk in diet increases irritation to the bowel and risk of obstruction.
4. Notify the physician immediately if unable to intubate the client.	4. Inability to intubate puts the client at high risk for bowel obstruction.

Documentation

Discharge summary record
    Client teaching and documentation of client and family understanding of education
    Response to teaching to ascertain if any counseling is needed or how much support will be required
      from the community health network
    Outcome achievement or status

Laminectomy

Surgery of the spine is performed for several reasons, such as trauma, removal of tumors/lesions, and for disk disease when diagnostic tests point out a herniation is not responding to conservative treatment, consistent pain, and/or a persistent neurologic deficit. There are several different approaches used but it depends on the disease/injury process that surgery is indicated for (Lewis et al., 2004). The surgical excision can be done with one of the following techniques:

- *Discectomy* is the removal of a herniated or fragmented inter-vertebral disk. This can include an anterior or posterior approach, with or without fusion involved. Anterior cervical discectomy with fusion (ACDF) is used to treat various pathologic conditions such as spondylosis and forminal stenosis. A discectomy with fusion is a small discectomy with a bone graft (donor or from client) to fuse the spinous process to stabilize the spine. Anterior cervical discectomy without fusion (ACD) is not advocated for by modern neurosurgeons and is considered antiquated (Bader & Littlejohns, 2004).

  Anterior corpectomy with fusion is indicated when a large anterior decompression of the spinal canal is required; often multiple spinal segments are involved, such as in severe spondylosis and or stenosis with associated reversal of normal lordosis. This method is more often used in trauma, tumors, or osteomyelitis. Interbody fusion options for anterior corpectomy are the same as for ACDF: allograft, autologous graft, or titanium cage. Anterior plating is desirable to promote osseous fusion (Bader & Littlejohns, 2004).

- *Laminectomy* is the surgical procedure which removes a part of the posterior arch of a vertebra (lamina) to provide access to the spinal canal and to remove pathology and relieve compression (Bader & Littlejohns, 2004; Lewis et al., 2004).

- *Hemilaminectomy* is the surgical removal of part of a lamina and part of the posterior arch (usually one side of a vertebral lamina) (Bhardwaj, Mirski, & Ulatowski, 2004).

- *Foraminotomy* is the surgical removal of the intervertebral foramen to increase space for a spinal nerve and to reduce compression.

- *Laminoplasty* is performed to decompress the cord when multiple vertebral segments are compressing (e.g., central cord syndrome from cervical stenosis). It requires normal lordotic curvature of the cervical spine (Bhardwaj, Mirski, & Ulatowski, 2004; Bader & Littlejohns, 2004).

- *Laminotomy*, bilateral or unilateral, is performed when a client has decreased functional ability, especially ambulation, associated with pain. A laminotomy preserves the central ligamentous structure and allows for adequate central foraminal decompression (Bhardwaj, Mirski, & Ulatowski, 2004; Bader & Littlejohns, 2004).

Microsurgical techniques make removal of tissue more precise with less damage to normal tissue.

 Time Frame
Preoperative and postoperative periods

■■■■■■ DIAGNOSTIC CLUSTER

Preoperative Period

Nursing Diagnoses

▲ High Risk for Injury related to lack of knowledge of postoperative position restrictions and log-rolling technique

Postoperative Period

Collaborative Problems

▲ PC: Neurological Sensory and Motor Impairments
▲ PC: Urinary Retention
▲ PC: Paralytic Ileus
△ PC: Cerebrospinal Fistula

(continued on page 607)

Nursing Diagnoses

▲ Acute Pain related to muscle spasms (back, thigh) secondary to nerve irritation during surgery, edema, skeletal malalignment, or bladder distention

▲ High Risk for Ineffective Therapeutic Regimen Management related to insufficient knowledge of home care, activity restrictions, and exercise program

Related Care Plan

General Surgery Generic care plan

▲ This diagnosis was reported to be monitored for or managed frequently (75%–100%).
△ This diagnosis was reported to be monitored for or managed often (50%–74%).

Discharge Criteria

Before discharge, the client or family will

1. Describe proper wound care at home.
2. Verbalize necessary activity precautions, including those regarding time frames for sitting, standing, lifting, and twisting, and the correct procedure in applying a brace, if ordered by the surgeon.
3. State signs and symptoms that must be reported to a health care professional, no matter how insignificant they may appear, especially neurologic deficits, wound leakage, and bulging at the incision site.

Preoperative: Nursing Diagnosis

High Risk for Injury Related to Lack of Knowledge of Postoperative Position Restrictions and Log-rolling Technique

NOC Risk Control, Safety Status: Falls Occurrence

Goal

The client will demonstrate correct positioning and log-rolling technique.

Indicators

- State why precautions are needed.
- State necessary restrictions.

NIC Fall Prevention, Environmental Management: Safety, Health Education, Surveillance: Safety, Risk Identification

Interventions	Rationale
1. Teach the client the correct body alignment to maintain while lying in bed, sitting, and standing. Teach the correct log-rolling technique to use to get in and out of bed; show the client how to do the following: a. Roll to the edge of the bed, keeping the lower back flat and the spine straight. b. Raise the head and simultaneously swing both legs (bent at the knees) over the side of the bed. c. Use the upper hand to support the stomach muscles and the lower arm to push away from the mattress (Wagner, Johnson, & Kidd, 2006; Bhardwaj, Mirski, & Ulatowski, 2004).	1. Maintaining proper positioning, good posture, and using proper procedure for getting in and out of bed will minimize back strain, muscle spasms, and discomfort.

Documentation

Discharge summary record
Client teaching
Outcome achievement or status

Postoperative: Collaborative Problems

Potential Complication: Neurological Sensory and/or Motor Impairment
Potential Complication: Urinary Retention
Potential Complication: Paralytic Ileus
Potential Complication: Cerebrospinal Fistula

Nursing Goal

The nurse will detect early signs and symptoms of (a) sensory and/or motor impairment, (b) urinary retention, (c) paralytic ileus, and (d) cerebrospinal fistula, and collaboratively intervene to stabilize the client.

Indicators

- Motor function equal and intact (a)
- Sensory function equal and intact (a)
- Strength equal and intact (a)
- Urinary output >5 mL/kg/h (a, b)
- Can verbalize bladder fullness (a, b)
- No complaints of lower abdominal pain (a, b)
- Bowel sounds present and all quadrants (c)
- Reports flatus (c)
- Bowel movement by third day (c)
- Minimal or no drainage (d)
- Negative glucose test of drainage (d)
- No complaints of headache (d)

Interventions	Rationales
1. Monitor symmetry of sensory and motor function in extremities: a. To touch, pin scratch b. Strength (have the client push your hand away with his or her soles, then pull his or her feet up against resistance). Compare findings from right side to left side and preoperative baseline.	1. Cord or nerve root edema, pressure on a nerve root from herniated disk fragments, or hematoma at the operative site can cause or exacerbate deficits in motor and sensory functions postoperatively. Surgical manipulation can result in nerve damage causing paresthesias, paralysis, and possibly respiratory insufficiency.
2. Monitor bladder function: a. Ability to void sufficient quantities, and to empty the bladder completely b. Ability to sense bladder fullness	2. Cord edema or disruption of autonomic pathways during surgery can cause a temporary loss of bladder tone (Hickey, 2003; Bader & Littlejohns, 2004; Bhardwaj, Mirski, & Ulatowski, 2004).
3. If possible, stand a male client 8–12 hours after surgery to void (mobilize as soon as possible either by nursing staff or physical therapy) (Bader & Littlejohns, 2004).	3. Urinary retention, especially when client lies flat, may be due to difficulty voiding in a horizontal position, the depressant effects of perioperative drugs, or sympathetic fiber stimulation during surgery (Hickey, 2003).
4. Monitor bowel function: a. Bowel sounds in all quadrants returning within 24 hours of surgery b. Flatus and defecation resuming by the second or third postoperative day	4. Surgery on the lumbosacral spine decreases innervation of the bowels, reducing peristalsis and possibly leading to transient paralytic ileus.

(continued on page 609)

Interventions	Rationales

5. Monitor for signs and symptoms of cerebrospinal fistula:
  a. Clear or pink ring around bloody drainage
  b. Positive glucose test of drainage
  c. Severe headache
	5. Incomplete closure of the dura causes CSF drainage. Glucose is present in CSF, but not in normal wound drainage. Changes in CSF volume cause headache.

6. Monitor and report incisional dressing for drainage.	6. There should be little or no drainage. Suspect bleeding or cerebrospinal fluid leakage if drainage occurs.
7. If the client smokes, advise him or her of increased risks. Discuss the possibility of quitting or cutting back.	7. Smokers are at high risk for postoperative cardiopulmonary complications and risk of developing pseudoarthrosis or delayed healing.
8. Monitor output from drains. Expect 20–250 mL/8 h during the first 24 hours with fusions (Bader & Littlejohns, 2004).	8. Hypovolemia can cause decreased cardiac output.

9. Monitor for and report the following:
  a. Restlessness, confusion, apprehension, tachypnea
 	
  b. Progressive weakness of lower extremities
 	
  c. Increased numbness and tingling in limbs (Bhardwaj, Mirski, & Ulatowski, 2004).
	9.
	  a. Symptoms of fat embolism can occur during surgery or 72 hours postoperatively.
	  b. Surgical trauma, hematoma formation, or vascular injury can cause cauda equina syndrome.

 ### Related Physician-Prescribed Interventions

Medications. Corticosteroids, non-steroidal anti-inflammatory drugs, muscle relaxants, narcotics
Intravenous Therapy. Refer to the General Surgery care plan
Laboratory Studies. Refer to the General Surgery care plan
Diagnostic Studies. CT scan, spinal x-ray film, myelography
Therapies. Brace, refer to the General Surgery care plan, electromyelography, MRI

Documentation

Flow records
  Vital signs (hemodynamics, neurologic, and neurovascular)
Intake and output
  Circulation (color, peripheral pulses)
    Neurologic sensory and motor status (reflexes, sensory, and motor function)
    Bowel function (bowel sounds, defecation)
    Wound condition (color, drainage, swelling)
Progress notes
  Changes in status

Postoperative: Nursing Diagnoses

Acute Pain Related to Muscle Spasms (Back or Thigh) Secondary to Nerve Irritation During Surgery, Edema, Skeletal Misalignment, or Bladder Distention

 NOC Comfort Level, Pain Control

Goal

The client will report progressive pain reduction and relief after pain-relief interventions.

Indicators

• Describe and/or demonstrate pharmacologic and non-pharmacologic techniques to reduce pain,
• Report movements to avoid, ensuring that the client and family understand the limitations and expectations required postsurgery.

NIC   Pain Management, Medication Management, Emotional Support, Teaching: Individual, Heat/Cold Application, Simple Massage

Interventions	Rationales
1. Explain to client that muscle spasms and paresthesias commonly occur after surgery.	1. Surgical trauma and edema cause pain and muscle spasms. Spasms may begin on the third or fourth postoperative day. Postoperative paresthesias in the affected leg and back may result from impaired neural function due to edema. As edema subsides, normal sensation returns.
2. Teach the importance of complying with the brace regimen.	2. Wearing a brace can prevent future hardware failure and pseudoarthrosis.
3. Evaluate if casts or brace fits properly.	3. Mobilizing devices can cause sustained pressure on tissues leading to ischemia and tissue necrosis.
4. Teach the client the need to evaluate if pressure areas are present.	4. Low pressure for long periods can cause damage and may not be noticed by the client.
5. Teach the client to use arms and legs to transfer weight properly when getting out of bed.	5. Using the stronger muscles of the arms and legs can reduce strain on the back.
6. Encourage walking, standing, and sitting for short periods from the first postoperative day or as soon as possible after surgery, ensuring that client understands that the nurse or physiotherapist will ambulate him or her the first time and continue to do so until he or she is deemed at low risk for falls (Bader & Littlejohns, 2004; Bhardwaj, Mirski, & Ulatowski, 2004). Assess carefully in the first few days after surgery to ensure proper use of body mechanics and to detect any gait or posture problems.	6. Activity goals depend on the client's pain level and functional ability. Gait or posture problems can contribute to pain on walking, standing, or sitting.
7. Teach the client the following precautions to maintain proper body alignment: a. Use the log-rolling technique with the help of two persons for the first 48 hours after surgery. (Refer to the nursing diagnosis High Risk for Injury in this care plan for details.) b. Avoid stress or strain on the operative site. c. Use the side-lying position in bed with the legs bent up evenly and the abdomen and back supported by pillows. d. Teach the client to keep her or his spine straight and when on side to place a pillow between the legs. Place pillow to support upper arm as well and to prevent the shoulder from sagging. e. Sit with knees higher than hips. f. When standing, regularly shift weight-bearing from one foot to the other.	7. Proper body alignment avoids tension on the operative site and reduces spasms. Techniques are taught to keep the lower spine as flat as possible and prevent twisting, flexing, or hyperextending.
8. Ask the client to rate pain from 0–10 before and after medication administration. Consult with the physician or advanced practice nurse if relief is unsatisfactory.	8. An objective rating scale can help to evaluate the subjective experience of pain.
9. Refer to the General Surgery care plan for general pain-relief techniques.	

Documentation

Medication administration record
  Type, dose, route, frequency of all medications
Progress notes
  Activity level
  Client's response to pain medication

High Risk for Ineffective Therapeutic Regimen Management Related to Insufficient Knowledge of Home Care, Activity Restrictions, and Exercise Program

Goals

The goals for this diagnosis represent those associated with discharge planning. Refer to the discharge criteria.

NIC Anticipatory Guidance, Learning Facilitation, Risk Management, Health Education, Teaching: Procedure/Treatment, Health System Guidance

Interventions	Rationales
1. Explain the rationale for activity restrictions and for gradual activity progression as tolerance increases.	1. Activity restrictions allow the spinal supporting structures time to heal. Complete healing of ligaments and muscles takes approximately 6 weeks.
2. Teach the client to avoid the following: a. Prolonged sitting b. Twisting the spine c. Bending at the waist d. Climbing stairs e. Automobile trips	2. These activities increase spinal flexion and create tension at the surgical site.
3. Teach the client the proper use of a back brace, if indicated.	3. A brace may be indicated to stabilize the spine and reduce pain; instruction in proper use is necessary.
4. Explain the importance of following a regular exercise program after recovery.	4. Regular, safe exercise increases spinal muscle strength and flexibility, helping protect against future injury.
5. Encourage the use of heat on the operative area, as indicated.	5. Heat increases circulation to the operative site; this promotes healing and removal of wound exudate.
6. Teach the client the postrecovery precautions, such as the following: a. Sleeping on a firm mattress b. Maintaining proper body mechanics c. Wearing only moderately high-heeled shoes d. Avoiding lifting objects over 10 lbs e. Sitting in a straight-backed chair with feet on a stool and knees flexed slightly higher than the hips f. For at least 3 weeks postsurgery, limit sitting time to 15–20 minutes	6. Techniques that reduce stress and strain on the lumbosacral spine can decrease spasms and help to prevent other disk herniations.
7. As appropriate, explain the connection between obesity and lower back problems; encourage weight loss.	7. Excess weight, particularly in the abdomen, strains and stretches muscles that support the spine, predisposing the client to spinal injury. Explaining these effects may encourage the client to lose weight.

(continued on page 612)

Interventions	Rationales
8. Explain that normal neurologic status may not return immediately.	8. Irritation of the nerve root during surgery may increase deficits temporarily (Hickey, 2002; Bhardwaj, Mirski, & Ulatowski, 2004).

9. Teach the client and family to report the following:
  a. Change in mobility, sensation, color, or pain in extremities
  b. Increased pain at the operative site
  c. Persistent headaches
  d. Elevated temperature
  e. Change in bowel or bladder function
  f. Drainage at incision site
	9. Early detection and reporting enable prompt intervention to prevent or minimize serious complications such as infection (marked by headache, fever, and increased pain) and cord compression (indicated by changes in bowel and bladder functions, movement, and sensation).

Documentation

Discharge summary record
    Client and family teaching, including the understanding of the teaching from both client and family (Lewis et al., 2004)
    Outcome achievement or status

Laryngectomy

Laryngectomy is the surgical excision of the larynx and the removal of affected structures, and is indicated for advanced-stage cancer of the vocal cords and surrounding area. The removal of the larynx causes loss of voice and speech, altered respirations via tracheostomy, and diminished sense of smell and taste (Carr, 2005).

 Time Frame
Preoperative and postoperative periods

■■■■■■ DIAGNOSTIC CLUSTER*

Preoperative Period

Nursing Diagnoses

Anxiety related to lack of knowledge of impending surgical experience and implications of condition on life style

Postoperative Period

Collaborative Problems

Refer to Tracheostomy care plan
Refer to Radical Neck Dissection care plan

Related Care Plans

Enteral Nutrition
General Surgery

✴ This surgical procedure was not included in the validation study.

Discharge Criteria

Before discharge, the client and family will

1. Describe and demonstrate proper wound care techniques.
2. Discuss strategies for performing ADLs.
3. State the signs and symptoms that must be reported to a health care professional.
4. Verbalize an intent to share feelings and concerns with significant others.
5. Identify appropriate community resources and self-help groups.

Postoperative: Nursing Diagnosis

Anxiety Related to Lack of Knowledge of Impending Surgical Experience and Implications of Condition on Life Style

NOC Anxiety Level, Coping

Goal

The client will

1. State the reason for surgery and its expected outcome.
2. Describe expected limitations on speech and swallowing.
3. Describe immediate postoperative care and self-care measures.

NIC Anxiety Reduction, Anticipatory Guidance

Interventions	Rationales
1. Explain commonly used terms and procedures. Provide written information to reinforce teaching, and introduce actual equipment. Cover these topics: a. Laryngectomy tube b. Stoma c. Drains, suctioning, and suction catheter d. Mucus e. Humidity collar f. Pharynx g. Laryngectomy ties h. Trachea	1. Effective client teaching enhances positive coping mechanisms, provides an opportunity for the client to express concerns and ask questions, and enables the nurse to correct misconceptions—all of which can help to decrease preoperative anxiety.
2. Explain the postoperative changes in appearance and body function that the client can expect (e.g., loss of ability to blow nose, suck, gargle, and whistle; diminished smell and taste sensations). If possible, after discussion with the client, arrange for a visit by a person who has already undergone laryngectomy. Inform the client and significant others of any support groups and community resources available for laryngeal clients (e.g., International Association of Laryngectomees) and Web-based support groups (e.g., www.webwhispers.org).	2. Research reports this information and contact with a person who has successfully adapted to the postoperative changes in appearance and functioning may help to reduce the client's anxiety associated with fear of the unknown (List, 1995).
3. Instruct the client in alternative communication techniques (e.g., flip chart, picture board, electrolarynx, and esophageal speech). Request return demonstration to ensure the client's mastery of the chosen technique(s).	3,4. Learning alternative communication techniques to speech lets the client maintain the ability to communicate. This can help to decrease the client's sense of alienation, isolation, and anxiety while enhancing his or her sense of control over the situation. Evaluating the client's performance of these techniques can also alert the nurse to possible cognitive or

(continued on page 614)

Interventions	Rationales
4. Explain various methods of voice restoration:	motor deficits (e.g., vision or hearing problems, facial nerve impairment, altered mentation) that may require further evaluation by a specialist.
a. Artificial larynx	a. A hand-held artificial larynx (electronic or pneumatic) transforms tone articulated by the tongue, lips, and teeth into fluent, intelligible speech.
b. Esophageal speech	b. The client ingests air into the esophagus and releases it to produce a pseudovoice.
c. Tracheoesophageal puncture (TEP)	c. A valved "voice" prosthesis (a hollow French silicone tube with a one-way flags valve) produces a voice when the user inhales, occludes the tracheostomal neck opening with the thumb, and exhales. Vibrations along the pharyngoesophagus produce a husky or hoarse voice. An alternative prosthesis (tracheostoma) has a valve that closes when the person exhales to speak, eliminating the need to use a finger to occlude.
5. Explain effects of surgery on eating, taste, and smell. Refer to care plan on Neck Dissection, Risk for Imbalanced Nutrition related to swallowing difficulties and decreased sense of smell and taste.	

Documentation

Progress notes
    Current knowledge level
    Ability to use alternative communication technique
    Response to laryngectomy visit
Discharge summary record
    Client teaching

Neck Dissection

Surgical removal of specific cervical lymph node groups and anatomic structures in the treatment of head and neck cancer is called a neck dissection. In 2001, the American Head and Neck Society (AHNS) and the American Academy of Otolaryngology—Head and Neck Surgery (AAO-HNS) revised the previous neck dissection classifications; as a result one more was added to total four procedures.

1. *Radical Neck Dissection* (RND) is the removal of all ipsilateral cervical lymph node groups from levels I through V, together with spinal accessory nerve (SAN), sternocleidomastoid muscle (SCM), and internal jugular vein (IJV).
2. *Modified Radical Neck Dissection* (MRND) is the removal of all lymph node groups routinely removed in a RND, but with preservation of one or more non-lymphatic structures (SAN, SCM, and IJV).
3. *Selective Neck Dissection* (SND) (together with the use of parentheses to denote the levels or sublevels removed) is a cervical lymphadenectomy with preservation of one or more lymph node groups that are routinely removed with a RND. For oral cavity cancers, SND (I-III) is commonly performed. For oropharyngeal, hypopharyngeal, and laryngeal cancers, SND (II-IV) is the procedure of choice.
4. *Extended Neck Dissection* (END) is the removal of one or more additional lymph node groups or non-lymphatic structures, or both, not encompassed by the RND (e.g., paratracheal or retropharyngeal nodes) or structures not routinely removed (e.g., the carotid artery or levator scapulae) (American Head and Neck Society, 2007; American Academy of Otolaryngology—Head and Neck Surgery, 2007;

Lewis et al., 2004). The spinal accessory innervates the trapezius muscle, one of the most important shoulder abductors. Neck dissections that preserve the nerve typically do not result in scapular destabilization with progressive drooping as well as anterior and lateral rotation of the scapular (AHNS, 2007; AAO-HNS, 2007; Lewis et al., 2004).

The neck has six levels, some with sublevels:

(1) Includes the *submental* and *submandibular* lymph nodes. The *submental triangle* (1A) is bounded by the anterior belly of the digastric muscles (laterally) and the hyoid (inferiorly). The *submandibular triangle* (1B) is bounded by the body of the mandible (superiorly), the stylohyoid (posteriorly), and the anterior belly of the digastric (anteriorly) (AHNS, 2007; AAO-HNS, 2007; Lewis et al., 2004).

(2) Includes lymph nodes of the upper jugular group, and is divided into sublevels: (Level II A) is bounded by the inferior border of the hyoid (inferiorly), the base of the skull (superiorly), the stylohyoid muscle (anteriorly), and the posterior border of the SCM (posteriorly). Sublevel II A nodes lie anterior to the SAN (Level II B) nodes lie posterior to the SAN (AHNS, 2007; AAO-HNS, 2007; Lewis et al., 2004).

(3) Includes lymph nodes of the middle jugular group. This level is bounded by the inferior border of the hyoid (superiorly), the inferior border of the cricoid (inferiorly), the posterior border of the sternohyoid (anteriorly), and the posterior border of the SCM (posteriorly) (AHNS, 2007; AAO-HNS, 2007; Lewis et al., 2004).

(4) This level includes the lymph nodes of the lower jugular group. It is bounded by the inferior border of the cricoid (superiorly), the clavicle/sternal notch (inferiorly), and the posterior border of the SCM (posteriorly) (AHNS, 2007; AAO-HNS, 2007; Lewis et al., 2004).

(5) Level V includes the posterior compartment lymph nodes. This compartment is bounded by the clavicle (inferiorly), the anterior border of the trapezius (posteriorly), and the posterior border of the SCM (anteriorly). It is divided into sublevels VA (lying above a transverse plane marking the inferior border of the anterior cricoid arch) and VB (below the aforementioned plane) (AHNS, 2007; AAO-HNS, 2007; Lewis et al., 2004).

(6) Level VI includes the anterior compartment lymph nodes. This compartment is bounded by the common carotid arteries (laterally), the hyoid (superiorly), and the suprasternal notch (inferiorly) (AHNS, 2007; AAO-HNS, 2007; Lewis et al., 2004).

 Time Frame
Preoperative and postoperative periods
Postintensive care

■■■■■■ **DIAGNOSTIC CLUSTER**

Preoperative Period

Nursing Diagnoses (refer to Laryngectomy and Cancer: Initial Diagnosis Care Plans)

Anxiety related to lack of knowledge of impending surgical experience and implications of condition on life style

Grieving related to losses associated with surgery and perceived effects on life style

Collaborative Problems

▲ PC: Flap Rejection (development of a hematoma, seroma, or infection with resulting flap necrosis)
✳ PC: Fistula Formation
✳ PC: Facial and CNS Edema (particularly after bilateral neck dissection)
▲ PC: Carotid Artery Rupture
▲ PC: Hemorrhage

Nursing Diagnoses

▲ High Risk for Impaired Physical Mobility: Shoulder, Head, related to removal of muscles, nerves, flap graft reconstruction, trauma secondary to surgery

(continued on page 616)

▲ High Risk for Disturbed Self-Concept related to change in appearance

Risk for Imbalanced Nutrition related to swallowing difficulties, decreased salivation, decreased sense of smell and taste, and impaired tongue movement

▲ High Risk for Ineffective Therapeutic Regimen Management related to insufficient knowledge of wound care, signs and symptoms of complications, exercises, and follow-up care

Related Care Plans

General Surgery Generic care plan
Tracheostomy
Laryngectomy
Chemotherapy
Radiation
Cancer: Initial Diagnosis

▲ This diagnosis was reported to be monitored for or managed frequently (75%–100%).
✱ This diagnosis was not included in the validation study.

Discharge Criteria

Before discharge, the client and family will

1. Demonstrate wound care.
2. Verbalize the need to continue exercises and follow-up care.
3. Discuss management of activities of daily living (ADLs).
4. State signs and symptoms that must be reported to a health care professional.
5. Verbalize an intent to share feelings and concerns related to appearance with significant others.
6. Identify available community resources and self-help groups.

Collaborative Problems

Potential Complication: Flap Rejection (development of a hematoma, seroma, or infection with resulting flap necrosis)

Potential Complication: Fistula Formation

Potential Complication: Facial and Central Nervous System Edema (particularly after bilateral neck dissection)

Potential Complication: Carotid Artery Rupture

Potential Complication: Hemorrhage

Potential Complication: Neurological Deficits

Nursing Goal

The nurse will monitor to detect early signs and symptoms of (a) flap rejection, (b) fistula formation, (c) facial/central nervous system edema, (d) carotid artery rupture, (e) hemorrhage, and (f) neurologic deficits (e.g., stroke), and collaboratively intervene to stabilize the client.

Indicators

- Pink, warm skin flap (a)
- Capillary refill <3 seconds (a)
- Minimal or no edema (a, c, f)
- Temperature 98.5–99°F (a, b, e)
- Pulse 60–100 beats/min (a, d, e, f)
- BP >90/60, <140/90 mmHg (a, d, e, f)

- Respirations 16–20 breaths/min (a, d, e)
- Oxygen saturation (pulse oximeter) >95% (a, d, e, f)
- Continuous drainage of clear or pinkish fluid (200–300 mL the first 24 h) (a, b, c)
- No bloody sputum (a, b, e)
- No epigastric distress (d, e)
- No decrease in level of consciousness (c, d, e, f)
- No slurring of speech (c, d, e, f)
- Full range of motion for upper extremities (c, d, e, f)
- No tongue deviation (c, d, e, f)

Interventions	Rationales
1. Monitor the pectoralis myocutaneous flap and surrounding tissue every hour for the first 48 hours postsurgery, then every 4 hours until postop day 5 for the following (Lewis et al., 2004; Baird, Keen, & Swearingen, 2005; Wagner, Johnson, & Kidd, 2006): a. Color: redness, pallor, blackness, cyanosis b. Increased capillary refill (>3 seconds); blanching c. Temperature changes, edema	1. Abnormal findings may indicate impending flap rejection and requires immediate medical evaluation. Maximum redness should occur within the first 8–12 hours postsurgery, and slowly decrease over the next 2–3 days. A healthy flap is pink and warm to the touch, has minimal edema, and recovers color slowly after exposure to blanching. Increasing edema and erythema of the skin flap in postoperative days 3–5 or later, associated with odor, fever, and elevated WBC, is indicative of infection; when associated with salivary drainage, it indicates fistula (American Head and Neck Society, 2007).
2. Report assessment changes promptly to the surgeon.	2. Flaps can tolerate only 4 hours of ischemia before irreversible tissue necrosis results (Lewis et al., 2004; Baird, Keen, & Swearingen, 2005).
3. Monitor vital signs and pulse oximetry.	3. Vital signs are monitored to determine circulatory, respiratory, and neurologic status (Lewis et al., 2004; Baird, Keen, & Swearingen, 2005; Wagner, Johnson, & Kidd, 2006).
4. Monitor surgical drainage tubes for presence of air; foul-smelling, bloody, milky, or opaque drainage; or absence of drainage. Record amount every hour.	4. Drains prevent development of dead space (air or fluid accumulation between flap and underlying tissue) and help to prevent approximation. Air in the drains indicates dead space. Milky drainage may point to a chylous fistula. Opaque or chyle leaks, particularly from the thoracic duct, can lead to severe fluid and electrolyte imbalance. Continuous bloody drainage may indicate small vessel rupture, requiring surgical ligation. Over the first 24 hours postsurgery, drainage should be between 200 and 300 mL and should decline daily thereafter.
5. Report increased drainage immediately.	5. Increased drainage may indicate development of a hematoma. It must be drained immediately to preserve viability of the flaps.
6. If grafts are used, monitor graft site for bleeding and infection.	6. Prompt attention to bleeding or infection can prevent systemic hypovolemia and sepsis.
7. Maintain proper body positioning. a. Elevate the head of bed 30–45 degrees. b. Use pillows or sandbags to maintain proper alignment. c. Instruct the client not to lie on the operative side.	7. Semi-Fowler's and high-Fowler's positions prevent hyperextension of the neck and they position the base of the flap inferior to the tip of the flap. This positioning limits tension of the flap and incision line and promotes venous drainage through the flap to minimize/alleviate flap, facial, cerebral, and laryngeal edemas (Lewis et al., 2004; Baird, Keen, & Swearingen, 2005; Wagner, Johnson, & Kidd, 2006). The position is dependent on flap location.

(continued on page 618)

Interventions	Rationales

8. Monitor for external pressure on the reconstruction/flap from any of these:
  a. IV lines
  b. Feeding tubes
  c. Drainage tubes
  d. Tracheostomy or laryngectomy ties
	8. External pressure on the flap compromises circulation, promotes venous congestion, and may lead to increased permeability and occlusion of the lymphatics. Fluid accumulation may result in dehiscence of the incision and failure of the graft to adhere to the underlying tissue; this provides a medium for bacterial growth potentiating abscess formation. Both circulatory compromise and problems resulting from accumulating fluid within the flap may potentiate wound and flap necrosis.

9. Monitor for signs of carotid artery rupture:
  a. Evidence of arterial erosion
  b. Change in color: redness, pallor, blackness
  c. Evidence of bleeding or bruising, pulsations, arterial exposure
  d. Temperature changes
  e. Neurologic deficits (e.g., decreased level of consciousness, tongue deviation, slurred speech) (Lewis et al., 2004; Baird, Keen, & Swearingen, 2005; Wagner, Johnson, & Kidd, 2006)
	9. Exposure of the adventitial layer of the artery to the atmosphere causes drying and interrupts blood supply to the flap. Once the artery is exposed to air, arterial destruction occurs in approximately 6–10 days. Factors contributing to arterial erosion include poor wound healing, exposure of the artery during surgery, tumor growth or invasion, radiation therapy, fistula formation, and infection.

10. Observe strict aseptic dressing technique using nonocclusive, fine-mesh, non-adherent gauze dressings with non-porous tape.	10. Dressings protect the wound from trauma and contamination, absorb drainage, and provide an aesthetic covering. Fine-mesh gauze inhibits interweaving of granulation tissue into dressing material, thus preventing mechanical debridement. Non-adherent dressings prevent growth of fungus and yeast infections that require a dark, moist environment.

11. If the carotid artery is exposed, do the following:
  a. Keep the wound moistened (e.g., with loosely packed saline-moistened gauze or Vaseline gauze). If gauze dries while in the wound, it should be moistened with sterile saline before removal.
  b. Keep the following emergency supplies available at the bedside:
    • Two to three clean towels
    • Box of 4 × 4's
    • Vaginal packing or fluffs
    • Cuffed tracheostomy tube or a No. 8 endotracheal tube
    • 10-mL syringe to inflate cuff, as needed
  c. Type and hold for 2 units of packed red blood cells.
  d. Suction apparatus and catheters
	11. Removal of a dry dressing from an exposed artery with inadvertent debridement of the arterial wall can precipitate an acute bleed.

12. When initial postoperative dressing is removed, change a saturated external dressing over draining wounds every 24 hours, per prescribed orders. Initial dressing may remain several days.	12. Secretion-saturated dressings over wounds with extensive tissue loss should be changed frequently, because lack of a skin barrier increases the risk of infection. Drains and initial dressings are placed in a manner to protect blood supply to flaps yet maximize drainage away from the surgical site to prevent hematoma and seroma formation (AHNS, 2007; AAO-HNS, 2007; Lewis et al., 2004).

13. Promote efforts to clear secretions without coughing.
  a. Position to maximize respiratory excursion.
  b. Encourage deep breathing.
  c. Provide gentle nasotracheal, tracheal, or oropharyngeal suctioning only when absolutely needed.
	13. Coughing increases intrathoracic pressure, which stresses the wound. Because suctioning also increases intrathoracic pressure, suction only when the presence of secretions is identified on chest auscultation.

(continued on page 619)

Interventions	Rationales
14. Monitor for nausea and vomiting.	14. Contraction of the diaphragm and abdominal muscles during vomiting raises intra-abdominal and intrathoracic pressure that stresses the wound.
15. Monitor for constipation/abdominal distention and take steps to prevent or treat constipation: a. Administer stool softener with wetting agent or glycerin suppository or gentle laxative. b. Encourage adequate dietary fiber and fluid intake.	15. a. Valsalva maneuver, which accompanies straining on defecation related to constipation or fecal impaction, increases intrathoracic pressure that stresses the wound. b. Adequate fiber and fluid intake helps to decrease the potential for constipation.
16. Monitor for bleeding at the wound site, a sudden increase in the output from external drainage apparatus, or an acute development of bloody sputum.	16. A small amount of blood or pink-tinged drainage at the wound site or on the dressing may herald major rupture. Typically a small prodromal bleed occurs 24–48 hours before a major rupture (Baird, Keen, & Swearingen, 2005).
17. Monitor for complaints of sternal or high epigastric distress.	17. These complaints may indicate carotid rupture.
18. During episodes of bleeding, maintain a patent airway, prevent aspiration, and stop the hemorrhage. a. For external hemorrhage: • Apply firm pressure directly to the bleed site or secondary over the artery that is the source of the bleed. • Position the client in high-Fowler's position with the head turned to the affected side. If unable to turn the head to the side, turn the entire body. • Provide continuous suctioning. b. For internal hemorrhage: • Pack site with absorptive pressure dressing. • Position the client to facilitate drainage from the airway. • Provide continuous suctioning. • If a tracheostomy is in place, inflate the cuff.	18. These measures aim to facilitate drainage, prevent aspiration, and suppress the hemorrhage (Carr, 2005; Wagner, Johnson, & Kidd, 2006).

 ### Related Physician-Prescribed Interventions

Medications. Chemotherapy; also refer to the General Surgery care plan

Intravenous Therapy. Refer to the General Surgery care plan

Laboratory Studies. Arterial blood gas analysis; CBC with differential; also refer to the General Surgery care plan

Diagnostic Studies. Pulmonary function studies, chest x-ray film

Therapies. Oxygen with humidification, speech therapy, donor site care, respiratory therapy, physical therapy, psychiatric or social work counseling, nasogastric intubation, CT scan, irrigations, Doppler scanning, bradytherapy, external-beam radiotherapy, interstitial implantation, hyperbaric oxygen

Documentation

Flow records
   Vital signs
   Intake and output
   Wound site and drainage tube assessment
   Progressive notes
Neurologic flow sheet

Nursing Diagnoses

High Risk for Impaired Physical Mobility: Shoulder, Head, Related to Removal of Muscles, Nerves, Flap Graft Reconstruction, Trauma Secondary to Surgery

NOC Ambulation: Walking, Joint Movement: Active, Mobility Level

Goal

The client will demonstrate measures to prevent complications of decreased mobility.

Indicators

* State limitations on shoulder and head mobility and surgical factors that influence mobility postoperatively.
* Demonstrate optimal head and shoulder mobility postoperatively.

NIC Exercise Therapy: Joint Mobility, Exercise Promotion: Strength Training, Exercise Therapy: Ambulation, Positioning, Teaching: Prescribed Activity/Exercise

Interventions	Rationales
1. Consult with the physician regarding an exercise program.	1. The physician determines when the exercise program should be initiated and recommends a program based on the extent of tissue excision and reconstruction and on the progression of healing. Generally, exercise is initiated after drains are removed, the suture line is intact, and postoperative edema resolves.
2. Teach the client to do the following: a. Maintain good posture at all times; pull shoulders back frequently. b. Avoid sitting for prolonged periods. c. Avoid putting pressure on the arm of the operative side; use other arm to lift, pull, and press. d. When reclining, lie in the supine position (avoid lying on the operative side); place the involved arm to the side of the body with the elbow bent and support the arm with pillows. e. Avoid lifting or carrying objects weighing more than 3 lbs. with the involved arm until approved by physician. f. Avoid injury to the involved side.	2. Positioning and activity instructions are the following. a. Good posture is essential to prevent chest muscles from tightening and pulling against weaker muscles on the back of the shoulder (e.g., rhomboids and levator). b. Prolonged sitting tires the muscles that provide good posture. c. These measures decrease stress on the remaining neuromuscular structures. d. Maintaining neutral alignment helps to prevent contractures. e. This restriction can prevent strain and pain in the involved arm. f. Minor injuries to the involved arm can compromise circulation and lymph drainage.
3. Provide pain medication as ordered before the client begins the prescribed exercises.	3. Pain can make the client reluctant to perform prescribed exercises. Adequate pain relief can increase compliance with the therapeutic regimen.
4. Consult with physical therapy, as appropriate.	4. A physical therapist can suggest specific exercises to strengthen remaining musculature and increase support and stability of the shoulder joint.

Documentation

Teaching flow records
Progress notes
    Client teaching
    Therapeutic exercises performed

High Risk for Disturbed Self-Concept Related to Change in Appearance

NOC Quality of Life, Depression Level, Self-Esteem, Coping

Goal

The client will communicate feelings about the surgery and its outcome.

Indicators

- Acknowledge changes in body structure and function.
- Participate in self-care.

NIC Hope Instillation, Mood Management, Values Certification, Counseling, Referral, Support Group, Coping Enhancement

Interventions	Rationales

1. Identify clients at high risk for unsuccessful adjustment (AHNS, 2007; AAO-HNS, 2007).
  a. Previous history of psychiatric problems
  b. Poor ego strength
  c. Unrealistic expectations concerning surgery
  d. Exhibition of too much or too little concern in the preoperative period
  e. Ineffective problem-solving ability
  f. Difficulty learning new skills
  g. Lack of motivation
  h. External focus of control
  i. Poor health
  j. Unsatisfactory preoperative sex life
  k. Lack of effective support systems
  l. Unstable economic status
  m. Rejection of counseling
	1. Successful adjustment to appearance changes is influenced by factors such as these:
	  • Previous coping success
	  • Achievement of developmental tasks before surgery
	  • Extent to which the change interferes with goal-directed activity
	  • Sense of control
	  • Realistic perception of the change by the client and others (AHNS, 2007; AAO-HNS, 2007).

2. Contact the client frequently and treat him or her with warm, positive regard.	2. Frequent contact by caregiver indicates acceptance and may facilitate trust. The client may be hesitant to approach staff because of a negative self-concept.
3. Incorporate emotional support into technical care teaching sessions (e.g., wound care, bathing).	3. This encourages resolution of emotional issues while teaching technical skills.
4. Encourage the client to look at the operative site.	4. Accepting the reality of the body change is the first step in successful adjustment to it.
5. Encourage the client to verbalize feelings about the surgery and perceptions of how life style has been affected. Validate his or her perceptions and reassure him or her that the responses are normal and appropriate.	5. Sharing concerns and ventilating feelings provide an opportunity for the nurse to correct any misinformation. Validating the client's perceptions increases his or her self-awareness.
6. Encourage the client to participate in self-care. Give feedback and reinforce positive techniques and progress.	6. Participation in self-care is a sign of successful adjustment and facilitates acceptance of body changes by providing the client with some control over his or her environment. For many clients it can provide the first sense of control over their well-being since diagnosis (AHNS, 2007; AAO-HNS, 2007; Lewis et al., 2004).
7. Have the client demonstrate proper wound care and teach the procedure to a support person.	7. Successful return demonstration and ability to teach the skill to others indicate mastery.

(continued on page 622)

Interventions	Rationales
8. Encourage the support persons to become involved with wound care and to provide emotional support.	8. Support persons' acceptance is a critical factor in the client's own acceptance and adjustment.
9. Encourage the client to identify and verbalize personal strengths and positive self-attributes and to verbalize intent to resume normal activities as soon as possible.	9. Evidence of positive self-concept and desire to pursue goals and life style reflect successful adjustment.
10. Provide information about measures to help improve appearance: a. Wearing clothes with high collars (e.g., turtleneck sweaters) b. Wearing ascots or scarves c. Wearing clothing with shoulder padding d. Wearing accessories that draw attention away from the neck (e.g., hats)	10. Improving appearance can boost self-confidence and aid successful adjustment.
11. Refer a client at high risk for unsuccessful adjustment for professional counseling.	11. Follow-up therapy may be indicated to assist with effective adjustment.

Documentation

Progress notes
  Present emotional status
  Interventions
  Response to interventions

Risk for Imbalanced Nutrition Related to Swallowing Difficulties, Decreased Salivation, and Decreased Sense of Smell and Taste

NOC Nutritional Status

Goal

The client will use methods to increase intake and maintain weight.

Indicators

- Demonstrate methods to improve swallowing.
- Relate reasons for decreased sense of taste and smell.
- Name resources available after discharge.

NIC Nutrition Management, Nutritional Monitoring

Interventions	Rationales
1. Administer tube feedings as prescribed. Refer to Enteral Nutrition care plan for additional interventions.	
2. Consult with a speech or swallowing therapist for a thorough evaluation. Prepare for a video fluoroscopy and a modified "cookie" swallow barium.	2. A thorough evaluation is needed to determine mobility of the tongue and pharynx.
3. Explain the effects of surgery on eating and nutrition: a. Loss of sense of smell	3. a. A permanent tracheostomy prevents air from passing over receptors in the nasal passages—a process necessary for smell.

(continued on page 623)

Interventions	Rationales
b. Decreased sense of taste	b. Receptors in the tongue are bypassed, which decreases the sense of taste.
c. Swallowing	c. Surgery can damage any of the cranial nerves needed for swallowing (e.g., trigeminal, facial, glossopharyngeal, vagus, spinal accessory, hypoglossal).
d. Decreased salivation	d. Surgical trauma to the salivary glands can reduce salivation.

4. Advise how these changes will affect nutrition:
  a. Food choices
 	
  b. Time required for eating
 	
  c. Social eating (e.g., restaurants)
	4.
	  a. Foods easier to swallow are selected regardless of their nutritional value.
	  b. The time required to eat is longer (e.g., 10–15 minutes more).
	  c. Social talking and eating are not easy.

5. Explain what foods are reported to improve enjoyment (fish, vegetables, pasta, potatoes, and milk) and what foods are less enjoyed (red meat, bitter foods, breads, sweets, cheese).	5. Post-laryngectomy clients reported these food preferences (Lennie, Christman, & Jadack, 2001).
6. Advise that these alterations do not occur in enzyme; any that do may diminish over time.	6. In one study, 89% of participants rated their sense of smell as less affected and 63% reported a diminished sense of taste (Lennie et al., 2001).

7. Provide written instructions about how to improve eating and nutritional status.
  a. Chew food thoroughly.
  b. Provide enough time to eat.
  c. Drink fluids while eating.
  d. Add more spices to food.
  e. Supplement meals with protein drinks.
	7. Postoperatively, the client and family will be overwhelmed, so information retention will be limited.
	  a. This will help to prevent aspiration.
	  b. The client must alternate breathing, chewing, and talking.
	  c. This will moisten foods and help swallowing.
	  d. This will enhance taste.
	  e. Supplements will provide proteins, vitamins, and minerals

8. Encourage the client, after discharge, to access information and join a support group such as the International Association of Laryngectomees (www.larynxlink.com) and Web Whispers (www.webwhispers.org) (AHNS, 2007, AAO-HNS, 2007).	8. Clients reported that they were unprepared for changes when they were home (Lennie et al., 2001).

High Risk for Ineffective Therapeutic Regimen Management Related to Insufficient Knowledge of Wound Care, Signs and Symptoms of Complications, Exercises, and Follow-up Care

NOC Compliance Behavior, Knowledge: Treatment Regimen, Participation: Health Care Decisions, Treatment Behavior: Illness or Injury

Goals

The goals for this diagnosis represent those associated with discharge planning. Refer to the discharge criteria.

NIC Anticipatory Guidance, Learning Facilitation, Risk Management, Health Education, Teaching: Procedure/Treatment, Health System Guidance

Interventions	Rationales
1. Teach wound-care measures. (Refer to the General Surgery care plan for specific interventions.)	
2. Explain the normal functions of neuromuscular structures and how they have been disrupted by surgery.	2. The client's understanding of the impairment can encourage compliance with postoperative instructions.

(continued on page 624)

Interventions	Rationales
3. Discuss the importance of complying with the prescribed exercise regimen. Reinforce teaching and provide written instructions.	3. The postoperative exercise program aims to strengthen the levator scapulae and rhomboid muscles to compensate for loss of the trapezius. If these muscles are not strengthened, the pectoralis muscle will pull the shoulder forward and down and cause pain. Explanations and written instructions can encourage compliance.

4. Instruct the client to report the following promptly:
  a. Increased temperature
  b. New or increasing pain
  c. Change in amount, consistency, or color of drainage
  d. Leakage of food or fluid from incision line
	4. Early detection of complications enables prompt intervention to reduce their severity. Increased temperature, pain, and a change in drainage typically point to infection. Perincisional erythema with leakage of purulent drainage, food, or other fluids indicates a fistula (Lewis et al., 2004; Baird, Keen, & Swearingen, 2005; Wagner, Johnson, & Kidd, 2006).

Documentation

Discharge summary record
    Client and family teaching
    Outcome achievement or status

Nephrectomy

Nephrectomy is the surgical procedure of removing a kidney or a section of a kidney. A nephrectomy is performed on clients with cancer of the kidney (renal cell carcinoma); a disease in which cysts (sac-like structures) displace healthy kidney tissue (polycystic kidney disease); massive trauma to the kidney, serious kidney infections, and renal failure. It is also used to remove a healthy kidney from a donor for the purposes of kidney transplantation (National Kidney Foundation, 2007; Parekattil, Gill, & Castle, et al., 2005).

    The removal of the kidney can be classified in various ways: a *simple nephrectomy* is the removal of the kidney while a *radical nephrectomy* is removal of the kidney and possibly the surrounding perinephritic fat, Gerota's fascia, and lymph nodes. Laparoscopic techniques are also utilized for *partial nephrectomies*, which are referred to as a (nephron-sparing nephrectomy) (Parekattil, Gill, & Castle, 2005; Mattar & Finelli, 2007).

 Time Frame
Preoperative and postoperative periods

▪▪▪▪ DIAGNOSTIC CLUSTER

Preoperative Period

Collaborative Problems	Refer to
▲ PC: Hemorrhage/Shock	
▲ PC: Paralytic Ileus	
▲ PC: Renal Insufficiency	
△ PC: Pyelonephritis	
△ PC: Pneumothorax Secondary to Thoracic Approach	Thoracic Surgery

(continued on page 625)

Nursing Diagnoses	Refer to
▲ High Risk for Ineffective Therapeutic Regimen Management related to insufficient knowledge of hydration requirements, nephrostomy care, and signs and symptoms of complications	
△ Acute Pain related to distention of renal capsule and incision	General Surgery
▲ High Risk for Ineffective Respiratory Function related to pain on breathing and coughing secondary to location of incision	General Surgery

Related Care Plans

General Surgery Generic care plan
Cancer (Initial Diagnosis)

▲ This diagnosis was reported to be monitored for or managed frequently (75%–100%).
△ This diagnosis was reported to be monitored for or managed often (50%–74%).

Discharge Criteria

Before discharge, the client and family will

1. Demonstrate nephrostomy tube care.
2. State measures for at-home wound care.
3. Share feelings regarding loss of kidney.
4. State signs and symptoms that must be reported to a health care professional.
5. Explain the difference between incisional pain and the pain of infection.

Postoperative: Collaborative Problems

Potential Complication: Hemorrhage/Shock
Potential Complication: Paralytic Ileus
Potential Complication: Renal Insufficiency
Potential Complication: Pyelonephritis

Nursing Goal

The nurse will detect early signs and symptoms of (a) hemorrhage/shock, (b) paralytic ileus, (c) renal insufficiency (partial nephrectomy), and (d) pyelonephritis (partial nephrectomy), and will collaboratively intervene to stabilize the client.

Indicators

- Calm, oriented, alert (a)
- Pulse 60–100 beats/min (a)
- Respirations 16–20 breaths/min (a)
- BP >90/60, <120–129/80–84 mmHg (a) (JNC, 2007).
- No chills (d)
- Temperature 98.5–99°F (d)
- Urine specific gravity 1.005–1.030 (c, d)
- Urine output >5 mL/h (a, c, d)
- Full peripheral pulses (a)

- Capillary refill <3 seconds (a)
- Dry, warm skin (a)
- Pinkish, brownish, or olive skin tones (a)
- Hemoglobin (a)
  - Male 13–18 gm/dL
  - Female 12–16 gm/dL
- Hematocrit (a)
  - Male 42%–50%
  - Female 40%–48%
- Bowel sounds present all quadrants (b)
- No abdominal distention (b)
- White blood cells 5000–10,000/mm³ (d)
- Urine sodium 130–200 mEq/24h (c)
- Blood urea nitrogen 10–20 mg/dL (c)
- Potassium 3.8–5 mEq/L (c)
- Serum sodium 135–145 mEq/L (c)
- Phosphorus 2.5–4.5 mg/dL (c)
- Creatinine clearance 100–150 mL of blood cleared per mm (c)
- No costovertebral angle (CVA) tenderness (d)
- Urine negative bacteria (d)
- No complaints of dysuria or frequency (d)
- No bladder distention (d)

Interventions	Rationales

1. Monitor for signs and symptoms of hemorrhage/shock every hour for the first 24 hours, then every 4 hours:
  a. Increasing pulse rate with normal or slightly decreased blood pressure
  b. Decreased oxygen saturation (pulse oximetry) <94%
  c. Urine output <5 mL/kg/h (normal value for urine output is 0.5 to 1.0 mL/kg/h) (Wagner, Johnson, & Kidd, 2006, p. 228)
  d. Restlessness, agitation, change in mentation
  e. Increasing respiratory rate
  f. Diminished peripheral pulses
  g. Cool, pale, or cyanotic skin
  h. Thirst
	1. Because the renal capsule is very vascular, massive blood loss can occur. The compensatory response to decreased circulatory volume is to increase blood oxygen by increasing the heart and respiratory rates and decreasing circulation to extremities (manifested by decreased pulses and cool skin). Diminished cerebral oxygenation can cause changes in mentation. Decreased oxygen to kidneys results in decreased urine output.

2. Monitor fluid status hourly:
  a. Intake (parenteral, oral)
  b. Output and loss (urinary, drainage, vomiting)
  c. Weigh daily at same time in same clothes, if needed.
	2. Fluid loss due to surgery and nothing-by-mouth (NPO) status can disrupt fluid balance in some clients. Stress can produce sodium and water retention.
	  Accurate daily assessment of body weight is more reliable in measuring fluid loss than intake-vs-output, because it accounts for water loss during fever, diaphoresis, and respiration: one liter (1000 mL) of water weighs one kilogram or 2.2 pounds (Wagner, Johnson, & Kidd, 2006).

3. Monitor surgical site for bleeding, dehiscence, and evisceration.	3. Frequent monitoring enables early detection of complications. Hypotension and vasospasm during surgery can cause temporary hemostasis, and can result in delayed bleeding.
4. Teach the client to splint the incision site with a pillow when coughing and deep breathing (to decrease/prevent occurrences of postoperative pneumonia secondary to the inability to breathe deeply due to pain).	4. Splinting reduces stress on suture lines by equalizing the pressure across the incision site.

(continued on page 627)

Interventions	Rationales

5. Monitor for signs and symptoms of paralytic ileus:
  a. Decreased or absent bowel sounds
  b. Abdominal distention
  c. Abdominal discomfort
 	
6. Do not initiate fluids until bowel sounds are present. Begin with small amounts. Note the client's response and the type and amount of emesis, if any.
	5,6. Reflex paralysis of intestinal peristalsis and manipulation of the colon to gain access place the client at high risk for ileus. The depressive effects of narcotics, and anesthetics on peristalsis, as well as the handling of the bowel during surgery, can also cause paralytic ileus. Ileus can occur between the third and fifth postoperative day. Pain can be localized, sharp, and intermittent (Wagner, Johnson, & Kidd, 2006, pp. 722–723).

7. Monitor for early signs and symptoms of renal insufficiency:
 	
  a. Sustained elevated urine specific gravity
  b. Elevated urine sodium level
  c. Sustained insufficient urine output (<30 mL/h)
  d. Elevated blood pressure
 	
  e. Elevated BUN and serum creatinine, potassium, phosphorus, and ammonia; decreased creatinine clearance
	7. Renal insufficiency can result from edema caused by surgical manipulation (partial nephrectomy) or by a nonpatent nephrostomy tube.
	a,b. Ability of renal tubules to reabsorb electrolytes results in increased urine sodium levels and urine specific gravity.
	c,d. Decreased glomerular filtration rate eventually leads to insufficient urine output and increased renin production, resulting in elevated blood pressure in the body's attempt to increase renal blood flow.
	e. These changes result from decreased excretion of urea and creatinine in urine.

8. Monitor the client for signs and symptoms of infection:
 	
  a. Chills and fever
 	
  b. Change in the type of pain
 	
  c. Costovertebral angle (CVA) pain (a dull, constant backache below the 12th rib)
  d. Leukocytosis
 	
  e. Bacteria and pus in urine
  f. Dysuria and frequency
	8. Microorganisms can be introduced into the body during surgery or through the incision. Urinary tract infections can be caused by urinary stasis (e.g., from a nonpatent nephrostomy tube) or by irritation of tissue by calculi.
	a. Endogenous pyrogens are released and they reset the hypothalamic setpoint to febrile levels. The body temperature is sensed as "too cool"; shivering and vasoconstriction result, to generate and consume heat. The core temperature rises to the new setpoint level, resulting in fever. The leukocytes (WBCs), are the circulating cells of the immune system; although their quantities are limited, they are an extremely quick and powerful defense system and respond immediately to foreign invaders by going to the site of involvement (Wagner, Johnson, & Kidd, 2006, p. 524; Kee, 2004, p. 352). Wound redness, tenderness, and edema result from lymphocyte migration to the area (Wagner, Johnson, & Kidd, 2006, p. 802).
	b. The literature states that a patient may experience considerable discomfort in the area around the incision and may need to be taught the difference between incisional pain and infection pain. Incisional pain will decrease each day while infection pain will increase and is usually accompanied by fever (Kok, Alwayn, Tran, Hop, Weimar, & Ijzermans, 2006).
	c. CVA pain results from distention of the renal capsule.
	
	d. Leukocytosis reflects an increase in WBCs to fight infection through phagocytosis.
	e. Bacteria and pus in urine indicate a urinary tract infection
	f. Bacteria irritate bladder tissue, causing spasms and frequency.

9. Monitor for signs of urinary retention:
  a. Bladder distention
  b. Urine overflow (30–60 mL of urine every 15–30 minutes)
	9. Trauma to the detrusor muscle and injury to the pelvic nerves during surgery can inhibit bladder function. Anxiety and pain can cause spasms of the reflex sphincters. Bladder neck edema can also cause retention. Sedatives and narcotics can affect the central nervous system and the effectiveness of the smooth muscles (Gillenwater et al., 1996).

10. Instruct the client to report bladder discomfort or inability to void.	10. Overdistention of the bladder can aggravate a client's ability to empty the bladder (Gillenwater et al., 1996).

Related Physician-Prescribed Interventions

Refer to the Surgical Client care plan.

Documentation

Flow records
   Vital signs
   Circulatory status
   Intake (oral, parenteral)
   Output (urinary drainage color, clarity, sediment, drainage tubes)
   Bowel function (bowel sounds, defecation pattern, abdominal distention)
   Wound status (color, drainage, pain around incision, tenderness)

Postoperative: Nursing Diagnosis

High Risk for Ineffective Therapeutic Regimen Management Related to Insufficient Knowledge of Hydration Requirements, Nephrostomy Care, and Signs and Symptoms of Complications

Goals

The goals for this diagnosis represent those associated with discharge planning. Refer to the discharge criteria.

NIC Anticipatory Guidance, Risk Identification, Health Education, Learning Facilitation

Interventions	Rationales
1. Explain the need to maintain optimal hydration.	1. Optimal hydration reduces urinary stasis, decreasing the risk of infection and calculi formation.
2. Teach and have the client perform a return demonstration of nephrostomy care measures, including: a. Aseptic technique b. Skin care c. Tube stabilization	2. Proper techniques can reduce the risk of infection. Movement of the tube can cause dislodgement or tissue trauma.
3. Teach the client to use pillows to support the back when lying on side.	3. Certain positions will decrease tension on the incisional area.
4. Explain why the pain is severe, as well as other discomforts. Teach the client to avoid lifting any weight more than 10 lbs for 6 weeks.	4. The client's position and the incision's size cause severe pain. The client's position on the operating room table will cause muscular aches and pains.
5. Teach the client to report the following: a. Decreased urine output b. Fever or malaise c. Purulent, cloudy drainage from or around the tube	5. Early detection enables prompt intervention to prevent serious complications such as renal insufficiency and infection.
6. Refer the client and family to a home health care agency for follow-up care.	6. A home care nurse evaluates the client's ability for home care and provides periodic assessment of renal function and development of infection.

Documentation

Discharge summary record
   Client and family teaching, and clarification of understanding towards education
   Outcome achievement or status
   Referrals

Radical Prostatectomy

Radical prostatectomy is the surgical removal of the prostate gland, ejaculatory ducts, seminal vesicles, some pelvic fasciae and sometimes the pelvic lymph nodes due to cancer of the prostate (James, 2007). There are three generations of radical prostate surgery: open, laparoscopic, and robot-assisted. The open approach can be performed via a perineal, suprapubic, or retropubic incision. Laparoscopic surgery involves smaller incisions and the use of a scope, but the equipment is difficult to manipulate accurately. Robot-assisted laparoscopic approaches provide improved dexterity for surgeons (Rigdon, 2006). Forty percent of laparoscopic approaches are now robot-assisted, also known as the da Vinci Surgical System, allowing nerve-sparing outcomes and reducing complications, blood loss, and surgical time (Challacombe & Dasgupta, 2007; Tewari, Peabody, Sarle, Balakrishnan, Hemal, Shrivastava, et al., 2002; Vattikuti Urology Institute, 2007).

 Time Frame
Preoperative and postoperative periods

■■■■■■ DIAGNOSTIC CLUSTER

Preoperative Period

Nursing Diagnoses

▲ Anxiety related to upcoming surgery and insufficient knowledge of routine and postoperative activities

Postoperative Period

Collaborative Problems

▲ PC: Hemorrhage
▲ PC: Clot Formation
△ PC: Thrombophlebitis

Nursing Diagnoses

▲ Grieving related to potential loss of body function and perceived effects on life style (refer to Cancer: Initial Diagnosis care plan)

Acute Pain related to bladder spasms; clot retention; and back, leg, and incisional pain

△ High Risk for Ineffective Sexuality Patterns related to fear of impotence resulting from surgical intervention

▲ High Risk for Ineffective Therapeutic Regimen Management related to insufficient knowledge of fluid restrictions, catheter care, activity restrictions, urinary control, and signs and symptoms of complications

Related Care Plan

General Surgery Generic care plan

▲ This diagnosis was reported to be monitored for or managed frequently (75%–100%).
△ This diagnosis was reported to be monitored for or managed often (50%–74%).

Discharge Criteria

Before discharge, the client and family will

1. Identify the need for increased oral fluid intake.
2. Demonstrate care of the indwelling (Foley) catheter.
3. Explain wound care at home.
4. Verbalize necessary precautions for activity and urination.
5. State the signs and symptoms that must be reported to a health care professional.
6. Verbalize an intent to share feelings and concerns related to sexual function with significant others.

Preoperative: Nursing Diagnosis

Anxiety Related to Upcoming Surgery and Insufficient Knowledge of Routine and Postoperative Activities

> **NOC** Anxiety Reduction, Coping, Impulse Control
>
> **Goal**
>
> The client will state the reasons for activity restrictions, indwelling catheterization, and increased fluid intake.
>
> **NIC** Anxiety Reduction, Impulse Control Training, Anticipatory Guidance

Interventions	Rationales
1. Reinforce the physician's explanation of the scheduled surgery and answer any questions.	1–3. The client's understanding can help to allay anxiety related to fear of the unknown. Preoperative education has been shown to reduce anxiety and also helps to improve compliance (Redman & Thomas, 1996). Immobilization on the operating room table for several hours will increase risk of pneumonia and venous stasis.
2. Explain expected postoperative procedures, such as the following: a. Indwelling (Foley) catheterization in the hospital and at home b. Continuous and manual irrigation c. IV infusions d. Drains	
3. Explain the expected activity restrictions and activities to prevent complications: a. Bed rest for the first postoperative day b. Progressive ambulation beginning on first post-operative day c. Avoiding activities that put strain on the bladder area d. Coughing and deep breathing exercises	
4. Explain that transient hematuria is normal in the immediate postoperative period.	4. Preparing the client for postoperative hematuria prevents him from being shocked at its appearance.
5. Explain the need for increased fluid intake.	5. Dilute urine deters clot formation.
6. Provide teaching aids (e.g., pamphlets or video tapes), as available.	6. A multisensory approach to teaching enhances learning and retention (Redman & Thomas, 1996).
7. Encourage the client to share fears.	7. Clients are extremely anxious with major concerns regarding sexual competence and urinary control (Butler, Downe-Wambolt, Marsh, Bell, Jarvi, 2000). Between 20%–70% of men report sexual dysfunction (James, 2007).
8. Elicit from the client what the surgeon has explained regarding effects of surgery on sexual function.	8. The nurse should not assume that the client understands the ramifications of surgery just because he asks no questions. Many clients are reluctant to discuss sexual concerns. Privacy may encourage sharing.

Documentation

Discharge summary record
    Client teaching
        Outcome achievement or status

Postoperative: Collaborative Problems

Potential Complication: Hemorrhage
Potential Complication: Clot Formation
Potential Complication: Thrombophlebitis

Nursing Goal

The nurse will detect early signs and symptoms of (a) hemorrhage, (b) clot formation, (c) urinary retention, and (d) thrombophlebitis, and will collaborative intervene to stabilize the client.

Indicators

- Calm, oriented, alert (a)
- Pulse 60–100 beats/min (a)
- Respirations 16–20 breaths/min (a)
- BP >90/60, <140–90 mmHg (a)
- Temperature 98–99.5°F (d)
- Urine output >5 mL/h (a, d)
- Pink or clear red urine in the first 24 h (a, d)
- Amber→pink urine after 24 h (a, d)
- Clots in urine (a, b, c)
- Warm, dry skin (a)
- Pinkish, brownish, or olive skin tones (a)
- Hemoglobin (a)
    - Male 13–18 gm/dL
    - Female 12–16 gm/dL
- Hematocrit (a)
    - Male 42%–50%
    - Female 40%–48%
- Continuous flowing bladder irrigation (b, c)
- No bladder distention (c)
- Positive Homans sign (calf pain when foot is flexed upward) (d)
- No complaints of calf tenderness, warmth, or redness (d)
- No leg edema (d)

Interventions	Rationales

1. Monitor for signs and symptoms of hemorrhage:
  a. Abnormal urine characteristics (e.g., highly viscous, clots, bright red or burgundy color)
  b. Increased pulse rate
  c. Urine output <30 mL/h
  d. Restlessness, agitation
  e. Cool, pale, or cyanotic skin
  f. Hemoglobin and hematocrit values
	1. The prostate gland is highly vascular, receiving its blood supply from the internal iliac artery. Elderly clients and those who have had prolonged urinary retention are vulnerable to rapid changes in bladder contents and fluid volume. During the first 24 hours after surgery, urine should be pink or clear red, gradually becoming amber to pink-tinged by the fourth day. Bright red urine with clots indicates arterial bleeding. Burgundy-colored urine indicates venous bleeding, which usually resolves spontaneously. Clots are expected; their absence may point to blood dyscrasias. Hemoglobin and hematocrit values decline if significant postoperative bleeding occurs (Kantaff, Carroll, D'Amico, Isaacs, Ross, & Scherett, 2001).

2. Monitor dressings, catheters, and drains that vary depending on the type of surgery performed:
  a. Suprapubic approach:
    • Urethral catheter
    • Suprapubic tube
    • Abdominal drain
	2. Heavy venous bleeding is expected the first 24 hours for all approaches except the perineal approach. Blood loss can occur from the catheter or incision (Kantaff et al., 2001).

(continued on page 632)

Interventions	Rationales

b. Retropubic approach:
  • Urethral catheter
  • Abdominal drain
c. Perineal approach:
  • Urethral catheter
  • Perineal drain	

3. Instruct the client to do the following:
  a. Avoid straining for bowel elimination.
  b. Do not sit in a firm, upright chair.
  c. Recline slightly while on the toilet.
	3. Increased pressure on the rectum can trigger bleeding and perforated rectal tissue.

4. Provide bladder irrigation as ordered; maintain aseptic technique:
  a. Continuous (closed)
  b. Manual: Using a bulb syringe, irrigate the catheter with 30–60 mL normal saline solution every 3–4 hours, as needed
	4. Continuous bladder irrigation with normal saline dilutes blood in the urine to prevent clot formation. Manual irrigation provides the negative pressure needed to remove obstructive clots or tissue particles.

5. Ensure adequate fluid intake (oral, parenteral).	5. Optimal hydration dilutes urine and prevents clot formation.

6. Monitor for signs and symptoms of thrombophlebitis:
  a. Positive Homans sign (pain on dorsiflexion of the foot resulting from insufficient circulation)
  b. Calf tenderness, unusual warmth, or redness
  c. Low-grade fever
  d. Extremity edema
	6. Initiation of the stress response during surgery results in hypercoagulability by inhibiting the fibrinolytic system. Pain, malignant disease, systemic infection, and cigarette smoking also cause hypercoagulability (Caswell, 1993).

7. Have the client ambulate as soon as possible with at least five minutes of walking per hour, and avoid sitting on a chair, with legs dependent.	7. Walking contracts the leg muscles, stimulates the venous pump, and reduces stasis (Carroll, 1993). Laparoscopic clients may experience "gas pain" from unabsorbed carbon dioxide (Rigdon, 2006), walking aids in dispersing the gas.
8. Ensure that the client uses sequential compression device, as prescribed, followed by antiembolic stockings.	8. These stockings reduce venous stasis by applying a graded degree of compression to the ankle and calf (Carroll, 1993).

 ### Related Physician-Prescribed Interventions

Medications. Antispasmodics (oral: oxybutynin, belladonna; suppository: belladonna & opium [B&O]); analgesics; antibiotics (Rigdon, 2006)

Intravenous Therapy. Refer to the General Surgery care plan, Appendix II, prostatic fluid, cytology, urine cytology

Laboratory Studies. CBC, PTT, BC, magnesium, electrolytes, prostate-specific antigen (PSA), urine culture, serum prostatic acid phosphatase level

Diagnostic Studies. Cystourethroscopy, bone scans, prostatic biopsy, transrectal ultrasound, CT, flow cytometry, MRI (abdomen, pelvis), voiding cystourethrogram

Therapies. Indwelling catheterization, wound drains, catheter traction, bladder irrigation (manual or continuous), radiotherapy, sitz baths, endocrine manipulation, sequential compression stocking device, chemotherapy, nasogastric tube

Documentation

Flow records
  Vital signs
  Intake and output
  Urine (color, viscosity, presence of clots)
  Continuous irrigations
  Manual irrigations (times, amounts)

Postoperative: Nursing Diagnoses

Acute Pain Related to Bladder Spasms; Clot Retention; and Back, Leg, and Incisional Pain

NOC Comfort Level, Pain Control

Goal

The client will report decreased pain after pain relief interventions.

Indicators

- Can do leg exercises.
- Increase activity progressively.

NIC Pain Management, Medication Management, Emotional Support, Teaching: Individual, Heat/Cold Application, Simple Massage

Interventions	Rationales
1. Monitor for intermittent suprapubic pain: bladder spasms, burning sensation at the tip of the penis.	1. Irritation from an indwelling catheter can cause bladder spasms and pain in the penis.
2. Monitor for persistent suprapubic pain: bladder distention with sensations of fullness and tightness, inability to void.	2. Catheter obstruction can cause urinary retention, leading to increased bladder spasms and increased risk of infection.
3. Monitor for lower back and leg pain. Provide gentle massage to the back and heat to the legs, if necessary.	3. During surgery, the client lies in the lithotomy position that can stretch and aggravate muscles that normally may be underused.
4. Anchor the catheter to the leg with a catheter leg strap.	4. Pressure from a dangling catheter can damage the urinary sphincter, resulting in urinary incontinence after catheter removal. Catheter movement also increases the likelihood of bladder spasms.
5. Monitor for testicular pain.	5. Clipping the vas deferens causes congestion of seminal fluid and blood. This congestion resolves over several weeks.
6. Administer medication, as ordered, for pain and spasms.	6. Antispasmodic medications (i.e., opium and belladonna suppositories) prevent bladder spasms. Analgesic medication diminishes the incisional pain.
7. Encourage adequate oral fluid intake (at least 2000 mL/day, unless contraindicated).	7. Adequate hydration dilutes urine that helps to flush out clots.
8. Manually irrigate the indwelling catheter only when prescribed.	8. Each time the closed system is opened for manual irrigation, risk of bacterial contamination increases.
9. Monitor output of wound drains (Rigdon, 2006).	9. Increased wound drainage may suggest a urine leak, lymph leak, or pelvic bleeding (Rigdon, 2006).

Documentation

Medication administration record
  Type, dose, route of all medications
Progress notes
  Complaints of pain (type, site, duration)
  Unsatisfactory pain relief

High Risk for Ineffective Sexuality Patterns Related to Fear of Impotence Resulting from Surgical Intervention

NOC Body Image, Self-Esteem, Role Performance, Sexual Identity: Acceptance

Goals

The client will discuss his and his partner's feelings and concerns regarding the effects of surgery on sexuality and sexual functioning.

Indicators

- Verbalize an intention to discuss concerns with partner after discharge from hospital.
- Explain effects of surgery on sexual function and expected course of resolution.

NIC Behavior Management: Sexual, Sexual Counseling, Emotional Support, Active Listening, Teaching: Sexuality

Interventions	Rationales
1. Explain the effects of surgery on sexual function (orgasms, erections, fertility, ejaculations).	1. If one or both nerve bundles responsible for erections are spared during surgery, erections will return. Orgasms will occur without ejaculations. It may take up to two years after wound healing and all edema from surgery subsides for full function to return. Men older than 70 years probably will not regain erections; ejaculate will be reduced but will still contain sperm. Robot-assisted laparoscopic approaches report 90% return to good sexual function after surgery (Vattikuti Urology Institute, 2007).
2. Use familiar terms, when possible, and explain unfamiliar terms.	2. Unfamiliar medical terminology may cause confusion and misunderstanding.
3. Explain that the surgeon's permission to resume sexual activity is needed. Clearly state that cancer of the prostate is not transmitted sexually.	3. Complete healing is needed to prevent bleeding and to resolve edema, which usually takes six weeks to three months.
4. Encourage the client to ask the physician questions during hospitalization and follow-up visits.	4. An open dialogue with the physician is encouraged to clarify concerns and to provide access to specific explanations.
5. Encourage open communication between the client and partner regarding limitations and alternative methods of pleasure.	5. Partners of men with prostate cancer clearly see themselves as partners in managing the effects of cancer on their partner's lives (Butler, Downe-Wannbolt, Marsh, Bell, & Jarvi, 2000).
6. Provide opportunities for the partner to share concerns and questions.	6. Partners are crucial to the recovery process. They manage their own anxiety and also assist their partner in managing his (Maliski, Heilemann, & McCorkle, 2001). Cultural and religious beliefs may affect the spouse's participation and queries (Sublett, 2007).
7. Encourage the client to continue to discuss concerns with significant others and professionals postdischarge.	
8. Determine the person's expectations of effects of surgery on urinary continence.	8. Damage to the muscle controlling the urethral sphincter or its nerve supply can cause incontinence. The retropubic approach can result in lower rates of incontinence. About 15%–50% of clients report incidence of urinary problems (James, 2007) and 30% report permanent incontinence (Moore, Truong, Estey, & Voaklander, 2007).

Documentation

Progress notes
   Usual sexual patterns
   Expressed concerns
Discharge summary record
   Client teaching
   Response to teaching

High Risk for Ineffective Therapeutic Regimen Management Related to Insufficient Knowledge of Fluid Restrictions, Catheter Care, Activity Restrictions, Urinary Control, and Signs and Symptoms of Complications

NOC Compliance Behavior, Knowledge: Treatment Regimen, Participation: Health Care Decisions, Treatment Behavior: Illness or Injury

Goals

The goals for this diagnosis represent those associated with discharge planning. Refer to the discharge criteria.

NIC Anticipatory Guidance, Risk Identification, Health Education, Learning Facilitation

Interventions	Rationales
1. Reinforce the need for adequate oral fluid intake (at least 2000 mL/day, unless contraindicated).	1. Optimal hydration helps to reestablish bladder tone after catheter removal by stimulating voiding, diluting urine, and decreasing susceptibility to urinary tract infections and clot formation.
2. Teach indwelling catheter care. a. Wash the urinary meatus with soap and water twice a day. b. Increase the frequency of cleansing if drainage is evident around the catheter insertion site.	2. The indwelling catheter provides a route for bacteria that are normally found on the urinary meatus to enter the urinary tract. These measures help to reduce risk of urinary tract infection.
3. Reinforce activity restrictions that may include the following: a. Avoid straining with bowel movements; increase intake of dietary fiber or take stool softeners, if indicated. b. Do not use suppositories or enemas. c. Avoid sitting with legs dependent. d. Avoid heavy lifting and strenuous activity. e. Avoid sexual intercourse until the physician advises otherwise (usually within 6–8 weeks after surgery).	3. These restrictions are necessary to reduce the risk of internal bleeding.
4. Advise that the client may do the following: a. Take long walks. b. Use stairs. c. Drive three weeks after surgery if power steering is used.	4. These activities do not impede healing of surgical site.
5. Explain expectations for urinary control after the catheter is removed: a. Dribbling, frequency, and urgency may occur initially, but will gradually subside over weeks.	5. a. Difficulty resuming normal voiding patterns may be related to bladder neck trauma, urinary tract infection, or catheter irritation. While the indwelling catheter is in place, constant urine drainage decreases muscle control and increases flaccidity.

(continued on page 636)

Interventions	Rationales
b. Perineal exercises (tense buttocks, hold, and release): • Tighten and hold for 10 seconds, then relax for 10 seconds; repeat 10 times. • Do exercises frequently (6–12 times a day; 10 at a time). c. Avoiding caffeine and alcohol can help to prevent problems. d. Transient hematuria is normal and should decrease with increased fluid intake. e. Wear a pants liner or diaper initially, if needed.	b. Regular contracture of the sphincter muscles will strengthen the pelvic floor muscles and decrease incontinence in 4–6 weeks. Use of biofeedback or anal electrical stimulation may help prevent continued incontinence (Hunter, Moore, & Glazener, 2007). c. Caffeine acts as a mild diuretic and makes it more difficult to control urine. Alcohol may increase the burning sensations on urination. e. Robot-assisted laparoscopic approaches report 93% continence rate three weeks after surgery (Vattikuti Urology Institute, 2007).
6. Review signs and symptoms of complications and the need to report them: a. Inability to void for more than 6 hours b. Fever, chills, flank pain c. Increased hematuria	6. Early detection enables prompt intervention to minimize severity of complications. a. Inability to void may indicate clot or tissue blockage. b. These symptoms may indicate urinary tract infection. c. Increased hematuria points to bleeding or hemorrhage.
7. Refer to community services (e.g., home care, counseling) and sources of information (e.g., www.cancer-prostate.com).	

Documentation

Discharge summary record
    Client teaching
    Outcome achievement or status
    Referrals, if indicated

Thoracic Pulmonary Surgery

A term encompassing various procedures involving a surgical opening into the chest cavity, thoracic surgery may be a pneumonectomy (removal of entire lung), lobectomy (removal of a lobe), segmentectomy (removal of a segment), wedge resection (small localized section of lung removed), sleeve resection with bronchoplastic reconstruction (partial removal of bronchus), or exploratory thoracotomy (internal view of the lung). Thoracic surgery usually is indicated for lung cancer but also may be indicated to repair a traumatized lung, treat pleural and interstitial lung diseases, and to isolate tuberculosis, abscesses, bronchiectasis, blebs, and bulla caused by emphysema (Khraim, 2007; "Respiratory Function and Therapy," 2006).

Thoracic surgery may be open or endoscopic, also known as video-assisted, or minimally invasive. Both require general anesthesia and possibly single lung ventilation, using a double-lumen endotracheal tube (Khraim, 2007; Stanbridge, Hon, Bateman, & Roberts, 2007; "Surgical Procedures," 2004). However, video-assisted thoracic surgery [VATS] can also be performed under local anesthesia ("Thoracoscopy [Pleuroscopy]," 2004) with less postoperative pain, decreased morbidity, shorter hospitalization, reduced postoperative shoulder dysfunction, and quicker return to preoperative activities/functions (Khraim, 2007; Stanbridge et al., 2007). VATS provides real-time, two-dimensional video images of the thoracic cavity (Khraim, 2007).

 Time Frame
Preoperative and postoperative periods

▪▪▪▪▪▪ DIAGNOSTIC CLUSTER

Preoperative Period

Nursing Diagnoses

△ Anxiety related to impending surgery and insufficient knowledge of preoperative routines, intraoperative activities, and postoperative self-care activities

Postoperative Period

Collaborative Problems	Refer to
△ PC: Mediastinal Shift	
▲ PC: Subcutaneous Emphysema	
▲ PC: Acute Pulmonary Edema	
▲ PC: Dysrhythmias	
✳ PC: Acute Lung Injury	
✳ PC: Bronchopleural Fistula	
▲ PC: Respiratory Insufficiency	Coronary Artery Bypass Grafting
▲ PC: Pneumothorax, Hemothorax	Abdominal Aortic Aneurysm Resection
▲ PC: Pulmonary Embolism	Abdominal Aortic Aneurysm Resection
△ PC: Thrombophlebitis	Abdominal Aortic Aneurysm Resection

Nursing Diagnoses	Refer to
▲ Ineffective Airway Clearance related to increased secretions and diminished cough secondary to pain and fatigue	
▲ Impaired Physical Mobility related to restricted arm and shoulder movement secondary to pain and muscle dissection and imposed position restrictions	
▲ Acute Pain related to surgical incision, chest tube sites, and immobility secondary to lengthy surgery	
Grieving related to loss of body part and its perceived effects on life style	Enucleation
Risk for Ineffective Therapeutic Regimen Management Related to Insufficient Knowledge of Activity Restrictions, see p. 646	

Related Care Plans

General Surgery Generic care plan
Mechanical Ventilation
Cancer: Initial Diagnosis

▲ This diagnosis was reported to be monitored for or managed frequently (75%–100%).
△ This diagnosis was reported to be monitored for or managed often (50%–74%).
✳ This diagnosis was not included in the validation study.

Discharge Criteria

Before discharge, the client or family will

1. Describe at-home wound care.
2. Relate the need to continue exercises at home.

3. Verbalize precautions for activities.
4. State signs and symptoms that must be reported to a health care professional.
5. Identify appropriate community resources and self-help groups.
6. Describe at-home pain management.

Preoperative: Nursing Diagnoses

Anxiety Related to Impending Surgery and Insufficient Knowledge of Preoperative Routines, Intraoperative Activities, and Postoperative Self-care Activities

NOC Anxiety Reduction, Coping, Impulse Control

Goal

The client will

1. Verbalize knowledge of routines and care before, during, and after surgery.
2. Share concerns and fears and demonstrate evidence of physical and psychosocial preparation for surgery.

NIC Anxiety Reduction, Impulse Control Training, Anticipatory Guidance

Interventions	Rationales
1. Provide information regarding what to expect before, during, and after surgery; use appropriate client education materials (e.g., booklets, video, one-on-one instruction). Explain the expected events, such as the following:	1. Preoperative education improves the client's ability to participate postoperatively and decreases anxiety associated with the unknown (Khraim, 2007). Research has shown that clients who stop smoking several weeks before surgery have fewer postoperative complications (Khraim, 2007).
a. Presence of chest tubes, drainage tubes, and indwelling catheter	a. Drainage tubes remove liquids and gas from the surgical site (thoracic cavity, pleural space, mediastinal cavity). Chest tubes reexpand the lungs by reestablishing negative intrapleural pressures. Chest tubes are not indicated after a pneumonectomy because it is desirable that the space accumulates fluid (Shah, Sharma, Mehta, Rau, & Solanki, 2002; Walker, 2002).
b. Need for oxygen therapy and oximetry monitoring	b. Supplemental oxygen is indicated to compensate for impaired ventilation.
c. Pain and available relief measures, such as	c. Moderate to severe pain is expected; the client should be aware of this possibility. Accurate expectations of pain lead to lower levels of anxiety. Splinting and decreased breath sounds indicate poor lung expansion and the need for improved pain control. Pain will cause ineffective coughing and deep breathing (Roman, Weinstein, & Macalusa, 2003).
• Client-controlled analgesia (PCA)	• Clients who are able to self-medicate with small IV doses of opioids by a programmable infusion pump have demonstrated less pain, anxiety, increased satisfaction, and early recovery and discharge.
• Epidural analgesia (Stanbridge et al., 2007)	• Pain control in the form of epidural analgesia after thoracic surgery provides excellent pain relief, improved pulmonary function, and overall recovery (Agency for Health Care Policy and Research (AHCPR), 1992). Although epidural is the choice for pain control, it may negatively influence respiratory muscle function (Bauer, Hents, Ducrocq, Nicolas, Oswald-Mammosser, Steib et al., 2007).
d. Location and extent of incision e. Progression from ICU/recovery room to stepdown unit and average length of stay postoperatively	d,e. Research reports explaining what to expect can help to reduce fears associated with the unknown (Johnson, Rice, Fuller, & Endress, 1978). Preoperative education reduces anxiety and promotes cooperation with postoperative interventions (Khraim, 2007).

(continued on page 639)

Interventions	Rationales
2. Teach the client postoperative respiratory exercises and routines, including the following: a. Coughing and deep breathing b. "Huff breathing" • Take a deep diaphragmatic breath and exhale forcefully against the hand with a "huff." • Start with small huffs and progress to one strong huff. c. Positioning d. Incentive spirometry e. Chest physiotherapy Reinforce their importance. Refer to General Surgery care plan, Appendix II.	2. Surgery on the lung reduces surface area for oxygen exchange, and trauma to the tracheobronchial tree produces excessive secretions and a diminished cough reflex. Respiratory exercises, including chest physiotherapy (CPT), incentive spirometry, and positioning, stimulate pulmonary expansion and assist in alveolar inflation (Nettina, 2006).
3. Instruct the client to refrain from smoking postoperatively.	3. Irritants from smoking increase pulmonary secretions.
4. Implement strategies to relieve anxiety, such as distraction, relaxation, and emotional support, if necessary.	4. Psychologic interventions for surgery intended to offer emotional support and relieve anxiety are often more effective than purely informational approaches.

Documentation

Teaching record
    Instructional method used
    Outcome achievement or status

Postoperative: Collaborative Problems

Potential Complication: Acute Pulmonary Edema

Potential Complication: Mediastinal Shift

Potential Complication: Subcutaneous Emphysema

Potential Complication: Dysrhythmias

Potential Complication: Acute Lung Injury [ALI]

Potential Complication: Bronchopleural Fistula

Nursing Goal

The nurse will detect early signs and symptoms of (a) increased pneumothorax, (b) pulmonary edema, (c) mediastinal shift, (d) subcutaneous emphysema, and (e) dysrhythmias, and collaboratively intervene to stabilize the client.

Indicators

- Alert, calm, oriented (a, b, c, d)
- Respirations 16–20 breaths/min (a, b, c)
- Symmetrical, easy, rhythmic respirations (a, b, c)
- Warm, dry skin (a, b, c)
- Breath sounds all lobes (a, b, c)
- No crackles or wheezing (a, b, c)
- Usual color (pinkish, brownish, or olive skin tones) (a, b, c)
- Capillary refill <3 sec (a, b, c)
- Oxygen saturation (PaO_2) >94% (a, b, c)
- pH 7.35–7.45 (a, b, c)
- Carbon dioxide ($PaCO_2$) 35–45 mmHg (a, b, c)
- Pulse 60–100 beats/min (a, b, c)

- BP >90/60, <140/90 mmHg (a, b, c)
- Peripheral pulses equal full (a, b, c)
- Pulmonary artery pressure 25/9 mmHg (a, b, c)
- Central venous pressure 0–8 mmHg (a, b, c)
- Normal EKG (e)
- Larynx/trachea midline (c)
- No neck vein distention (c)
- Minimal subcutaneous air (d)

Interventions	Rationales
1. Maintain a closed intact chest drainage system. Inspect hourly during the first 24 hours.	1. Malfunction or disconnection of the chest drainage system will cause air to enter the pleural system, resulting in pneumothorax.
2. Monitor for malfunction of system and report signs and symptoms immediately: • No fluctuation in water seal chamber • Respiratory distress (excessive bubbling in water seal chamber) • Subcutaneous air under skin (e.g., neck, chest, face) • Vital signs at least every two hours; especially rate, depth, and pattern of respirations with SpO_2 readings (Coughlin & Parchinsky, 2006)	2. Malfunction of the chest drainage system causes air accumulation in the pleural space, compromising respirations and forcing air into the subcutaneous tissue (subcutaneous emphysema).
3. If a tube disconnects, reattach or place end under water as the client exhales. Do not clamp the tube. Notify the surgeon and plan for a stat chest x-ray (Coughlin & Parchinsky, 2006).	3. Exhalation prior to reconnection will force excess air from pleural space. Clamping the tube can cause a tension pneumothorax.
4. Assess chest tube insertion site every 2 hours: a. Evidence of bleeding b. Intact occlusive dressing c. Correct position of chest tubes d. Evidence of subcutaneous emphysema (Coughlin & Parchinsky, 2006)	4. a. Recent bleeding can be detected early. b. An occlusive dressing is needed to prevent air from entering pleural space. c. Improper positioning of tubes can increase air and drainage in pleural space.
5. Position tubing with the excess tubing coiled on bed. Drain the fluid in the coiled tubing into the collection device (Coughlin & Parchinsky, 2006).	5. Proper positioning will promote drainage. Coiling the tubing can prevent accidental disconnection.
6. Observe fluctuation of water level during respirations; this is called tidaling (Coughlin & Parchinsky, 2006).	6. Tidaling indicates an airtight drainage system. When lung expansion is complete, tidaling stops.
7. Document amount, consistency, and color of chest tube drainage every hour according to protocol. Notify the surgeon if drainage increases. Color and consistency of drainage in the chamber may be mixed and not appear accurately; assess drainage in the tubing for changes (Coughlin & Parchinsky, 2006).	7. Increased drainage can indicate bleeding; no drainage can indicate a non-patent tube that can cause an increase in intrapleural pressure.
8. Prior to removal of chest tubes (3–4 days postop), assess for absence of chest tube drainage, no tidaling with respirations, and breath sounds in affected area (Coughlin & Parchinsky, 2006).	8. These clinical findings indicate lung reexpansion.

(continued on page 641)

Interventions	Rationales

9. Assist the surgeon to remove the tubes.
  a. Medicate prior to removal (½–1 hour), per order (Allibone, 2003).
  b. Position in high-Fowler's.
  c. Instruct the client to take a deep breath and cough (Allibone, 2003).
  d. Apply an occlusive dressing.
 	
  e. Post removal chest x-ray (Allibone, 2003; Coughlin & Parchinsky, 2006).
	9.
	  a. This will reduce the pain of removal.
	
	  b,c. High-Fowler position and a deep breath provide for maximum lung expansion and positive intrapleural pressure
	  d. An occlusive dressing is needed to prevent air leaks and infection.
	  e. Pneumothorax is the most common complication after removing a chest tube (Allibone, 2003).

10. After tube removal, evaluate respiratory status:
  a. No distress
  b. Breath sounds present in all lobes
  c. Even chest movement
  d. Calm
  e. No dysrhythmias
	10. Complications after tube removal can be pneumothorax, hemothorax, or mediastinal shift. Early changes in respiratory or cardiac function can prevent serious complications.

11. Instruct the client to use a spirometer 3–4 times an hour.	11. Frequent use of a spirometer increases lung volumes and prevents pneumonia.
12. Monitor vital signs, pulse oximetry, pulmonary artery catheter readings, and arterial blood gases, according to protocol.	12. Careful monitoring can detect early signs and symptoms of hypoxia.
13. Monitor respiratory function (rate, rhythm, capillary refill, breath sounds, skin color).	13. Frequent respiratory assessments are needed to evaluate early signs and symptoms of atelectasis, pneumothorax, and hemothorax.
14. Provide oxygen and position the client in semi-Fowlers or full-Fowlers.	14. The semi-Fowler position aids in lung expansion. Oxygen may be needed until lungs are fully reexpanded.

15. Monitor for signs of acute pulmonary edema:
  a. Severe dyspnea
  b. Tachycardia
  c. Adventitious breath sounds
  d. Persistent cough
  e. Cough productive of frothy sputum
  f. Cyanosis
	15. Circulatory overload can result from the reduced size of the pulmonary vascular bed caused by removal of pulmonary tissue and the yet-unexpanded lung postoperatively. Hypoxia produces increased capillary permeability, causing fluid to enter pulmonary tissue and triggering signs and symptoms.

16. Cautiously administer IV fluids.	16. Caution is needed to prevent circulatory overload.
17. Encourage and assist the client to get adequate rest and conserve strength.	17. Rest reduces oxygen consumption and decreases hypoxia.

18. Monitor for signs of mediastinal shift:
  a. Increased weak, irregular pulse rate
  b. Severe dyspnea, cyanosis, and hypoxia
  c. Increased restlessness and agitation
  d. Deviation of larynx or trachea from midline
  e. Shift in the point of apical impulse
  f. Hypotension
  g. Asymmetric chest excursion
  h. Neck vein distention
	18. Increased intrapleural pressure on the operative side from fluid and air accumulations or excessive negative pressure on the operative side from inadequate fluid accumulation provides a space for the contents of the mediastinum (heart, trachea, esophagus, pulmonary vessels) to shift. Constriction of vessels (aorta, vena cava) creates hypoxia and its resultant signs and symptoms.

19. If signs and symptoms of a mediastinal shift occur, do the following:
  a. Position the client in a semi-Fowler's position.
	19.
	
	  a. Sitting upright reduces mediastinal shifting.

(continued on page 642)

Interventions	Rationales
b. Maintain oxygen therapy. c. Assist the client to clear present chest tube or reinsert a new one.	b. Oxygen therapy reduces hypoxia. c. The treatment of choice is insertion of a thoracic chest tube to release elevated intrapleural pressure.

20. Monitor for signs of pneumothorax (Khraim, 2007; Roman et al., 2003):
  a. Reduced or absent breath sounds in affected area
  b. Subcutaneous emphysema (also known as crepitus)
  c. Dyspnea
  d. Chest pain (pleuritic), usually increasing with respiratory effort
  e. Clinical signs of respiratory failure: cyanosis, tachycardia, tachypnea
  f. Reduced chest wall movement on affected side
  g. Clinical signs of mediastinal shift
	20. Pneumothorax can cause acute respiratory failure (Roman et al., 2003).

21. Monitor status of subcutaneous emphysema:
 	
  a. Mark periphery of the emphysematous tissue with a skin-marking pencil; reevaluate frequently.
  b. Monitor for neck involvement.
	21. Subcutaneous emphysema can occur after thoracic surgery as air leaks out of incised pulmonary tissue:
	  a. Serial markings help the nurse to evaluate the rate of progression.
	  b. Severe subcutaneous emphysema can indicate air leakage through the bronchial stump and can compress the trachea.

22. If subcutaneous emphysema worsens, check patency of the chest drainage system and notify the surgeon.	22. Some subcutaneous emphysema may be present. Severe manifestations need to be corrected.
23. Monitor for cardiac dysrhythmias. Report any changes immediately and initiate protocol.	23. Decreased oxygen to the myocardium causes cardiac dysrhythmias.

 Related Physician-Prescribed Interventions

Medications. Bronchodilators, opioids, expectorants, local anesthetics, narcotic, nonsteroidal anti-inflammatory

Intravenous Therapy. Refer to the General Surgery care plan

Laboratory Studies. Arterial blood gas analysis; also refer to the General Surgery care plan

Diagnostic Studies. Chest x-ray film, pulmonary function studies, fiberoptic bronchoscopy, computed tomography (CT) scan, continuous pulse oximetry, sputum cytology, fine-needle aspiration, gallium scan, MRI, pulse oximetry, pulmonary artery pressure monitoring, central venous pressure monitoring

Therapies. Intermittent positive-pressure breathing (IPPB) treatments, chest drainage system, client-controlled analgesia, chest physiotherapy, epidural analgesia, antiembolism devices, chemotherapy, radiation, and pleurodesis (Roman, Weinstein, & Macaluso, 2003).

Documentation

Flow records
  Vital signs
  Intake and output records

Postoperative: Nursing Diagnoses

Ineffective Airway Clearance Related to Increased Secretions and Diminished Cough Secondary to Pain and Fatigue

NOC Aspiration Prevention, Respiratory Status: Airway Patency

Goal

The client will demonstrate adequate oxygen and ventilation.

Indicators

- Demonstrate effective coughing and increased air exchange.
- Explain rationale for interventions.

NIC Cough Enhancement, Airway Suctioning, Positioning, Energy Management

Interventions	Rationales
1. Teach the client to sit as erect as possible; use pillows for support, if needed.	1. Slouching and cramping positions of the thorax and abdomen interfere with air exchange.
2. Teach the client the proper method of controlled coughing: a. Breathe deeply and slowly every 1–2 hours while sitting up as high as possible. b. Use diaphragmatic breathing. Hold breath for 3–5 seconds, then slowly exhale as much as possible through the mouth (the lower rib cage and abdomen should sink down). c. Take a second breath, hold, and cough forcefully from the chest (not from the back of the mouth or throat) using two short, forceful coughs. Splint the chest with hands or pillow. Check any tube connections. d. If indicated, use the "huffing" breathing technique as taught preoperatively. e. Use a spirometer 3–4 times per hour (Nettina, 2006).	2. Deep breathing dilates the airways, stimulates surfactant production, and expands the lung tissue surface; this improves respiratory gas exchange. Coughing loosens secretions and forces them into the bronchus to be expectorated or suctioned. In some clients, "huff" breathing may be effective and less painful.
3. Assess lung fields before and after coughing exercises.	3. Comparison assessments help to evaluate the effectiveness of coughing.
4. If breath sounds are moist-sounding, instruct the client to rest briefly, then repeat the exercises.	4. Crackles indicate trapped secretions.
5. Assess the current analgesic regimen: a. Administer pain medication, as needed. b. Assess its effectiveness: Is the client still in pain? If not, is he or she too lethargic? c. Note the times when the client seems to obtain the best pain relief with an optimal level of alertness and physical ability. This is the time to initiate breathing and coughing exercises.	5. Pain or fear of pain can inhibit participation in coughing and breathing exercises ("Major Postoperative Pulmonary Complications," 2004). Adequate pain relief is essential.
6. Provide emotional support: a. Stay with the client for the entire coughing session. b. Explain the importance of coughing after pain relief is obtained. c. Reassure the client that the suture lines are secure and that splinting by hand or pillow will minimize pain on movement.	6. Coughing exercises are fatiguing and painful. Emotional support provides encouragement; warm water can aid relaxation.
7. Maintain adequate hydration and humidity of inspired air (Nettina, 2006).	7. These measures help to decrease viscosity of secretions. Tenacious secretions are difficult to mobilize and expectorate (Nettina, 2006).
8. Move the client out of bed to chair on postoperative day 1 and begin ambulation as soon as possible.	8. Early ambulation promotes aeration and can help to minimize pulmonary complications.

(continued on page 644)

Interventions	Rationales
9. Provide motivation and plan strategies to avoid overexertion: a. Plan and bargain for adequate rest periods (e.g., "Work hard now, then I'll let you rest."). b. Vigorously coach and encourage coughing; use positive reinforcement. c. Plan coughing sessions for periods when the client is alert and obtaining optimal pain relief. d. Allow for rest after coughing sessions and before meals.	9. The client's cooperation enhances the exercises' effectiveness.
10. Evaluate the need for tracheobronchial suctioning.	10. Suctioning will be needed if the client is unable to cough effectively.

Documentation

Flow records
  Auscultation findings (before and after coughing exercises)
Progress notes
  Effectiveness of coughing
Teaching records
  Client teaching

Impaired Physical Mobility Related to Restricted Arm and Shoulder Movement Secondary to Pain and Muscle Dissection and Imposed Position Restrictions

NOC Ambulation: Walking, Joint Movement: Active, Mobility Level

Goal

The client will return or progress to preoperative arm and shoulder function.

Indicators

• Demonstrate knowledge of the need to maintain certain positions.
• Demonstrate ROM exercises.

NIC Exercise Therapy: Joint Mobility, Exercise Promotion: Strength Training, Exercise Therapy: Ambulation, Positioning, Teaching: Prescribed Activity/Exercise

Interventions	Rationales
1. Position the client as indicated or prescribed: a. Supine position until consciousness is regained b. Semi-Fowler position (30–45 degrees) thereafter	1. a. The supine position prevents aspiration. b. This position allows the diaphragm to resume its normal position, which reduces the effort of respiration.
2. Explain the need for frequent turning. Gently turn the client from side to side every 1–2 hours, unless contraindicated. Check with a thoracic surgeon or the institutional procedural manual.	2. Turning mobilizes drainage of secretions, promotes circulation, inhibits thrombus formation, and aerates all parts of the remaining lung tissue. Lying on the operative side can be contraindicated following a wedge resection and pneumonectomy.
3. Avoid extreme lateral turning following a pneumonectomy.	3. This can cause a mediastinal shift (refer to Potential Complication: Mediastinal Shift in this entry for more information).

(continued on page 645)

Interventions	Rationales
4. Avoid traction on chest tubes during movement; check for kinks after repositioning.	4. Traction can cause dislodgment; kinks can inhibit drainage or negative pressure.
5. Explain the need for frequent exercises of arms, shoulders, and trunk, even in the presence of some pain and discomfort.	5. The muscle groups transcended by a thoracotomy form the shoulder girdle and maintain the trunk's posture. Failure to perform exercises can result in muscle adhesions, contractures, and postural deformities.
6. Initiate passive ROM exercises on the operative arm and shoulder within 4 hours after recovery from anesthesia. Begin with two times every 4 hours for the first 24 hours; progress to 10–20 times every 2 hours.	6. Passive ROM exercises help to prevent ankylosis of the shoulder and contractures of the arm.
7. Consult with a physical therapist for active ROM exercises for the client to perform, starting 1–2 days after surgery: a. Hyperextending the arms to strengthen the latissimus dorsi b. Adducting and forward flexing the arms and shoulders to maintain shoulder girdle motion c. Adducting the scapula to strengthen the trapezius	7. Active ROM exercises help to prevent adhesions of two incised muscle layers.
8. Encourage use of the affected arm in ADLs and stress the need to continue exercises at home.	8. Regular use increases ROM and decreases contractures and shift (refer to Potential Complication: Mediastinal Shift in this entry for more information).

Documentation

Progress notes
 Limitations on performing activities
 Therapeutic exercises performed
Flow records
 Turning, positioning
Discharge summary record
 Client teaching
 Response to teaching

Acute Pain Related to Surgical Incision, Chest Tube Sites, and Immobility Secondary to Lengthy Surgery

NOC Comfort Level, Pain Control

Goal

The client will report satisfactory relief after pain-relief interventions.

Indicators

• Verbalize or demonstrate behaviors that indicate improved level of comfort.
• Demonstrate knowledge of measures to decrease pain or to cope appropriately with the pain.

NIC Pain Management, Medication Management, Emotional Support, Teaching: Individual, Heat/Cold Application, Simple Massage

Interventions	Rationales
1. Work with the client, physician, and family to develop a pain management plan. To alleviate fears and clarify misconceptions, communicate openly about pain-relief measures.	1. Collaboration and client involvement in the pain management plan help to minimize fears and feelings of loss of control.

2. Provide optimal pain relief with prescribed analgesia. See General Surgery care plan.
  a. Determine the client's ability to tolerate epidural analgesia and to comply with PCA therapy. Consult physician if appropriate.
  b. Assess the client's level of sedation, pain, and motor responses every 1–2 hours for 24–48 hours, then every 4 hours for the duration of pain therapy. Use pain scale (0–10).
  c. Assess the client on a regular basis for the following signs and symptoms:
    • Respiratory depression
    • Motor blocks
    • Change in level of consciousness
    • Pruritus
    • Nausea and vomiting
    • Dysphoria
    • Urinary retention
  d. Keep intravenous naloxone at the bedside at all times.
	2. The proper administration rate optimizes the efficacy of pain medications:
	  a. Pain after thoracic surgery initially is best managed with epidural analgesia, with a change to PCA after 2–3 days (AHCPR, 1992)
	  b. Frequent assessment and use of the pain scale will provide the nurse with objective data that can be used to prevent potential complications and allow appropriate intervention.
	  c. There are multiple potential risks of epidural and PCA analgesia using opioids and local anesthetics listed.
	
	  d. Narcotics can depress the brain's respiratory center. IV naloxone can quickly reverse these symptoms.

3. Explain and assist the client with noninvasive and nonpharmacologic pain-relief measures (see General Surgery care plan).	3. Music, imagery, relaxation, and other non-pharmacologic approaches have all shown effectiveness in reducing pain.
4. Provide a comfortable environment (e.g., close the door, pull curtains, dim the lights).	4. Privacy and a comfortable environment allow client to express pain in his or her own manner; this can help to reduce anxiety and pain.

Risk for Ineffective Therapeutic Regimen Management Related to Insufficient Knowledge of Activity Restrictions, Wound Care, Shoulder Exercises, Signs and Symptoms of Complications, and Follow-up Care

NOC Compliance Behavior, Knowledge: Treatment Regimen, Participation: Health Care Decisions, Treatment Behavior: Illness or Injury

Goals

The goals for this diagnosis represent those associated with the discharge planning. Refer to the discharge criteria.

NIC Anticipatory Guidance, Risk Identification, Health Education, Learning Facilitation

Interventions	Rationales

1. Explain restrictions:
  a. Avoid heavy lifting or moving heavy objects for 3–6 months.
  b. Avoid excessive fatigue.
  c. Avoid crowds and bronchial irritants (smoke, fumes, aerosol sprays).
	1.
	  a. Heavy lifting can increase tension on the incision, which can prolong healing.
	  b. Fatigue can prolong the healing process.
	  c. Attempts should be made to prevent infection and irritations.

(continued on page 647)

Interventions	Rationales
2. Practice breathing exercises and shoulder exercises (refer to Impaired Physical Mobility and Ineffective Airway Clearance for specifics). Provide written exercise instructions.	2. These will prevent complications of contractures, pneumonia, and atelectasis.
3. Apply local heat to the intracostal region. Use analgesics, as needed.	3. All attempts to relieve pain are needed to promote mobility and exercises.

4. Report to the surgeon:
  a. Chest pain
  b. Increasing shortness of breath
  c. Increasing fatigue
  d. Fever, chills
  e. Drainage from wound
  f. Increasing pain
	4. These signs and symptoms can indicate infection, bleeding, and/or respiratory insufficiency.

5. Provide information on community resources (e.g., American Cancer Society, smoking cessation programs, support groups, home health agencies, Meals-On-Wheels) and follow-up plan.	5. The client and/or family may need assistance after discharge.

Documentation

Discharge summary record
    Client teaching
    Outcome achievement or status
    Referrals (e.g., PT)
Progress notes
    Exercises done

Total Joint Replacement (Hip, Knee, Shoulder)

Joint replacement (arthroplasty) is the surgical replacement of all or part of a joint. This surgery is indicated for irreversibly damaged joints caused by osteoarthritis or rheumatoid arthritis, fractures of hip or femoral neck with avascular necrosis, trauma, and congenital deformity. Osteoarthritis remains the most common cause of arthroplasty (Branson & Goldstein, 2001).

For hip replacements, a ball and socket prosthesis is implanted, either with cement or uncemented. Uncemented prostheses have porous surfaces that allow the client's bone to grow into and stabilize the prosthesis.

For knee joint replacements, the prosthesis is tricompartmental, with femoral, tibial, and patellar components. As with hip prostheses, the knee prosthesis can be cemented or uncemented. Cemented fixation reduces blood loss because the cement seals open bone edges; it is therefore the most common fixation technique (Branson & Goldstein, 2001).

Knee and hip arthroplasty can now be done with minimally invasive and small-incision techniques. These techniques reduce postoperative pain, length of hospital stay, rehabilitation requirements, and complications. Clients are able to return to usual activities faster with less complications (McGrory et al., 2005).

 Time Frame
Preoperative and postoperative periods

Preoperative teaching is encouraged to reduce length of stay and complications. Medical, economic, social, and environmental issues should be identified before admission (Lopez-Bushnell, Gary, Mitchell, & Reil, 2004; Mauer, Abrahams, Arslanian, Schoenly, & Taggart, 2002; Thomas, Burton, Withrow, & Adkisson, 2004).

■■■■■ DIAGNOSTIC CLUSTER

Preoperative Period

Nursing Diagnoses	Refer to
▲ Anxiety related to scheduled surgery and lack of knowledge of preoperative and postoperative routines, postoperative sensations, and use of assistive devices	Fractured Hip and Femur

Postoperative Period

Collaborative Problems

▲ PC: Hemorrhage/Hematoma Formation	
▲ PC: Dislocation/Subluxation of Joint	
▲ PC: Neurovascular Compromise	Fractured Hip and Femur
▲ PC: Fat Emboli	Fractured Hip and Femur
▲ PC: Sepsis	Fractured Hip and Femur
▲ PC: Thromboemboli	

Nursing Diagnoses	Refer to
▲ Impaired Physical Mobility related to pain, stiffness, fatigue, restrictive equipment, and prescribed activity restrictions	
▲ High Risk for Impaired Skin Integrity related to pressure and decreased mobility secondary to pain and temporary restrictions	
△ High Risk for Ineffective Therapeutic Regimen Management related to insufficient knowledge of activity restrictions, use of assistive devices, signs of complications, and follow-up care	Amputation
▲ High Risk for Injury related to altered gait and use of assistive devices	Amputation

Related Care Plans

General Surgery Generic care plan
Anticoagulant Therapy
Amputation

▲ This diagnosis was reported to be monitored for or managed frequently (75%–100%).
△ This diagnosis was reported to be monitored for or managed often (50%–74%).

Discharge Criteria

Before discharge, the client and family will

1. Describe activity restrictions.
2. Describe a plan for resuming ADLs.
3. Regain mobility while adhering to weight-bearing restrictions.
4. State signs and symptoms that must be reported to a health care professional.

Postoperative: Collaborative Problems

Potential Complication: Hemorrhage/Hematoma
Potential Complication: Dislocation of Joint (Hip, Knee)
Potential Complication: Neurovascular Compromise

Nursing Goal

The nurse will detect early signs and symptoms of (a) hemorrhage/hematoma, (b) dislocation (hip, knee), and (c) neurovascular compromise, and will collaboratively intervene to stabilize the client.

Indicators

- Alert, oriented, calm (a)
- Pulse 60–100 beats/min (a)
- Respirations 16–20 breaths/min (a)
- BP >90/60, <140/90 mmHg (a)
- Capillary refill <3 sec (a, c)
- Peripheral pulses full, bilateral (a, c)
- Warm, dry skin, no blanching (a, c)
- Urine output 5 mL/kg/h (a)
- Hip in abduction or neutral rotation (b)
- Leg length even (b)
- Knee in neutral position (b)
- No complaints of tingling, numbness (c)
- Ability to move toes (c)
- Oxygen saturation >94% (a)
- Hemoglobin (a)
  - Male 13–18 gm/dL
  - Female 12–16 gm/dL
- Hematocrit (a)
  - Male 42%–50%
  - Female 40%–48%

If on anticoagulant therapy:

- Partial thromboplastin time 1.5 × control (a)
- Prothrombin time 1.5–2 × normal (a)
- International Normalized Ratio (INR) 2–3 (a)

Interventions	Rationales
1. Identify individuals at high risk for complications: a. History of cardiac problems b. Poor nutritional status c. Obesity d. Diabetes mellitus e. History of deep vein thrombosis (DVT) or pulmonary embolism (PE) f. Blood dyscrasias g. Deconditioned state h. Older adults	1. Wound healing is compromised by diabetes mellitus, inadequate nutrition, obesity, and impaired oxygen transport. Older adults, with associated comorbidities, are most vulnerable to postoperative complications and mortality. Preoperative identification of potential complications permits development of preventative strategies (Graul, 2002; Lopez-Bushnell et al., 2004).
2. Monitor drainage from suction device every hour.	2. The hip is a very vascular area and the use of anticoagulants creates a high risk for bleeding. Expect 200–500 mL in the first 24 hours reducing to approximately 50 mL in 48 hours. Some drainage systems permit salvage and autologous transfusion (Graul, 2002).

(continued on page 650)

Interventions	Rationales
3. Maintain pressure dressing and ice to surgical area as ordered.	3. Pressure can reduce bleeding at site, reducing hematoma formation.
4. Monitor for early signs and symptoms of bleeding and hypoxia: • Increased pulse • Increased respirations • Decreased oxygen saturation <94% • Urinary output >30 mL/kg/h	4. Early signs and symptoms of bleeding and hypoxia can prompt rapid interventions to prevent hemorrhage.
5. Monitor for hematoma: a. Increased pain at site b. Tense swelling in buttock and thigh	5. Bleeding into the surgical area can cause hematoma formation.
6. Notify the surgeon if signs and symptoms of bleeding and hypoxia occur.	6. The client may need to return to OR for repair of bleeding vessels.
7. Identify individuals at high risk for joint implant infection: a. Chronic urinary tract infections b. Gastrointestinal (GI) infection c. Dental infection or poor dentition	7. Joint implants can be infected through the hematogenous route anytime postoperatively or postdischarge (Altizer, 1998).
8. Determine whether or not antiinflammatory medications have been discontinued 7–10 days preoperatively.	8. Platelet function is inhibited by antiinflammatory medications (Altizer, 1998).
9. Maintain correct positioning: a. Hip: Maintain hip in abduction, neutral rotation, or slight external rotation. b. Hip: Avoid hip flexion over 60 degrees. c. Knee: Keep knees apart at all times and slightly elevated from hip; avoid gatching bed under knee or placing pillows under knee (to prevent flexion contractures); pillows should be placed under calf.	9. Specific positions are used to prevent prosthesis dislocation.
10. Assess for signs of joint (hip, knee) dislocation: a. Hip: • Acute groin pain in operative hip • Shortening of leg and in external rotation b. Hip, knee: • "Popping" sound heard by client • Inability to move • Bulge at surgical site	10. Until the surrounding muscles and joint capsule heal, joint dislocation may occur if positioning exceeds the limits of the prosthesis, such as when flexing or hyperextending the knee or abducting the hip more than 45 degrees.
11. Maintain bed rest, as ordered. Keep affected joint in a neutral position with rolls, pillows, or specified devices.	11. Bed rest typically is ordered for 1–3 days after surgery to allow stabilization of the prosthesis. Most clients transfer to chair or ambulate the first postoperative day (Branson & Goldstein, 2001; Mauer et al., 2002).
12. Client may be turned toward either side, unless contraindicated by the physician. Always maintain abduction pillow when turning; limit use of Fowler position.	12. If proper positioning is maintained including the abduction pillow, the client may safely be turned toward operative and nonoperative sides. This promotes circulation and decreases the potential for pressure ulcer formation as a result of immobility. Prolonged Fowler position can dislocate the prosthesis (Salmond, 1996; Graul, 2002).
13. Monitor for signs and symptoms of neurovascular compromise; compare findings with the unaffected limb: a. Diminished or absent pedal pulses	13. a. Surgical trauma causes swelling and edema that can compromise circulation and compress nerves.

(continued on page 651)

Interventions	Rationales
b. Capillary refill time >3 seconds	b. Prolonged capillary refill time points to diminished capillary perfusion.
c. Pallor, blanching, cyanosis, coolness of extremity	c. These signs may indicate compromised circulation.
d. Complaints of abnormal sensations (e.g., tingling and numbness)	d. These symptoms may result from nerve compression.
e. Increasing pain not controlled by medication	e. Tissue and nerve ischemia produce a deep, throbbing, unrelenting pain.
14. Instruct the client to report numbness, tingling, coolness, or change in skin color.	14. Early detection of neurovascular compromise enables prompt intervention to prevent serious complications.
15. Use elastic stockings or sequential compression device, as prescribed. Refer Thrombophlebitis in the Index for more interventions.	15. These aid in venous blood return and prevent stasis (Mauer et al., 2002).

 Related Physician-Prescribed Interventions

Medications. Anticoagulants (e.g., low-molecular-weight heparin, warfarin)

Intravenous Therapy. Refer to the General Surgery care plan

Laboratory Studies. Coagulant studies (PT, PTT, INR); also refer to the General Surgery care plan, Appendix II

Diagnostic Studies. x-ray films, bone scans, MRI, CT scan

Therapies. Antiembolic hose, sequential compression devices, continuous passive motion machines, client-controlled analgesia

Documentation

Flow records
  Positioning
  Peripheral circulation status
Surgical tracking information: name; size; serial, model and lot numbers; cement package (Branson & Goldstein, 2001).

Postoperative: Nursing Diagnoses

Impaired Physical Mobility Related to Pain, Stiffness, Fatigue, Restrictive Equipment, and Prescribed Activity Restrictions

NOC Ambulation: Walking, Joint Movement: Active, Mobility Level

Goal

The client will increase activity to a level consistent with abilities.

Indicators

- Demonstrate exercises.
- Report importance of continuing exercises at home.

NIC Exercise Therapy: Joint Mobility, Exercise Promotion: Strength Training, Exercise Therapy: Ambulation, Positioning, Teaching: Prescribed Activity/Exercise

Interventions	Rationales
1. Support an exercise program tailored to the client's ability; consult with physical therapist: a. For hip: Quadriceps and gluteal settings, plantar flexion of foot, and leg lifts b. For knee: Quadriceps setting, isometrics, and leg lifts	1. Exercises are needed to improve circulation and strengthen muscle groups needed for ambulation.
2. Develop a plan for ROM exercise at regular intervals, increasing the use of involved extremity as ordered.	2. Active ROM increases muscle mass, tone, and strength and improves cardiac and respiratory functioning. Studies show that postoperative rehabilitation beginning postoperative day 3 vs. postoperative day 7 reduces length of stay and increases speed in which functionality and range of motion are attained (Dillingham, 2007).
3. Collaborate with physical therapy and rehabilitation in teaching body mechanics and transfer techniques. Ensure proper body alignment.	3. Proper mechanics and alignment help to prevent dislocation of the prosthesis.
4. Encourage the client's independence and reward progress. Include the client in care planning and contracting. Assess cultural, religious, and language issues that may affect comprehension, compliance, and ability to maintain plan of care (Lopez-Bushnell et al., 2004).	4. The client's participation in decision-making about care increases self-esteem and can encourage compliance.
5. Schedule progressive and paced activities, as appropriate. Consult with physical therapist for weight-bearing regimen.	5. The amount of weight-bearing depends on the type of prosthesis used and the client's condition and abilities.
6. Reinforce use of ambulatory aids as taught by physical therapist and supervise client ambulation, as necessary. Encourage preoperative home preparation with modification equipment (Lopez-Bushnell et al., 2004).	6. Such devices must be used correctly and safely to ensure effectiveness and prevent injury.

Documentation

Progress notes
   Activity level
   Response to activity

High Risk for Impaired Skin Integrity Related to Pressure and Decreased Mobility Secondary to Pain and Temporary Restrictions

NOC Tissue Integrity: Skin & Mucous Membranes

Goal

The client will maintain intact skin.

Indicators

• Shift position every hour.
• Describe strategies to prevent pressure ulcers.

NIC Pressure Management, Pressure Ulcer Care, Skin Surveillance, Positioning

Interventions	Rationales
1. Use a pressure-relieving device (e.g., alternating mattress and heel protectors).	1. These and other devices can help to distribute pressure uniformly over the skin surface.
2. Turn and reposition the client every hour. Teach the client ways to shift position in bed (e.g., lifting buttocks and legs) and to use overhead trapeze.	2. Frequent repositioning allows circulation to return to tissues inhibited by pressure.
3. Assess pressure points—shoulder blades, heels, elbow, sacrum, and hips—each shift.	3. Bony prominences are covered with minimal skin and subcutaneous fat and are more prone to skin breakdown from pressure.
4. Lightly massage bony prominences with lotion. Protect vulnerable areas with film dressings.	4. Light massage stimulates circulation. Film dressings provide more structure to prevent injury from shearing force.
5. Stress the importance of optimal nutritional intake and hydration.	5. Inadequate nutrition and hydration reduce circulation and increase tissue wasting.
6. Encourage ambulation as indicated.	6. Ambulation improves circulation and reduces pressure on vessels.
7. Avoid elevating head of bed more than 30 degrees; support the feet with a footboard.	7. These interventions prevent shear pressure that causes decreased capillary perfusion when the feet are pinched, as bony prominences slide across subcutaneous tissue.

Documentation

Flow records
  Turning and repositioning
  Skin assessment

High Risk for Ineffective Therapeutic Regimen Management Related to Insufficient Knowledge of Activity Restrictions, Use of Assistive Devices, Signs of Complications, and Follow-up Care

NOC Compliance Behavior, Knowledge: Treatment Regimen, Participation: Health Care Decisions, Treatment Behavior: Illness or Injury

Goals

The goals for this diagnosis represent those associated with discharge planning. Refer to the discharge criteria.

NIC Anticipatory Guidance, Risk Identification, Health Education, Learning Facilitation

Interventions	Rationales

1. Explain restrictions that typically include avoiding the following:
  a. Excessive bending and lifting
  b. Crossing the legs
  c. Jogging, jumping, and kneeling
	1. These activities can put great stress on the implant.

2. Explain the need to continue prescribed exercises at home.	2. Exercises increase muscle strength and joint mobility.

(continued on page 654)

Interventions	Rationales
3. Teach wound care and assessment techniques.	3. Instructions are needed to prevent infection and to detect early signs of infection.
4. Reinforce and encourage the safe use of assistive devices and therapeutic aids; request return demonstration of correct use.	4. Assistive devices may be needed. Return demonstration allows nurse to evaluate proper, safe use.
5. Explain the need to continue leg exercises (5–10 times an hour) and use of antiembolic hose at home.	5. The risk of thrombophlebitis continues after discharge.
6. If continuous passive motion (CPM) will be used at home, teach the client and family the following: a. Correct application and use of the CPM. Reinforce limited time of CPM to maintain motion. b. Signs and symptoms of potential complications: • Joint swelling, redness, tenderness • Unusual pain • Reappearance of drainage that previously had ceased	6. Without properly learning CPM usage with daily reinforcement, the client may not fully use the benefits of CPM and may predispose him- or herself for future postjoint arthroplasty complications (adhesions or decreased range of motion). Only 15% of clients are discharged with CPM (Mauer et al., 2002).
7. Initiate (CPM) for knee arthroplasty per protocol: a. Focus neurovascular assessment on extremity using CPM. b. Assess skin integrity of extremity in CPM (pressure points, heel, upper thigh, or elbow). c. Assess involved joint for increased drainage, swelling, tenderness, and condition of surgical incision. d. Assess level of pain while using CPM; intervene with appropriate analgesia.	7. Passive motion has been shown to stimulate healing of articular cartilage and reduce potential for adhesion development. Continuous use is most effective to obtain and maintain desired degrees of flexion and extension (Salmond, 1996). This is usually started the day of surgery or postoperative day one (Mauer et al., 2002). a–d. Thorough assessment of extremity using CPM is necessary to monitor for potential complications associated with CPM. As degrees of flexion are increased on CPM, the client may initially experience increased discomfort and may require analgesic intervention (Salmond, 1996).
8. Explain risk of infection: early, delayed, or late.	8. Early infection occurs during the first 3 months. Delayed infection occurs between 3 months and 1 year. Late infection occurs after 1 year.
9. Teach the client to report signs and symptoms of complications: a. Increased temperature b. Red, swollen, draining incision c. Coolness of skin on affected limb or numbness d. Pain in calf or upper thigh	9. Early detection enables prompt interventions to prevent serious complications: a. Fever may indicate an infection or phlebitis. b. Incision changes may indicate infection. c. These signs indicate compromised circulation. d. Leg pain may point to thrombophlebitis.
10. If anticoagulants are prescribed, refer to the Anticoagulant Therapy care plan for specific interventions.	10. Up to 70% of postoperative orthopedic clients develop deep vein thrombosis (DVT) without prophylaxis; as much as 30% develop pulmonary embolus, particularly if there is excessive postoperative bleeding (Graul, 2002).
11. Explain to the client and family the importance of continuing therapy program at home for at least 6–12 months.	11. Clients with joint replacements should not be expected to regain full function for 6–12 months (Salmond, 1996). Range of motion (ROM) should be assessed at six and twelve weeks after surgery. If ROM is not at the anticipated range, then manipulation under anesthesia may be required. With knees, most clients resume all activities and are pain-free by the twelfth week (Branson & Goldstein, 2001).
12. Consult with community nursing service to prepare home and physical therapy environment for discharge.	12. Adaptations may be needed (e.g., commode, eliminate scatter rugs).

Documentation

Discharge summary record
  Client teaching
  Outcome achievement or status
Progress notes
  CPM usage
  Degree of flexion/extension

Urostomy

Urinary diversions, usually called urostomies or ileal conduits (Pullen, 2007), are performed when the bladder is bypassed or removed to divert urine from the ureters to a new exit site that is usually a stoma (opening in the skin). This procedure is most commonly performed because of bladder cancer, but may be necessary due to birth defects, neurogenic bladder dysfunction, intractable interstitial cystitis, and refractory radiation cystitis.

There are two types of urinary diversions: conventional or incontinent urostomy, and continent urinary reservoir (Clark & DuBois, 2004; Pontieri-Lewis, 2006; United Ostomy Association, 2006). The conventional incontinent urostomy is the creation of an ileal conduit. A segment of the ileum is excised; one end is sutured closed and the other end is brought through the abdominal wall to create a stoma. The ureters are detached from the bladder and implanted to the ileal segment. Urine drains freely into the ileal pouch, then out through the stoma into a collection bag (Clark & DuBois, 2004; United Ostomy Association, 2006). If the bladder is not cancerous and does not have to be removed, an alternative to the ileal conduit can be performed, called an ileovesicostomy. This procedure requires a small tube of ileum; one end is attached to the bladder and the other end is brought through the abdominal wall to create a stoma. This procedure is preferred for neurogenic bladder, because it avoids ureteroileal anastomosis decreasing complications; it is reversible, and it can be converted into an ileal conduit (Stamm & Tiemann, 2004).

There are four types of continent urostomies: Kock pouch, Indiana pouch, Mitrofanoff pouch and Ileal (or Orthotopic) Neobladder. All four pouches are made from portions of the intestine, usually the terminal ileum. All except the Ileal Neobladder require routine catheter drainage through a stoma. Catheterization is done four to five times per day. In the Ileal Neobladder, the original ureters and urethra are attached to a pouch, enabling normal urination (Clark & DuBois, 2004; Mathews & Courts, 2001). It may take several months for continence to return, but then daytime continence rates are at 86%–95%. Nighttime continence rates are higher for women than for men. A suprapubic catheter may be required for weeks after surgery (Mathews & Courts, 2001).

 Time Frame
Preoperative and postoperative periods

▪▪▪▪▪▪ DIAGNOSTIC CLUSTER

Preoperative Period

Nursing Diagnoses

▲ Anxiety related to lack of knowledge of urostomy care and perceived negative effects on life style

Postoperative Period

Collaborative Problems

△ PC: Internal Urine Leakage
▲ PC: Urinary Tract Infection/Urinary Calculi/Peritonitis

(continued on page 656)

▲ PC: Peristomal Ulceration/Herniation
▲ PC: Stomal Necrosis, Retraction, Prolapse, Stenosis, Obstruction

Nursing Diagnoses	Refer to
High Risk for Ineffective Sexuality Patterns related to erectile dysfunction (male) or inadequate vaginal lubrication (female)	
△ High Risk for Loneliness related to anxiety about possible odor and leakage from appliance	
▲ High Risk for Ineffective Therapeutic Regimen Management related to insufficient knowledge of stoma pouching procedure, colostomy irrigation, peristomal skin care, perineal wound care, and incorporation of ostomy care into activity of daily living (ADL)	
△ High Risk for Ineffective Therapeutic Regimen Management related to insufficient knowledge of intermittent self-catheterization of continent urostomy	
△ High Risk for Disturbed Self-Concept related to effects of ostomy on body image	Ileostomy
High Risk for Ineffective Sexuality Patterns related to perceived negative impact of ostomy on sexual functioning and attractiveness	Ileostomy

Related Care Plans

General Surgery Generic care plan
Cancer: Initial Diagnosis
Ileostomy

▲ This diagnosis was reported to be monitored for or managed frequently (75%–100%).
△ This diagnosis was reported to be monitored for or managed often (50%–74%).

Discharge Criteria

Before discharge, the client and family will

1. Describe routine ostomy care.
2. Demonstrate the proper stoma pouching procedure.
3. State measures to help maintain peristomal skin integrity.
4. Demonstrate intermittent self-catheterization.
5. State conditions of ostomy care at home: stoma, pouching, irrigation, skin care.
6. Discuss strategies for incorporating ostomy management into ADLs.
7. Verbalize precautions for medication use, fluid intake, and prevention of UTI and stone formation.
8. State signs and symptoms that must be reported to a health care professional.
9. Verbalize an intent to share with significant others feelings and concerns related to ostomy.
10. Identify available community resources and self-help groups:
    a. Visiting nurse
    b. UOA
    c. Recovery of Male Potency; Help for Impotent Male

d. American Cancer Society
e. Community supplier of ostomy equipment
f. Financial reimbursement for ostomy equipment

Preoperative Nursing Diagnoses

Anxiety Related to Lack of Knowledge of Urostomy Care and Perceived Negative Effects on Life Style

NOC Anxiety Level, Coping, Impulse Control

Goal

The client will verbalize decreased anxiety related to fear of the unknown.

Indicators

- State reason for urostomy.
- Describe anatomic changes following urostomy surgery.
- Identify the client's particular type of urostomy.

NIC Anticipatory Guidance, Risk Identification, Health Education, Learning Facilitation

Interventions	Rationales
1. Identify and dispel any misinformation or misconceptions the client may have regarding ostomy.	1. Replacing misinformation with facts can reduce anxiety.
2. Explain the normal anatomic structure and function of the genitourinary (GU) tract.	2. Knowledge increases confidence; confidence enhances control and reduces anxiety.
3. Explain the effects of the client's particular disorder on the affected organs.	3. Understanding the disorder can help the client accept the need for urostomy.
4. Use an anatomic diagram or model to show the resultant altered route of elimination.	4. Understanding how urine elimination occurs after the diversion and/or removal can help to allay anxiety related to altered body function.
5. Describe the appearance and anticipated location of the stoma. Explain the following facts about the stoma: a. It will be of the same color and moistness as the oral mucous membrane. b. It will not hurt when touched because it has no sensory endings. c. It may bleed slightly when wiped; this is normal and not of concern. d. It will become smaller as the surgical area heals; its color will remain the same. e. It may change in size depending on illness, hormone levels, and weight gain or loss.	5. Learning about expected events and sensations can help to reduce anxiety associated with the unknown and unexpected. Accurate descriptions of the stoma appearance help to ease shock at the first sight of it after ostomy surgery.
6. Discuss the function of the stoma pouch. Explain that it serves as an external receptacle for storage of urine, much as the bladder acts as an internal storage receptacle (Ewing, 1989).	6. Understanding the purpose and need for a pouch encourages the client to accept it and to participate in ostomy management.
7. Encourage the client to handle the stoma pouching equipment.	7. Many clients are relieved to see the actual size and material of a stoma pouch. Uninformed clients often envision large bags and complicated, difficult-to-manage equipment, leading to anxiety.

Documentation

Progress notes
    Presence of dysfunctional anxiety
Teaching records
    Client teaching

Collaborative Problems

Potential Complication: Internal Urine Leakage

Potential Complication: Urinary Tract Infection/Urinary Calculi, Peritonitis

Potential Complication: Peristomal Skin Ulceration

Potential Complication: Stomal Necrosis, Retraction, Prolapse, Stenosis, Obstruction

Nursing Goal

The nurse will detect early signs and symptoms of (a) internal urine leakage, (b) urinary tract infection/urinary calculi, peritonitis, (c) peristomal skin ulceration, and (d) stomal necrosis/retraction, and will collaboratively intervene to stabilize the client.

Indicators

- Temperature 98.5–99°F (a)
- Urinary output >30 mL/h (a)
- Pulse 60–100 beats/min (b)
- BP >90/60, <140/90 mmHg (b)
- Respirations 16–20 breaths/min (b)
- Capillary refill <3 sec (b)
- Oxygen saturation >94% (b)
- No sudden increase or decrease in drainage (a, b)
- Clear, light yellow urine (b)
- Urine pH 4.6–8.0 (b)
- No flank pain (b)
- No signs of peristomal ulceration or herniation (d)
- No abdominal distention (d)
- No complaints of nausea/vomiting (d)
- Stoma shrinking, with change in shape or color (d)

Interventions	Rationales
1. Monitor drainage amount and color every hour for the first 24 hours from: a. Incision b. Cecostomy catheter c. Urethral stents and bile catheters d. Stomal catheter e. Urethral catheter	1. A sudden decrease in urine flow may indicate obstruction (edema, mucus) or dehydration.
2. Irrigate cecostomy tube 2–3 times each day, as prescribed.	2. Irrigation removes mucus to prevent blockage.
3. Report a sudden change (increased or decreased) in drainage or bleeding from the stoma.	3. A change in drainage can indicate bleeding or infection (increased) or blockage (decreased).
4. Monitor every hour for the first 24 hours: a. Vital signs	4. Changes in vital signs (increased pulse, decreased BP, decreased urine output, decreased oxygen saturation, and

(continued on page 659)

Interventions	Rationales
b. Capillary refill <3 seconds c. Oxygen saturation (pulse oximetry) d. Urine output	increased capillary fill time) can indicate dehydration, bleeding, and/or hypoxia.
5. Monitor for signs of internal urine leakage: a. Abdominal distention with adynamic ileus b. Fever c. Elevated serum creatinine level d. Decreased urine output despite adequate hydration	5. Urine leakage either from the ureteroileal anastomosis or from the base of the conduit, occurs in as many as 8% of clients with a urostomy. Leakage is confirmed through fluoroscopy. Small leaks may seal themselves with continuous drainage of the conduit via a stomal catheter.
6. Explain the reason for cloudy urine.	6. Because the intestine produces mucus, mucus in the diversion will cause urine to appear cloudy (Early & Poquette, 2000; Clark & DuBois, 2004).
7. Monitor for signs and symptoms of urinary tract infection (Ewing, 1989): a. Fever b. Flank pain c. Malodorous, cloudy urine d. Alkaline urine pH	7. Between 10%–20% of clients with a urinary diversion develop pyelonephritis. The major cause is poor urine flow through the conduit, leading to urinary stasis and bacterial contamination through the stoma.
8. Consult with the physician for a urine culture from a double-lumen catheter specimen.	8. Cultures enable identification of the causative organism and guide pharmacologic therapy.
9. Monitor for signs of peristomal ulceration or herniation: a. Decreased peristomal muscle tone b. Bulging beyond normal skin surface and musculature c. Persistent ulceration d. Redness, skin breakdown or irritation, itching, warmth or pain in the peristomal area (Colwell & Beitz, 2007). Teach proper assessment of the peristomal area.	9. Early detection of ulcerations and herniation enables prompt intervention to prevent serious tissue damage.
10. Consult with a clinical specialist or ostomy therapist regarding persistent ulceration.	10. Expert assistance may be needed for persistent skin problems.
11. Monitor for stomal necrosis, prolapse, retraction, stenosis, and obstruction. Assess the following: a. Color, size, and shape of stoma b. Color and amount of urine from the urostomy or from each stent c. Complaints of cramping abdominal pain, nausea and vomiting, abdominal distention d. Ostomy appliance and appliance belt fit	11. Daily assessment is necessary to detect early changes in stoma condition. a. Changes can indicate inflammation, retraction, prolapse, edema. b. Changes can indicate bleeding or infection. Decreased output can indicate obstruction. c. These complaints may indicate obstruction. d. Improperly fitting appliance or belt can cause mechanical trauma to the stoma.

 ## Related Physician-Prescribed Interventions

Medications. Refer to the General Surgery care plan.
Intravenous Therapy. Refer to the General Surgery care plan.
Laboratory Studies. Refer to the General Surgery care plan.
Diagnostic Studies. Intravenous pyelography, CT scan, cystoscopy, conduitogram, bone scan, endoscopy, flow cytometry, pouchogram
Therapies. Sitz baths, urinary diversion collection appliances

Documentation

Flow records
    Vital signs
      Intake and output

Abdomen (girth, bowel sounds)
Condition of peristomal area

Postoperative: Nursing Diagnoses

High Risk for Ineffective Sexuality Patterns Related to Erectile Dysfunction (Male) or Inadequate Vaginal Lubrication (Female)

> **NOC** Body Image, Self-Esteem, Role Performance, Sexual Identity: Acceptance

> **Goal**

> The client will state the intent to discuss sexual concerns with partner after discharge.

> **Indicators**

> • Describe the possible effects of urostomy surgery on sexual function.
> • Identify available community resources, if necessary.

> **NIC** Behavior Management: Sexual, Counseling, Sexual Counseling, Emotional Support, Active Listening, Teaching: Sexuality

Interventions	Rationales
1. In men (Ofman, 1993; Junkin & Beitz, 2005): a. Suggest that sexual activity need not always culminate in vaginal intercourse and that orgasm can be reached through noncoital manual or oral stimulation. Remind the client that sexual expression is not limited to intercourse, but includes closeness, communication, touching, and giving and receiving pleasure. b. Explain the function of a penile prosthesis. Both semirigid and inflatable penile prostheses have high rates of success. c. Suggest counseling with a certified sex therapist.	1. a. Alternative methods of sexual expression and gratification promote positive sexual function. b. Penile implants provide the erection needed for intercourse and do not alter sensations or the ability to ejaculate. c. Certain sexual problems require continuing therapy and the advanced knowledge of therapists.
2. In women (Ofman, 1993): a. Suggest using a water-based vaginal lubricant for intercourse. b. Teach the client to perform Kegel exercises and instruct her to do them regularly. c. Suggest that she sit astride her partner during intercourse.	2. a. A water-based lubricant can help to prevent dyspareunia related to inadequate vaginal lubrication. b. Kegel exercises promote control of the pubococcygeal muscles around the vaginal entrance; this can ease dyspareunia. c. A woman on top can control the depth and rate of penetration; this can enhance vaginal lubrication and relaxation.

Documentation

Progress notes
  Interventions
  Response to interventions

High Risk for Loneliness Related to Anxiety About Possible Odor and Leakage From Appliance

> **NOC** Loneliness, Social Involvement

> **Goal**

> The client will state the intent to reestablish preoperative socialization pattern.

Indicators

- Discuss methods to control odor and appliance leakage.
- State the intent to dialogue with other persons in the same situation.

NIC Socialization Enhancement, Spiritual Support, Behavior Modification: Social Skills, Presence, Anticipatory Guidance

Interventions	Rationales
1. Select an appropriate odor-proof pouching system; explain to the client how it works.	1. Fear of accidents and odor can be reduced through effective management. Some pouches have charcoal filters that reduce urine odor.
2. Stress the need for good personal hygiene. 3. Teach the client the care of a reusable appliance.	2,3. Proper hygiene and appliance care remove odoriferous retained urine.

4. Discuss methods for reducing odor; such as:
  a. Avoid odor-producing foods, (e.g., asparagus, cabbage).
  b. Drink cranberry juice or use a liquid appliance deodorant.
  c. Empty or change the ostomy pouch regularly when one-third to one-half full.
	4. Minimizing odor improves self-confidence and can permit more effective socialization. Bacterial proliferation in retained urine increases odor over time. A full pouch also puts excessive pressure on seals, increasing the risk of leakage.

5. Encourage the client to reestablish his or her preoperative socialization pattern. Help with measures such as progressively increasing the client's socializing time in the hospital, role-playing possible situations that the client feels may cause anxiety, and encouraging the client to visualize and anticipate solutions to "worst-case scenarios" for social situations.	5. Encouraging and facilitating socialization helps to prevent isolation. Role-playing can help the client identify and learn to cope with potential anxiety-causing situations in a nonthreatening environment.
6. Suggest that the client meet with a person from the United Ostomy Association who can share similar experiences (Maklebust, 1985, Smith, 1992, Clark & DuBois, 2004; United Ostomy Association, 2006).	6. Others in a similar situation can provide a realistic appraisal of the condition and may provide information to answer the client's unasked questions.

Documentation

Progress notes
  Dialogues and interactions
Teaching record
  Client teaching

High Risk for Ineffective Therapeutic Regimen Management Related to Insufficient Knowledge of Stoma Pouching Procedure, Peristomal Skin Care, Perineal Wound Care, and Incorporation of Ostomy Care Into Activities of Daily Living (ADLs)

NOC Compliance Behavior, Knowledge: Treatment Regimen, Participation: Health Care Decisions, Treatment Behavior: Illness or Injury

Goals

The goals for this diagnosis represent those associated with discharge planning. Refer to the discharge criteria.

NIC Anticipatory Guidance, Risk Identification, Health Education, Learning Facilitation

Interventions	Rationales
1. Teach the client the basic stoma pouching principles. Make sure that teaching strategies are appropriate to the client's age (Zurakowski, Taylor, & Bradway, 2006):	1. Proper pouching techniques can prevent leakage and skin problems. Geriatric clients may have sensory deficits (e.g., poor vision), making skill acquisition more difficult (Zurakowski et al., 2006):
a. Keep the peristomal skin clean and dry.	a. This ensures that the appliance adheres to the skin.
b. Use a well-fitting antireflux appliance.	b. Proper fit protects the surrounding skin surface from contact with the drainage.
c. Change the pouch when the least amount of drainage is anticipated (usually on arising).	c. This prevents copious drainage from interfering with pouch changes
d. Empty the pouch when it is one-third to one-half full, and change it routinely before it leaks.	d. A pouch filled more than halfway exerts greater pressure on the seal, which increases the risk of leakage.
e. Change the pouch if the skin under the appliance gets wet or becomes painful.	e. Pain or wetness may indicate that urine has undermined the skin barrier; prompt intervention is necessary to prevent skin breakdown.
f. Observe the condition of the stoma and peristomal skin during pouch changes.	f. Regular observation enables early detection of skin problems.
2. Teach the client the procedure for preparing a stoma pouch (Pontieri-Lewis, 2006):	2. Preparing a new pouch beforehand ensures that the new pouch is ready to apply as soon as the used pouch is removed; this helps to minimize drainage on the skin surface.
a. Select the appropriate stoma pouching system.	
b. For urinary stomas, faceplates with convexity will lengthen wear time of the pouching system.	
c. Measure the stoma carefully.	
d. Use appliance manufacturer's stoma measuring card, if possible. If the card does not accommodate the stoma's size or shape, teach the client to make a customized stoma pattern: (1) place clear plastic wrap over the stoma; (2) trace the stoma with a marking pen; and (3) cut a hole in the plastic wrap to accommodate the stoma.	
e. Use this pattern to trace the opening onto the reverse side of a skin barrier wafer.	
f. Cut an opening in the center of the skin barrier slightly larger (approximately ⅛ inch) than the stoma.	
g. Secure an appropriate antireflux pouch onto the skin barrier wafer (if using a two-piece appliance system). The pouch should have an antireflux valve to prevent urine from bathing the stoma.	
3. Teach the client the procedure for changing a disposable stoma pouch:	3. Correct pouch removal and attachment techniques minimize irritation and injury of the peristomal skin and ensure a tight, reliable seal between the pouch and skin.
a. Remove the old pouch by gently pushing, rather than pulling, the skin away from the paper tape and skin barrier wafer (Pullen, 2007).	
b. Fold the old pouch over on itself and discard it in a plastic bag.	
c. Hold gauze or toilet paper over the stoma.	
d. Cleanse the peristomal skin with a wash cloth and warm tap water.	
e. Blot or pat the skin dry.	
f. Apply the new pouch to the abdomen, carefully centering the hole in the skin barrier wafer over the stoma. Press on the wafer for a few minutes.	
g. Secure the pouch by "picture framing" the wafer with four strips of hypoallergenic paper tape (if the wafer does not already have a tape attached).	

(continued on page 663)

Interventions	Rationales

4. Teach the client the procedure for emptying a stoma pouch:
  a. Put some toilet paper in the toilet bowl and sit on toilet seat.
  b. Remove the plug or turn the valve to open the pouch, and carefully empty the pouch contents into the toilet.
	4. Correct techniques can reduce spillage, soiling, and odor. Placing toilet paper in the bowl prevents water from splashing when the pouch contents are emptied into it. Add a mucus dispersant to the pouch or straight drainage tubing if it is connected to a secondary receptacle.

5. Connect the appliance to a straight drainage when the client is sleeping in bed.	5. Bacteria multiply rapidly as urine collects in the pouch. Bacterial contamination of the urinary tract can result from backflow of urine from a full pouch. Nighttime drainage systems hold large amounts of urine and drain urine away from the stoma.

6. Teach the client strategies for preventing and managing peristomal skin problems:
  a. Shave the peristomal skin with an electric razor rather than a blade.
  b. Evaluate all skin products for possible allergic reaction; patch-test all suspect products elsewhere on the abdomen.
  c. Do not change brands of skin barriers and adhesives casually; assess for allergic reaction before using a new brand.
  d. Avoid irritation from contact with urine; clean the skin regularly with warm water—if necessary, use mild soap, rinse well, and pat dry (Pullen, 2007; United Ostomy Association, 2006). Do not use oily soaps (Clark & DuBois, 2004) or lotions (Pullen, 2007) around the stoma.
  e. Avoid prolonged skin pressure, especially if the client is fair-skinned or has thin, atrophic skin due to long-term corticosteroid therapy.
  f. Use corticosteroid creams sparingly and briefly; they can cause dryness and irritation.
  g. If bacterial or fungal infection is suspected, use a specific antibacterial or antifungal cream or powder.
  h. Use a liquid film barrier; avoid a tincture of benzoin compound that can dry the skin.
  i. Avoid aluminum paste and greasy ointments that can mask skin problems and interfere with pouch adherence.
  j. Protect the skin with barriers.
  k. Expect the stoma to shrink slightly over time, especially during the first 6–8 weeks after surgery. This necessitates remeasuring the stoma to ensure proper appliance fit (Pontieri-Lewis, 2006).
	6. A client with a stoma is at increased risk for peristomal skin breakdown. Factors that influence skin integrity include allergies; mechanical trauma; the underlying disease and its treatment (including medications); the quality of ostomy and peristomal skin care; availability of proper supplies; nutritional status; overall health status; hygiene; and activity level. Allowing urine to remain in contact with the skin for prolonged periods can result in maceration and hyperplasia of the epidermis.

7. Promote measures to help the client incorporate ostomy care into ADLs:
 	
  a. *Fluid management:*
    • Drink 2–3 liters of fluids daily (Black, 2000).
 	
    • Consume cranberry juice, prune juice, plums, poultry, fish, whole grains.
    • Avoid excessive intake of milk, citrus fruits, and carbonated drinks.
	7. Successful incorporation of ostomy management into ADLs allows the client to resume pre-urostomy life style and pursue goals and interests:
	  a.
	    • Sufficient fluids flush urinary tract and prevent infection.
	    • These substances acidify urine and prevent bacteria growth.
	    • These substances create a more alkaline urine.

(continued on page 664)

Interventions	Rationales
b. *Working/traveling:* Keep extra supplies at work. When traveling, carry supplies, rather than pack them in a suitcase and risk losing them; keep in mind that pectin-based wafers melt in high temperatures. Take a list of ostomy supplies when traveling. c. *Exercise:* The only limits involve contact sports, during which trauma to the stoma may occur. Normal exercise is beneficial and may help to stimulate urine excretion. d. *Wardrobe:* Ostomy appliances are invisible under clothing. Any clothing worn preoperatively may be worn postoperatively. Dress comfortably. e. *Bathing/showering/swimming:* These activities may be done while wearing an ostomy appliance. "Picture-frame" the skin barrier with a paper tape to seal the edges and keep the barrier edge from getting wet. Showering may be done with or without an appliance. Soap does not harm the stoma; just rinse it well with warm water (Clark & DuBois, 2004; Hyland, 2002).	
8. Teach measures to help prevent urinary calculi: a. Ensure optimal hydration. b. Avoid sulfa drugs and vitamin C supplements. c. Engage in regular physical activity.	8. Inadequate hydration promotes urinary stasis and calculi formation. Certain drugs and inactivity can predispose to calculi formation (Gorshorn, 2000).
9. Prevent urostomy oxalate crystal formation (Collett, 2002): a. Stomal crystal encrustation is associated with alkaline urine. b. Crystal encrustation may lead to stomal bleeding, ulceration, and strong odor.	9. Manage crystal encrustation: a. Clean peristomal crystal encrustation with a 1:1 solution of white vinegar and warm water for 20–30 minutes. The solution may also be placed in the collection pouch and allowed to bathe over the stoma. b. Cranberry juice or capsules have also been reported to restore a more acidic pH to the urine (Collett, 2002).
10. Use appliance and teach stoma management methods that blend with the client's cultural and religious beliefs (Black, 2000).	10. Cultural and religious values affect the way clients perceive and manage their care (Black, 2000).
11. Investigate availability of long-term follow-up by an ostomy nurse after discharge (Richbourg, Thorpe, & Rapp, 2007).	11. Ostimates desire postdischarge assistance with difficulties related to ostomies and ostomy care. Access to assistance promotes improved confidence in ostomy self-management. It also provides an opportunity to ask new questions (Richbourg et al., 2007).

Documentation

Discharge summary record
  Client and family teaching
  Outcome achievement or status

High Risk for Ineffective Therapeutic Regimen Management Related to Insufficient Knowledge of Intermittent Self-catheterization of Continent Urostomy

NOC Compliance Behavior, Knowledge: Treatment Regimen, Participation: Health Care Decisions, Treatment Behavior: Illness or Injury

Goals

The goals for this diagnosis represent those associated with discharge planning. Refer to the discharge criteria.

NIC Anticipatory Guidance, Risk Identification, Health Education, Learning Facilitation

Interventions	Rationales
1. Explain the reasons for continuous drainage and frequent irrigations postoperatively. Discuss the frequency of irrigation with the physician (National Kidney and Urologic Diseases Information Clearinghouse, 2006).	1. Continuous drainage is needed to eliminate urine; irrigations help to keep the catheter from plugging up with mucus.
2. Instruct the client on how to perform intermittent self-catheterization (Early & Poquette, 2000) to drain the pouch: a. Wash hands. b. Clean the catheter with cleanser of choice. c. Lubricate the catheter. d. Insert the catheter into stoma until urine flows. e. When urine stops, move the catheter in or pull it out a little to drain more urine. f. Pinch the catheter and remove it. g. Place the covering over the stoma.	2. Proper technique prevents perforation and urinary stasis.
3. Supervise the client in self-catheterization.	3. Evaluation of skill performance is more accurate when observed.
4. Instruct the client to notify the physician immediately if he or she is unable to self-catheterize the stoma.	4. Inability to catheterize the stoma puts the client at high risk for obstruction.
5. Provide a written catheterization schedule after collaborating with the physician or advanced practice nurse (Early & Poquette, 2000): • 1st week—catheterization should be done every two hours during the day and every three hours at night. • 2nd week—catheterize every three hours during the day and every four hours at night. • 3rd week—catheterize every four hours during the day and every five hours at night. • 4th week—catheterize every five hours during the day and every six hours at night. • 5th week—catheterize every six hours during the day and not at all during the night.	5. This schedule will gradually increase the capacity for urination.
6. Teach irrigation of the pouch to clear it of excess mucus (National Kidney and Urologic Diseases Information Clearinghouse, 2006): a. Irrigate daily for two months, then only PRN if mucus increases. b. Use a 60-mL syringe or a new poultry baster to instill normal saline. c. Normal saline can be made by mixing two teaspoons of salt in one quart of distilled water.	6. Irrigation of the pouch removes mucus to prevent blockage.
7. Observe the client irrigating the pouch.	7. Direct observation is the best method to evaluate understanding.
8. Teach the client to clean used catheters in warm soapy water and rinse them with tap water. Air dry catheters on a paper towel and store them in a resealable plastic bag.	8. This procedure is clean, not sterile.
9. If urinary reservoir is attached to skin or urethra, teach care of the catheter. a. Flush with 60 mL normal saline every 4 hours during day.	9. Flushing prevents a plugged catheter.

(continued on page 666)

Interventions	Rationales
b. Shower with a clear plastic covering over the catheter or, if there is no drainage, remove the bag and wash the skin around the drain. c. Empty the bag when it is one-third to one-half full. d. Measure the amount of urine collected from the bag.	
10. If the continent urinary reservoir is to the urethra, after the catheter is removed (usually in 3 weeks), instruct the client how to self-catheterize: a. Wash hands. b. Sit on toilet or in front of the toilet. c. Clean the urethral opening; wash the tip of penis or separate the labia and wash it with soap and water in a circular motion; start at the urethra and move outward. d. Lubricate catheter with a water-soluble lubricant. e. Insert the catheter into the urethra until urine flows—for males, 6–8 inches in; for females, 1–1.5 inches; then 1 inch further in. f. Flush the catheter with 60 mL of saline solution. g. Withdraw the catheter slowly; pinch and remove it. h. Assess if the urine is cloudy, bloody, or foul smelling. i. Clean the catheter as outlined in Intervention 7.	10. Self-catheterization is needed to drain urine.
11. Arrange for professional supervision of self-catheterization at the surgeon's office or through home care.	11. Direct observation is needed to assure competency.
12. Advise the client to call the surgeon or advance practice nurse to report any changes or for questions.	12. After discharge, the client will need assistance to manage problems and assess for complications.

Documentation

Discharge summary record
    Client teaching
    Response to teaching
    Outcome achievement or status

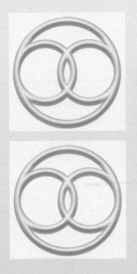

Diagnostic and Therapeutic Procedures

Anticoagulant Therapy

Anticoagulant therapy is treatment for a coagulation disorder (e.g., deep vein thrombosis, pulmonary embolism, atrial fibrillation, ischemic stroke) or prophylaxis for coagulation for people undergoing orthopedic surgery or receiving prosthetic cardiac valves.

Anticoagulants for therapy or prophylaxis include warfarin (Coumadin), heparin, low-molecular-weight heparin (Lovenox, Fragmin, Orgaran, Normiflo), all of which prevent clot extension and formation; antiplatelet agents (aspirin, Plavix, Ticlid) that interfere with platelet activity; and thrombolytic agents that dissolve existing thrombi. This care plan addresses the use of heparin and warfarin (Coumadin).

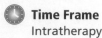 **Time Frame**
Intratherapy

■■■■■■ DIAGNOSTIC CLUSTER

Collaborative Problems

▲ PC: Hemorrhage

Nursing Diagnoses

△ High Risk for Ineffective Therapeutic Regimen Management related to insufficient knowledge of administration schedule, identification card/band, contraindications, risk factors, and signs and symptoms of bleeding

▲ This diagnosis was reported to be monitored for or managed frequently (75%–100%).
△ This diagnosis was reported to be monitored for or managed often (50%–74%).

Discharge Criteria

Before discharge, the client or family will

1. Describe proper medication use.
2. State indications for contacting a health care professional.
3. State intent to wear Medic-Alert identification.
4. Identify the need for follow-up care.

Collaborative Problems

Potential Complication: Hemorrhage

Nursing Goal

The nurse will detect early signs and symptoms of hemorrhage and collaboratively stabilize client.

Indicators

• Clear, light-yellow urine
• No bruises or nosebleeds
• No change in stool color
• No bleeding gums

Interventions	Rationales

1. Monitor for signs and symptoms of bleeding:
   a. Bruises
   b. Nosebleeds
   c. Bleeding gums
	1. The prolonged clotting time caused by anticoagulant therapy can cause spontaneous bleeding anywhere in the body. Hematuria is a common early sign.

(continued on page 669)

Interventions	Rationales
d. Hematuria e. Severe headaches f. Red or black stools	

2. Reduce hematomas and bleeding at injection sites.
  a. Use small-gauge needles.
  b. Do not massage sites.
  c. Rotate sites.
  d. Use subcutaneous route.
  e. Apply steady pressure for 1–2 minutes.
	2. These techniques will reduce trauma to tissues and avoid highly vascular areas (e.g., muscles).

3. Test stools daily for occult blood.	3. Signs of bleeding may be detected early.
4. Monitor lab results of activated partial thromboplastin time (aPTT) for heparin therapy and prothrombin time (PT) and International Normalized Ratio (INR) for oral therapy. Report values over target therapeutic range.	4. Anticoagulant therapy will prolong both times. The therapeutic range goal for PT is 1.3–1.5 × control, or INR of 2.0–3.0.
5. Carefully monitor older clients.	5. Older clients may be more susceptible to the effects of anticoagulants and may need a lower maintenance dose.
6. Report any signs of bleeding to prescribing practitioner.	6. The warfarin dose may be reduced or omitted and oral potassium given to reverse anticoagulant effects.

7. Determine if the client is taking any medications that can interfere with anticoagulant therapy:
  a. Substances that can potentiate anticoagulant action include the following:
    • Alcohol
    • Allopurinol or probenecid
    • Amiodarone
    • Antibiotics
    • Chloral hydrate
    • Chloramphenicol
    • Cimetidine
    • Erythromycin
    • Fluconazole
    • Isoniazid
    • Metronidazole
    • Miconazole
    • Mineral oil
    • Nonsteroidal antiinflammatory analgesics (NSAIAs)
    • Omeprazole
    • Tolbutamide (Orinase)
    • Phenylbutazone
    • Piroxicam
    • Propafenone
    • Propranolol
    • Salicylates
    • Sulfinpyrazone
    • Thrombolytics
    • Thyroid medications
  b. Substances that can inhibit anticoagulant action include the following:
    • Adrenal corticosteroids
    • Antacids
    • Barbiturates
    • Carbamazepine	

(continued on page 670)

Interventions	Rationales

- Colestipol
- Estrogens
- Griseofulvin
- Nafcillin
- Oral contraceptives
- Rifampin
- Sucralfate

8. Determine the medical history for conditions that can increase or decrease PT time
   a. Conditions associated with increased PT time include the following:
      - Cachexia
      - Cancer
      - Collagen disease
      - Congestive heart failure
      - Diarrhea
      - Fever
      - Hepatic disorders
      - Malnutrition
      - Pancreatic disorders
      - Radiation therapy
      - Renal insufficiency
      - Thyrotoxicosis
      - Vitamin K deficiency
   b. Conditions associated with decreased PT time include the following:
      - Diabetes mellitus
      - Edema
      - Hereditary resistance to anticoagulants
      - Hypercholesterolemia
      - Hyperlipidemia
      - Hypothyroidism
      - Visceral carcinoma

 ### Related Physician-Prescribed Interventions

Medications. Anticoagulant agents (dosage varies with daily coagulation test results)
Intravenous Therapy. For IV administration
Laboratory Studies. Activated partial thromboplastin time (aPTT), prothrombin time (PT), platelets, International Normalized Ratio (INR)

Documentation

Flow records
   Occult blood test results (urine and stool)
Progress notes
   Unusual complaints

Nursing Diagnosis

High Risk for Ineffective Therapeutic Regimen Management Related to Insufficient Knowledge of Administration Schedule, Identification Card/Band, Contraindications, and Signs and Symptoms of Bleeding

NOC Compliance Behavior, Knowledge: Treatment Regimen, Participation: Health Care Decisions, Treatment Behavior: Illness or Injury

Goals

The goals for this diagnosis represent those associated with discharge planning. Refer to the discharge criteria.

NIC Anticipatory Guidance, Learning Facilitation, Risk Identification, Medication Management

Interventions	Rationales
1. Instruct client to take medication exactly as prescribed. Stress the importance of regular laboratory tests to monitor effects.	1. Adherence to the prescribed dosage schedule can prevent under- or overmedication.
2. If low molecular weight heparin (LMWH) is prescribed for home use: a. Review actions and dosing schedule. b. Teach subcutaneous injection technique to client or family member. c. Observe injection technique of client or family member.	2. LMWH is given subcutaneously and can be administered at home.
3. If warfarin is prescribed for home use: a. Review actions and dosing schedule. b. Advise client about the risk of warfarin if client becomes pregnant.	3. Bleeding can occur if INR is prolonged or if another factor potentiates anticoagulant action. a. Understanding therapeutic goals can decrease adverse events. b. Warfarin causes fetal defects.
4. Instruct client and family to watch for and report signs and symptoms of bleeding immediately: a. Bruises b. Headaches c. Blood in stool or black stools d. Blood in urine e. Nosebleeds f. Bleeding gums g. Coughing or vomiting blood	4. Bleeding can occur if PT is prolonged or if another factor potentiates anticoagulant action.
5. Instruct client to avoid over-the-counter products that can affect coagulation: a. Alcohol b. Antacids c. Aspirin d. Nonsteroidal antiinflammatory agents e. Vitamin C	5. Certain substances prolong coagulation by inhibiting anti-coagulant metabolism (e.g., alcohol) or inhibiting procoagulant factors (e.g., aspirin and antacids).
6. Instruct client to avoid or limit intake of foods high in vitamin K, including the following: • Collard turnip greens • Broccoli, cauliflower, and brussel sprouts • Cabbage and lettuce • Asparagus and watercress • Beef liver and high-fat foods • Green tea, herbal tea, and coffee • Soy beans and olive oils • Beans • Dairy foods	6. Increased vitamin K intake (>500 mg/day) decreases anti-coagulant action by promoting synthesis of vitamin K-dependent clotting factors. A balanced diet with some foods containing vitamin K will not interfere with therapy. Herbal and green teas should be avoided because they have large quantities of vitamin K (>1400 µg/m).
7. Advise client to try to avoid large fluctuations in dietary vitamin K intake but to have a consistent intake of dietary sources of vitamin K.	

(continued on page 672)

Interventions	Rationales
8. Instruct client to alert all health care providers of his or her anticoagulant therapy before undergoing any procedures (e.g., dentist).	8. Precautions may be needed to prevent hemorrhage from routine medical procedures.
9. Instruct client to avoid potentially hazardous situations while on anticoagulant therapy (e.g., contact sports, use of razor, pregnancy).	9. Contact sports and razors put client at risk of bleeding from injury. Anticoagulants cross the placental barrier and can cause fatal fetal hemorrhage.
10. Encourage client to obtain and wear Medic-Alert identification if outpatient therapy is anticipated.	10. In an emergency, an ID alerts others that client is prone to bleeding.
11. Stress the importance of regular follow-up care and laboratory work.	11. Periodic laboratory blood work is needed to evaluate effects of therapy and risk of bleeding.
12. If home INR testing is prescribed: a. Teach client normal result ranges. b. Teach client action to take if results are above or below normal.	12. Home INR testing is being covered by insurance companies for mechanical valves, and possibly for other diagnoses if need is justified (Harvard Heart Letter, 2006): a. Clients will feel confident and in control of their own care when they can evaluate their levels against a baseline. b. Sliding scale anticoagulant adjustments can help to prevent bleeding problems or strokes.

Documentation

Discharge summary record
  Client and family teaching
  Outcome achievement or status

Casts

Casts are used to immobilize a fractured bone or dislocated joint, support injured tissues during the healing process, correct deformities, prevent movement of joints during healing, and provide traction force. Casting materials can be dehydrated gypsum that recrystallizes when reconstituted with water, fiberglass, and casting tape. The material used depends on the severity of the fracture's displacement. Plaster casts take 24–72 hours to dry; synthetic casts usually dry in 30 minutes.

 Time Frame
Intratherapy

◼◼◼◼◼ DIAGNOSTIC CLUSTER

Collaborative Problems
▲ PC: Compartment Syndrome
▲ PC: Infection/Sepsis

Nursing Diagnoses

▲ High Risk for Impaired Skin Integrity related to pressure of cast on skin surface

▲ (Specify) Self-Care Deficit related to limitation of movement secondary to cast

(continued on page 673)

Nursing Diagnoses

▲ High Risk for Ineffective Therapeutic Regimen Management related to insufficient knowledge of cast care, signs and symptoms of complications, use of assistive devices, and hazards

▲ This diagnosis was reported to be monitored for or managed frequently (75%–100%).

Discharge Criteria

Before discharge, the client or family will

1. Describe precautions to take with the cast.
2. Identify how to monitor for signs and symptoms of complications.
3. Identify barriers in the home environment and relate strategies for overcoming these barriers.
4. Identify a plan to meet role responsibilities.

Collaborative Problems

Potential Complication: Compartment Syndrome

Potential Complication: Infection/Sepsis

Nursing Goal

The nurse will monitor for early signs and symptoms of (a) compartment syndrome and (b) infection/sepsis, and will collaboratively intervene to stabilize client.

Indicators

- Alert, calm, oriented (b)
- Temperature 98.5–99°F (b)
- Heart rate 60–100 beats/min (b)
- Respirations 16–20 breaths/min (b)
- Deep, relaxed respirations (b)
- Blood pressure >90/60, 140/90 mmHg (b)
- Peripheral pulses full, equal, strong (a)
- Sensation intact (a)
- No pain with passive dorsiflexion (calf and toes) (a)
- Mild edema (a)
- Pain relieved by analgesics (a)
- No tingling in legs (a)
- Can move legs (a)
- White blood cells 4800–10,000/mm³ (b)
- Oxygen saturation 94%–100% (b)
- Capillary refill <3 sec (a)
- Blood urea nitrogen (BUN) 10–20 mg/dL (a)
- Creatinine 0.7–1.4 mg/dL (b)

Interventions	Rationales
1. Instruct client to report any changes however slight. Determine if these changes are new and different.	1. Nerve deficit is one of the earliest signs of compartment syndrome. Close monitoring and early detection can help save an extremity or prevent permanent deformity (Altizer, 2004).

2. Monitor for signs and symptoms of compartment syndrome.
  a. Deep, throbbing pain at fracture site
  b. Increasing pain with passive movement
  c. Decreased sensation to light touch
	2. These signs and symptoms are indicative of venous or arterial obstruction and nerve compression. Edema at the fracture site can compromise muscular vascular perfusion. Stretching damaged muscle causes pain. Sensory deficit is an

(continued on page 674)

Interventions	Rationales
d. Inability to distinguish between sharp and dull sensation in first web space of toes, sole, and dorsum and lateral aspect of foot e. Diminished or absent pedal pulses f. Increased edema and induration in extremity g. Increased capillary refill (toes or fingers) >3 seconds	early sign of nerve ischemia. Utilize the five "Ps" of assessment on both the affected and unaffected limb to determine a baseline; assess for pain, pallor, paresthesia, paralysis and pulselessness (Altizer, 2004).
3. Warn client not to mask pain with analgesics until the exact cause has been identified.	3. Identifying the location and nature of pain assists in differential diagnosis.
4. Investigate any complaints of pain, burning, or an offensive odor from inside the cast. Smell the cast to check for odors.	4. These signs and symptoms may indicate that a pressure sore is forming or has become infected. Pathologic tissue necrosis emits a musty, offensive odor that can easily be detected.
5. Feel cast surface to identify areas that are appreciably warmer than other areas ("hot spots"). Particularly evaluate areas over pressure points.	5. Areas of tissue necrosis or infection often cause the overlying area of the cast to feel warmer.
6. If drainage is noted on cast, draw a mark around drainage area and record date and time on cast. Notify surgeon if drainage increases.	6. Marking the initial drainage will provide a baseline for comparison.
7. When moving client or body part, support plaster cast during hardening with palms of hands. Avoid pressure or sharp edges on cast.	7. Maximum hardness of plaster cast takes 24–72 hours depending on thickness. Careful hardening will prevent dents that can cause pressure on underlying tissue.

 Related Physician-Prescribed Interventions

Diagnostic Studies. X-ray films (preapplication and postapplication)
Therapies. Assistive devices, physical therapy, casts (plaster, non-plaster)

Documentation

Flow records
   Skin color (distal to injury)
   Pulses (distal to injury)
   Sensations (pain, paresthesias, paralysis)
   Odor (under cast)
   Temperature of cast surface
   Temperature of distal digits
   Mobility of distal digits
   Elevation of casted limb, if applicable
   Progress notes
   Unusual complaints
   Any drainage noted
   Client's acceptance of cast

Nursing Diagnoses

High Risk for Impaired Skin Integrity Related to Pressure of Cast on Skin Surface

NOC Tissue Integrity: Skin & Mucous Membranes

Goal

The client will continue to have intact skin.

Indicators

- Relate instructions to prevent skin breakdown.
- Describe cast care and precautions.

NIC   Pressure Management, Pressure Ulcer Care, Skin Surveillance, Positioning

Interventions	Rationales
1. Monitor common pressure sites in relationship to cast application: a. Leg: heel, malleoli, dorsal aspect of foot, head of fibula, and anterior surface of patella b. Arm: medial epicondyle of humerus and ulnar styloid c. Plaster jackets or body spica casts: sacrum, anterior and superior iliac spines, and vertebral borders of scapulae To assess skin under the cast, pull skin taut and use a flashlight for illumination.	1. Prolonged pressure of cast on neurovascular structures and other body parts can cause necrosis, pressure sores, and nerve palsies (Redemann, 2002).
2. Inspect skin of uncasted body areas. Pad elbows and heels of unaffected extremities or the sacrum if applicable.	2. The heel on the unaffected side may become sore because client habitually pushes up in bed with the uninvolved leg. The elbows sometimes become sore because client braces him- or herself on elbows to see what is going on around him or her (Redemann, 2002).
3. Apply padding over bony prominences (when between cast and skin surface, padding should fit smoothly without wrinkles). Cover skin surface with stockinette or padding—usually both—before cast application.	3. Padding over bony prominences is essential to prevent pressure ulcers (Redemann, 2002).
4. Use proper technique in handling a wet or damp cast. Support cast with the open, flat palm of your hand at all times; avoid using fingertips.	4. Wrinkles or indentations caused by fingers produce pressure points on the skin under the cast (Redemann, 2002).
5. Avoid rapid cast drying with excessive heat.	5. A cast should dry from the inside out. Too-rapid drying with excessive heat can cause the inner portions of the cast to remain damp and become moldy (Redemann, 2002).
6. Explain the intense heat sensation that can occur as the cast dries and the need to avoid covering a damp cast.	6. Covering the cast can precipitate increased heat, which can cause skin damage.
7. After cast application, clean skin with a weak solution of vinegar on a cloth to remove excess plaster while it is still damp.	7. Unless removed, pieces of plaster can dry and get under the cast, causing skin damage.
8. While plaster cast is drying, use soft pillows to support it properly; avoid contact with hard surfaces (place padding between cast and plastic-covered pillows).	8. Plastic-covered pillows inhibit evaporation. A wet cast placed on a hard surface can become flattened over bony prominences; the resulting pressure causes decreased circulation to tissues enclosed in the cast (Redemann, 2002).
9. Keep cast edges smooth and away from skin surfaces. a. Petal the edges with moleskin or adhesive; place one side of the material on the inside surface of the cast (1–2 inches), then fold over to the outside surface of cast (1–2 inches). b. Bend cast edges slightly with a duck-billed cast bender. c. Elevate affected limb properly to prevent cast from pushing against skin surface.	9. Rough or improperly bent plaster edges may cause damage to surrounding skin by friction. When an extremity is not elevated properly, cast edges press into the skin and cause pain (Redemann, 2002).

(continued on page 676)

Interventions	Rationales

10. Provide and teach correct skin and cast care.
    a. Bathe only accessible skin and massage it with emollient lotion. Massage skin underneath the cast.
    b. Inspect for loose plaster. Avoid using powder in cast.
    c. Inspect position of padding.
    d. Avoid inserting any foreign object under cast.
	10.
	    a. Lotion or soap under the cast creates a film and can irritate skin.
	    b. Loose plaster and powder irritate skin under the cast.
	    c. Padding that slips down must be pulled up and petaled.
	    d. Foreign objects can cause skin injury.

11. Using proper technique, turn a bedridden client every 2–4 hours. Turn toward the unaffected limb; enlist one or more experienced staff members to help (number of persons needed depends on client's size and weight and type of cast).	11. Proper technique prevents damage to the cast and injury to joints.

Documentation

Flow records
    Skin assessment
    Positioning
Discharge summary record
    Client teaching
        Outcome achievement or status

(Specify) Self-Care Deficit Related to Limitation of Movement Secondary to Cast

NOC See Bathing/Hygiene, Feeding, Dressing, Toileting, and/or Instrumental Self-Care Deficit

Goals

The client will perform activities of daily living (ADLs) within the limitations of the cast. The client will perform muscle-strengthening exercises on a regular basis, as permitted.

Indicators

• Demonstrate correct use of assistive devices.

NIC See Feeding, Bathing, Dressing, Toileting, and/or Instrumental Self-Care Deficit

Interventions	Rationales
1. Teach proper crutch-walking technique, if indicated.	1. Proper technique is necessary to prevent injury.
2. Elevate a casted leg when client is not ambulatory. Elevate a casted arm with a sling when client is out of bed; teach client how to use the sling properly.	2. At rest, a dependent extremity develops venous pooling that causes pain and swelling. Elevation helps to prevent this problem.
3. Instruct client to use plastic bags to protect plaster cast during wet weather or while bathing.	3. Moisture weakens plaster casts. Moisture has no effect on fiberglass casts.
4. Teach client to use a blow dryer at home to dry small areas of a dampened cast.	4. Heat speeds drying.

5. Consult with physical therapist regarding actively exercising joints above and below the cast in the following ways:
    a. Raising a casted arm over head
    b. Moving each finger and thumb or toes
    c. Raising and lowering wrist
	5. Exercise helps to prevent complications, promotes healing, and aids the rehabilitation process after cast removal. Moving frequently stimulates circulation and promotes venous return.

(continued on page 677)

Interventions	Rationales
d. Quadricep-setting: tightening and relaxing muscles e. Gluteal-setting f. Abdominal tightening g. Deep breathing h. Opening and closing hand	
6. Teach isometric exercises, starting with unaffected limb.	6. Isometric exercises produce muscle contraction without bending joints or moving limbs; they help to maintain muscle strength and mass.
7. Teach client to put unaffected joints through their full range of motion (ROM) four times daily.	7. Performing full ROM helps to maintain muscle tone and mobility.
8. Consult with a home health coordinator, if indicated.	8. Referral can provide for needed services after discharge (e.g., transportation, housekeeping).

Documentation

Flow records
    Ability to perform ADLs

High Risk for Ineffective Therapeutic Regimen Management Related to Insufficient Knowledge of Cast Care, Signs and Symptoms of Complications, Use of Assistive Devices, and Hazards

NOC Compliance Behavior, Knowledge: Treatment Regimen, Participation: Health Care Decisions, Treatment Behavior: Illness or Injury

Goals

The goals for this diagnosis represent those associated with discharge planning. Refer to the discharge criteria.

NIC Anticipatory Guidance, Learning Facilitation, Health Education, Cast Care: Maintenance

Interventions	Rationales
1. Teach client and family to watch for and report the following symptoms: a. Severe pain b. Numbness or tingling c. Swelling d. Skin discoloration e. Paralysis or reduced movement f. Cool, white toes or fingertips g. Foul odor, warm spots, soft areas, or cracks in the cast	1. Early detection of possible problems enables prompt intervention to prevent serious complications such as infection or impaired circulation.
2. Instruct client never to insert objects down inside edges of cast.	2. Sharp objects used for scratching may cause breaks in skin continuity that provide an entry point for infectious microorganisms.
3. Teach client and family to handle a drying plaster cast with palms of hands only; using fingertips may cause indentations.	3. Cast indentations may lead to pressure sores.
4. Instruct client to keep cast uncovered until it is completely dry.	4. A damp, soiled cast can weaken and may cause skin irritation or promote bacteria growth.

(continued on page 678)

Interventions	Rationales
5. Instruct client to avoid weightbearing or other stress on cast for at least 24 hours after application.	5. Covers restrict escape of heat, especially in a large cast, and prolong the drying process.
6. Instruct client to avoid getting plaster cast wet; teach how to protect cast from moisture.	6. Ultimate cast strength is obtained after cast is dry—within 48–72 hours, depending on factors such as environmental temperature and humidity.
7. Encourage use of an orthopedic mattress or a mattress with a fracture board placed underneath.	7. A sagging or soft mattress tends to deform a green cast and may crack a dry cast.
8. Warn client against using cast braces or turnbuckles to lift a casted part.	8. These devices are not placed in casts to serve as handles. They may easily be broken, dislocated, or pulled out of casts.
9. Teach client what to expect with cast removal: a. Buzz of saw b. Vibrations c. Chalky dust d. Warmth on limbs as saw cuts; will not cut skin or burn e. Limb will be stiff f. Skin will be scaly	9. Explaining what the client can expect, why the procedures are done, and why certain sensations may occur, can help to reduce fears associated with the unknown and un-expected (Christman & Kirchhoff, 1992).
10. Staff and client should use eye protection during cast removal.	10. Cast particles can injure eyes.
11. Apply a cold water enzyme wash (e.g., Woolite, Delicare) for 20 minutes, then gently wash limb in warm water.	11. These solutions loosen dead cells and help to emulsify fatty and crusty lesions that can cause irritation.
12. Instruct client not to rub or scratch skin and to apply mois-turizing skin lotion.	

Documentation

Discharge summary record
    Client and family teaching
    Response to teaching
    Outcome achievement or status

Chemotherapy

This systemic cancer treatment modality aims to safely eradicate or control the growth of cancerous cells by producing maximum cancer cell death with minimum toxicity. Chemotherapy may be the sole treatment provided, as with leukemia, or it may be used in combination with surgery, radiation, or biologic response therapy. Chemotherapeutic agents may be given alone or in combination and may be administered either continuously or intermittently using various routes, techniques, and special equipment. Most agents affect proliferating cells and thus are most effective against rapidly dividing cancer cells. However, they also can damage rapidly dividing normal cells, such as blood cells, cells of the gastrointestinal (GI) epithelium, and hair follicles, producing adverse effects that require careful management.

 Time Frame
Pretherapy and intratherapy

◼◼◼◼◼ DIAGNOSTIC CLUSTER

Collaborative Problems

▲ PC: Anaphylactic Reaction
△ PC: Cardiotoxicity
▲ PC: Electrolyte Imbalance
▲ PC: Extravasation of Vesicant Drugs
△ PC: Hemorrhagic Cystitis
▲ PC: Bone Marrow Depression
▲ PC: Renal Insufficiency
△ PC: Pulmonary Toxicity
△ PC: Neurotoxicity
  PC: Renal Calculi

Nursing Diagnoses	Refer to
▲ Anxiety related to prescribed chemotherapy, insufficient knowledge of chemotherapy, and self-care measures	
▲ Nausea related to gastrointestinal cell damage, stimulation of vomiting center, fear, and anxiety	
▲ Imbalanced Nutrition: Less Than Body Requirements, related to anorexia, taste changes, persistent nausea/vomiting, and increased metabolic rate	
▲ Impaired Oral Mucous Membrane related to dryness and epithelial cell damage secondary to chemotherapy	
▲ Fatigue related to effects of anemia, malnutrition, persistent vomiting, and sleep pattern disturbance	Inflammatory Joint Disease
△ High Risk for Constipation related to autonomic nerve dysfunction secondary to *Vinca* alkaloid administration and inactivity	Immobility or Unconsciousness
▲ Diarrhea related to intestinal cell damage, inflammation, and increased intestinal mobility	Inflammatory Intestinal Disease
▲ High Risk for Impaired Skin Integrity related to persistent diarrhea, malnutrition, prolonged sedation, and fatigue	Immobility or Unconsciousness
△ Disturbed Self-Concept related to change in life style, role, alopecia, and weight loss or gain	Cancer (Initial Diagnosis)

▲ This diagnosis was reported to be monitored for or managed frequently (75%–100%).
△ This diagnosis was reported to be monitored for or managed often (50%–74%).

Discharge Planning

Before discharge, the client and family will

1. Explain treatment plan.
2. Describe signs and symptoms that must be reported to a health care professional.
3. Relate an intent to share feelings and concerns with significant others and health care professionals.
4. Identify available community resources.

Collaborative Problems

Potential Complication: Anaphylactic Reaction
Potential Complication: Cardiotoxicity
Potential Complication: Electrolyte Imbalance
Potential Complication: Extravasation of Vesicant Drugs
Potential Complication: Hemorrhagic Cystitis
Potential Complication: Bone Marrow Depression
Potential Complication: Renal Insufficiency
Potential Complication: Pulmonary Toxicity
Potential Complication: Neurotoxicity
Potential Complication: Renal Calculi

Nursing Goal

The nurse will detect early signs and symptoms of (a) anaphylactic reaction, (b) cardiotoxicity, (c) electrolyte imbalance, (d) extravasation of vesicant drugs, (e) hemorrhagic cystitis, (f) bone marrow depression, (g) renal insufficiency, (h) pulmonary toxicity, (i) neurotoxicity, and (j) renal calculi, and collaboratively intervene to stabilize client.

Indicators

- Calm, alert, oriented (a, i)
- No complaints of urticaria or pruritus (a)
- No complaints of tightness in throat (a)
- No complaints of shortness of breath or wheezing (a, h)
- Temperature 98.5–99°F (h)
- Pulse 60–100 beats/min (b, h)
- BP >90/160, <140/90 mmHg (b, g)
- Normal sinus rhythm (b)
- Flat neck veins (b)
- Serum sodium 135–145 mEq/L (c, g)
- Serum potassium 3.8–5 mEq/L (c, g)
- Serum magnesium 1.3–2.4 mEq/L (c, g)
- Serum phosphorous 2.5–4.5 mEq/L (c, g)
- Serum calcium 8.5–10.5 mEq/L (c, g)
- Urine output >5 mL/kg/h (c, g, j)
- Intact strength (c, i)
- Intact sensation (c, i)
- Stable gait (c, i)
- No seizures (c, i)
- No complaints of headache (c)
- No muscle cramps or twitching (c)
- No nausea or vomiting (c, j)
- Stools soft and formed (c, i)
- No swelling at IV site (d)
- No erythema or pain at IV site (d)
- No dysuria, frequency or urgency (e, j)
- Urine clear yellow (e, j)
- Urine specific gravity 1.005–1.030 (e, g)
- Urine sodium 130–2000 mEq/24h (g)
- White blood cells 4800–10,000/mm³ (f)
- Red blood cells (f)
  - Male 4,600,000–6,200,000
  - Female 4,200,000–5,400,000/mm³

- Platelet 100,000–400,000/mm³ (f)
- Monocytes 2%–6% (f)
- Blood urea nitrogen 10–20 mg/dL (g)
- Serum creatinine 0.7–1.4 mg/dL (g)
- Skin color (pinkish, brownish, olive tones) (g)
- Serum pH 7.35–7.45 (h)
- Oxygen saturation (SaO₂) 94% (h)
- Carbon dioxide (PaCO₂) 34–45 mm/Hg (h)
- Normal chest x-ray (h)
- Normal pulmonary function tests (h)
- No complaints of flank or abdominal pain (j)

Interventions	Rationales
1. Inquire about previous drug reactions; record baseline vital signs and mental status before administering chemotherapy. a. Skin tests or test dose should be given when administering a drug known to have increased incidence of hypersensitivity.	1. Any cytotoxic drug—including cisplatin, teniposide, nitrogen mustard, doxorubicin, bleomycin, methotrexate, L-asparaginase, and melphalan—can precipitate anaphylaxis. Release of histamine in an antigen–antibody reaction results in cutaneous symptoms (urticaria or pruritus) and systemic symptoms (laryngeal edema, bronchospasm, and dyspnea) (Porth, 2005).
2. Monitor for symptoms of anaphylactic reaction: a. Urticaria, pruritus b. Sensation of lump in throat c. Shortness of breath/wheezing	2. These assessment steps help to determine risk of complications and provide a baseline against which to compare subsequent findings.
3. If symptoms of anaphylaxis develop, discontinue chemotherapy and apply a tourniquet proximal to the injection site. Administer emergency drugs as ordered by physician (epinephrine, diphenhydramine, hydrocortisone), following institutional policy.	3. Prompt discontinuation prevents possible serious response; tourniquet application retards drug absorption. Emergency drugs reduce histamine release, relieve edema and spasm, and prevent shock.
4. Monitor vital signs every 15 minutes until client is stable.	4. Careful monitoring can detect early signs of hypotension and shock.
5. Monitor for signs and symptoms of cardiotoxicity. Report promptly: a. Gradual increase in heart rate b. Increased shortness of breath c. Diminished breath sound, rales d. Decreased systolic blood pressure e. Presence of or increase in S₃ or S₄ gallop f. Peripheral edema g. Distended neck veins h. Arrhythmia i. Asymptomatic ECG changes 6. Assess for preexisting conditions (myocardial damage, radiation to mediastinum).	5,6. Cardiotoxicity can be (1) acute, occurring soon after administration of chemotherapy; (2) subacute, associated with pericarditis and myocardial dysfunction that occur 4–5 weeks after treatment; and (3) cardiomyopathy, which occurs within months of treatment. Anthracyclines, such as doxorubicin and daunorubicin, are known for their potential to cause cardiotoxicity. In high doses, anthracyclines damage heart cells, causing loss of pumping ability and increased oxygen need. A QRS voltage change in an ECG may signal a life-threatening condition (Simbre, Duffy, Dadlani, Miller, & Lipshultz, 2005).
7. Monitor for electrolyte imbalances. a. Hyponatremia or hypernatremia	7. Chemotherapeutic agents, as well as cancers themselves, often precipitate electrolyte imbalance (Astle, 2005). a. Hyponatremia is caused by secretion of antidiuretic hormone secondary to vincristine or cyclophosphamide therapy, excessive hydration, or decrease in peripheral blast count secondary to daunorubicin or cytosine therapy. Hypernatremia may result from renal failure secondary to drug nephrotoxicity.

(continued on page 682)

Interventions	Rationales
b. Hypokalemia or hyperkalemia	b. Hypokalemia may be due to intercellular shift, excessive diarrhea, or renal tubular injury. Hyperkalemia is caused by cell lysis and renal damage.
c. Hypomagnesemia	c. Hypomagnesemia can result from vomiting, diarrhea, or cisplatin therapy, which causes excretion of divalent ions.
d. Hypophosphatemia	d. Hypophosphatemia is associated with hypercalcemia, hypokalemia, and hypomagnesemia.
e. Hypocalcemia or hypercalcemia (refer to the Collaborative Problems section of the Chronic Renal Failure care plan for specific signs and symptoms of each electrolyte imbalance).	e. Hypercalcemia is secondary to hypophosphatemia, renal failure, or mithramycin therapy; hypocalcemia is secondary to hyperphosphatemia or renal failure.
8. Monitor and teach client and family to monitor for and report the following: a. Excessive fluid loss or gain b. Change in orientation or level of consciousness c. Changes in vital signs d. Weakness or ataxia e. Paresthesias f. Seizure activity g. Persistent headache h. Muscle cramps, twitching, or tetany i. Nausea and vomiting j. Diarrhea	8. Electrolyte imbalances affect neurotransmission, muscle activity, and fluid balance.
9. Take steps to reduce extravasation of vesicant medications—agents that cause severe necrosis if they leak from blood vessels into tissue. Examples of vesicant medications are the following: amsacrine, bisantrene, dactinomycin, dacarbazine, daunomycin, daunorubicin, estramustine, maytansine, mithramycin, mitomycin, nitrogen mustard, pyrazofurin, vinblastine, vincristine, and vindesine. a. Preventive measures are as follows: • Avoid infusing vesicants over joints, bony prominences, tendons, neurovascular bundles, or the antecubital fossa. • Avoid multiple punctures of the same vein within 24 hours. • Administer drug through a long-term venous catheter. • Do not administer drug if edema is present or blood return is absent. • If peripheral IV site is used, evaluate its status and if it is less than 24 hours old. • Observe peripheral infusion continuously. • Provide infusion through a central line and check every 1–2 hours. • Infuse vesicant before any other medication, even antiemetics.	9. Extravasation may occur secondary to improper placement, damaged vein, or obstructed venous drainage secondary to superior vena cava syndrome, edema, or tumor. • The venous integrity is greatest earlier in the procedure.
10. Monitor during drug infusion. a. Assess patency of intravenous (IV) infusion line. b. Observe tissue at the IV site every 30 minutes for the following: • Swelling (most common) • Leakage • Burning/pain (not always present) • Inflammation • Erythema (not seen initially) • Hyperpigmentation	10,11. Detecting signs of extravasation early enables prompt intervention to prevent serious complications, including tissue necrosis.

(continued on page 683)

Interventions	Rationales

11. If extravasation occurs, take the following steps with gloves on:
a. Stop administration of drug.
b. Leave needle in place.
c. Gently aspirate residual drug and blood in tubing or needle.
d. Avoid applying direct pressure on site.
e. Give antidote as ordered by physician or institutional policy.
f. If plant alkaloid extravasation, apply warm compresses 15–20 minutes QID for 24 hours.
g. If anthracycline extravasation, apply ice for 15–20 minutes every 3–4 hours for 24–48 hours.
h. Monitor site:
  • Elevate limb above heart for 48 hours.
  • After 48 hours, encourage client to use limb normally.
  * Outline area of extravasation with pen.	

12. Monitor for erythema, pain, and indication every hour for 4 hours and then every 4–8 hours according to protocol. • For future intravenous sites, avoid sites that infuse vesicants over joints, bony prominences, tendons, neurovascular bundles, and antecubital fossa. • Avoid multiple punctures in the same vein within 24 hours.	12. Extravasation can cause underlying tissue damage resulting in permanent damage. • This will reduce the concentration of drug at site and will serve as a baseline for subsequent assessments. Necrosis of tissue can occur. These sites, if extravasated, into can cause permanent damage or deformity. • Multiple punctures make the vessel more vulnerable to infiltration.
13. When administering cyclophosphamide, monitor for signs and symptoms of hemorrhagic cystitis: a. Dysuria b. Frequency c. Urgency d. Hematuria	13. Cyclophosphamide administration is associated with the development of hemorrhagic cystitis.
14. Administer cyclophosphamide early in the day.	14. Administration early in the day reduces the high drug concentration that can occur during the night secondary to reduced intake.
15. Teach client to do the following: a. Void every 2 hours. b. Increase fluid intake to 2500–3000 mL/day unless contraindicated.	15. Frequent voiding and optimal hydration reduce drug concentration in the bladder.
16. Monitor for signs of bone marrow depression: a. Decreased WBC and RBC counts b. Decreased platelet count c. Decreased granulocyte count	16. Cytotoxic chemotherapy often yields untoward side effects such as bone marrow depression. The earlier the symptoms are realized, the faster they can be treated (Forsythe & Faulkner, 2004). Chemotherapy interferes with cell division of bone marrow stem cells that form blood cells. Granulocytes are mainly neutrophils that are the first line of defense against infection.
17. Explain risks of bleeding and infection. (Refer to the Corticosteroid Therapy care plan for strategies to reduce these risks.)	17. Radiation therapy may cause a depression in bone marrow production, especially when the bone marrow of skeletal sites is irradiated. Leukocytes, thrombocytes, and RBCs are decreased, predisposing the client to infection, bleeding, and anemia, in that order (Twite, 2005).

(continued on page 684)

Interventions	Rationales

18. Monitor for signs of renal insufficiency.
  a. Sustained elevated urine specific gravity
  b. Elevated urine sodium levels
  c. Sustained insufficient urine output (<30 mL/h)
  d. Elevated blood pressure
  e. Hypomagnesemia or hypocalcemia
  f. Increasing BUN and serum creatinine, potassium, phosphorus, ammonia, and decreased creatinine clearance
	18. Chemotherapy-induced renal toxicity can occur (1) directly, as with cisplatin, methotrexate, and mitomycin, which can produce toxic effects on renal glomeruli and tubules, and (2) indirectly because of rapid tumor cell lysis, causing hyperuricemia and nephropathy (Camp-Sorrell, 2005).

19. Monitor for pulmonary toxicity (pneumonitis or fibrosis) when administering bleomycin and nitrosoureas; signs and symptoms include the following:
  a. Cough
  b. Fever
  c. Tachycardia
  d. Dyspnea
  e. Rales
  f. Weakness
  g. Cyanosis
  h. Abnormal arterial blood gas analysis
  i. Abnormal chest x-ray film
  j. Abnormal pulmonary function tests
	19. Lung inflammation and fibrosis are associated with administration of bleomycin and nitrosoureas (e.g., carmustine and busulfan). The extent of fibrosis determines the severity of respiratory dysfunction.

20. Instruct client to cough and do deep breathing every 2 hours.	20. These activities help to reduce retention of secretions and dilate alveoli.

21. Monitor for signs and symptoms of neurotoxicity when administering *Vinca* alkaloids and L-asparaginase, procarbazine, and intrathecal methotrexate:
  a. Paresthesias
  b. Gait disturbance
  c. Altered fine motor activity
  d. Constipation
  e. Lethargy
  f. Numbness
  g. Muscle weakness
  h. Foot or wrist drop
  i. Somnolence
  j. Disorientation
  k. Impotence
  l. Confusion
	21. Chemotherapy may cause peripheral or central neurotoxicity. Peripheral neurotoxicity is usually noted as a peripheral neuropathy, while central neurotoxicity might range from minor cognitive impairments to encephalopathy accompanied by dementia, or even a coma (Verstappen, Heimans, Hoekman, & Postma, 2003).

22. If dysfunction results from neurotoxicity, refer to the Immobility care plan for interventions to prevent complications.	22. Prompt intervention is necessary to prevent serious complications.

23. Monitor for signs and symptoms of renal calculi.
  a. Flank pain
  b. Nausea and vomiting
  c. Abdominal pain
	23. Renal calculi may result from chemotherapy because rapid cell lysis of tumor cells produces hyperuricemia. Pain is caused by pressure of calculi on the renal tubules. Afferent stimuli in renal capsule may cause pylorospasm of the smooth muscle of the enteric tract and adjacent structures.

24. Refer to the Urolithiasis care plan for specific interventions to reduce risk of renal calculi.	

Related Physician-Prescribed Interventions

Medications. Antiemetics, antianxiety, dexamethasone, chemotherapeutic agents
Laboratory Studies. Complete blood count, urinalysis, electrolytes, BUN, serum albumin, pulmonary function test
Diagnostic Studies. Chest x-ray, pulse oximetry

Documentation

Flow records
   Vital signs
   Abnormal laboratory values (electrolytes, complete blood count (CBC), platelets, and BUN)
   Condition of injection sites
   Intake and output
   Urine specific gravity
   Client teaching
Progress notes
   Complaints of rashes or unusual sensations

Nursing Diagnoses

Anxiety Related to Prescribed Chemotherapy, Insufficient Knowledge of Chemotherapy, and Self-Care Measures

NOC Anxiety Level, Coping, Impulse Control

Goal

The client will share feelings regarding scheduled chemotherapy.

Indicators

- Describe the anticipated effects of chemotherapy.
- Relate signs and symptoms of toxicity.
- Identify important self-care measures.

NIC Anxiety Reduction, Impulse Control Training, Anticipatory Guidance

Interventions	Rationales
1. Encourage client to share feelings and beliefs regarding chemotherapy. Delay teaching if high levels of anxiety are present.	1. Verbalization can identify sources of client anxiety and allow the nurse to correct misinformation. High anxiety impairs learning.
2. Reinforce physician's explanations of the chemotherapeutic regimen—the drugs, dosage schedules, and management of side effects.	2,3,4. Specific explanations provide information to help reduce anxiety associated with fear of the unknown and loss of control.
3. Explain the therapeutic effects of cytotoxic drugs; provide written information. (*Note:* Client education booklets are available from the National Cancer Institute and the American Cancer Society.)	
4. Explain the common side effects and toxicities of chemotherapy: a. Decreased WBC count b. Decreased platelet count c. Infection d. GI alterations	

(*continued on page 686*)

Interventions	Rationales
e. Hair loss f. Fatigue g. Emotional responses	
5. Discuss self-care measures to reduce risk of toxicities: a. Nutrition b. Hygiene c. Rest d. Activity e. Managing bowel elimination problems f. Managing hair loss g. Monitoring for infection h. Prioritizing activities	5. Research reports individuals who receive side-effect management report a higher degree of perceived effectiveness than those who did not receive this information (Dadd, 1983).
6. Refer also to the Cancer (Initial Diagnosis) care plan for additional information.	

Documentation

Discharge summary record or teaching record
  Client teaching
  Outcome achievement or status
Progress notes
  Dialogues

Nausea Related to Gastrointestinal Cell Damage, Stimulation of Vomiting Center, Fear, and Anxiety

NOC Comfort Level, Nutritional Status, Hydration

Goal

The client will report decreased nausea.

Indicators

• Name foods or beverages that do not increase nausea
• Describe factors that increase nausea

NIC Medication Management, Nausea Management, Fluid/Electrolyte Management, Nutrition Management

Interventions	Rationales
1. Promote a positive attitude about chemotherapy; reinforce its cancer cell-killing effects.	1. Frank discussions can increase motivation to reduce and tolerate nausea.
2. Explain possible reasons for nausea and vomiting.	2. Chemotherapy-induced nausea and vomiting is thought to be due to a stimulation of the chemoreceptor trigger zone located in the medulla. This area of the brain reacts according to the level of circulating chemicals found in the blood (Porth, 2005). Cytotoxic drugs damage GI cells, which can produce a vagal response. They also can stimulate the vomiting center in the brain. Anxiety and fear contribute to the problem. Chemotherapy effects can lead to marked disruption in self-care, requiring more family support.

(continued on page 687)

Interventions	Rationales
3. Explain the rationale for antiemetic agents; administer them before initiating chemotherapy and during the time chemotherapy drugs are most likely to cause nausea and vomiting.	3. Antiemetics are given before chemotherapy to reduce nausea.
4. Infuse cytotoxic drugs slowly.	4. Slow infusion can decrease stimulation of the vomiting center.
5. Eat only lightly before therapy.	5. This will avoid gastric overstimulation.
6. Administer nightly emetic and cytotoxic drugs at night (during sleep if possible) or have client lie quietly for 2 hours after administration.	6. Activity stimulates the GI tract, which can increase nausea and vomiting.
7. If delayed nausea develops 3–4 days after treatment, consult with nurse or physician.	7. Delayed nausea is usually unresponsive to standard antiemetics. Antianxiety agents (e.g., lorazepam), are often as effective as dexamethasone.
8. If taste alterations occur, suggest that the client suck on hard candy during chemotherapy.	8. Hard candy can reduce the metallic or bitter taste that client may experience from chemotherapy.
9. Encourage client to eat small, frequent meals and to eat slowly. Cool, bland foods and liquids are usually well tolerated. Vary diet.	9. Intake of small amounts prevents gastric distention from stimulating vomiting.
10. Eliminate unpleasant sights and odors from the eating area.	10. Eliminating noxious stimuli can decrease stimulation of the vomiting center.
11. Instruct client to avoid the following: a. Hot or cold liquids b. Foods containing fat and fiber c. Spicy foods d. Caffeine	11. Certain foods increase peristalsis and provoke nausea and vomiting: a. Cold liquids can induce cramping; hot liquids can stimulate peristalsis. b. High-fat and high-fiber food and drinks increase peristalsis. c. Caffeine stimulates intestinal motility.
12. Encourage client to rest in semi-Fowler position after eating and to change position slowly.	12. Muscle relaxation can reduce peristalsis.
13. Teach stress reduction techniques such as these: a. Relaxation exercises b. Visual imagery	13. These techniques reduce muscle tension and decrease client's focus on nausea.

Documentation

Flow records
    Intake and output
    Tolerance of intake

Imbalanced Nutrition: Less Than Body Requirements Related to Anorexia, Taste Changes, Persistent Nausea/Vomiting, and Increased Metabolic Rate

NOC Nutritional Status

Goal

The client will increase oral intake as evidence by (specify).

Indicators

• Maintain or gain weight with minimal further weight loss.
• Describe strategies to increase nutritional intake.

NIC   Nutrition Management, Nutritional Monitoring

Interventions	Rationales
1. Help client to identify reasons for inadequate nutrition and explain possible causes: a. Increased metabolic rate b. GI tract alterations c. Stimulation of vomiting d. Decreased appetite e. Taste changes f. Anxiety and fear	1. Nutritional deficits associated with chemotherapy can have many causes. Cytotoxic drugs can stimulate the vomiting center in the brain (see the nursing diagnosis Altered Comfort: Nausea/Vomiting in this entry for more information). They also can alter GI cells, causing anorexia, taste changes, nausea and vomiting, and altered protein metabolism. Damage to the absorptive surface of the GI mucosa can lead to nutrient malabsorption. Research shows that while in this state, the hypothalamus releases anorexigenic substances, further compounding the nutritional deficit. Chemotherapy-induced mucositis also inhibits intake and absorption of nutrients. Finally, anxiety and stress can inhibit appetite and lead to decreased intake (Twite, 2005).
2. Stress the need to increase caloric intake.	2. Malignant disease increases the metabolic rate and alters the metabolism of nutrients. Caloric intake must be increased to avoid a further debilitated state (Twite, 2005). Cytotoxic drugs raise the metabolic rate through destruction of rapidly proliferating cells. This factor, coupled with the body's increased nutritional needs resulting from GI damage or other factors, necessitates increased caloric intake to maintain adequate nutritional status.
3. Encourage resting before meals.	3. Fatigue further decreases appetite.
4. Offer small, frequent meals (optimally six per day plus snacks).	4. Increased intra-abdominal pressure from fluid accumulation (ascites) compresses the GI tract and decreases capacity.
5. Restrict liquids with meals and avoid fluids 1 hour before and after meals.	5. Fluid restrictions at meals can help to prevent gastric overdistention and can enhance appetite.
6. Maintain good oral hygiene before and after eating.	6. Poor oral hygiene can result in foul odors or taste, which diminishes appetite.
7. Arrange to have foods with the greatest protein and caloric value served at times the client feels most like eating.	7. This strategy increases client's chance of consuming more protein and calories.
8. Teach techniques to reduce nausea: a. Avoid the smell of food preparation and other noxious stimuli. b. Loosen clothing before eating. c. Sit in fresh air. d. Avoid lying flat for at least 2 hours after eating (a client who must rest should sit or recline with head elevated at least 4 inches higher than feet).	8. Nausea can be reduced by controlling environmental conditions and promoting positions that minimize abdominal pressure.
9. Instruct client to limit foods and fluids high in fat.	9. Fatty foods are difficult to absorb.

(continued on page 689)

Interventions	Rationales

10. Suggest dietary modifications such as these:
   a. Eat fish, chicken, eggs, and cheese if pork and beef taste bitter
   b. Eat meat for breakfast rather than later in the day
   c. Experiment with different flavorings and seasonings
	10. These measures can help to make food more palatable and encourage increased intake.

11. Teach techniques to enhance protein and calorie content when preparing meals at home:
   a. Add powdered milk or egg to milkshakes, gravies, sauces, puddings, cereals, meatballs, or milk to increase protein and calorie content.
   b. Add blenderized or baby foods to meat juices or soups.
   c. Use fortified milk (i.e., 1 cup instant nonfat milk added to 1 quart fresh milk).
   d. Use milk or half-and-half instead of water when making soups and sauces; soy formulas can also be used.
   e. Add cheese or diced meat whenever able.
   f. Add cream cheese or peanut butter to toast, crackers, celery sticks.
   g. Add extra butter or margarine to soups, sauces, vegetables.
   h. Use mayonnaise (100 cal/tbsp) instead of salad dressing.
   i. Add sour cream or yogurt to vegetables or as dip.
   j. Use whipped cream (60 cal/tbsp) as much as possible.
   k. Add raisins, dates, nuts, and brown sugar to hot or cold cereals.
   l. Have snacks readily available.
	11. These simple measures can increase the nutritional content of foods even when intake is limited.

12. Refer client to dietitian for further nutritional information.	12. Additional nutritional information can be acquired from an expert.
13. Give client copy of *Eating Hints*, a National Cancer Institute publication.	

Documentation

Flow records
   Weight
   Intake (type and amount)
Progress notes
   Complaints of nausea and vomiting

Impaired Oral Mucous Membrane Related to Dryness and Epithelial Cell Damage Secondary to Chemotherapy

NOC Oral Hygiene

Goal

The client will exhibit signs of healing with decreased inflammation.

Indicators

- Relate the need for optimal oral hygiene.
- Report decreased discomfort.
- Describe how to prevent oral injury.

NIC Oral Health Restoration, Chemotherapy Management, Oral Health Maintenance

Interventions	Rationales
1. Explain the need for regular, meticulous oral hygiene. 2. Dental work should be done before chemotherapy begins.	1,2. Chemotherapy increases the mucosal cells' susceptibility to infection. Frequent oral hygiene removes microorganisms and reduces risk.

3. Instruct client to do the following:
  a. Perform oral care regimen after meals and before bedtime (and before breakfast if necessary).
  b. Avoid mouthwashes high in alcohol, lemon/glycerine swabs, and prolonged use of hydrogen peroxide.
  c. Use an oxidizing agent to loosen thick, tenacious mucus; gargle and expectorate. For example, use hydrogen peroxide and water ¼ strength (avoid prolonged use) or 1 tbsp sodium bicarbonate mixed in 8 oz warm water (flavored with mouthwash, oil of wintergreen, etc., if desired).
  d. Rinse mouth with saline solution after gargling.
  e. Apply a lubricant to lips every 2 hours and as needed (e.g., lanolin, A & D ointment, petroleum jelly).
  f. Inspect mouth daily for lesions and inflammation; report any alterations.
	3. These practices can eliminate sources of microorganism growth and prevent mucosal drying and damage.

4. If client cannot tolerate brushing or swabbing, teach mouth irrigation:
  a. Use a baking soda solution (4 tbsp in 1 L warm water) in an enema bag (labeled for oral use only) with a soft irrigation catheter tip.
  b. Place catheter in the mouth and slowly increase flow while standing over a basin or having someone hold a basin under chin.
  c. Remove dentures before irrigation; do not replace them if client has severe stomatitis.
  d. Perform irrigation every 2 hours or as needed.
	4. Brushing can further damage irritated mucosa. These measures enable maintenance of good hygiene in client who cannot brush.

5. Teach precautionary measures:
  a. Breathe through nose rather than mouth.
  b. Consume cool, soothing liquids and semisolids such as gelatin.
  c. Avoid smoking.
  d. Avoid hot and spicy or acidic food and fluids.
  e. Omit flossing if excessive bleeding occurs.
	5. These practices can reduce oral irritation.

6. Explain the importance of hydration and good nutrition.	6. Optimal nutritional status can increase healing ability.
7. Consult with physician for an oral pain relief solution (e.g., lidocaine [Xylocaine], diphenhydramine, and antimicrobial agents).	7. Medications may be needed to reduce pain and enable adequate nutritional intake.

Documentation

Flow records
  Oral assessments
  Treatments

Corticosteroid Therapy

Corticosteroid is the generic name for commercial adrenocortical hormones and synthetic analogues. Corticosteroids are indicated as replacement therapy for adrenal insufficiency, inflammation suppression, allergic reaction control, and reducing the risk of graft rejection in transplantation. A client on long-term corticosteroid therapy has suppressed pituitary and adrenal functions. Some indications for corticosteroid therapy are severe autoimmune diseases, rheumatoid arthritis, severe asthma, cancer, multiple sclerosis, and psoriasis.

 Time Frame
Pretherapy and intratherapy

■■■■■■ DIAGNOSTIC CLUSTER

Collaborative Problems

▲ PC: Steroid-Induced Diabetes
△ PC: Hypertension
△ PC: Osteoporosis
△ PC: Peptic Ulcer
△ PC: Thromboembolism
△ PC: Hypokalemia
✱ PC: Pseudotumor Cerebri
✱ PC: Hypocalcemia

Nursing Diagnoses

▲ High Risk for Excess Fluid Volume related to sodium and water retention

---

△ High Risk for Imbalanced Nutrition: More Than Body Requirements related to increased appetite

---

▲ High Risk for Infection related to immunosuppression

△ High Risk for Disturbed Body Image related to changes in appearance

---

△ High Risk for Ineffective Therapeutic Regimen Management related to insufficient knowledge of administration schedule, adverse reactions, signs and symptoms of complications, hazards of adrenal insufficiency, and potential causes of adrenal insufficiency

▲ This diagnosis was reported to be monitored for or managed frequently (75%–100%).
△ This diagnosis was reported to be monitored for or managed often (50%–74%).
✱ This diagnosis was not included in the validation study.

Discharge Criteria

Before discharge, the client or family will

1. Relate proper use of the medication.
2. Identify circumstances that require notification of a health care professional.
3. Relate dietary sodium restrictions.
4. Identify signs and symptoms of side effects and adverse reactions.
5. Describe practices that can reduce the side effects of corticosteroid therapy.
6. Verbalize the intent to seek ongoing follow-up care.
7. Verbalize the intent to wear Medic-alert identification.

Collaborative Problems

Potential Complication: Steroid-Induced Diabetes

Potential Complication: Hypertension

Potential Complication: Osteoporosis

Potential Complication: Peptic Ulcer
Potential Complication: Thromboembolism
Potential Complication: Hypokalemia
Potential Complication: Pseudotumor Cerebri
Potential Complication: Hypocalcemia

Nursing Goal

The nurse will detect early signs and symptoms of (a) steroid-induced diabetes, (b) hypertension, (c) osteoporosis, (d) peptic ulcer, (e) thromboembolism, (f) hypokalemia, (g) pseudotumor cerebri, and (h) hypocalcemia and collaboratively intervene to stabilize client.

Indicators

- Alert, oriented (f, g, h)
- Urine output >5 mL/kg/h (a)
- Specific gravity 1.005–1.030 (a)
- Urine negative for protein (a)
- Urine negative for glucose (a)
- Stool negative blood (guaiac) (d)
- BP >90/60, <140/90 mmHg (b)
- No complaints of bone pain (c)
- No complaints of muscle cramps (b)
- No complaints of numbness/tingling in fingers or toes (h)
- Muscle strength—intact (f)
- No seizure activity (h)
- No complaints of gastric pain (d)
- No complaints of headaches (g)
- No complaints of visual changes (g)
- No complaints of nausea or vomiting (f, g)
- Normal sinus rhythm (EKG) (f, h)
- Serum potassium 3.8–5 mEq/L (f)
- Serum calcium 8.5–10.5 mg/dL (h)

Interventions	Rationales

1. Monitor for signs and symptoms of diabetes mellitus:
  a. Polyuria, polydipsia
  b. Glycosuria
  c. Proteinuria
	1. Excessive glucocorticoid level antagonizes insulin and promotes glyconeogenesis, resulting in hyperglycemia (Porth, 2005).

2. Monitor for hypertension.	2. Mineralocorticoids increase sodium reabsorption, with resulting fluid retention that can adversely affect clients with preexisting hypertension or congestive heart failure (CHF).

3. Monitor for signs and symptoms of osteoporosis, especially in ribs and vertebrae:
  a. Pain
  b. Localized tenderness
4. Monitor for hypocalcemia:
  a. Altered mental status
  b. Muscle cramps
  c. Numbness/tingling in fingers and toes
  d. ECG changes
  e. Seizures
	3,4. Corticosteroids oppose the effects of vitamin D, thus reducing calcium absorption and increasing urinary excretion of calcium. The release of growth hormone is inhibited, which decreases osteoblast function and thinning of epiphyseal plates (Porth, 2005).

(continued on page 693)

Interventions	Rationales
5. Teach client about measures to reduce risk of pathologic fractures. (Refer to the Osteoporosis care plan in the index for more details.)	5. A client on long-term corticosteroid therapy—especially an older client—is at increased risk for fractures owing to loss of bone density.
6. Teach client the relationship of increased calcium and vitamin D intake and weightbearing exercise to reduced risk of osteoporosis.	6. Increase in vitamin D and calcium intake increases their availability to bone. Weightbearing exercise (e.g., walking) slows rate of calcium loss from bone.

7. Monitor for signs and symptoms of peptic ulcer:
  a. Positive guaiac stool test
  b. Gastric pain (rhythmic, gnawing, burning, cramplike)
	7. Clients with cirrhosis, nephrotic syndrome, or connective tissue disorders receiving over 1 g of steroids, or those taking potentially ulcerogenic medications concurrently, are susceptible to peptic ulcers.

8. Teach client to take prescribed medication with food or milk.	8. Food or milk can help to neutralize gastric hydrochloric acid; this minimizes gastric upset.

9. Monitor for signs and symptoms of hypokalemia:
  a. Weakness
  b. Lethargy
  c. Serum potassium level <3.5 mEq/L
  d. Nausea and vomiting
  e. Characteristic ECG changes
	9. Excessive mineralocorticoids increase sodium retention and potassium excretion.

10. Monitor for pseudotumor cerebri:
  a. Headaches
  b. Visual changes
  c. Nausea
	10. This is a well-recognized complication of unknown pathophysiology manifested by intracranial hypertension and papilledema. It occurs when therapy is decreased or the preparation changed, is self-limiting, and reverses when therapy is discontinued.

 Related Physician-Prescribed Interventions

Symptom-specific

Documentation

Flow records
Vital signs
Urine glucose and other laboratory values
Pain and numbness in extremities
Gastric pain
Intake and output
Stool guaiac results

Nursing Diagnoses

High Risk for Excess Fluid Volume Related to Sodium and Water Retention

NOC Electrolyte & Acid–Base Balance, Fluid Balance, Hydration

Goal

The client will report no or minimal edema.

Indicators

- Relate causative factors of edema.
- State controllable factors for edema prevention.

NIC Electrolyte Management, Fluid Management, Fluid Monitoring, Skin Surveillance

Interventions	Rationales

1. Encourage client to decrease salt intake; limit sodium to 6 g/day. Teach client to take the following actions:
  a. Read food labels for sodium content. Review foods high in sodium: mineral water, club soda, crackers, snacks (chips, nuts, and pretzels), muffins, instant cooked foods (cereals, potato soup, sauces, entrees, and vegetables), granola, buttermilk, regular cheese, regular salad dressing, smoked or cured products, sauerkraut, tomato juice, V-8, olives, pickles, and certain seasonings (Accent® Flavor Enhancer, soy sauce, mustard, catsup, horseradish, steak sauces, and seasoned salt).
  b. Cook without salt and use spices (e.g., lemon, basil, tarragon, and mint) to add flavor.
  c. Use vinegar in place of salt to flavor soups, stews, and so on (e.g., 2–3 teaspoons of vinegar to 4–6 quarts, according to taste).
  d. Foods low in sodium are poultry, pumpkin, turnips, egg yolks, cooked vegetables, fruits, grits, honey, jams, jellies, lean meats, potatoes, puffed wheat and rice, red kidney beans, lima beans, sherbet, and unsalted nuts.
	1. Corticosteroids contain both glucocorticoid and mineralocorticoid elements. The mineralocorticoid element promotes sodium reabsorption and potassium excretion from distal renal tubules. Resultant sodium retention expands extracellular fluid volume by preventing water excretion.

2. Identify strategies to decrease dependent edema:
  a. Changing positions frequently
  b. Avoiding constrictive clothing
  c. Elevating legs when sitting
  d. Wearing elastic support stockings
	2. Edema develops as increased extracellular fluid enters interstitial spaces and the blood; this increases interstitial fluid and blood volume.

3. Teach the importance of a daily walking program.	3. Lymph flow is propelled by contracting skeletal muscles (Hillman, Hedrick, Withers, & Drewes, 2004). Exercise increases muscle efficiency.

4. Explain measures to protect skin from injury:
  a. Avoid walking barefoot.
  b. Break in new shoes slowly.
  c. Avoid contact sports.
  d. Prevent dry skin with lubricants.
	4. Besides increased risk of skin injury due to edema, loss of perivascular collagen in the skin's small vessels makes them more susceptible to damage.

Documentation

Flow records
  Weight
  Presence and degree of edema

High Risk for Imbalanced Nutrition: More Than Body Requirements Related to Increased Appetite

NOC Nutritional Status, Weight Control

Goal

The client will maintain present weight.

Indicators

- Relate factors that contribute to weight gain.
- Identify behaviors that remain under his or her control.

NIC Nutrition Management, Weight Management, Teaching: Individual, Behavior Modification, Exercise Promotion

Interventions	Rationales

1. Increase client's awareness of actions that contribute to excessive food intake:
  a. Request that client write down all the food eaten in the past 24 hours.
  b. Instruct client to keep a diet diary for 1 week that specifies the following:
    • What, when, where, and why eaten
    • Whether he or she was doing anything else (e.g., watching television or cooking) while eating
    • Emotions before eating
    • Others present (e.g., snacking with spouse and children)
  c. Review diet diary to point out patterns (e.g., time, place, emotions, foods, and persons) that affect food intake.
  d. Review high- and low-calorie food items.
	1. The ability to lose weight while on corticosteroid therapy likely depends on limiting sodium intake and maintaining a reasonable caloric intake.

2. Teach client behavior modification techniques to decrease caloric intake:
  a. Eat only at a specific spot at home (e.g., the kitchen table).
  b. Do not eat while performing other activities.
  c. Drink an 8-oz glass of water immediately before a meal.
  d. Decrease second helpings, fatty foods, sweets, and alcohol.
  e. Prepare small portions that are just enough for one meal; discard leftovers.
  f. Use small plates to make portions look bigger.
  g. Never eat from another person's plate.
  h. Eat slowly and chew food thoroughly.
  i. Put down utensils and wait 15 seconds between bites.
  j. Eat low-calorie snacks that must be chewed to satisfy oral needs (e.g., carrots, celery, and apples).
  k. Decrease liquid calories by drinking low-sodium diet soda or water.
  l. Plan eating splurges (save a number of calories each day and have a treat once a week) but eat only a small amount of "splurge" foods.
	2. These measures can help to control caloric intake. Obesity is often promoted by an inappropriate response to external cues—most often, stressors. This response triggers an ineffective coping mechanism in which client eats in response to stress rather than physiologic hunger.

3. Instruct client to increase activity level to burn calories; encourage her or him to do the following:
  a. Use stairs instead of elevators.
  b. Park at the farthest point in parking lots and walk to buildings.
  c. Plan a daily walking program with a progressive increase in distance and pace.
Urge client to consult with physician before beginning any exercise program.
	3. Increased activity can promote weight loss. Keep in mind, however, that the client's ability to exercise may be limited by the pathologic condition that necessitates corticosteroid therapy, as well as by the drug's adverse effects (e.g., osteoporosis or muscle wasting).

4. Refer to Obesity care plan in index for more information.	

Documentation

Flow records
  Weight
  Intake
  Activity level

High Risk for Infection Related to Immunosuppression

NOC Infection Status, Wound Healing: Primary Intention, Immune Status

Goal

The client will be infection free or report early signs or symptoms.

Indicators

- Relate risk factors associated with potential for infection.
- Practice appropriate precautions to prevent infection.

NIC   Infection Control, Wound Care, Incision Site Care, Health Education

Interventions	Rationales
1. Explain the increased risk of infection; stress the importance of reporting promptly any change in status.	1. High doses (50 mg or more) of prednisone for more than 2 weeks may increase opportunistic infections. Corticosteroids can mask the usual signs and symptoms of infection such as fever and increased WBC count; this necessitates increased vigilance for subtle changes.
2. Instruct client to avoid persons with infections and large crowds in close quarters.	2. These precautions can help to limit exposure to infectious microorganisms.
3. Explain the vulnerability of skin and risk for injury.	3. Glucocorticoids promote mobilization of fatty acids from adipose tissue, resulting in thin, fragile skin.
4. Instruct client to discuss use of echinacea with provider.	4. Studies have shown that echinacea may overstimulate and then suppress the immune system, altering the effects of the corticosteroids (Schmidt, 2004).

Documentation

Flow records
    Temperature
Progress notes
    Change in health status

High Risk for Disturbed Body Image Related to Changes in Appearance

NOC   Body Image, Child Development: (specify age), Grief Resolution, Psychosocial Adjustment: Life Change, Self-Esteem

Goal

The client will demonstrate movement toward reconstruction of an altered body image.

Indicators

- Relate factors contributing to disturbed body image.
- Describe changes related to corticosteroid therapy.

NIC   Self-Esteem Enhancement, Counseling, Presence, Active Listening, Body Image Enhancement, Grief Work Facilitation, Support Group, Referral

Interventions	Rationales
1. Explain that appearance changes are drug-induced and will diminish or resolve with discontinuation or dosage reduction.	1. This explanation can reduce the fear of permanent appearance changes and help to preserve positive self-concept.

(continued on page 697)

Interventions	Rationales
2. Encourage client to express feelings about appearance changes.	2. Sharing concerns promotes trust and enables clarification of misconceptions.
3. Promote social interaction.	3. Social isolation can promote fear and unrealistic perceptions.
4. Refer to Disturbed Body Image in index for additional interventions.	

Documentation

Progress notes
Interactions

High Risk for Ineffective Therapeutic Regimen Management Related to Insufficient Knowledge of Administration Schedule, Adverse Reactions, Signs and Symptoms of Complications, Hazards of Adrenal Insufficiency, and Potential Causes of Adrenal Insufficiency

NOC Compliance Behavior, Knowledge: Treatment Regimen, Participation: Health Care Decisions, Treatment Behavior: Illness or Injury

Goals

The goals for this diagnosis represent those associated with discharge planning. Refer to the discharge criteria.

NIC Anticipatory Guidance, Learning Facilitation, Risk Identification, Health Education

Interventions	Rationales
1. Instruct client to take drug dose exactly as prescribed in the morning; keeping in mind these considerations: a. Do not discontinue administration because of adverse effects; if unable to tolerate oral medication, contact physician for instructions. b. If possible, take daily dose in the morning. c. Take the daily B_{12} dose before 4 PM.	1. Abrupt cessation of medication after 2 weeks of therapy may precipitate an adrenal crisis. Early morning doses stimulate the body's natural peak excretion. Taking the medication in the morning can reduce hyperactivity at bedtime.
2. Provide written instructions on dosage schedule if appropriate.	2. A printed schedule may help to improve compliance and avoid under- or overdosing.
3. Teach client to watch for and report serious adverse effects, such as the following: a. Altered mood such as euphoria or even psychosis b. Increased susceptibility to skin injury c. Weight gain d. Increase in BP e. Excessive thirst, urination f. Severe edema g. Change in vision, eye pain h. Weakness i. Leg pain j. Change in stool color k. Change in appetite l. Rash	3. The client's vigilance can aid in early detection of serious side effects such as hypokalemia, cataracts, diabetes mellitus, thromboembolism, and peptic ulcer.

(continued on page 698)

Interventions	Rationales
4. Teach client to recognize and report signs and symptoms of adrenal insufficiency: a. Hypoglycemia b. Nausea and vomiting c. Diarrhea d. Decreased mental acuity e. Fatigue, weakness, and malaise f. Hyponatremia g. Orthostatic hypotension h. Palpitations i. Decreased appetite j. Weight loss	4. Corticosteroid therapy inhibits pituitary function, resulting in inhibited adrenal function. Early detection enables prompt intervention to prevent serious complications.
5. Encourage client scheduled for long-term corticosteroid therapy to obtain and wear Medic-alert identification.	5. A visible identification bracelet or necklace can aid early detection of adrenal insufficiency.
6. Inform client that he or she should notify physician about a possible increase in corticosteroid dosage before undergoing invasive procedures or vaccinations or when experiencing infection.	6. Additional stress normally triggers an increased adrenal response; however, corticosteroid therapy interferes with adrenal function, possibly necessitating increased corticosteroid dosage to maintain homeostasis. When vaccinated for a disease, a client whose immune system is compromised can get the disease.
7. Teach client that corticosteroids can increase or decrease the effectiveness of certain medications. Other medications can influence the effectiveness of corticosteroids. Instruct client to consult with pharmacist before taking a medication. a. Medications affected by corticosteroids are digitalis products, salicylates, amphotericin B, diuretics, potassium supplements, ritodrine, somatrem, tacrolimus, vaccines, and immunizations. b. Medications that affect corticosteroid effects are antacids, mitotane, oral contraceptives, liver-enzyme–inducing agents, phenobarbital, rifampin, phenytoin, and aminoglutethimide.	7. The chemical effects of corticosteroids on the body can influence the effects of other chemicals.
8. Teach client to have regular eye examinations.	8. Systemic corticosteroid use can cause posterior subcapsular cataracts and increased intraocular pressure (glaucoma).
9. Advise client to a. Start smoking cessation program. b. Limit alcohol intake. c. Engage in weight-bearing exercises for 30–60 minutes per day.	9. These measures increase the effectiveness of corticosteroids.
10. Discuss the addition of 1500 mg calcium with 800 mg of Vitamin D a day.	10. Corticosteroid therapy inhibits calcium mobilization and causes decreased calcium levels.
11. Advise client of the effects on triglyceride levels and the need for follow-up lipid profiles.	11. Corticosteroids promote glyconeogenesis, which raises blood glucose and triglyceride levels.
12. Advise client to wear a Medic-alert bracelet.	12. Abrupt cessation of corticosteroids can precipitate an adrenal crisis.
13. Encourage client to keep regular follow-up appointments.	13. Because of the seriousness of adverse effects, careful monitoring is needed.

Documentation

Discharge summary record
Client teaching
Outcome achievement or status

Enteral Nutrition

Enteral nutrition is the administration of an elemental liquid diet (calories, minerals, and vitamins) to the GI tract through a nasogastric, nasojejunostomy, gastric, or jejunostomy tube. Enteral nutrition can include both oral supplements and tube-feeding techniques. The client with a functioning intestine but who is unable to eat sufficient calories is a candidate. Enteral nutrition is not recommended in clients experiencing severe diarrhea, intensive chemotherapy, immediate postoperative stress period, severe acute pancreatitis, shock, ileus, intestinal obstruction, or high-output external fistulas, or when the client or legal guardian does not desire aggressive nutritional support (if in accordance with agency policy and existing law).

Time Frame
Preprocedure and postprocedure

DIAGNOSTIC CLUSTER

Collaborative Problems

▲ PC: Hypoglycemia/Hyperglycemia
▲ PC: Hypervolemia
△ PC: Hypertonic Dehydration
▲ PC: Electrolyte Imbalances
△ PC: Mucosal Erosion

Nursing Diagnoses

▲ High Risk for Infection related to gastrostomy incision and enzymatic action of gastric juices on skin

▲ Impaired Comfort: Cramping, Distention, Nausea, Vomiting related to type of formula, administration rate, route, or formula temperature

▲ Diarrhea related to adverse response to formula, rate, or temperature

▲ Risk for Aspiration related to position of tube and client

△ High Risk for Ineffective Therapeutic Regimen Management related to lack of knowledge of nutritional indications/requirements, home care, and signs and symptoms of complications

▲ This diagnosis was reported to be monitored for or managed frequently (75%–100%).
△ This diagnosis was reported to be monitored for or managed often (50%–74%).

Discharge Criteria

Before discharge, the client or family will

1. Identify therapeutic indications and nutritional requirements.
2. Demonstrate tube feeding administration and management.
3. Discuss strategies for incorporating enteral management into ADLs.
4. State signs and symptoms that must be reported to a health care professional.

Collaborative Problems

Potential Complication: Hypoglycemia or Hyperglycemia

Potential Complication: Hypervolemia

Potential Complication: Hypertonic Dehydration

Potential Complication: Electrolyte and Trace Mineral Imbalance

Potential Complication: Mucosal Erosion

Nursing Goal

The nurse will detect early signs and symptoms of (a) hypoglycemia/hyperglycemia, (b) hypervolemia, (c) hypertonic dehydration, (d) electrolyte imbalances, and mucosal erosion, and will collaboratively intervene to stabilize client.

Indicators

- Alert, oriented, calm (a)
- Pulse 60–100 beats/min (a, b)
- Respirations easy, rhythmic 16–20 breaths/min (b)
- Respiratory, no rales or wheezing (b)
- BP >90/60, <140/90 mmHg (b)
- No complaints of dizziness (a)
- Intact muscle strength (a)
- Warm, dry skin (a)
- Urine output 5 mL/kg/h (a)
- Urine specific gravity 1.005–1.030 (c)
- Serum potassium 3.8–5 mEq/L (c, d)
- Serum sodium 135–145 mEq/L (c, d)
- Serum osmolality 280–300 mOsm/kg H_2O (c, d)
- No peripheral edema (b)
- Moist mucous membranes (oral) (c)
- Intact mucosa at tube exit site (d)
- No complaints of fatigue (a)
- No complaints of nausea (a)

Interventions	Rationales
1. Monitor for symptoms of hypoglycemia after completion of tube feeding: a. Tachycardia b. Diaphoresis c. Confusion d. Dizziness e. Generalized weakness	1. Sudden cessation of enteral feedings in a physiologically stressed client may trigger a hypoglycemic reaction.
2. Monitor for symptoms of hyperglycemia during formula administration: a. Thirst b. Increased urination c. Fatigue d. Generalized weakness e. Increased respirations f. Increased pulse g. Nausea	2. Hyperglycemia most commonly occurs in clients with inadequate insulin reserves. Enteral formulas with a higher fat percentage are less likely to contribute to hyperglycemic reaction.

(continued on page 701)

Interventions	Rationales
3. Monitor for signs and symptoms of overhydration during formula administration: a. Tachycardia b. Elevated blood pressure c. Pulmonary edema d. Shortness of breath e. Peripheral edema	3. Hypervolemia usually is associated with the high water and sodium contents of the enteral formula. This complication most often occurs as feeding is initiated or reintroduced in a client with compromised cardiac, renal, or hepatic function.
4. Monitor for signs and symptoms of hypertonic dehydration during formula administration. a. Dry mucous membranes b. Thirst c. Decreased serum sodium d. Circulatory overload (increased BP, increased respirations) e. Decreasing urine output f. Concentrated urine	4. Hypertonic dehydration most often results when a formula of high osmolarity and protein content is administered to a client unable to recognize or respond to thirst. It causes circulatory overload and cellular dehydration.
5. Monitor tube exit and entrance sites for: a. Mucosal erosion b. Pain and tenderness c. Bleeding d. Ulceration 6. Take steps to reduce tube irritation: a. Tape tubes securely without causing pressure or tension. b. Prepare skin prior to taping with a skin protective agent. c. Use a PVC tube only if the feeding is needed for 10 days or less. Fine-bore polyurethane tubes are preferable for longer term nasogastric enteral therapy (Best, 2007). d. All tubes should be clearly marked in centimeters or line markers (Best, 2007).	5,6. External pressure or tension on delicate structures can produce mucosal erosion. Prolonged use of large-bore polyvinyl chloride (PVC) catheters has been linked to the development of rhinitis, pharyngitis, nasal cartilage destruction, and esophageal erosion (Best, 2007). After 10 days PVC tubes begin to break down and lose their flexibility, increasing the risk of complications. Graded tubes improve the accuracy of measurement during insertion, and at subsequent client assessments.

 Related Physician-Prescribed Interventions

Medications. Formula (frequency and dilution) and flush or free water amount
Intravenous Therapy. Not applicable
Laboratory Studies. Serum prealbumin, electrolytes, serum glucose, serum transferrin
Diagnostic Studies. Radiogram (verification)
Therapies. Dependent on the type of tube used, weights

Documentation

Flow records
  Vital signs
  Intake and output
  Urine specific gravity
  Serum glucose
  Tube site condition

Nursing Diagnoses

High Risk for Infection Related to Gastrostomy Incision and Enzymatic Action of Gastric Juices on Skin

NOC Infection Status, Wound Healing: Primary Intention, Immune Status

Goal

The client or family will report risk factors.

Indicators

1. Describe measures for infection prevention.
2. Report any discomfort/drainage around the gastrostomy site.

NIC Infection Control, Wound Care, Incision Site Care, Health Education

Interventions	Rationales
1. Cleanse incision and tube insertion site regularly following standard protocol.	1. Cleaning removes microorganisms and reduces risk of infection.
2. Protect skin around the external feeding tube with a protective barrier film. Apply a loose dressing cover and change it when moist. For excessive drainage, protect skin with an adhesive barrier square and ostomy pouch to capture drainage; change the barrier when nonadherent or soiled.	2. The catheter can irritate skin and mucosa. Gastric juices can cause severe skin breakdown.
3. For a temporary gastrostomy or jejunostomy tube, anchor tube to an external surface to minimize tube migration and retraction.	3. Movement can cause tissue trauma and create entry points for opportunistic microorganisms.
4. Teach client to promptly report discomfort around incision or tube.	4. Early detection and reporting enables prompt intervention to prevent serious inflammation.
5. If skin problems persist, consult clinical nurse specialist or enterostomal therapist for assistance.	5. The expertise of a skin care specialist may be needed.

Documentation

Flow records
    Vital signs
    Drainage (characteristics, amount)
    Site condition

Impaired Comfort: Cramping, Distention, Nausea, Vomiting Related to Type of Formula, Administration Rate, Route, or Formula Temperature

NOC Symptom Control

Goal

The client will tolerate enteral feedings.

Indicators

Will report no episodes of cramping, distention, nausea, or vomiting.

NIC Pruritus Management, Fever Treatment, Environmental Management: Comfort

Interventions	Rationales
1. Review enteral product information for formula characteristics (i.e., lactose, osmolarity, calories, fiber). Consult with nutritional expert.	1. Many current enteral products have a significantly lower osmolarity and are now lactose free. Specialty formulas (i.e., specific for renal or liver conditions) tend to have higher osmolarities because of their increased calorie-to-milliliter ratio.
2. Initiate feedings slowly; gradually increase rate based on tolerance. Begin with an isotonic, lactose-free formula or alternately dilute other types of feedings with water to decrease osmolarity. 3. Instill formula at room temperature directly from the can whenever possible.	2,3. The feeding regimen itself may cause problems. For example, a bolus feeding of high osmolarity at cold temperature can provoke gastric and digestive problems. Uncontrolled feedings by jejunal route are particularly prone to these complications because the feeding is not processed in the stomach before it reaches the intestines.
4. Discard unused portions or store in a tightly sealed container. 5. For continuous feeding, fill container with enough formula for a 4-hour feeding. Do not overfill or allow formula to stand for a longer period.	4,5. Extended exposure of a feeding to room temperature promotes microorganism growth.
6. For intermittent feeding, instill formula gradually over a 15- to 45-minute period. Do not administer as a bolus or at a rapid rate.	6. Slow administration can reduce cramping, nausea, and vomiting.

Documentation

Flow records
    Intake and output
Progress notes
    Unusual events or problems

Diarrhea Related to Adverse Response to Formula Rate or Temperature

NOC Bowel Elimination, Electrolyte & Acid–Base Balance, Fluid Balance, Hydration, Symptom Control

Goal

The client will report less diarrhea.

Indicators

Demonstrate a tolerable, consistent bowel pattern with no episodes of diarrhea

NIC Bowel Management, Diarrhea Management, Fluid/Electrolyte Management, Nutrition Management, Enteral Tube Feeding

Interventions	Rationales
1. Initiate feedings slowly; progress gradually as tolerated. Begin with an isotonic, lactose-free, fiber-enriched supplement.	1. Diminished intestinal absorption must be compensated for through gradual, progressive introduction of enteral supplements.

(continued on page 704)

Interventions	Rationales
2. Instill formula at room temperature directly from the can when possible.	2. Administering cold formula can cause cramping and possibly lead to elimination problems.
3. Discard unused portions or store in a tightly sealed container.	3. These precautions can minimize growth of microorganisms.
4. For continuous feeding, fill container with enough formula for a 4-hour feeding. Do not overfill or allow formula to stand for a longer period.	4. Each type of formula has an individual shelf-life after opening. Formula should be protected from environmental contaminants to prevent bacterial growth and possible resultant diarrhea. Jejunal intestinal feedings are particularly sensitive to diarrhea because they lack hydrochloric acid.
5. For intermittent feeding, instill formula gradually over a 15- to 45-minute period. Do not administer as a bolus or at a rapid rate.	5. Intermittent feedings simulate a normal feeding regimen and allow for stomach digestion and emptying. Intermittent stomach feedings also allow for unencumbered physical care between feedings.
6. Consult with physician for antidiarrheal medications as necessary.	6. Medications may be needed to control severe diarrhea.

Documentation

Flow records
> Intake and output

High Risk for Aspiration Related to Position of Tube and Client

NOC Aspiration Control

Goal

The client will not experience aspiration.

Indicators

Relate measures to prevent aspiration

NIC Aspiration Precautions, Airway Management, Positioning, Airway Suctioning

Interventions	Rationales
1. All at-risk clients should be placed in a semi-recumbent position during feedings; if not possible, place client in reverse Trendelenburg (Methany, 2005).	1. Upper body elevation can prevent reflux through use of gravity.
2. For a gastric tube, the preferred method to verify proper tube placement is to check pH of aspirate (Huffman, 2004), or, if additional verification is necessary, by air auscultation and aspirating for residual contents.	2,3. Proper tube position must be verified before feeding to prevent introducing formula into the respiratory tract.
3. For a tube positioned intestinally (jejunally), measuring pH of aspirate is still preferable, but can be more difficult to obtain a measurable sample. The secondary recommendation is to verify placement by auscultation (Huffman, 2004).	

(continued on page 705)

Interventions	Rationales
4. If using pH aspirate, administer a scheduled intermittent tube feeding only if gastric pH is 4.0 or less (intrinsically higher in neonates), or postpyloric pH is greater than 6. (*Note:* continuous feedings and pH altering medications will affect accuracy of pH testing) (Huffman, 2004). When aspirating for residual contents, administer a scheduled intermittent tube feeding only if residual contents are less than residual limit set by physician or policy. When a high residual is identified, return it to the stomach. Delay feeding if it is intermittent; stop it for 1 hour if it is continuous. Recheck the residual in 1 hour; if it is still high, notify physician. A different rate, method, route, or formula change may be indicated.	4. Although there is no one volume of gastric residual determined to be a cutoff point, administering feedings in the presence of excessive residual contents increases risks of reflux and aspiration (Serna, 2006).
5. Regulate intermittent gastric feedings to allow gastric emptying between feedings. 6. Regulate continuous feedings to allow periods of rest so client can ambulate unencumbered by feeding apparatus.	5,6. Such regulation is necessary to prevent overfeeding and increased risk of reflux and aspiration. Gastric feedings should be administered intermittently when the potential for aspiration is high. When clients are predisposed to aspiration, jejunal tube placement for continual feeding is preferred (Methany, 2004).
7. Flush feeding tube with water after completion of feeding.	7. Flushing is necessary to remove formula that can provide a medium for microorganism growth.

Documentation

Flow records
   Vital signs
   Breath sounds
   Intake and output
Progress notes
   Unusual complaints

High Risk for Ineffective Therapeutic Regimen Management Related to Lack of Knowledge of Nutritional Indications/Requirements, Home Care, and Signs and Symptoms of Complications

NOC Compliance Behavior, Knowledge: Treatment Regimen, Participation: Health Care Decisions, Treatment Behavior: Illness or Injury

Goals

The goals for this diagnosis represent those associated with discharge planning. Refer to the discharge criteria.

NIC Anticipatory Guidance, Learning Facilitation, Risk Identification, Health Education, Teaching: Procedure/Treatment, Health System Guidance

Interventions	Rationales
1. Explain rationale for, and aspects of, enteral nutrition therapy. Discuss client's specific nutritional requirements and specific indications for therapy.	1. Explaining the need for optimal nutrition and the advantages of enteral feedings can reduce misconceptions and encourage compliance.

(*continued on page 706*)

Interventions	Rationales
2. Explain rationale for continued diagnostic tests (e.g., routine weighing, intake and output measurements, urine tests, serum evaluation).	2. Careful monitoring is needed to evaluate the effectiveness and safety of enteral therapy and enable early detection of problems or complications.

3. Review potential problems and complications such as these:
  a. Vomiting
  b. Diarrhea/constipation
  c. Improper tube placement
  d. Aspiration
	3. Client's and family's understanding of potential complications enables them to detect and report signs and symptoms soon after they develop.

4. Refer client to a home care agency for follow-up home visits.	4. A home health care agency can provide ongoing assistance and support.
5. Teach client to do enteral tube care and maintenance. In certain cases, nasogastric tube insertion may be taught.	5. Some clients and families can be taught insertion of gastric feeding tubes. Tubes positioned to feed specific areas of the GI tract are generally more complex and require radiologic confirmation.

6. Teach client aspects of the enteral feeding regimen; cover these elements:
  a. Handwashing
  b. Work surface preparation
  c. Formula preparation
  d. Administration procedure
  e. Completion of feeding
  f. Dressing changes and skin protection measures
  g. Equipment operation and care
	6. Certain knowledge is needed for proper administration and prevention of complications.

7. Have client or support person perform return demonstration of selected care measures.	7. Return demonstration lets nurse evaluate client's and family's abilities to perform feedings safely.
8. Explain measures to prevent aspiration. (Refer to the nursing diagnosis Potential for Aspiration in this entry for more information)	8. Aspiration is a potential complication of all types of tube feedings.

9. Teach other self-care measures including these:
  a. Use tap water to irrigate feeding tube before and after instilling formula.
  b. Chew gum, if indicated.
  c. Brush teeth and use mouthwash three to four times a day.
  d. Review client medications and teach proper administration to ensure correct dosing and absorption. Medications should not be added to formula container.
  e. Mark tube when it is in the correct position.
	9.
	  a. Irrigation allows evaluation of tube patency, clears tubes, and ensures delivery of a full dose of formula.
	  b. Gum can help to keep the mouth moist.
	  c. Frequent mouth care can maintain moist mucous membranes and remove microorganisms.
	  d. Medications added directly to the formula container can alter dosages, block the feeding tube, or decrease medication effectiveness.
	  e. Markings provide a visible cue of a tube position change.

10. Provide client with a written list of required equipment and supplies and sources for these items.	10. Advance planning can prevent shortages and improper substitutions.

Documentation

Discharge summary record
  Client and family teaching
  Outcome achievement or status
  Referrals, if indicated

Hemodialysis

Hemodialysis is the removal of metabolic wastes and excess electrolytes and fluids from the blood to treat acute or chronic kidney disease. The procedure uses the principles of diffusion, osmosis, and filtration. Blood is pumped into an artificial kidney through a semi-permeable, cellophane-like membrane surrounded by a flow of dialysate, which is a solution composed of water, glucose, sodium, chloride, potassium, calcium, and acetate or bicarbonate. The amounts of these constituents vary depending on the amount of water, waste products, or electrolytes to be removed. Hemodialysis does not correct renal dysfunction; it only corrects metabolic waste, fluid, electrolyte, and acid–base imbalances (Wagner, Johnson, & Kidd, 2006).

Time Frame
Pretherapy, intratherapy, and posttherapy

■■■■■■ DIAGNOSTIC CLUSTER

Collaborative Problems	Refer to
▲ PC: Electrolyte Imbalance (Potassium, Sodium, and Magnesium)	
✳ PC: Hemolysis	
△ PC: Dialysis Disequilibrium Syndrome	
▲ PC: Clotting	
▲ PC: Air Embolism	
▲ PC: Pyrogen Reaction	
▲ PC: Fluid Imbalances	Peritoneal Dialysis
▲ PC: Anemia	Chronic Kidney Disease
✳ PC: Sepsis	
✳ PC: Anaphylaxis/Allergies	

Nursing Diagnoses	Refer to
▲ High Risk for Infection Transmission related to frequent contacts with blood and high risk of hepatitis B and C	
△ Powerlessness related to need for treatments to live despite effects on life style	Chronic Kidney Disease
△ Interrupted Family Processes related to the disruption in role responsibilities caused by the treatment schedule	Chronic Kidney Disease

Related Care Plans

Chronic Kidney Disease or Acute Kidney Failure
External Arteriovenous Shunting

▲ This diagnosis was reported to be monitored for or managed frequently (75%–100%).
△ This diagnosis was reported to be monitored for or managed often (50%–74%).
✳ This diagnosis was not included in the validation study.

Discharge Criteria

Before discharge, the client and/or family will

1. Describe the purpose of hemodialysis.
2. Discuss feelings and concerns regarding the effects of long-term therapy on self and family.
3. State signs and symptoms that must be reported to a health care professional.

Collaborative Problems

Potential Complication: Electrolyte Imbalance (Potassium, Sodium, Magnesium)

Potential Complication: Hemolysis

Potential Complication: Dialysis Disequilibrium Syndrome

Potential Complication: Clotting

Potential Complication: Air Embolism

Potential Complication: Fluid Imbalances

Potential Complication: Anemia

Potential Complication: Sepsis

Potential Complication: Anaphylaxis or Allergies

Nursing Goal

The nurse will monitor to detect early signs and symptoms of (a) electrolyte imbalance, (b) hemolysis, (c) dialysis disequilibrium syndrome, (d) clotting, (e) air embolism, (f) fluid imbalances, (g) anemia, (h) sepsis, and (i) anaphylaxis/allergies, and will intervene collaboratively to stabilize the client.

Indicators

- Alert, oriented, calm (c, h)
- Skin warm, dry, usual color, and no itching/hives (e, h, i)
- No or minimal edema (f)
- BP >90–60, <140/90 mmHg (c, e, h, i)
- Pulse pressure (40 mmHg difference in systolic or diastolic) (c, e, h, i)
- Pulse 60–100 beats/min (c, e, h, i)
- Respirations 16–20 breaths/min (e, h, i)
- Respirations relaxed, rhythmic (e, h, i)
- No rales or wheezing (e, h, i)
- No weight change (f)
- No headache (c)
- No chest pain (e, i)
- No change in vision (e)
- No complaints of nausea/vomiting (c)
- No seizures (c)
- Serum potassium 3.5–5 mEq/L (a)
- Hemoglobin (g)
  - Male 13.5–17.5 g/dL
  - Female 13–16 g/dL
- Hematocrit (g)
  - Male 40%–54%
  - Female 37%–47%
- Serum sodium 135–148 mm/dL (a)
- Serum creatinine 0.6–1.2 mg/dL (a)
- Blood urea nitrogen 7–18 mg/dL (a)
- Intact access site (d)
- Intact connections (d)
- No burning at site (b)
- No blood in venous line (b)
- Urine output 5 mL/kg/h (i),
- White Blood cells >4000 cells/mms or <12,000 cells/mms or <10% bands
- Temperature >96.8°F or <100.4°F

Interventions	Rationales

1. Assess the following:
 	
  a. Skin (color, turgor, temperature, moisture, and edema)
 	
  b. Blood pressure (lying and sitting)
 	
  c. Apical pulse (rhythm and rate)
 	
  d. Respirations (rate, effort, and abnormal sounds)
 	
  e. Weight (gain or loss)
 	
  f. Vascular access (site and patency)
 	
  g. Pretreatment BUN, serum creatinine, sodium, and potassium levels
	1. Predialysis assessment and documentation of client's status are mandatory before initiation of the hemodialysis procedure to establish a baseline and to identify problems.
	  a. Skin assessment can provide data to evaluate circulation, level of hydration, fluid retention, and uremia.
	  b. Low blood pressure may indicate intolerance to transmembrane pressure, hypovolemia, or the effects of antihypertensive medication given predialysis. High blood pressure may indicate overhydration, increased renin production, or dietary and fluid indiscretion.
	  c. Cardiac assessment evaluates the heart's ability to compensate for changes in fluid volume.
	  d. Respiratory assessment evaluates compensatory ability of the system and presence of infection.
	  e. Predialysis weight indicating gain or loss may necessitate a need to reevaluate dry weight.
	  f. The vascular access site is assessed for signs of infection or abnormal drainage. Patency is evaluated by assessment of bruits and thrills.
	  g. Pretreatment serum levels are used as a baseline for evaluation of the effectiveness of the dialysis (Wagner, Johnson, & Kidd, 2006; Baird, Keen, & Swearingen, 2005).

2. Assess the client's complaints of the following symptoms:
  a. Chest pain
  b. Shortness of breath
  c. Cramps
  d. Headache
  e. Dizziness
  f. Blurred vision
  g. Nausea and vomiting
  h. Change in mentation or speech
	2. These assessment data help to determine if there has been a change in the client's condition since last treatment or if a change in treatment is indicated. When a client presents with problems predialysis, underlying etiology needs to be determined before initiation of treatment.

3. Check the dialysis machine set-up for the following:
  a. Evidence of air in line
  b. Secure connections
  c. Armed air detector
  d. Poor connection or crack around the hub of the vascular needles
  e. Fluid in normal saline bag
  f. Arterial needle site collapse, allowing air to enter around the needle
	3. Careful checking can detect air or leaks.

4. Intradialysis—monitor for signs and symptoms of potassium and sodium imbalance. (Refer to the Peritoneal Dialysis care plan for more information.)	4. Dialysate fluid composition and rates of inflow and outflow determine electrolyte imbalances.
5. Do not leave the client unattended at any time during dialysis.	5. A complication such as hemorrhage, transfusion reaction, or clotting can become serious quickly if not detected and treated promptly. Early detection can prevent substantial blood loss.
6. Alternate puncture sites with every treatment and question the client regarding pain in the area of access.	6. Repeated needle punctures at the same site can cause an aneurysm.

(continued on page 710)

Interventions	Rationales
7. Apply pinpoint pressure to fistula sticks postdialysis to control bleeding. When cannulating a new shunt, maintain pressure for 20 minutes, and then apply pressure dressings after bleeding is controlled.	7. These measures can help to prevent exsanguination from access site.
8. Check the shunt dressing every 2 hours for bleeding or disconnection.	8. Bleeding can be a sign of disconnected or clotted shunt tubing.
9. Monitor for manifestations of hemolysis: a. Bright red blood in venous line b. Burning at the circulatory return site c. Pink- to red-tinged dialysate	9. Rupture of red blood cells can result from the hypotonic dialysate, high dialysate temperature, or chloramines, nitrates, copper, zinc, or formaldehyde in the dialysate.
10. Monitor for seizure activity.	10. Hypotension caused by rapid fluid loss can precipitate a seizure.
11. Monitor for signs and symptoms of dialysis/disequilibrium syndrome: a. Headache b. Nausea c. Vomiting d. Restlessness e. Hypertension f. Increased pulse pressures g. Altered sensorium h. Convulsions i. Coma	11. As a result of hemodialysis, the concentration of BUN is reduced more rapidly than the urea nitrogen level in cerebrospinal fluid and brain tissue, because of the slow transport of urea across the blood–brain barrier. Urea acts as an osmotic agent, drawing water from the plasma and extracellular fluid into the cerebral cells and producing cerebral edema. Other factors, such as rapid pH changes and electrolyte shifts, also can cause cerebral edema (Wagner, Johnson, & Kidd, 2006; Baird, Keen, & Swearingen, 2005).
12. Monitor for clotting: a. Observe for clot formation in kidney and drip chambers. b. Monitor pressure readings every 15 minutes. c. Observe for clots when aspirating fistula needles, arteriovenous shunt, or subclavian catheter.	12. Blood contacting the nonvascular surface of the extracorporeal circuit activates the normal clotting mechanism. During dialysis, fibrin formation within the venous trap and a gradual increase in the circuit's venous pressure (resulting from clotting in the venous trap or needle) may indicate inadequate heparinization. Clot formation elevates blood pressure readings (Baird, Keen, & Swearingen, 2005).
13. Monitor for signs and symptoms of air embolism: a. Cyanosis b. Shortness of breath c. Chest pain d. Visual changes: diplopia, "seeing stars," and blindness e. Anxiety f. Persistent cough	13. As little as 10 mL of air introduced into the venous circulation is clinically significant. Large air bubbles are changed to foam as they enter the heart. Foam can decrease the volume of blood entering the lungs, decreasing left heart blood flow and cardiac output. Entry of air into the respiratory circulatory system causes a profound negative response.
14. If signs and symptoms of air embolism occur, take these steps: a. Clamp the venous line and stop the blood pump. b. Position client on his or her left side with feet elevated for 30 minutes.	14 a. Clamping the line and stopping the pump can halt infusion of air. b. This prevents air from going to the head and traps air in the right atrium and in the right ventricle away from the pulmonic valve.
15. Monitor for signs and symptoms of sepsis: a. WBC <4000 cells/mms or >12,000 cells/mms or greater than 10% bands forms	15. a. WBC count may be normal, elevated, or decreased; the presence of greater than 10% banding indicates an inflammatory response.

(continued on page 711)

Interventions	Rationales
b. Temperature <96.8°F or >100.4°F c. Tachycardia d. Dyspnea e. BP >90–60, <140/90 mmHg f. Disorientation and decreased level of consciousness	b,c,d. A temperature change above or below the normal range, tachycardia, and dyspnea can be early signs of the body's natural defense to fight infection. e. Hypotension can be as a direct result of central dilation of the vessels while the cardiac function is hyperdynamic (Baird, Keen, & Swearingen, 2005). f. Disorientation can be an indirect result of hypoperfusion of major organs such as the neurologic, circulatory, and respiratory systems (Baird, Keen, & Swearingen, 2005).

16. Monitor for signs and symptoms of anaphylaxis:
  a. Polyuria
  b. Respiratory distress
  c. Hypotension
  d. Urticaria
  e. Angio-edema
  f. Vomiting
  g. Diarrhea
  h. Anxiety
  i. Abdominal pain
	16. This is due to an allergic response to the ingredients in the dialysate which involves the interaction between immunoglobin E (IgE) and mast cells. Anaphylaxis is a severe hypersensitivity response caused by a massive release of chemical mediators and other substances. The cardiovascular, respiratory, cutaneous, and gastrointestinal systems are generally involved in anaphylaxis. The IgE antibodies interact with mast cells, triggering the release of histamine, which, because of its potent vasodilator effect, causes widespread edema and vascular congestion (Wagner, Johnson, & Kidd, 2006).

Related Physician-Prescribed Interventions

Medications. Refer to the Chronic Kidney Disease care plan
Laboratory Studies. Refer to the Chronic Kidney Disease care plan
Diagnostic Studies. Refer to the Chronic Kidney Disease care plan
Therapies. Dialysate solution

Documentation

Flow records
  Vital signs
  Weight
  Vascular access site
  Dialysis (time, solution)
Progress notes
  Predialysis complaints
  Intradialysis complaints

Nursing Diagnoses

High Risk for Infection Transmission Related to Frequent Contacts with Blood and People at High Risk for Hepatitis B and C

NOC Infection Status, Risk Control, Risk Detection

Goal

The client will relate the risks of hepatitis B virus (HBV) transmission.

Indicators

- Have antibodies to HBV.
- Take precautions to prevent transmission of HBV.

NIC   Teaching: Disease Process, Infection Protection

Interventions	Rationales
1. Observe strict isolation procedure: a. Wear an isolation gown and mask during dialysis treatment. b. Dialysis should be performed in client's private room or a dialysis unit isolation area. c. All blood or dialysis effluent spills must be cleaned up immediately with antimicrobial soap and water. d. Observe isolation disposal procedure for all needles, syringes, and effluent. e. Do not permit staff and other personnel or visitors to eat or drink anything within the dialysis treatment area. f. Ensure that all specimens for laboratory analysis are labeled "Isolation" and placed in bags also labeled "Isolation." g. Use special disposable thermometers to assess temperature. h. Avoid contact with other dialysis clients, if staffing level permits. If contact is necessary, change isolation gowns and wash hands carefully. i. Avoid any skin contact with the client's blood. j. Follow isolation procedure for waste and linen disposal per institutional protocol. k. Follow the recommended sterilization procedure for the hemodialysis machine after use.	1. HBV/HCV is found in the blood, saliva, semen, and vaginal secretions. Transmission is usually through blood (percutaneous or permucosal). Regularly practicing certain precautions provides protection (Lewis et al., 2004).
2. Administer immunizations, as appropriate, following facility policies.	2. High-risk clients and others should be immunized.
3. Explain that there is no prophylaxis for hepatitis C virus (HCV) and that it can go unnoticed for years.	3. Only 10% of people report an acute illness.
4. Minimize use of anticoagulants in clients with liver disease. 5. Collaborate with physician and/or advanced practice nurse to adjust medications with potential hepatotoxicity, including immunosuppressants. 6. Reinforce to client and family the serious nature of HBV/HCV, precautions, and risks.	4–6. Reiterating the seriousness of HBV/HCV and its possible sequelae may encourage compliance with instructions and precautions.

Documentation

Teaching record
    Client and family teaching
Flow records
    Monthly HBV screening results

Long-Term Venous Access Devices

Long-term venous access devices (VADs) are used for clients who have a need for frequent venous access to deliver chemotherapy, intravenous fluids, and blood products. They also provide access for blood samples.

There are four groups of central venous access devices: nontunneled (percutaneous) central catheters; peripherally inserted central catheters (PICC); tunneled catheters (e.g., Groshong, Hickman-Broviac); and implanted ports. These devices can last weeks, months, or years. Percutaneous central catheters have the shortest duration.

The risks and possible complications differ according to the choice of VAD and the vessel in which it is placed. Both the catheter choice and placement site should be tailored to the needs of the client.

 Time Frame
Preprocedure and postprocedure

■■■■■ DIAGNOSTIC CLUSTER

Collaborative Problems

▲ PC: Hemorrhage
△ PC: Embolism/Thrombosis
▲ PC: Sepsis
　PC: Phlebitis (site)
　PC: Extravasation (site)

Nursing Diagnoses

▲ Anxiety related to upcoming insertion of catheter/port and insufficient knowledge of procedure

△ High Risk for Ineffective Therapeutic Regimen Management related to insufficient knowledge of home care, signs and symptoms of complications, and community resources

▲ High Risk for Infection related to catheter's direct access to bloodstream (Refer to Total Parenteral Nutrition)

Related Care Plans

Cancer: Initial Diagnosis
Chemotherapy

▲ This diagnosis was reported to be monitored for or managed frequently (75%–100%).
△ This diagnosis was reported to be monitored for or managed often (50%–74%).

Discharge Criteria

Before discharge, the client and/or family will

1. Demonstrate procedure and discuss conditions of catheter care and administration at home.
2. Discuss strategies for incorporating catheter management in activities of daily living (ADLs).
3. Verbalize necessary precautions.
4. State signs and symptoms that must be reported to a health care professional.
5. Identify available community resources.

Collaborative Problems

Potential Complication: Hemorrhage

Potential Complication: Embolism/Thrombosis

Potential Complication: Sepsis

Potential Complication: Phlebitis (site)

Potential Complication: Extravasation (site)

Nursing Goal

The nurse will monitor for early signs and symptoms of (a) hemorrhage, (b) embolism/thrombosis, (c) sepsis, (d) phlebitis (site), and (e) extravasation (site), and collaboratively intervene to stabilize the client.

Indicators

- Calm, alert, oriented (b, c)
- Warm, dry, skin (a, c)
- BP >90/60, <140/90 mmHg (a, b, c)
- Pulse 60–100 beats/min (a, b, c)
- Respirations 16–20 breaths/min (a, b, c)
- Respirations easy, rhythmic (a, b, c)
- Temperature 98.5–99°F (c, d)
- Urine output >5 mL/kg/h (a, c)
- Urine negative for bacteria, WBC (c)
- Negative blood culture (c)
- Intact insertion site (d, e)
- Client catheter with blood return (d, e)
- No swelling, tenderness, drainage at site (d, e)
- No complaints of stinging, pain, or burning at insertion site (d, e)

Interventions	Rationales
1. Follow agency protocols for insertion, maintenance and management of local complications. If chemotherapeutic agents are administered, refer to Chemotherapy care plan.	1. Institutional policies will specifically outline monitoring and interventions for catheter care and local complications (e.g., phlebitis, extravasation [leakage of chemotherapeutic or other caustic agents into surrounding tissues]).
2. Monitor for signs and symptoms of hemorrhage: a. Hypotension b. Tachycardia c. Evidence of bleeding d. Hematoma around insertion site (Hamilton, 2006) e. Cool, clammy skin (Hamilton, 2006)	2. Hemorrhage is a serious surgical complication of long-term venous access catheter placement. It can occur within several hours of insertion after blood pressure returns to pre-insertion levels and puts increased pressure on a newly formed clot. It also can develop later, secondary to vascular erosion due to infection.
3. Monitor for signs and symptoms of air embolism. Report changes to physician and advanced nurse practitioner: a. Anxiety, restlessness b. Altered level of consciousness c. Shortness of breath (SOB), cyanosis d. Tachycardia e. Shoulder or back pain (Hamilton, 2006)	3. A client with a long-term VAD is at increased risk for air embolism. Accidental leakage of air from catheter can occlude a major pulmonary artery; obstruction of blood flow to the alveoli decreases alveolar perfusion, shunts air to patent alveoli, and leads to bronchial constriction and possible collapse of pulmonary tissue. There is an increased risk of air embolism in those individuals with compromised circulation from hemorrhage or dehydration, and in dyspneic clients due to fluctuations in chest pressures (Hamilton, 2006).
4. Monitor for signs and symptoms of hematoma: a. Tenderness and swelling at insertion site b. Discoloration at insertion site	4. Long-term VAD placement can cause soft tissue injury resulting in rupture of small vessels. As blood collects at insertion site, hematoma forms.
5. Monitor for signs of sepsis. Report changes to physicians or advanced nurse practitioners: a. Temperature >101°F or <98.6°F b. Decreased urine output c. Tachycardia, tachypnea d. Pale, cool skin	5. The invasive nature of a VAD puts client at risk for opportunistic infection and septicemia. If the VAD is used to instill chemotherapy, the possibility of chemotherapy-induced leukopenia further increases risk. Sepsis causes massive vasodilation and resultant hypovolemia, leading to tissue hypoxia and decreased renal and cardiac function. The

(continued on page 715)

Interventions	Rationales
e. WBCs and bacteria in urine f. Positive blood culture	body's compensatory response increases respiratory and heart rates in an attempt to correct hypoxia and acidosis.

6. Monitor for phlebitis:
  a. Redness or streak of red at insertion site
  b. Purulent drainage at insertion site
  c. Tenderness
  d. Elevated temperature
  e. Elevated WBC
	6. Phlebitis is inflammation of a vein, usually from chemical or mechanical infiltration. An infective phlebitis is the inflammation of the intima from a bacterial infection. The incidence of phlebitis increases with the length of time the IV line is in place.

7. Monitor for catheter displacement, damage, infiltration, extravasation, and obstruction:
  a. Superior vena cava syndrome (facial edema, distention of thoracic and neck veins)
  b. Swelling, redness, tenderness or drainage from insertion site (extravasation)
  c. Leakage of fluid from catheter
  d. Inaccurate infusion rate
  e. Inability to infuse or draw blood
  f. Bulging of catheter during infusion
  g. Chest or infraclavicular pain, paresthesia of the arm, dysrhythmias, palpitations, or an extra heart sound (Schummer, Schummer, & Schelenz, 2003)
	7. Catheters can malfunction, obstruct, or displace from misuse or defects.

8. If signs of skin infection are assessed, remove needle from the port and do not reaccess until infection is cleared.	8. To prevent systematic infections, treatment is required before nurse reaccesses.

 Related Physician-Prescribed Interventions

Refer to the care plan for the underlying condition necessitating VAD use (e.g., Cancer: Initial Diagnosis)

Documentation

Flow records
Vital signs
Respiratory assessment
Catheter site/patency assessment

Nursing Diagnoses

Anxiety Related to Upcoming Insertion of Catheter/Port and Insufficient Knowledge of Procedure

NOC Anxiety Reduction, Coping, Impulse Control

Goal

The client will report decreased anxiety after explanations.

Indicators

• Share feelings regarding scheduled catheter insertion.
• Relate what to expect during insertion.

NIC Anxiety Reduction, Impulse Control Training, Anticipatory Guidance

Interventions	Rationales
1. Reinforce physician's explanation of surgical diagnostic procedure. Notify physician if additional explanations are indicated.	1. The physician is legally responsible for explanations for an informed consent; the nurse is legally responsible for clarifying information, evaluating client's understanding, and notifying physician if more information is necessary.
2. Provide an opportunity for client to share fears and beliefs regarding chemotherapy. Delay teaching if a high level of anxiety is present.	2. Sharing helps nurse identify sources of anxiety and correct misinformation. High anxiety prevents retention of information.
3. Explain what to expect: a. Preprocedure (e.g., site preparation and draping) b. During insertion (e.g., positioning and sensations)	3. Perception of an event is gained through all senses. Providing sensory information along with procedural information gives the client more data to use to accurately interpret and master the event.
4. Instruct client on how he or she can assist during the procedure. a. Communicate any sensations felt to physician. b. Following physician's instructions (e.g., holding breath and lying still during insertion; coughing, deep breathing, and exercising legs postprocedure).	4. Eliciting client's cooperation with the procedure can help to improve compliance and reduce risk of complications.
5. Explain that nursing staff monitor the following at frequent intervals: a. Blood pressure b. Pulse rate and rhythm c. Condition of catheter insertion site d. Condition of limb distal to insertion site. Also, explain that a chest x-ray film will be obtained.	5. Instructions about specific procedures can help to reduce anxiety associated with the unknown and the unexpected.
6. Instruct client about the need to immobilize the limb used for the procedure for the prescribed length of time.	6. Immobilization helps to reduce complications of hemorrhage or thrombosis.
7. Refer to the Cancer: Initial Diagnosis care plan for additional specific strategies to reduce anxiety.	

Documentation

Teaching record
Client teaching
Outcome achievement or status

High Risk for Ineffective Therapeutic Regimen Management Related to Insufficient Knowledge of Home Care, Signs and Symptoms of Complications, and Community Resources

NOC Compliance Behavior, Knowledge: Treatment Regimen, Participation: Health Care Decisions, Treatment Behavior: Illness or Injury

Goals

The goals for this diagnosis represent those associated with discharge planning. Refer to the discharge criteria.

NIC Anticipatory Guidance, Learning Facilitation, Risk Identification, Health Education, Teaching: Procedure/Treatment

Interventions	Rationales
1. Reinforce physician's explanation of the catheterization procedure, including line placement; incorporate individually oriented media when possible.	1. Explanations can reduce misconceptions and increase participation.

2. Explain advantages and disadvantages of atrial catheters and vascular access ports.
 	
  a. Atrial catheters (open and closed)—advantages:
  • Provide unlimited venous access
  • Eliminate need for painful needle sticks
  • Can be used for continuous infusion in both hospital and home
  • Carry a reduced risk of extravasation
  • Cause little discomfort
 	
  b. Atrial catheters (open and closed)—disadvantages:
  • Require dressing changes
  • Require heparin (open) or saline (closed) flushes
  • Require cap changes (usually weekly)
  c. PICC lines are silastic or polyurethane catheters that are placed antecubitally and advanced to a large central vein:
  • PICC advantages include the following:
  PICC lines are less expensive and easier to insert. They are placed by specially trained nurses and can be inserted at the bedside or in the home setting.
  There is less risk for air embolism because insertion site is well below the heart.
  No possibility of pneumothorax exists.
  • PICC disadvantages include the following:
  Phlebitis incidence is higher than with other VADs.
  Smaller lumen does not lend itself to blood sampling. If blood aspiration is done, it must be done slowly, with a syringe, to prevent catheter collapse.
  Catheter is easily displaced because it is held in place with steristrips (arm exercise contraindicated).
  Catheter may be easily ruptured if irrigated with high pressure.
  d. Vascular access ports—advantage:
  • Free client from most responsibility for routine dressing changes and flushing
  • When not in use, port virtually undetectable
  e. Vascular access ports—disadvantages:
  • Require needle sticks through the skin to gain access
  • Allow a limited number of accesses, depending on needle size (typically 1000–2000)
  • Require surgery to implant and remove
	2. Discussing different devices can help client to better understand how the decision was made about which type to use. Knowing the logic behind the decision may encourage compliance.
	  a. Open catheter method provides a catheter at the skin surface for medication administration. Single- and double-lumen catheters are available. Double-lumen catheters provide greater flexibility with treatment (e.g., chemotherapy and total parenteral nutrition [TPN] can be administered simultaneously). Both the open and closed catheters require surgical insertion.
	
	  e. Vascular access ports consist of a chamber with a septum attached to a catheter. Chamber and catheter are surgically implanted under the skin. Drugs and fluids are administered by injecting a noncoring needle through the skin and into the chamber. Fluid flows through the needle into the chamber and through the catheter into the right atrium.

3. Explain reasons for continued assessment procedures and diagnostic tests (e.g., daily weights, intake and output monitoring, and urine and serum evaluations)	3. The client's understanding that careful monitoring is needed to assess status and to detect problems early promotes cooperation with procedures.
4. Explain aseptic technique; obtain return demonstration of handwashing and preparation of work surface.	4. Understanding enables compliance with infection-prevention measures.

(continued on page 718)

Interventions	Rationales
5. Explain home care measures and discuss roles and expectations of all concerned—client, family members, visiting nurse, and others, as appropriate.	5. Expectations should be clear to prevent misunderstanding.
6. Teach manipulation of syringe and needle and method of drawing up solution. Obtain return demonstrations from client and family members to demonstrate understanding and mastery.	6. These skills are needed for home management.
7. Teach catheter care according to protocols; obtain return demonstrations of care measures as necessary. Provide written material for the following: a. Dressing change b. Site care c. Emergency measures d. Changing injection cap e. Catheter repair	7. Understanding protocols and techniques for home care is critical to prevent infection and clotting and to manage problems or emergencies.
8. Discuss strategies for keeping the home environment safe and conducive to good care: a. Store supplies in a clean, dry place. b. Do not tell others that syringes are stored in the home. c. Use a shoebox with a small hole in the top for discarding used syringes. d. Tape and discard the box when filled. e. Keep clean syringes, the used syringe box, and heparin out of reach and sight of children and confused adults. f. Perform catheter care in a clean area where a sink is available for hand-washing. g. Thoroughly clean the work area before laying out supplies.	8. These measures help to reduce risk of injury and infection transmission.
9. Explain signs and symptoms of VAD complications: a. Fever b. Tenderness, swelling, and drainage at site c. VAD occlusion d. Inability to infuse e. Facial edema and distended neck veins f. Phlebitis management	9. Understanding signs and symptoms of complications enables early detection and reporting to a health care professional for timely intervention: a,b. Fever and changes at the insertion site may indicate infection. c,d. Inaccurate infusion rate or inability to infuse points to obstruction or catheter damage. e. Facial edema and neck vein distention may indicate superior vena caval syndrome. f. Early intervention can limit the effects of the phlebitis, decrease discomfort, and extend use of catheter.
10. Provide a list of required equipment and supplies.	10. Planning can prevent shortages and improper substitutions.
11. Instruct client or family about whom to call with questions day or night (e.g., nurses' station or physician).	11. Questions are likely to arise after discharge.

Documentation

Discharge summary record
Client and family teaching
Outcome achievement or status

Mechanical Ventilation

Mechanical ventilation is indicated for a variety of clinical conditions that lead to an inadequate ventilation or oxygenation (Newmarch, 2006). Negative pressure ventilators, such as the iron lung, are rarely used today (Pruitt & Jacobs, 2006). Most positive pressure ventilators are pressure, time, or volume cycled (Newmarch, 2006). These ventilators force air into the lungs during inspiration, generating positive alveolar pressure. Exhalation is passive. For continuous use, endotracheal intubation or tracheostomy is required. Conditions that necessitate continuous mechanical ventilation include central nervous system disorders that compromise the respiratory center in the medulla; musculoskeletal conditions that limit chest expansion; neuromuscular disorders; heart failure; respiratory disorders; upper airway obstruction; and ineffective breathing pattern (Pruitt & Jacobs, 2006) or inability to maintain patent/effective airway (Scales & Pilsworth, 2007).

 Time Frame
During acute therapy in facility

■■■■■ **DIAGNOSTIC CLUSTER**

Collaborative Problems

▲ PC: Respiratory Insufficiency
▲ PC: Atelectasis
△ PC: Oxygen Toxicity
△ PC: Decreased Cardiac Output
△ PC: GI Bleeding
✱ PC: Ventilator Acquired Pneumonia (VAP)
✱ PC: Barotrauma

Nursing Diagnoses	Refer to
△ High Risk for Dysfunctional Weaning Response related to weaning attempts, respiratory muscle fatigue secondary to mechanical ventilation, increased work of breathing, supine position, protein–calorie malnutrition, inactivity, and fatigue	
△ Disuse Syndrome	Immobility or Unconsciousness
△ Fear related to the nature of the situation, uncertain prognosis of ventilator dependence, or weaning	Chronic Obstructive Pulmonary Disease
▲ Impaired Verbal Communication related to effects of intubation on ability to speak	Tracheostomy
▲ High Risk for Infection related to disruption of skin layer secondary to tracheostomy	
▲ High Risk for Ineffective Airway Clearance related to increased secretions secondary to tracheostomy, obstruction of inner cannula, or displacement of tracheostomy tube	
△ Powerlessness related to dependency on respirator, inability to talk, and loss of mobility	Chronic Obstructive Pulmonary Disease

▲ This diagnosis was reported to be monitored for or managed frequently (75%–100%).
△ This diagnosis was reported to be monitored for or managed often (50%–74%).
✱ This diagnosis was not included in the validation study.

Discharge Criteria

Because mechanical ventilation in this care plan is discontinued before discharge, no discharge criteria are applicable.

Collaborative Problems

Potential Complication: Respiratory Insufficiency

Potential Complication: Atelectasis

Potential Complication: Oxygen Toxicity

Potential Complication: Decreased Cardiac Output

Potential Complication: GI Bleeding

Potential Complication: Ventilator Acquired Pneumonia (VAP)

Potential Complications: Barotrauma

Nursing Goal

The nurse will monitor for early signs and symptoms of (a) respiratory insufficiency, (b) atelectasis, (c) oxygen toxicity, (d) decreased cardiac output, (e) GI bleeding, (f) ventilator acquired pneumonia (VAP), and (g) barotraumas, and will collaboratively intervene to stabilize the client.

Indicators

- Alert, calm, oriented (a, b, c, g)
- Respiratory rate 16–20 breaths/min (a, c, g)
- Respirations easy, rhythmic (a, c, g)
- Symmetrical chest movements (a, g)
- Pulse 60–100 beats/min (a, d, f, g)
- BP >90/60, <140/90 mmHg (a, d, f, g)
- Temperature 98.5–99°F (b, f)
- Oxygen saturation (SaO_2) >94% (a, f, g)
- Carbon dioxide ($PaCO_2$) 35–45 mmHg (a)
- Arterial pH 7.35–7.45 (a)
- Warm, dry skin (a, d)
- No change in usual skin color (a, b, d, g)
- No complaints of numbness, tingling in extremities (c)
- No complaints of substernal distress (c)
- Stool negative for occult blood (e)
- Gastric pH >4 (e)
- No change in sputum character or color (f)
- Sputum cultures negative (f)
- No confusion or agitation (a, g)
- No leukocytosis (f)
- No new radiographic infiltrates or free air (f, g)
- No subcutaneous emphysema (g)

Interventions	Rationales
1. Follow agency protocols for management and documentation of ventilator (settings, alarms, maintenance) (Newmarch, 2006); consult with respiratory therapist.	1. The type of ventilator and mode used will have specific nursing responsibilities.
2. Monitor respiratory status (Lynn-McHale Wiegand & Carlson, 2005): a. Respiratory rate b. Breath sounds c. Chest movements symmetry d. Pulse oximetry	2. These criteria will serve to determine the effectiveness of mechanical ventilation. Asymmetrical chest movements can indicate improper tube placement, atelectasis, or pneumothorax (Lynn-McHale Wiegand & Carlson, 2005).

(continued on page 721)

Interventions	Rationales
e. Arterial blood gases f. Peripheral pulses g. Capillary refill h. Nasal flaring i. Tracheal tug j. Intractable cough k. Use of accessory muscles l. Air leaks m. Amount and character of sputum	
3. Monitor for signs of respiratory insufficiency (Lynn-McHale Wiegand & Carlson, 2005): a. Increased respiratory rate b. Labored respirations c. Restlessness, agitation, confusion d. Increased pulse and BP e. Decreased SaO_2; increased $PaCO_2$	3. Respiratory insufficiency can result from airway obstruction, ventilator problems, atelectasis, bronchospasm, or pneumothorax.
4. Monitor for signs of atelectasis (Lynn-McHale Wiegand & Carlson, 2005): a. Marked dyspnea b. Anxiety c. Cyanosis d. Tachycardia e. Increase or decrease in bronchial breath sounds f. Dull percussion g. Localized consolidation on chest x-ray h. Increased peak and plateau pressures	4. Atelectasis can result from bronchial obstruction due to a mucous plug or from upward diaphragmatic displacement due to increased intraabdominal pressure. Resulting signs and symptoms reflect decreased alveolar exchange and circulating oxygen.
5. Monitor for barotrauma (e.g., pneumothorax) (Lynn-McHale Wiegand & Carlson, 2005): a. Sudden decrease in oxygen saturation b. Sudden onset of respiratory distress c. Limited lung movement d. High pressure alarms on ventilator (peak/plateau) e. Restlessness and agitation f. Decreased or absent breath sounds g. Subcutaneous emphysema h. Absent lung markings on chest x-ray i. Tracheal deviation	5. Excessive positive pressure from ventilator can cause trauma to alveoli and result in pneumothorax (Lynn-McHale Wiegand & Carlson, 2005).
6. Initiate emergency measures (e.g., chest tube insertion).	6. Pneumothorax can be a life-threatening event (Lynn-McHale Wiegand & Carlson, 2005).
7. Maintain a patent airway; suction as needed.	7. Airway obstruction causes respiratory insufficiency. An intubated client who has ineffective cough reflex or fatigue is dependent on suctioning to remove secretions.
8. Maintain proper cuff inflation of tracheostomy. Refer to Tracheostomy or Endotracheal Tube care plans.	8. Underinflation allows aspiration of gastric or respiratory secretions. Overinflation can cause tracheal tissue compression, resulting in ulceration. Maintaining cuff pressures 20–25 mmHg minimizes aspiration risks and tracheal wall injury (DePew & McCarthy, 2007). A secure airway is imperative for successful ventilation (Pruitt & Jacobs, 2006).

(continued on page 722)

Interventions	Rationales

9. Monitor for signs and symptoms of oxygen toxicity:
  a. Substernal distress
  b. Paresthesias in extremities
  c. Progressive dyspnea
  d. Restlessness
	9. Oxygen toxicity, resulting from prolonged administration of excessive oxygen concentrations, leads to decreased surfactant secretion. This causes decreased lung compliance and colloid degeneration, leading to hyaline membrane formation in the lung lining and the development of pulmonary edema.

10. Monitor for signs of decreased cardiac output (Lynn-McHale Wiegand & Carlson, 2005):
  a. Dysrhythmias
  b. Diminished peripheral pulses
  c. Acute or gradual decrease in arterial blood pressure with altered hemodynamics.
  d. Cold, clammy skin
  e. Dyspnea
  f. Decreased urine output
  g. Decreased mixed venous oxygen tension
	10. Positive-pressure ventilation increases intrathoracic pressure, which can reduce venous return and cardiac output. The resulting signs reflect decreased venous return and hypoxemia.

11. Monitor for GI bleeding:
 	
  a. Stool positive for occult blood
  b. Acid gastric pH
 	
  c. Bloody nasogastric drainage
	11. Profound stimulation of the vagus nerve causes hypersecretion of gastric secretions and possible ulcer formation.
	  a. Microscopic bleeding can be detected.
	  b. The pH of stomach is 2. To prevent ulcer formation, pH is maintained above 4.

 ### Related Physician-Prescribed Interventions

Medications. Bronchodilators, short-acting hypnotics, antacids, H₂ blockers, inotropes, sedatives, paralytics/neuromuscular blockade agents, analgesics

Intravenous Therapy. Total parenteral nutrition, fluid/electrolyte replacement, volume expanders

Laboratory Studies. Arterial blood gases, serum electrolytes, albumin, blood urea nitrogen, CBC, creatinine, sputum cultures

Diagnostic Studies. Chest x-ray film, pulse oximetry, capnography, bispectral index (BIS) monitoring, peripheral nerve stimulation

Therapies. Type and operation of ventilator (volume, pressure, rate, control mode, percentage of oxygen), positive end-expiratory pressure; type and size of endotracheal/tracheostomy tube; enteral feeding

Documentation

Flow records
  Vital signs
  Respiratory assessment
  Cuff pressure
  Proximal inspiratory pressure (PIP)

Nursing Diagnoses

High Risk for Dysfunctional Weaning Response Related to Weaning Attempts, Respiratory Muscle Fatigue Secondary to Mechanical Ventilation, Increased Work of Breathing, Supine Position, Protein–Calorie Malnutrition, Inactivity, and Fatigue

 NOC Anxiety Control, Respiratory Status: Ventilation, Vital Signs Status, Knowledge: Treatment Procedure, Energy Conservation, Endurance

Goal

The client will achieve progressive weaning goals.

Indicators

- Demonstrate required protein and calorie intake.
- Participate in activities to reduce inactivity.
- Demonstrate required fluid intake.

NIC Anxiety Reduction, Preparatory Sensory Information, Respiratory Monitoring, Ventilation Assistance, Presence

Interventions	Rationales
1. Remove secretions, as necessary. Preoxygenate before suctioning (Newmarch, 2006). Instillation of saline should not be a routine procedure (Kuriakose, 2008).	1. A tube partially obstructed with secretions increases resistance to flow, which increases the work of breathing. Indications for suctioning are high airway pressures, adventitious breath sounds, and reduced oxygen saturation levels. Suctioning should be performed as needed, not on a routine basis due to risk of mucosal damage. Suction pressures should be 80–120 mmHg. Preoxygenation can prevent hypoxia, arrhythmias and atelectasis (Lynn-McHale Wiegand & Carlson, 2005; Newmarch, 2006; Pruitt & Jacobs, 2006). There is no evidence substantiating the benefits of routinely instilling saline for endotracheal suctioning; in fact it may cause compromise in multiple body systems (Kuriakose, 2008).
2. Promote chest expansion.	2. Any impediment to chest expansion increases the work of breathing.
3. Assess for tube-related causes of resistance to flow such as these: a. Too-small endotracheal or tracheostomy tube b. Too long endotracheal or tracheostomy tube c. Inflated cuff d. T-piece weaning	3. An endotracheal tube's caliber and length influence flow resistance. Continuous positive airway pressure decreases the work of breathing as compared to T-piece weaning. For every 1-mm decrease in the endotracheal tube diameter, the work of breathing increases 34%–152% (Porth, 2007).
4. Assess for dyspnea.	4. Dyspnea interferes with successful weaning. A weaning schedule that reduces tidal volume slowly and increases endurance is recommended.
5. Position client to optimize oxygenation and prevent aspiration: a. Head of bed (HOB) at least 30 degrees b. Prone positioning (de Leon & Spiegler, 2005; Fineman, LaBrecque, Shih, & Curley, 2006)	5. An upright position maximizes diaphragm excursion, increasing lung volume and gas exchange. Maintaining HOB at least 30 degrees reduces aspiration risk. Prone positioning improves oxygenation in acute lung injury (ALI) or adult respiratory distress syndrome (ARDS) by recruiting alveoli and improving ventilation-perfusion mismatching (de Leon & Spiegler, 2005; Fineman et al., 2006).
6. Plan adequate rest periods before and after activity and during weaning efforts (Lynn-McHale Wiegand & Carlson, 2005).	6. Respiratory muscle fatigue can result from prolonged artificial ventilation, increased work of breathing, and reduction in energy reserves. a. Rest periods help to replenish energy expended in activity. b. Alternating weaning with rest periods on mechanical ventilation rests fatigued muscles.
7. Take precautions to prevent infection. Implement VAP bundle (Evans, 2005): a. Change tubing every 24–48 hours. b. Remove invasive lines as early as possible.	7. A client on long-term ventilation is at increased risk of infection owing to altered defense mechanisms and microorganisms on equipment and in the environment. Incidence of VAP can run as high as 65%, increase length

(continued on page 724)

Interventions	Rationales

c. Reduce endogenous organisms through frequent hand-washing, careful housekeeping, universal precautions, and other measures.
d. Remove Foley catheter early.
e. Ventilatory Acquired Pneumonia Protocol:
  • HOB elevated at least 30 degrees
  • Deep vein thrombosis (DVT) prophylaxis, peptic ulcer prophylaxis
  • Daily "sedation vacation"
  • Daily assessment for weaning readiness
  • Comprehensive oral care (Evans, 2005; Institute for Healthcare Improvement, n.d.; Pruitt & Jacobs, 2006).
  • Use of endotracheal tube capable of subglottic suction (CASS [continuous aspiration of subglottic secretions] tube) (DePew & McCarthy, 2007)
	of stay by 4.3 days, and have mortality rates from 20%–70% (Evans, 2005). Pathogens enter the lower respiratory tract by colonization of digestive and airways tracts and micro-aspiration of secretions. Subglottic suction evacuates secretions that are difficult to manually suction, lowering aspiration risk. Microaspiration occurs in 20%–40% of intubated clients, progressively increasing after three days of intubation (DePew & McCarthy, 2007).

8. Promote optimal nutrition:
 	
a. Consult nutritionist to calculate specific protein and calorie needs.
 	
b. Weigh client daily.
 	
c. Monitor laboratory study results:
  • Serum albumin and transferrin
  • CBC
  • Creatinine index
d. Maintain adequate hydration.
	8. In most cases, a client with an artificial airway is unable to meet his or her nutritional needs solely through oral ingestion. When supplemental feeding is required, the enteral route is preferred over the parenteral route because of the parenteral route's greater risk of catheter-related sepsis. Enteral feeding decreases the chances of GI bleeding and GI problems. Motility agents can promote gastric emptying and improve absorption (Newmarch, 2006).
	    Malnutrition has a negative effect on respiratory function, which depends on adequate muscle function and uses energy continuously. A malnourished client has a decreased response to hypoxia, expiratory muscle weakness, reduced muscle endurance, decrease surfactant, impaired immune responses, and fluid imbalances from electrolyte changes:
	a. Nurse may need assistance to calculate client's specific nutritional requirements according to metabolic demands. Caloric intake should be 1.4–1.6 times the energy expenditure. Underfeeding can increase risk of pulmonary complications; overfeeding can increase metabolic rate and carbon dioxide production.
	b. Actual weight on a properly calibrated scale can provide a reflection of overall nutritional status. Weekly weight loss of 1%–2% of total body weight is significant.
	c. Laboratory data can provide information on nutritional status, especially when weight fluctuates with fluid retention or loss.
	
	d. This reduces viscosity of secretions, decreasing airway resistance.

9. Take steps to reduce pain and anxiety to tolerable levels (e.g., analgesics, sedatives or nonpharmacologic pain relief measures such as relaxation, distraction, and guided imagery) to prevent ventilator asynchrony and reduce oxygen requirements (Kress & Hall, 2006; Newmarch, 2006; Pruitt & Jacobs, 2006). Use of neuromuscular blockade agents require careful monitoring and must include sedation.	9. Pain can contribute to anxiety, inhibit chest excursion on respiration, and increase oxygen consumption by 15%. Oversedation or prolonged sedation may lead to extended intubation times and ICU stay, and increased reintubation rates; oversedation can be prevented with the use of sedation scoring systems (Newmarch, 2006) or bispectral image monitoring. Peripheral nerve stimulation must be used with neuromuscular blockade to prevent excessive paralysis.

(continued on page 725)

Interventions	Rationales
10. Consult with physician to delay weaning if any of these factors occur: a. Metabolic alkalosis or acidosis b. Multisystem failure c. Clinical instability (Scales & Pilsworth, 2007) d. Decreased maximal inspiratory pressure (MIP) during weaning e. Rapid, shallow breathing during weaning (Scales & Pilsworth, 2007) f. Pain not controlled (Scales & Pilsworth, 2007) g. Client not awake enough to maintain airway or breathing (Scales & Pilsworth, 2007) h. Temperature elevates (Lynn-McHale Wiegand & Carlson, 2005)	10. a–d. A client who is not improving or is not clinically stable does not have the reserves to accommodate successfully to weaning. e. A malnourished client is unable to produce sufficient energy supplies to allow weaning. f,g. A decrease in MIP or rapid, shallow breathing in response to weaning indicates poor respiratory muscle strength.
11. Before weaning, discuss the process with client and family.	11. Adequate preparation is needed to reduce fears. Emphasizing the client's improvement, explain the procedure and provide constant supervision to improve motivation and decrease anxiety. Delayed weaning increases risk of complications and traumatic self-extubation by client (Scales & Pilsworth, 2007).
12. Before, during, and after weaning attempts, assess the following factors: a. Vital capacity b. Negative inspiratory pressure (Lynn-McHale Wiegand & Carlson, 2005) c. Vital signs d. Arterial blood gas values or SaO_2 (Scales & Pilsworth, 2007) e. Need/benefits for changing from endotracheal tube to tracheostomy tube (Scales & Pilsworth, 2007) f. Spontaneous tidal volume (Lynn-McHale Wiegand & Carlson, 2005) g. Positive end-expiratory pressure (Lynn-McHale Wiegand & Carlson, 2005)	12. The client's ventilator capacities and perfusion serve as criteria for evaluating whether or not to progress weaning.
13. Provide communication aids (e.g., letter boards, paper & pencil, lip reading, gestures, etc.) (Newmarch, 2006; Pruitt & Jacobs, 2006).	13. Ventilated clients are unable to speak because air bypasses the larynx. The inability to communicate can lead to discomfort and frustration (Newmarch, 2006; Pruitt & Jacobs, 2006).
14. Provide psychological support (e.g., explain procedures and alarms; assess if constant family presence during weaning is advantageous) (Happ et al., 2007; Newmarch, 2006; Pruitt & Jacobs, 2006).	14. Unaddressed psychosocial needs increase pain and anxiety (Pruitt & Jacobs, 2006).
15. Protect from skin breakdown.	15. Ventilated clients are often unstable and critically ill; inability to turn or mobilize increases opportunity for skin breakdown.

Documentation

Flow records
    Vital signs
    Ventilator settings

Type of tube (inflation)
Respiratory assessment
Intake and output
Bowel sounds
Rest and activity patterns
Suctioning provided and results
Pre-, intra-, and postweaning assessments
Client teaching
Progress notes
Psychological status

Pacemaker Insertion (Permanent)

A pacemaker is an electrical device implanted to help maintain normal cardiac rate and sometimes rhythm in the presence of sinoatrial (SA), atrioventricular (AV) node, or His-Purkinje system conduction disturbances (e.g., any bradycardia such as heart block, junctional rhythm, atrial fibrillation with a slow ventricular response, or asystole) and certain tachyarrhythmias (Hayes, 2006). In the implantation procedure, a bipolar or unipolar electrode is inserted through the subclavian vein into the right atrium or right ventricle under fluoroscopy. Biventricular pacing (cardiac resynchronization therapy) contains a third wire to the left ventricle, synchronizing the activity of both ventricles and improving cardiac function for congestive heart failure clients (Foo & Lin, 2005; Saxon, Kumar, & DeMarco, 2007). Permanent pacemakers may also come with a cardioversion/defibrillator mode that is initiated during lethal or tachycardic arrhythmias. Permanent pacemakers have a pulse generator implanted in a subcutaneous pouch in the upper right or left chest. Pacemaker generators also can be placed in a subcutaneous pouch in the abdomen with the pacemaker wires placed in the epicardial surface of the heart. This is done in conjunction with open-heart surgery or via a thoracotomy approach. The pulse generator houses the batteries, which eventually become depleted. When this occurs, the old generator is removed and a new one is implanted.

The Inter-Society Commission for Heart Disease has a code system for pacemakers to provide a method of communicating their functions. The code system has five letters but usually only three are used, except with permanent pacemakers. The code system is as follows (Hayes, 2007; Lynn-McHale Wiegand & Carlson, 2005):

1st letter—chamber being paced
    A-Atrium, V-Ventricle, D-Dual (both)
2nd letter—chamber being sensed
    A-Atrium, V-Ventricle, D-Dual, O-Off
3rd letter—type of response by pacemaker to sensory
    I-Inhibited (pacemaker will not function when the client's heart beats)
    T-Triggered, D-Dual, O-None
4th letter—Rate modulation (rate responsiveness)
    O-Unavailable or disabled
    R-Rate modulation present; sensor present that adapts to client activity
5th letter—ability for multisite pacing
    A-Atrium, V-Ventricle, D-Dual (A+V), O-None

 Time Frame
Preprocedure and postprocedure

■■■■■ DIAGNOSTIC CLUSTER

Preprocedure Period

Nursing Diagnoses

▲ Anxiety related to impending pacemaker insertion and prognosis

Postprocedure Period

Collaborative Problems

❋ PC: Perforation of the Right Ventricle
▲ PC: Cardiac Dysrhythmias
❋ PC: Pneumothorax
▲ PC: Pacemaker Malfunction (failure to sense, failure to fire, or failure to capture)
❋ PC: Infection
△ PC: Necrosis over Pulse Generator

Nursing Diagnoses

△ Impaired Physical Mobility related to incisional site pain, activity restrictions, and fear of lead displacement

△ High Risk for Ineffective Therapeutic Regimen Management related to insufficient knowledge of activity restrictions, precautions, signs and symptoms of complications, and follow-up care

▲ This diagnosis was reported to be monitored for or managed frequently (75%–100%).
△ This diagnosis was reported to be monitored for or managed often (50%–74%).
❋ This diagnosis was not included in the validation study.

Discharge Criteria

Before discharge, the client or family will

1. Demonstrate accuracy in counting a pulse.
2. Verbalize precautions to take with regard to the pacemaker.
3. State signs and symptoms that must be reported to a health care professional.
4. Verbalize an intent to share feelings and concerns related to the pacemaker with significant others.
5. Demonstrate site care.
6. Relate activity restrictions.

Preprocedure: Nursing Diagnoses

Anxiety Related to Impending Pacemaker Insertion and Prognosis

NOC Anxiety Level, Coping, Impulse Control

Goal

The client will

1. Verbalize the goal of pacemaker implantation as treatment, not cure.
2. Verbalize accurate information about the procedure and postprocedure care.

NIC Anxiety Reduction, Impulse Control, Anticipatory Guidance

Interventions	Rationales
1. Reinforce physician's explanation of the surgical procedure.	1. If anxiety impedes client's ability to assimilate information, repeated exposure to this or any other information may be helpful.
2. Assess client's understanding and notify physician if additional explanations are needed.	2. The physician is legally responsible for explaining the surgery to client and family; the nurse for determining the level of client understanding and notifying the physician if additional explanations are required.
3. Have client recall symptoms leading to the present point. Explain that symptoms are the manifestation of a heart-rhythm disturbance.	3. Recognition of symptoms as a manifestation of an underlying problem helps client to understand and accept the need for a pacemaker.
4. Show client a pulse generator, if available. Explain its functions (see description of letter codes).	4. Handling actual equipment provides visual and tactile information and helps client better understand the device and its operation.
5. If client is on cardiac monitor preprocedure, avoid placing ECG electrodes over potential incision sites on upper right or left chest.	5. Pulling off electrodes can cause potential skin breakdown and lead to possible infection postprocedure (Karchmer, 2007).
6. Describe preprocedural routine (as appropriate for client) of blood tests, ECG, chest x-ray film, and food and fluid restrictions.	6–9. Explaining what to expect may help to reduce client's anxiety related to fear of the unknown and unexpected, and may enhance his or her sense of control over the situation.
7. Explain that client will be awake during insertion, but that a sedative will be given to aid relaxation and a local anesthetic will be given to numb incisional area (Cotter et al., 2006; Foo & Lin, 2005).	
8. Explain physical appearance of catheterization laboratory or operating room, wherever the procedure will be done.	
9. Instruct client concerning pacemaker insertion and associated sensations; cover the following: a. Time of procedure b. Approximate length of procedure c. Attachment of telemetry leads to monitor cardiac rate and rhythm d. Insertion of intravenous lines to provide direct IV access, if needed e. Preparation of skin with a cold solution where incision is to be made f. Injection of local anesthetic into entire area where generator will be placed; explain that initial injection may burn slightly (Foo & Lin, 2005) g. Expected sensations of pressure and pulling during lead insertion, with no sensation after insertion is complete h. The need to notify nurse or physician of pain experienced during procedure i. Positioning x-ray machine over the body and loud clicking sounds from x-ray machine j. Possibility of palpitations during assessment of lead placement k. Creation of a small pocket underneath skin and closure with sutures (internal or external, depending on physician preference) (Foo & Lin, 2005)	

(continued on page 729)

Interventions	Rationales
l. Return to recovery room or unit on telemetry (Foo & Lin, 2005) m. Likelihood that he or she will notice the pulse generator under the skin for about 2 months; at this point conscious awareness of the implant should diminish and edema should be gone n. When client will be able to see family and other support persons postprocedure	
10. Instruct client on postprocedure routine; cover these factors (Cotter et al., 2006; Foo & Lin, 2005): a. Frequent monitoring of blood pressure, pulse and temperature, pulse oximetry b. Telemetry ECG c. Frequent assessment of insertion site d. Presence of pressure dressing over incision for about 24–48 hours after procedure	10. The client's understanding that careful monitoring is necessary to evaluate her or his response to the pacemaker can ease anxiety and encourage cooperation. d. The pressure dressing is to prevent bleeding into pacemaker pocket.
11. Instruct client not to use affected arm while transferring from or to the bed or pushing her- or himself up in bed for the first 24–48 hours. A sling may be applied to affected arm to help restrict movement.	11. Movement restrictions aim to prevent displacement of leads.
12. Instruct client to report the following immediately (Cotter et al., 2006): a. Pain at insertion site b. Palpitations c. Dizziness d. Hiccups or chest muscle twitching	12. Early detection enables prompt intervention to reduce the severity of complications. a. Pain at site may indicate compression from hemorrhage or edema. b. Palpitations can indicate failure of pacemaker to control heart rate. c. Dizziness may result from decreased cardiac output with resultant cerebral hypoxia resulting from pacemaker failure. d. Hiccups or chest muscle twitching may point to perforation of ventricle and stimulation of diaphragm or intercostal muscle by the lead.
13. Provide written materials that reinforce teaching.	13. Client and family can retain and refer to written materials after discharge. Such materials also can provide information to support persons not accompanying the client for teaching.
14. If possible, arrange for client to talk with a person who has successfully gone through pacemaker implantation.	14. A person who has had a pacemaker implanted successfully can provide a role model for the client and promote a relaxed, healthy attitude toward the procedure.
15. Refer client to clinical nurse specialist, social worker, or clergy if anxiety is dysfunctional.	15. For some clients, referrals may be necessary for intensive interventions and consultation.

Documentation

Teaching record
Client teaching
Outcome achievement or status
Progress notes
Unusual responses
Referrals, if indicated

Postprocedure: Collaborative Problems

Potential Complication: Perforation of the Right Ventricle

Potential Complication: Cardiac Dysrhythmias

Potential Complication: Pneumothorax

Potential Complication: Pacemaker Malfunction (failure to sense, failure to fire, or failure to capture)

Potential Complication: Infection

Potential Complication: Necrosis over Pulse Generator

Potential Complication: Lead Dislodgement

Potential Complication: Deep Vein Thrombosis

Potential Complication: Bleeding

Nursing Goal

The nurse will detect early signs and symptoms of (a) perforation of the right ventricle, (b) cardiac dysrhythmias, (c) pneumothorax, (d) pacemaker malfunction, (e) infection (site), and (f) necrosis over pulse generator, and will collaboratively intervene to stabilize the client.

Indicators

- Calm, alert, oriented (a, c)
- BP >90/60, <140/90 mmHg (a)
- Pulse 60–100 beats/min (a, b)
- Respirations 16–20 breaths/min (a, c)
- Respirations relaxed, rhythmic (a, c)
- Symmetrical chest movements (c)
- Breath sounds in all lobes (c)
- Flat neck veins (a)
- No complaints of chest pain (a, c)
- Stable pulse pressure (approximately 40 mm/Hg difference between diastolic and systolic pressure) (a, c)
- ECG—normal sinus rhythm implantation (b)
- Intact wound (site) (e, f)
- Minimal drainage or bleeding (e, f)
- Oxygen saturation (SaO_2) >94% (a, b, c)
- Carbon dioxide ($PaCO_2$) 35–45 mmHg (a, b, c)
- Arterial pH 7.35–7.45 (a, b, c)

Interventions	Rationales
1. Monitor for signs of perforation of right ventricle: a. Distended neck veins b. Hepatic engorgement c. Narrow pulse pressure d. Decreased blood pressure 2. Initiate emergency measures for cardiac arrest.	1,2. Perforation of right ventricle into left ventricle or pericardium results in decreased cardiac output, circulatory congestion (particularly in hepatic and neck areas), and shock.
3. Monitor for dysrhythmias.	3. Rhythm disturbances are common for 48–72 hours after implantation, owing to myocardial irritability and injury from lead insertion.
4. Monitor for signs and symptoms of pneumothorax (Lynn-McHale Wiegand & Carlson, 2005):	4. Placement of any catheter into the subclavian vein can potentially cause puncture of the lung on the affected side.

(continued on page 731)

Interventions	Rationales
a. Sudden shortness of breath b. Decreased or absent breath sounds c. Sudden stabbing chest pain d. Asymmetric chest movement e. Decreased arterial oxygen saturation f. Increased arterial carbon dioxide	
5. Monitor for electromagnetic interference marked by onset of pacemaker symptoms when near a source of electromagnetic interference (e.g., Transcutaneous Electrical Nerve Stimulator (TENS) units, electromagnets, MRI scanners or lithotripsy) or by intermittent failure to pace with an artifact absent. If this occurs, move client away from source of interference (Foo & Lin, 2005).	5. Electromagnetic interference can inhibit pacemaker function or cause it to revert to a fixed mode of pacing (Foo & Lin, 2005).
6. Monitor for sensing problems (Lynn-McHale Wiegand & Carlson, 2005). a. Monitor for undersensing (failure to sense). The pacemaker is not sensitive enough to the heart's own electrical signals and will pace as though there were no intrinsic signals. b. Monitor for oversensing. Pacemaker is too aware of the heart's intrinsic electrical signals or of other electrical signals such as skeletal muscle electrical signals. In this case, pacemaker will not pace if it senses these "false" electrical signals.	6. a. The danger of undersensing is that the pacemaker may deliver an unnecessary stimulus during ventricular repolarization (T-wave on the ECG) because it cannot sense intrinsic beats properly. Ventricular repolarization is the most vulnerable phase of the cardiac cycle and any electrical stimulus during this time can cause ventricular tachycardia or ventricular fibrillation. b. The danger of oversensing is that the pacemaker may interpret an inappropriate electrical signal as a QRS complex and will not pace when it should, thus reducing cardiac output and causing potential hemodynamic compromise.
7. Monitor for failure to fire. Pacemaker fails to deliver a stimulus, so there will be no pacer spike and no ventricular depolarization (no pacemaker spike and no QRS complex on the ECG) (Lynn-McHale Wiegand & Carlson, 2005).	7. Fractured lead wires, circuitry failure, or faulty lead connections can cause pacemaker to fail to fire. This can lead to slow heart rates, decreased cardiac output, and potential hemodynamic compromise.
8. Monitor for failure to capture. Pacemaker will deliver a stimulus at the appropriate pacing interval but it will not be followed by a ventricular depolarization (there will be a pacemaker spike at the appropriate time but no QRS complex on the ECG) (Lynn-McHale Wiegand & Carlson, 2005).	8. Failure to capture may be caused by lead displacement (lead is no longer in contact with endocardial surface), or by high thresholds of the myocardium from fibrosis, or ischemia at the lead tip. This can lead to slow heart rates, decreased cardiac output, and potential hemodynamic compromise (Lynn-McHale Wiegand & Carlson, 2005).
9. Monitor for pacemaker-mediated tachycardia with dual chamber pacemakers. This tachycardia is marked by sustained ventricular upper-rate limit pacing caused by loss of AV synchrony and retrograde conduction from ventricle to atrium.	9. Sustained upper rate ventricular pacing may cause hemodynamic compromise in some clients or feelings of palpitations.
10. Monitor for diaphragmatic or phrenic nerve pacing—diaphragmatic contractions or hiccups at the pacemaker rate with pacemaker artifact.	10. Lead placement near diaphragmatic portion of the right ventricle or tip of the atrial lead may be too close to the phrenic nerve, leading to stimulation of these nerves.
11. Monitor for chest muscle stimulation around the pulse generator; if it occurs, verify that client is not moving the pulse generator.	11. Chest muscle stimulation may result from high pacemaker output, high current density, lead fracture, flipped pulse generator, or low threshold to muscle pacing.

(continued on page 732)

Interventions	Rationales
12. Monitor the pulse generator implantation site for the following (Cotter et al., 2006): a. Hemorrhage b. Signs and symptoms of infection c. Skin inflammation or necrosis over and around pulse generator	12. The surgical implantation and the presence of a foreign body increase risk of hemorrhage, necrosis, and infection. Careful monitoring can help to ensure early detection of problems. Antibiotics are prescribed preprocedure and postprocedure prophylactically.
13. Obtain chest x-ray after insertion (Cotter et al., 2006).	13. Chest x-rays confirm lead placement and diagnose complications such as pneumothorax (Cotter et al., 2006).
14. No showering or bathing for 5–10 days (Cotter et al., 2006).	14. Bathing increases potential for incision infection that can spread to generator and pacing system (Cotter et al., 2006; Karchmer, 2007).

 Related Physician-Prescribed Interventions

Medications. Antibiotics (preprocedure and postprocedure)
Intravenous Therapy. Intravenous line for direct venous access
Laboratory Studies. Electrolytes, arterial blood gases
Diagnostic Studies. ECG, electrophysiology studies, chest x-ray film, echocardiogram, exercise stress test, Holter monitoring
Therapies. Pacemaker setting, site care, pulse counting, activity restrictions, pulse oximetry

Documentation

Flow records
Vital signs
Rhythm strips
Wound and dressing status
Unusual symptoms

Postprocedure: Nursing Diagnoses

Impaired Physical Mobility Related to Incisional Site Pain, Activity Restrictions, and Fear of Lead Displacement

NOC Ambulation: Walking, Joint Movement: Active, Mobility Level

Goal

The client will demonstrate the ability to perform activities of daily living (ADLs).

Indicator

- Demonstrate the ability to maintain arm restriction limitations.
- Verbalize prescribed restrictions.

NIC Exercise Therapy: Joint Mobility, Exercise Promotion: Strength Training, Exercise Therapy: Ambulation, Positioning, Teaching: Prescribed Activity/Exercise

Interventions	Rationales
1. Explain the need to remain on bed rest for up to 24 hours postprocedure (or as prescribed).	1. Bed rest is prescribed to allow fibrosis to occur around the pacemaker and electrodes; this helps to prevent dislodgement.
2. Medicate with prescribed analgesics before client engages in any activity (Cotter et al., 2006).	2. Judicious use of pain medication keeps pain signals from discouraging use of affected arm.
3. Explain that incision and subcutaneous pocket should feel sore for 3–4 weeks but that discomfort eventually disappears.	3. Understanding that discomfort is temporary encourages client to accept the pacemaker and participate in activity.
4. Explain that affected arm and shoulder should not be moved in an overzealous manner (i.e., over the head) for 48 hours, or as prescribed. Encourage client to perform active ROM (except for overzealous movements) in affected arm following physician's instructions.	4. Overzealous arm movements may potentially cause lead dislodgement, but regular active ROM exercise maintains joint function and prevents muscle contractures.
5. Encourage early and complete participation in ADLs.	5. Self-care increases independence and a sense of well-being.
6. Reinforce physician-prescribed postoperative activity restrictions; these may include no driving, lifting, golfing, bowling, etc., for 4–6 weeks after surgery (Cotter et al., 2006; Foo & Lin, 2005).	6. Activity restrictions allow continued fibrosis around pacemaker and electrodes to provide increased stabilization.
7. Provide written information on activity instructions and restrictions.	7. Written materials can serve as a valuable resource for post-discharge care at home.

Documentation

Discharge summary record
Level of activity
Client teaching
Outcome achievement or status
Referrals if indicated

High Risk for Ineffective Therapeutic Regimen Management Related to Insufficient Knowledge of Activity Restrictions, Precautions, Signs and Symptoms of Complications, and Follow-up Care

NOC Compliance Behavior, Knowledge: Treatment Regimen, Participation: Health Care Decisions, Treatment Behavior: Illness or Injury

Goals

The goals for this diagnosis represent those associated with discharge planning. Refer to the discharge criteria.

NIC Anticipatory Guidance, Learning Facilitation, Risk Identification, Health Education, Teaching: Procedure/Treatment, Health System Guidance

Interventions	Rationales
1. Review postprocedural routine, as needed (Cotter et al., 2006).	1. Reviewing enables nurse to evaluate whether or not client needs additional teaching.
2. Instruct on incisional care including the following (Cotter et al., 2006): a. Wound cleansing b. Suture removal, if present (usually after 7 days) c. Expected swelling for 2–4 weeks d. Recognizing signs and symptoms of infection e. For a woman, wearing a brassiere for support, with a gauze pad over the pulse generator to decrease rubbing over the suture line	2. Proper incision care helps to prevent infection and other complications.
3. Instruct client on home care measures (Cotter et al., 2006): a. Keep affected arm immobile for 24–48 hours post-procedure. b. Continue taking prescribed cardiac medication until otherwise instructed by physician.	3. Understanding home care enables client to comply with the regimen: a. Arm movement could cause traction on the lead and possible lead displacement. b. Pacemaker implantation does not preclude the need for medication.
4. Teach client and family to watch for and promptly report the following: a. Redness, swelling, warmth, drainage, or pain at the surgical wound, or temperature greater than 101°F b. Join stiffness, pain, and muscle weakness in affected arm c. Light-headedness, fainting, dizzy spells, or chronic fatigue d. Very rapid or very slow pulse e. Chronic hiccups or chest muscle twitching f. Swollen ankles or hands	4. Early detection enables prompt treatment to prevent serious complications. a. These signs and symptoms point to wound infection. b. Joint stiffness, pain, and muscle weakness may indicate neurovascular compression. c. Light-headedness, fainting, dizzy spells, or chronic fatigue may result from cerebral hypoxia owing to insufficient cardiac output secondary to pacemaker malfunction. d. Pulse changes may indicate pacemaker failure. e. Chronic hiccups or chest muscle twitching may indicate lead displacement and electrical stimulation of diaphragm or intercostal muscles. f. Swelling ankles or hands may indicate congestive heart failure related to insufficient cardiac output.
5. Instruct client to check with physician before engaging in the following activities: a. Driving b. Lifting anything weighing more than 25 lb c. Using an ax by lifting it over the head and dropping it to cut d. Participating in contact sports or sports such as golf or bowling e. Using an air hammer f. Firing a rifle from the affected side g. Serving overhead-style when playing tennis h. Diving head first into water	5. These activities could potentially damage either the pulse generator or leads.
6. Reassure that pacemaker should not interfere with sexual activity.	6. Specifically discussing sexual activity can reduce fears and let client share concerns.
7. Instruct client to carry a pacemaker identification card at all times (he or she will receive a temporary card before going home; pacemaker manufacturer will mail a permanent card later). Encourage client to apply for a Medic-Alert bracelet (Foo & Lin, 2005).	7. A pacemaker identification card and Medic-Alert bracelet provide important information to caregivers in emergency situations.

(continued on page 735)

Interventions	Rationales
8. Instruct client to notify physicians, nurses, and dentists about his or her pacemaker so that prophylactic antibiotics may be given before invasive procedures, if needed.	8. Because the pulse generator increases tissue susceptibility to infection, prophylactic therapy is indicated before many invasive procedures.
9. Instruct client to avoid strong electromagnetic fields, including magnetic resonance imaging equipment, arc welding equipment, high-intensity power lines, dental ultrasonic cleaners, drills, internal combustion engines, and poorly shielded microwave ovens (older microwave ovens): a. Instruct client to avoid leaning over open hood of a running car engine.	9. Electromagnetic fields can interfere with pacemaker function. A client with any anxiety about using a microwave oven should stand about 6 feet away from oven when it is operating: a. Anything that revolves at high revolutions can cause an electromagnetic field; therefore, this could lead to pacemaker malfunction.
10. Warn that pacemaker triggers magnetic detection alarms such as those found at airports. Instruct client to carry pacemaker identification card to verify pacemaker placement with airport security personnel.	10. This information allows client to inform airport security personnel at detectors to avoid misunderstanding and embarrassment.
11. Emphasize the necessity of long-term follow-up care; reinforce physician's instructions.	11. Regular follow-up care is essential for ongoing evaluation.
12. Explain that the battery is not lifelong and replacement might be necessary (average battery life is 5–10 years) (Foo & Lin, 2005).	12. Understanding the need for battery replacement assists with coping should replacement be needed.
13. Teach pulse-taking, if appropriate, and instruct client to notify physician if pulse rate falls below pacemaker set rate.	13. Pulse taking may help to enhance client's sense of control over the situation (although some studies show that clients can become anxious about pulse counting).
14. Instruct client on functions of pacemaker (refer to codes at the beginning of this care plan). Advise client to carry a card or wear an ID bracelet indicating pacemaker and functions of codes.	14. Pacemakers have varied options. In an emergency the specific options need to be known.
15. Explain the importance of seeking medical care or advice (phone) if shock function occurs.	15. Further evaluation may be needed.
16. Provide written instructional materials at discharge.	16. Written information reinforces teaching and serves as a resource at home.
17. Provide client with names and phone numbers of persons to call should questions or an emergency arise (day or night).	17. This can help to reassure client that direct access for assistance is always available.
18. Explain transtelephonic follow-up care, a system in which client uses a transmitter at home to have the pacemaker checked over the telephone.	18. Knowing what to expect after discharge may decrease client's anxiety. Transtelephone monitoring provides reassurance to client that the pacemaker is working properly and can determine the need for battery replacement. It does not preclude the need for physician follow-up visits.

Documentation

Discharge summary record
Client and family teaching
Outcome achievement or status

Peritoneal Dialysis

Peritoneal dialysis (PD)—the repetitive instillation and drainage of dialysis solution into and from the peritoneal cavity—uses the processes of osmosis, ultrafiltration, and diffusion to remove wastes, toxins, and fluid from the blood. PD uses the client's own peritoneal lining to serve as the semi permeable membrane through which diffusion, osmosis, and filtration occur (Wagner, Johnson, & Kidd, 2006). The procedure is indicated for acute or chronic kidney disease and severe fluid or electrolyte imbalances unresponsive to other treatments.

Numerous techniques for instillation and drainage of dialysis fluid have been developed. These methods are both manual and automated. Therapy can be continuous or automated.

Continuous therapies include continuous ambulatory peritoneal dialysis (CAPD), carried out manually by the client or carer, and automated peritoneal dialysis (APD) carried out by a PD machine. The variations of APD include continuous cycling peritoneal dialysis (CCPD), nocturnal peritoneal dialysis (NPD), optimized cycling peritoneal dialysis (OCPD), intermittent peritoneal dialysis (IPD), and tidal peritoneal dialysis (TPD) (Redmond & Doherty, 2005). CAPD is most commonly used and provides dialysate inflow with the disposable bag and tubing remaining connected, folded, and secured to the torso during dwell time. Exchanges are done four times per day with 2.0–2.5 liters. CCPD uses an automated cycler to perform exchanges during sleep and the abdomen is left full during the day. IPD consists of treatment periods with dwell time and alternates with periods of peritoneal cavity draining. Intermittent techniques use multiple short dwell exchanges three or four times a week. Automated intermittent exchanges may occur with repeated small TPD or at night. NPD. Manual IPD also may be done in hospitals for a prescribed number of cycles and length of time based on client requirements. Manual peritoneal dialysis requires careful control of dialysate instillation (2 liters), dwell time, and outflow (see Table 1).

 Time Frame
Pretherapy and intratherapy

■■■■■ DIAGNOSTIC CLUSTER

Collaborative Problems

▲ PC: Fluid Imbalances
▲ PC: Electrolyte Imbalances
▲ PC: Uremia
△ PC: Hemorrhage
△ PC: Hyperglycemia
△ PC: Bladder/Bowel Perforation
▲ PC: Inflow/Outflow Problems
✳ PC: Sepsis

Nursing Diagnoses	Refer to
▲ High Risk for Infection related to access to peritoneal cavity	
△ High Risk for Ineffective Breathing Pattern related to immobility, pressure, and pain	
△ Altered Comfort related to catheter insertion, instillation of dialysis solution, outflow, suction, and chemical irritation of peritoneum	
△ High Risk for Ineffective Therapeutic Regimen Management related to insufficient knowledge of rationale of treatment, medications, home dialysis procedure, signs and symptoms of complications, community resources, and follow-up care	
△ Imbalanced Nutrition: Less Than Body Requirements related to anorexia	Chronic Kidney Disease

(continued on page 737)

TABLE 1 Variations of Automated Peritoneal Dialysis Treatments

Type	Procedure
Continuous cycling peritoneal dialysis (CCPD)	Fluid is in contact with the peritoneum for 24 hours, the cycler machine is used at night and the client has a final fill of fluid which stays in the abdomen all day.
Nocturnal peritoneal dialysis (NPD)	Similar to CCPD, but with a dry day.
Optimized cycling peritoneal dialysis (OCPD)	An additional day exchange is carried out using the APD machine.
Intermittent peritoneal dialysis	12–20 hours each session, two to three times per week. Usually used in hospital, but not widely used because of low clearance rates.
Tidal peritoneal dialysis (TPD)	A reserve volume of dialysate is left in the abdomen at the end of each cycle to achieve greater solute clearance or prevent pain at the end of each drain.

(Adapted from Thomas 2002).

Nursing Diagnoses	Refer to
△ Interrupted Family Processes related to the effects of interruptions of the treatment schedule on role responsibilities	Chronic Kidney Disease
△ Powerlessness related to chronic illness and the need for continuous treatment	Chronic Kidney Disease

▲ This diagnosis was reported to be monitored for or managed frequently (75%–100%).
△ This diagnosis was reported to be monitored for or managed often (50%–74%).
✳ This diagnosis was not included in the validation study.

Discharge Criteria

Before discharge, the client or family will

1. Be able to demonstrate home peritoneal dialysis procedures, if appropriate.
2. State signs and symptoms of infection.
3. Discuss the expected effects of long-term dialysis on the client and family.
4. State signs and symptoms that must be reported to a health care professional.

Collaborative Problems

Potential Complication: Fluid Imbalances
Potential Complication: Electrolyte Imbalances
Potential Complication: Uremia
Potential Complication: Hemorrhage
Potential Complication: Hyperglycemia
Potential Complication: Bladder or Bowel Perforation
Potential Complication: Inflow or Outflow Problems
Potential Complication: Sepsis

Nursing Goal

The nurse will detect early signs and symptoms of (a) fluid imbalances, (b) electrolyte imbalances, (c) uremia, (d) hemorrhage, (e) hyperglycemia, (f) bladder or bowel perforation, (g) inflow or outflow problems, and (h) sepsis, and will intervene collaboratively to stabilize the client.

Indicators

- Alert, oriented, calm (a, b, c, g)
- Skin warm, dry, usual color, no lesions (a, c, d, e, g)
- No or minimal edema (a)
- BP >90/60, <140/90 mmHg (a, b, d, g)
- Pulse pressure (40 mmHg difference in systolic or diastolic) (a, b, d, g)
- Pulse 60–100 beats/min (a, b, d, g)
- Respirations 16–20 breaths/min (a, g)
- Respirations relaxed, rhythmic (a, g)
- No rales or wheezing (a)
- No weight change (a)
- Flat neck veins (a)
- No headache (b, g)
- Bowel sounds present (b)
- No chest pain (c)
- No abdominal pain (b, e, g)
- Intact reflexes (b)
- No change in vision (c)
- No complaints of nausea/vomiting (c, g)
- Intact muscle strength (b, c)
- No seizures (b)
- Serum potassium 3.5–5 mEq/L (b, c)
- Fasting blood glucose 70–110 mg/dL (e)
- Hemoglobin (d)
  - Male 13.5–17.5 g/dL
  - Female 13–16 g/dL
- Hematocrit (d)
  - Male 40%–54%
  - Female 37%–47%
- Serum sodium 135–148 mm/dL (c)
- Serum creatinine 0.6–1.2 mg/dL (c)
- Blood urea nitrogen 7–18 mg/dL (c)
- Patent inflow and outflow (g)
- Intact connections, no kinks (g)
- No urinary urgency (f)
- No glucose in urine (e, f)
- No bowel urgency (f)
- No diarrhea (c, f)
- No fecal material in dialysate (f)
  - White blood cell count >4000 cells/mms or <12,000 with bands <10% (g)
  - Temperature >96.8°F or <100.4°F (g)

Interventions	Rationales
1. Monitor for signs and symptoms of hypervolemia: a. Edema b. Dyspnea or tachypnea c. Rales or frothy secretions d. Rapid, bounding pulse e. Hypertension f. Jugular vein distention g. S_3 heart sounds	1. Hypervolemia may occur if dialysate does not drain freely or if excess IV or oral fluids have been infused or injected (Wagner, Johnson, & Kidd, 2006). Excess fluid greater than 5% of body weight is needed to produce edema. Fluid in lungs produces signs and symptoms of hypoxia. Increasing flow rate will increase fluid removal with little change in clearance of solutes.
2. Monitor for signs and symptoms of hypovolemia: a. Dry skin and mucous membranes	2. Hypovolemia may occur from excessive or too-rapid removal of dialysate fluid, inadequate salt and fluid intake,

(continued on page 739)

Interventions	Rationales
b. Poor skin turgor c. Thirst d. Tachycardia e. Tachypnea f. Hypotension with orthostatic changes g. Narrowed pulse pressure h. Altered level of consciousness	increased insensible loss, or overuse of hypertonic solution. Decreasing dextrose concentration to 1.5% may remove solutes without fluid (Wagner, Johnson, & Kidd, 2006; Baird, Keen, & Swearingen, 2005).
3. Monitor intake and output.	3. Urine output varies depending on renal status.
4. Enforce fluid restrictions, as ordered.	4. Physician may restrict fluid intake to insensible losses or the previous day's urine output.
5. Weigh daily or before and after each dialysis treatment.	5. Daily weights help to evaluate fluid balance.
6. Add medications to dialysate, as ordered.	6. Heparin commonly is added to decrease fibrin clots in the catheter. Potassium is added to prevent hypokalemia.
7. Monitor peritoneal dialysis inflow, dwell time, and outflow.	7. *Inflow* (usually taking less than 15 minutes) is the infusion of dialysis solution by gravity into the peritoneal cavity. *Dwell time* (0–20 minutes) is the length of time that the dialysis solution remains in the peritoneal cavity, which determines the amount of diffusion and osmosis that occurs. *Outflow* (usually less than 20 minutes) is the emptying of the peritoneal cavity by gravity.
8. Monitor for signs and symptoms of hypernatremia with fluid overload: a. Thirst b. Agitation c. Convulsions	8. Dialysate solution >4.25% or rapid outflow can cause hypernatremia (Redmond & Doherty, 2005).
9. Monitor for signs and symptoms of hyponatremia: a. Lethargy or coma b. Weakness c. Abdominal pain d. Muscle twitching or convulsions	9. Hyponatremia results from the dilutional effects of hypervolemia. Extracellular volume decrease lowers blood pressure and leads to hypoxia.
10. Monitor for signs and symptoms of hyperkalemia: a. Weakness or paralysis b. Muscle irritability c. Paresthesias d. Nausea, vomiting, abdominal cramping, or diarrhea e. Irregular pulse	10. Prolonged dwell time can increase potassium fluctuations that can affect neuromuscular transmission, reduce action of GI smooth muscles, and impair electrical conduction of the heart. Infusing dialysate with lower potassium than that of the plasma can decrease overall potassium.
11. Monitor for signs and symptoms of hypokalemia: a. Weakness or paralysis b. Decreased or absent tendon reflexes c. Hypoventilation d. Polyuria e. Hypotension f. Paralytic ileus	11. Hypokalemia impairs neuromuscular transmission and reduces action of respiratory muscles and GI smooth muscles. The kidneys become less sensitive to the effects of antidiuretic hormone and thus excrete large quantities of dilute urine.
12. Monitor for signs and symptoms of uremia: a. Skin and mucous membrane lesions b. Pericardial friction rub c. Pleural friction rub d. GI disturbances	12. A multisystem syndrome, uremia is a manifestation of end-stage renal disease resulting from waste products of protein metabolism including urea, creatinine, and uric acid. To increase removal of wastes, the number of exchanges can be increased.

(continued on page 740)

Interventions	Rationales

    e. Peripheral neuropathy
    f. Vision changes
    g. Central nervous system impairment
    h. Tachypnea
    i. Musculoskeletal changes

13. Monitor for vessel perforation and hemorrhage marked by increasingly bloody dialysate return.	13. Perforation of a blood vessel during catheter insertion can cause bloody dialysate, urine, or stool, or bleeding at insertion site.
14. Explain procedure and expected sensations and provide support during temporary catheter insertion.	14. Explanations encourage client to avoid sudden movement during catheter insertion.
15. If bleeding persists, apply a pressure dressing and carefully monitor vital signs.	15. Pressure may stop bleeding.

16. Monitor for signs and symptoms of hyperglycemia:
  a. Elevated or depressed blood glucose level
  b. Polyuria
  c. Polyphagia
  d. Polydipsia
  e. Abdominal pain
  f. Diaphoresis
	16. The amount of dextrose absorbed from the dialysate varies with dextrose concentration and number of cycles. In two cycles of 1.5% solution, 41 kcal are absorbed. After dialysis is complete, hypoglycemia may occur because of increased insulin production during instillation of high dextrose concentrations.

17. Monitor for signs and symptoms of bladder or bowel perforation:
  a. Fecal material in dialysate
  b. Complaints of urgency
  c. Increased urine output with high glucose concentrations
  d. Complaints of pressure in the sensation to defecate
  e. Watery diarrhea
	17. Catheter insertion may perforate bowel or bladder, allowing dialysate to infuse into bowel or bladder.

18. Have client empty bladder and bowel before insertion of peritoneal dialysis catheter.	18. Emptying bladder and bowel decreases risk of perforation during catheter insertion.
19. Monitor drug levels during dialysis to maintain therapeutic treatment (Tapasi & Harmeet, 2007).	19. Drugs may be added to the dialysate.

20. If inflow or outflow problems occur, do the following:
 	
  a. Increase height of the dialysate bag and lower the bed.
 	
  b. Reposition client and instruct him or her to cough.
 	
  c. Check for kinks and closed clamps.
  d. Remove a nontransparent dressing to check for catheter obstruction.
  e. Check dressing for wetness. Dialysate leaking from exit site presents as a clear fluid testing strongly for glucose.
  f. Assess abdominal pain on outflow.
 	
  g. Assess amount of dialysate return. Notify physician if >50% of inflow is retained (Tapasi & Harmeet, 2007; Pearce, 2007).
  h. Ascertain if heparin has been added to dialysate.
  i. If ordered, irrigate with heparinized saline (Redmond & Doherty, 2005).
	20. These measures can enhance the effectiveness of dialysis and prevent complications:
	  a. Raising the bag and lowering the bed can help to maximize gravity drainage.
	  b. Repositioning and coughing may help to clear a blocked or kinked catheter.
	
	  d. Dressing can obscure an external obstruction or kink.
	
	  e. Leakage at site may be from poor insertion technique or delayed healing and infection.
	  f. Abdominal pain may result from excessive suction on abdominal viscera or incorrect catheter position.
	  g. If catheter does not drain, omentum may be obstructing or fibrin may have formed in the catheter.
	
	  h,i. Heparin can help to prevent catheter blockage from fibrin or blood clots.

(continued on page 741)

Interventions	Rationales
j. If ordered, irrigate with fibrinolytic agents.	j. Fibrinolytic agents may be effective in removing blockage.
k. Assess for constipation.	k. Constipation may lead to shifting of catheter position, drainage failure, and catheter loss.
21. Calculate inflow and outflow volume at the end of each dialysis cycle. Report discrepancies in accordance with hospital protocol (Pearce, 2007).	21. Accurate inflow and outflow records determine fluid loss or retention by client.

 Related Physician-Prescribed Interventions

Medications. Heparinized saline, fibrinolytic agents
Laboratory Studies. Refer to either the Acute Kidney Failure or Chronic Kidney Disease care plan.
Therapies. Dialysate solution, dwell time, number of cycles

Documentation

Flow records
   Vital signs
   Intake and output
   Weight and medications
   Dialysate color
   Abdominal girth
   Serum glucose
   Urine specific gravity
   Other laboratory values
Progress notes
   Changes in status
   Inflow or outflow problems
   Interventions

Nursing Diagnoses

High Risk for Infection Related to Access to Peritoneal Cavity

NOC Infection Status, Wound Healing: Primary Intention, Immune Status

Goal

The client will be infection free at catheter site and will not develop peritonitis or a systemic infection.

Indicators

• Temperature >96.8°F or <100.4°F (Seaward-Hersh, 2004; Baird, Keen, & Swearingen, 2005).
• No edema or drainage at site.

NIC Infection Control, Wound Care, Incision Site Care, Health Education

Interventions	Rationales
1. Ensure use of sterile technique when setting up equipment.	1–5. Aseptic technique reduces microorganisms and helps prevent their introduction into the system.
2. Ensure complete skin preparation before catheter insertion.	

(continued on page 742)

Interventions	Rationales
3. Use sterile technique when assisting with catheter insertion or removal and when performing dialysis. Wear gloves to examine exit site.	
4. Apply masks to all staff and the client during catheter insertion, removal, and dressing changes.	
5. Minimize catheter movement at exit site (not to be used until site healed postinsertion, approximately 7 days) (Seaward-Hersh, 2004).	
6. Warm dialysate solution in a dedicated peritoneal dialysis microwave oven for the institution's recommended time frame. Agitate bag before infusing.	6. Because microwave ovens vary in rate, consistency, and method of heating, each institution needs to establish its own time frame (Seaward-Hersh, 2004; Baird, Keen, & Swearingen, 2005).
7. Determine that dialysate is between 36.5°C to 37.5°C (97.7 to 99.5°F) before infusing.	7. External temperature may be measured by folding the bag over an electronic thermometer (Seaward-Hersh, 2004; Baird, Keen, & Swearingen, 2005).
8. When performing manual peritoneal dialysis, prevent contamination of spikes when changing dialysate bags.	8. Peritoneal dialysate may be done manually with a manifold setup or by an automatic cycler (Redmond & Doherty, 2005). Use of bags allows the peritoneal dialysis system to remain closed except when spiking.
9. Monitor dialysate return for color and clarity. Obtain culture of any drainage.	9–13. Turbidity may indicate infection (Redmond & Doherty, 2005).
10. Perform routine exit site care using aseptic technique.	
11. Increase frequency of exit site care, as needed.	
12. Change cleansing agent for exit site care, as indicated.	
13. Teach alternative methods of exit site care.	

Documentation

Progress notes
    Signs and symptoms of infection
Flow records
    Dressing changes

High Risk for Ineffective Breathing Pattern Related to Immobility, Pressure, and Pain

NOC Respiratory Status: Gas Exchange, Vital Sign Status, Anxiety Control

Goal

The client will demonstrate optimal respiratory function.

Indicators

• Bilateral breath sounds, clear lung fields globally with no rales or crepitus
• Arterial blood gases

NIC Respiratory Monitoring, Progressive Muscle Relaxation, Teaching, Anxiety Reduction

Interventions	Rationales
1. Encourage regular coughing and deep-breathing exercises.	1. Hypoventilation may result from increased pressure on the diaphragm as a result of dialysate instillation and position during cycle. Pulmonary edema, pleuritis, infection, or uremic lung also may contribute to respiratory distress.
2. Evaluate effect of smaller dialysate solution volumes on adequacy and initiate if appropriate.	2–6. Stopping flow reduces pressure on the diaphragm, possibly relieving distress.
3. If client experiences respiratory distress, immediately stop inflow or begin outflow.	
4. Evaluate potential for PD modality change to cycling therapy.	
5. Support physical therapy, exercise, and weight loss program, as indicated.	
6. Administer analgesics, as indicated.	

Documentation

Progress notes
　Abnormal respiratory status

Altered Comfort Related to Catheter Insertion, Instillation of Dialysis Solution, Outflow Suction, and Chemical Irritation of Peritoneum

NOC Comfort Level, Pain Control

Goal

The client will be as comfortable as possible during peritoneal dialysis.

Indicators

Explain reason for discomforts

• No pressure or pain during the procedure
• Report measures used that reduced pain

NIC Respiratory Monitoring, Progressive Muscle Relaxation, Pain Management, Anxiety Reduction

Interventions	Rationales
1. Instruct client to report excessive pain on catheter insertion or dialysate installation. Have client describe pain's severity on a scale of 0–10 (0 = no pain; 10 = most severe pain).	1. Pain on catheter insertion calls for catheter repositioning; pain during dialysate installation may result from various factors including too-rapid inflow rate, cool dialysate temperature, and complications of treatment.
2. Position client to minimize pain while maintaining good air exchange and free-flowing dialysate.	2. Certain positions can reduce abdominal discomfort during instillation.
3. Drain effluent to assess for cloudy or bloody fluid. Initiate protocol for peritonitis, if indicated.	3. Lidocaine may be used as an intra-peritoneal analgesic (Wagner, Johnson, & Kidd, 2006; Baird, Keen, & Swearingen, 2005).

(continued on page 744)

Interventions	Rationales
4. As necessary, use nonpharmacologic pain relief techniques such as distraction, massage, guided imagery, and relaxation exercises.	4. Nonpharmacologic pain relief techniques can offer effective, safe alternatives to medication in some clients.
5. Check temperature of dialysate before and during instillation.	5. A too-cool dialysate temperature can cause abdominal cramps; too warm a temperature can cause tissue damage.
6. If client reports extreme pain during dialysis, decrease inflow rate and consult with physician to decrease temporarily the amount of dialysate instilled (Wagner, Johnson, & Kidd, 2006; Baird, Keen, & Swearingen, 2005).	6. A slower instillation rate reduces intra-abdominal pressure and may decrease pain. A decrease in volume reduces degree of abdominal distention, especially on initiation of dialysis.
7. Investigate carefully any client reports of pain in the shoulder blades.	7. Referred pain to the shoulders may be from diaphragmatic irritation or from air infused on insertion (Redmond & Doherty, 2005).

Documentation

Progress notes
　　Pain
　　Relief measures instituted
　　Client's response

High Risk for Ineffective Therapeutic Regimen Management Related to Insufficient Knowledge of Rationale of Treatment, Medications, Home Dialysis Procedure, Signs and Symptoms of Complications, Community Resources, and Follow-up Care

NOC Compliance Behavior, Knowledge: Treatment Regimen, Participation: Health Care Decisions, Treatment Behavior: Illness or Injury

Goals

The goals for this diagnosis represent those associated with discharge planning. Refer to the discharge criteria.

NIC Anticipatory Guidance, Learning Facilitation, Risk Identification, Health Education, Teaching: Procedure/Treatment, Health System Guidance

Interventions	Rationales
1. Reinforce physician's explanations of renal disease and of peritoneal dialysis procedure and its effects.	1,2. Client's understanding can help to increase compliance and tolerance of treatment.
2. Discuss all prescribed medications, covering purpose, dosage, and side effects.	
3. As appropriate, teach client the following and ask client to perform return demonstrations so nurse can evaluate client's ability to do procedures safely and effectively: a. Aseptic technique b. Catheter care and insertion c. Dialysate preparation d. Positioning during treatment e. Instilling additives to dialysate f. Inflow and outflow procedure	3. Many clients can perform home peritoneal dialysis without assistance. Proper technique can help to prevent infection and inflow and outflow problems (Swanson, 2004; Redmond & Doherty, 2005).

(continued on page 745)

Interventions	Rationales
4. Discuss how to manage inflow pain by ensuring proper temperature and flow rate of dialysate.	4. Cold dialysate, too-rapid inflow, acid dialysate, and stretching of diaphragm can cause inflow pain.
5. Teach client to maintain adequate protein and calorie intake.	5. Low serum albumin levels are known to be associated with an increased risk of death (Wagner, Johnson, & Kidd, 2006; Baird, Keen, & Swearingen, 2005).
6. Teach client to prevent constipation through adequate diet, fluid intake, and physical activity.	6. Constipation or bowel distention impedes dialysate outflow. Large protein losses occur with peritoneal dialysis (Wagner, Johnson, & Kidd, 2006; Baird, Keen, & Swearingen, 2005).
7. Teach client to watch for and promptly report: a. Unresolved pain from inflow b. Outflow failure c. Low-grade fever, cloudy outflow, malaise, and catheter site changes (redness, inflammation, drainage, tenderness, warmth, and leaks). d. Signs of fluid/electrolyte imbalance (see PC: Fluid Imbalance, PC: Electrolyte Imbalances for specific signs and symptoms of various imbalances) e. Abdominal pain, stool changes, constipation	7. Early detection of complications enables prompt intervention to minimize their seriousness (Wagner, Johnson, & Kidd, 2006; Baird, Keen, & Swearingen, 2005; Lewis et al., 2004): a. This finding can indicate intra-peritoneal infection. b. This finding may result from catheter obstruction, peritonitis, dislodged catheter, or a full colon. c. These signs can point to infection. d. Dialysis alters fluid and electrolyte levels, possibly resulting in imbalance. e. Bowel distention impedes outflow.
8. Provide information on where to purchase necessary supplies.	8. Knowledge of sources of supplies can prevent incorrect substitutions.
9. Teach client to record the following: a. Vital signs and weight before and after dialysis b. Percent of dialysate and amount of inflow c. Amount of outflow d. Number of exchanges required e. Medications taken f. Problems g. Urine output and number and character of stools	9. Accurate records aid in evaluating effectiveness of treatment.
10. Initiate referral to a home health care agency for necessary follow-up.	10. The initial home care visit is needed to evaluate client's suitability for home dialysis and takes into account factors such as physical condition, ability, environment, financial needs, and support system. Subsequent visits are indicated to assess client for signs of infection, improper procedures, and complications (e.g., electrolyte, fluid, and nutritional imbalances).
11. Provide information on available community resources and self-help groups (e.g., National Kidney Foundation).	11. Access to resources and self-help groups may ease difficulties of home dialysis and help to minimize its effects on home life.

Documentation

Discharge summary record
    Client and family teaching
    Outcome achievement or status
    Referrals, if indicated

Radiation Therapy

Radiation therapy is the use of high-energy ionizing radiation to destroy cancer cells. It also can serve as palliative treatment to relieve pain, prevent fracture, or mobilize a client following cord compression. When used in cancer treatment, radiation therapy aims to kill maximum cancer cells while causing minimal damage to normal tissue.

The ionizing radiation can be delivered in two ways. In *external beam radiation (teletherapy)*, a radioactive source or electromagnetic energy from a machine placed at some distance from the target site delivers the treatment. The distance is advantageous because the dose is relatively uniform across a given volume and allows for dose-shaping or modifying devices to be interposed between the source and the client. In *internal therapy (brachytherapy)*, the radioactive sources are placed directly into the tumor or tumor bed. A high dose is near the sources in the tumor bed and a much lower dose in the normal tissues. Combination teletherapy and brachytherapy is used in the treatment of many neoplasms. *Radiation sensitizers* are compounds that enhance the damaging effects of ionizing radiation. *Radioprotector* compounds protect cells and tissues from the damaging effects of radiation. A *radiolabeled antibody* is an antibody with a radioactive substance attached to its molecular structure that binds the antibody and radioisotope.

Tissues with a rapid rate of cellular division are more sensitive to the effects of radiation therapy. Some examples of radiosensitive tissues include bone marrow, epithelial cells lining the GI and genitourinary (GU) tracts, gonads, and hair follicles. Radioresistant tissues with a slow generation time, such as muscles, tendons, and nerves, have a less dramatic response. The response of tissues to radiation is divided into three specific time periods: *acute*, *subacute*, and *chronic*. Acute response period is the first 6 months after exposure to radiation. Subacute response period occurs 6 months to 1 year after exposure, and late or chronic response occurs 1–5 years longer after exposure to radiation.

General side effects include fatigue, anorexia, and skin alterations. The remaining side effects depend on the site treated (refer to site-specific chart) (Hilderley, 2000; Maher, 2005).

Site	Acute Effects	Late Effects

Head and neck	Eye
	  Dryness
	  Itching
	Other
	  Mucositis
	  Xerostomia
	  Dysphagia
	  Taste alterations
	  Pharyngitis
		Eye
		  Cataracts
		  Optic nerve
		  Keratitis
		  Glaucoma
		  Retinal hemorrhage
		  Sicca
		Other
		  Xerostomia or dental caries
		  Osteoradionecrosis
		  Taste changes
		  Trismus
		  Soft tissue edema
		  Subcutaneous fistula
		  Flap necrosis
		  Hypothyroidism

Chest	Esophagus
	  Esophagitis
	
	Lung
	  Pneumonitis
	  Dysphagia
	  Dyspnea
	
	Breast
	  Breast Edema
	  Lymphedema
		Esophagus
		  Stricture
		  Fistula
		
		Lung
		  Pneumonitis
		  Fibrosis
		  Alveolar type II pneumocytes
		
		Heart
		  Coronary artery disease
		  Pericarditis

(continued on page 747)

Abdomen	Stomach	Stomach
	Retching	Atrophy
	Nausea	Ulcer
	Vomiting	Liver
	Indigestion	Hepatitis
		Cirrhosis
Pelvis	Bowel	Bowel
	Diarrhea	Adhesions
		Enteritis
		Proctitis
	Bladder	Bladder
	Cystitis	Contracted bladder
	Dysuria	Cystitis
	Urinary frequency/urgency	
	Hematuria	
	Urinary incontinence	
	Urinary retention	
	Vagina	Vagina
	Vaginal discharge	Fibrosis
	Amenorrhea	Loss of lubrication
	Vaginal dryness	Gonadal effects
	Dyspareunia	Impotence
		Loss of fertility
		Ovary—menstrual irregularity or cessation
		Testis—oligospermia; aspermia
		Genetic effects
		Alopecia
Brain and central nervous system	Cerebral edema	
	Motor deficits	
	Nausea/vomiting	
	Neurologic deficits	
	Sensory deficits	

 Time Frame
Pretherapy and intratherapy

■■■■■ DIAGNOSTIC CLUSTER

Collaborative Problems	Refer to
▲ PC: Myelosuppression (Infection, Bleeding)	
PC: Malabsorption	
PC: Pleural Effusion	
PC: Cerebral Edema	
△ PC: Cystitis, Urethritis, and Tenesmus	
△ PC: Mucositis, Esophagitis, Pneumonitis	
△ PC: Myelitis and Parotitis	
△ PC: Fluid and Electrolyte Imbalance	Renal Failure

(continued on page 748)

Nursing Diagnoses	Refer to
▲ Anxiety related to prescribed radiation therapy and insufficient knowledge of treatments and self-care measures	
△ High Risk for Impaired Oral Mucous Membrane related to dry mouth or inadequate oral hygiene	
▲ Impaired Skin Integrity related to effects of radiation on epithelial and basal cells and effects of diarrhea on perineal area	
△ Impaired Comfort related to stimulation of the vomiting center and damage to the gastrointestinal mucosa cells secondary to radiation	Gastroenteritis
▲ Fatigue related to systemic effects of radiation therapy	
Impaired Comfort related to damage to sebaceous and sweat glands secondary to radiation	Inflammatory Joint Disease Cirrhosis
▲ Imbalanced Nutrition: Less Than Body Requirements related to decreased oral intake, reduced salivation, mouth discomfort, dysphasia, nausea/vomiting, increased metabolic rate, and diarrhea	Chemotherapy
△ Disturbed Self-Concept related to alopecia, skin changes, weight loss, sterility, and changes in role, relationships and life styles	Cancer: Initial Diagnosis
△ Grieving related to changes in life style, role, finances, functional capacity, body image, and health losses	Cancer: Initial Diagnosis
△ Interrupted Family Processes related to imposed changes in family roles, relationships, and responsibilities	Cancer: Initial Diagnosis

▲ This diagnosis was reported to be monitored for or managed frequently (75%–100%).
△ This diagnosis was reported to be monitored for or managed often (50%–74%).

Discharge Criteria

Before discharge, the client or family will

1. Relate skin care, oral care, and rest requirements.
2. State the intent to discuss fears and concerns with a trusted friend.
3. Relate signs and symptoms that must be reported to a health care professional.

Collaborative Problems

Potential Complication: Myelosuppression (Infection, Bleeding)

Potential Complication: Malabsorption

Potential Complication: Pleural Effusion

Potential Complication: Cerebral Edema

Potential Complication: Cystitis, Urethritis, and Tenesmus

Potential Complication: Mucositis, Esophagitis, Pneumonitis
Potential Complication: Myelitis and Parotitis

Nursing Goal

The nurse will monitor to detect early signs and symptoms of (a) myelosuppression (infection, bleeding), (b) malabsorption, (c) pleural effusion, (d) cerebral edema, (e) mucositis (esophagitis, pneumonitis), (f) cystitis, urethritis, and tenesmus, and (g) myelitis and parotitis, and collaboratively intervene to stabilize client.

Indicators

- Calm, alert oriented (a, c, d)
- Temperature 98.5–99°F (a, c, d)
- Pulse 60–100 beats/min (a, c, d)
- Stable pulse pressure (approximately 40 mmHg difference between diastolic and systolic pressures) (d)
- BP >90/60, <140/90 mmHg (a, c, d)
- Respirations 16–20 breaths/min (a, c, d, e)
- No rales or wheezing (a, c, d, e)
- Respirations relaxed, rhythmic (a, c, e)
- Breath sound in all lobes (a, d)
- Clear sputum (a, d)
- No abdominal pain (b)
- No chest pain (c)
- No rectal, abnormal vaginal, or nasal bleeding (a)
- No prolonged bleeding after invasive procedure (e.g., IV, IM) (a)
- No evidence of petechiae or ecchymoses (pinpoint or more diffuse bleeding under skin) (a, b)
- Clear, yellow urine (a)
- Urine output >5 mL/kg/h (a)
- Urine specific gravity 1.005–1.030 (e)
- Sensation intact (b)
- Strength intact (d)
- Range of motion intact (d)
- No change in vision (d)
- Pupils equal and reactive to light (d)
- Pinkish or brownish oral mucous membranes (e)
- Oral mucous membranes intact (e)
- No swallowing difficulties (e)
- Stable weight (b, e)
- No nausea and vomiting (d)
- No change in urge to void or defecate (f)
- No edema in parotid glands (g)
- White blood cell count 4800–10,000/mm³ (a)
- Red blood cell count (a)
  - Male 4,600,000–6,200,000/mm³
  - Female 4,200,000–5,400,000/mm³
- Platelet count 100,000–400,000/mm³ (a)
- Hemoglobin (a, b)
  - Male 13–18 g/dL
  - Female 12–16 g/dL
- Hematocrit (a, b)
  - Male 42%–50%
  - Female 40%–48%
- Serum iron 50–160 µg/dL (b)
- Vitamin B$_6$ 3.6–1.8 mg/mL (b)
- Folic acid 2.5–20 ng/mL (b)
- Prothrombin time 9.5–12 (b)
- INR 1.0 (b)
- No change at radiation site (f)
- No change in bowel function (b)
- Normal chest x-ray (c)

Interventions	Rationales
1. Monitor for signs of myelosuppression: a. Decreased WBC and RBC counts b. Decreased platelet count	1. Myelosuppression (bone marrow depression) occurs when large volumes of active bone marrow are irradiated (e.g., pelvis, brain, chest, long bones). The results are decreased production of WBCs and platelet cells. RBCs are less affected because of their longer life span (Hilderley, 2000, Maher, 2005).
2. Monitor for signs and symptoms of spontaneous or excessive bleeding: a. Petechiae, ecchymoses, or hematomas b. Bleeding from nose or gums c. Prolonged bleeding from invasive procedures d. Hemoptysis e. Hematuria f. Vaginal bleeding g. Rectal bleeding h. Change in vital signs i. Change in neurologic status j. Change in respiratory status	2. Platelets are most important for hemostasis or the formation of a hemostatic mechanical plug. They also facilitate the action of clotting factors of the intrinsic system when needed. Platelets are required for lysis of the fibrin clot and vessel repair. When platelet levels are decreased, clotting is impaired and uncontrolled bleeding can occur (Gobel, 2005).
3. Instruct client to: a. Use soft toothbrushes. b. Use electric razors. c. Avoid injections. d. Avoid medications that interfere with hemostasis/platelet function. e. Avoid venipuncture. If necessary, avoid prolonged tourniquet use. Apply direct pressure 3–5 minutes after. f. Avoid forceful coughing, sneezing, nose blowing. g. Avoid straining during defecation.	3. Clients with diminished clotting ability and at risk for infection are taught methods to prevent trauma, which can initiate bleeding or be a site for infection (Gobel, 2005).
4. Monitor for signs and symptoms of infection: a. Fever b. Redness/swelling at site c. Pus formation d. Pain/discomfort	4. Lymphocytes provide long-term protection against various microorganisms. They produce antibodies that neutralize foreign proteins and facilitate phagocytosis (Ellerhorst-Ryan, 2000; Shelton, 2005).
5. Explain risks of bleeding and infection. (Refer to the Corticosteroid Therapy care plan for strategies to reduce the risk of infection.)	5. Refer to rationales 2 and 4.
6. Monitor for signs and symptoms of malabsorption: a. Diarrhea b. Steatorrhea c. Abdominal pain d. Iron deficiency anemia e. Easy bleeding or bruising f. Paresthesias g. Skin and vision changes h. Weight loss i. Abnormal laboratory study results: vitamin B_{12}, folic acid, hemoglobin, hematocrit, electrolytes, and prothrombin time and International Normalized Ratio (INR)	6. Radiation damage to the small intestine results in shortening of intestinal villi and loss of absorptive surface. Radiation doses >5000 rads to the pelvis or abdomen can denude intestinal mucosa, impairing absorption of amino acids, carbohydrates, fats, fat-soluble vitamins (A, E, D, K), folic acid, vitamin B, and iron (Foltz, 2000; Cunningham & Huhmana, 2005).
7. Monitor for signs and symptoms of pleural effusion: a. Dyspnea b. Cough c. Chest pain	7. High-dose radiation therapy to the lungs can cause lung inflammation (pneumonitis) and changes in membrane transfer capability, leading to fluid leakage into the interpleural space (Hilderley, 2000; Maher, 2005).

(continued on page 751)

Interventions	Rationales
d. Tachycardia e. Tachypnea f. Bulging of intercostal spaces g. Decreased breath sounds h. Abnormal chest x-ray film	
8. Monitor for signs and symptoms of cerebral edema: a. Restlessness, irritability, memory loss b. Somnolence c. Headache d. Vomiting e. Seizure activity f. Increased systolic blood pressure with widening pulse pressure g. Bradycardia h. Depressed respirations i. Weakness j. Hemiparesis k. Vision changes l. Abnormal pupillary response to light	8. Radiation therapy administered to treat radiosensitive brain tumors such as medulloblastomas or metastatic brain tumors can cause cerebral edema. Effects mimic those of increased intracranial pressure (Hilderley, 2000; Maher, 2005).
9. Monitor for signs and symptoms of mucositis: a. White patches on oral mucosa b. Reddened, swollen mucous membranes c. Ulcerated, bleeding lesions	9. Radiation therapy commonly causes tissue inflammation; higher doses generally produce more damage. Severe mucositis may necessitate interruption of radiation therapy (Hilderley, 2000).
10. Instruct client to do the following: a. Perform diphenhydramine (Benadryl) mouth irrigations every 4 hours. b. Avoid alcohol, smoking, and spicy or acidic foods. c. Avoid very hot or cold liquids and foods.	10. These agents can help to reduce or ease pain of local inflammation. Alcohol, smoking, hydrogen peroxide, spicy or acidic foods, and very hot or cold foods and liquids can irritate mucosa (Hilderley, 2000; Maher, 2005).
11. Monitor for signs and symptoms of pneumonitis: a. Shortness of breath b. Hemoptysis c. Dry cough 12. Monitor for signs and symptoms of esophagitis: a. Difficulty swallowing b. Sore throat c. Nausea and vomiting	11,12. Radiation to the chest or back can cause pneumonitis or esophagitis (Hilderley, 2000; Maher, 2005).
13. Monitor for signs and symptoms of cystitis or urethritis. a. Urinary urgency and frequency b. Hematuria c. Dysuria d. Negative urine cultures	13. Irradiation of the pelvic area can cause cystitis or urethritis. Symptoms mimic those of urinary tract or bladder infection except with negative urine cultures (Hilderley, 2000; Maher, 2005).
14. Monitor for tenesmus: a. Persistent sensation of need to void or defecate	14. Radiation to the anal or urinary sphincter area can cause mucositis of sites (Hilderley, 2000; Maher, 2005).
15. Monitor for signs and symptoms of myelitis: a. Paresthesias in back or extremities b. Shocklike sensation on neck flexion 16. Monitor for signs and symptoms of parotitis: a. Painful, swollen parotid glands	15,16. Radiation therapy to head and neck can cause myelitis or parotitis. These problems usually are transient, not serious, and resolve spontaneously (Hilderley, 2000; Maher, 2005).

Related Physician-Prescribed Interventions

Depend on cancer site, stage, and extent

Documentation

Flow records
Intake and output
Abnormal laboratory values
Assessments (skin, oral, respiratory, neurologic)
Stool for occult blood
Daily weights

Nursing Diagnoses

Anxiety Related to Prescribed Radiation Therapy and Insufficient Knowledge of Treatment and Self-Care Measures

 Anxiety Level, Coping, Impulse Control

Goal

The client will report less anxiety after teaching.

Indicators

• Verbalize rationale for radiation treatment and treatment plan.
• Identify expected side effects and their management.
• Describe self-care measures to reduce fatigue, promote nutrition, manage skin problems, and prevent infection and bleeding.

NIC Energy Management, Exercise Promotion, Sleep Enhancement, Mutual Goal Setting

Interventions	Rationales
1. Encourage client to share fears and beliefs regarding radiation therapy. Delay teaching if client is experiencing severe anxiety.	1. Sharing enables nurse to identify sources of client anxiety and to correct misinformation. Severe anxiety prevents retention of learning.
2. Review general principles of radiation therapy, as necessary. Provide written materials such as a client education booklet from the National Cancer Institute.	2. A client undergoing radiation therapy is likely to have many questions about the treatment and its effects. Reinforcing information provided by the physician and radiologist and answering questions can help to reduce client's anxiety related to lack of knowledge (Hilderley, 2000; Maher, 2005).
3. Reinforce physician's explanation of the treatment plan; cover the following items: a. Area to be irradiated b. Treatment schedule c. Dose to be administered d. Simulation to compute dose and delivery of radiation e. Markings and tattoos f. Shielding of vital organs	3. This information can help to reduce client's anxiety associated with fear of the unknown and the unexpected.
4. Explain the fatigue that accompanies radiation therapy.	4. Several factors can contribute to fatigue: recent surgery, chemotherapy, pain, malnourishment, medications, frequency of treatments, tumor burden, anemia, and respiratory compromise (Hilderley, 2000; Maher, 2005).

(continued on page 753)

Interventions	Rationales
5. Refer to Fatigue in index for additional interventions.	
6. Explain skin reactions and precautions. (Refer to Impaired Skin Integrity in this care plan.)	

7. Explain site-specific radiation side effects:
  a. Neck:
    • Mucositis
    • Dry mouth
    • Altered taste
    • Dental problems
    • Hoarseness
    • Dysphagia
  b. Head:
    • Headache
    • Alopecia
    • Nausea and vomiting
  c. Chest and back:
    • Pneumonitis
    • Esophagitis
  d. Abdomen and pelvis:
    • Nausea and vomiting
    • Cystitis
    • Tenesmus
    • Diarrhea
    • Abdominal cramps
	7. Understanding what to expect can decrease anxiety related to fear of the unknown and the unexpected and can help client to recognize and report adverse effects.

Documentation

Progress notes
Anxiety level
Client teaching
Outcome achievement or status

High Risk for Impaired Oral Mucous Membrane Related to Dry Mouth or Inadequate Oral Hygiene

NOC Oral Hygiene

Goal

The client will maintain intact oral mucosa.

Indicators

• Describe the possible effects of radiation on the oral cavity.
• Explain proper techniques for oral care.

NIC Oral Health Restoration, Chemotherapy Management, Oral Health Maintenance

Interventions	Rationales
1. Explain signs and symptoms of mucositis and stomatitis.	1. Client's understanding can help to ensure early detection and prompt intervention to minimize problems.
2. Stress the need to have caries filled and bad or loose teeth extracted before initiation of radiation therapy to the head and neck.	2. Preexisting dental problems increase risk of radiation-induced infection.

(continued on page 754)

Interventions	Rationales
3. Emphasize the need for regular oral hygiene during and after therapy. Instruct client to do the following: a. Brush with fluoridated toothpaste after meals. b. Use a soft-bristle toothbrush. c. Rinse mouth with topical fluoride solution after each brushing. d. Use a molded dental carrier and fluoride gel daily.	3. Proper oral hygiene eliminates microorganisms and reduces risk of infection.
4. If gingival tissue becomes inflamed, suggest an oral rinse.	4. Rinsing removes debris and microorganisms without causing trauma to mucosal tissue.
5. Teach client to avoid the following: a. Commercial mouthwashes b. Very hot foods/drinks c. Alcoholic beverages d. Tobacco e. Highly seasoned foods f. Acidic foods (grapefruit, tomatoes, and oranges)	5. These substances are irritating to oral mucosa and can increase inflammation (Hilderley, 2000; Maher, 2005).
6. Explain the need for dental examinations during and after course of treatment.	6. Increased risk of dental caries and gum disease persists for months to years after completion of radiation therapy. Long-term follow-up dental care decreases the risk.

Documentation

Flow records
    Mouth assessment
    Oral care
Teaching record
    Client teaching
    Outcome achievement or status

Impaired Skin Integrity Related to Effects of Radiation on Epithelial and Basal Cells and Effects of Diarrhea on Perineal Area

NOC Tissue Integrity: Skin & Mucous Membranes

Goal

The client will demonstrate healing of tissue.

Indicators

* Relate strategies to reduce skin damage.
* Relate importance of good nutrition.

NIC Pressure Management, Pressure Ulcer Care, Skin Surveillance, Positioning

Interventions	Rationales
1. Explain the effects of radiation on skin (e.g., redness, tanning, peeling, itching, hair loss, decreased perspiration), and monitor skin in the irradiated area(s).	1. Radiation damages epithelial, sebaceous, and hair follicle cells, causing localized skin reactions. Understanding the reason for these effects can promote compliance with protective and preventive measures (Hilderley, 2000; Maher, 2005).

(continued on page 755)

Interventions	Rationales
2. Explain the need for optimal nutritional intake; provide instruction.	2. During radiation treatments, the body must build and repair tissue and protect itself from infection. This process requires increased intake of protein, carbohydrates, vitamins, and minerals (Hilderley, 2000).

3. Teach client the precautions to protect skin integrity:
  a. Do not wash treated area until therapist allows.
  b. If tattoos are used for skin markings, wash irradiated skin with a mild soap and tepid water; do not remove markings.
 	
  c. Avoid harsh soap, ointments, creams, cosmetics, and deodorants on treated skin unless approved by health care professionals.
  d. Avoid exposure of radiated skin to sun, chlorinated pools, wind, and shaving.
  e. Wear loose-fitting cotton clothing over treated skin.
 	
  f. Apply a thin layer of vitamin A and D ointment for dry skin if needed.
  g. Apply cool air to the affected area; avoid heat lamps and warmth.
  h. Use an electric razor only—no blades—to shave irradiated area.
  i. If moist desquamation is present, shower or irrigate the area frequently; use a moist wound healing dressing.
	3. These measures can help to maintain skin integrity:
	  a. Moisture enhances skin reactions.
	  b. To reduce irritation, harsh soaps and hot water should be avoided. The tattoo must remain to guide evaluation and subsequent therapy, if necessary.
	  c. Harsh substances may increase skin's vulnerability to damage.
	
	  d. This exposure can cause additional damage.
	
	  e. Loose-fitting cotton clothing can minimize irritation and injury to the epithelial surface.
	  f. Vitamin A and D ointment can prevent or treat dry skin.
	
	  g. Coldness reduces irritating sensory stimulation (e.g., pruritus) and prevents moist desquamation.
	  h. An electric razor can protect sensitive skin from razor cuts.
	
	  i. Showering or irrigation and moist wound dressings can help to debride the area and aid healing.

4. Instruct client to report any skin changes promptly.	4. Early detection of moist desquamation with shedding of surface epithelium enables prompt intervention to prevent severe skin damage and subsequent fibrosis.
5. Teach client to keep rectal and perineal areas clean and to apply protective ointment after each cleaning.	5. Good hygiene and application of non–water-soluble ointments reduce erosion of acidic excreta on perineal area.

6. After skin is completely healed, teach client sun precautions:
  a. Use no. 15 sun block.
  b. Increase exposure time very slowly.
  c. Discontinue sun exposure if redness occurs.
  d. Protect treated skin with hats and long sleeves.
	6. Radiation will temporarily deter the protective capacity of the epidermis, so specific precautions are required (Hilderley, 2000).

Documentation

Flow records
    Skin assessments
Teaching record
    Client teaching
    Outcome achievement or status

Total Parenteral Nutrition

Total parenteral nutrition (TPN) involves intravenous (IV) administration of an elemental diet (dextrose, amino acids, and lipids) in a hypertonic solution to a client who cannot ingest or assimilate sufficient calories or who has increased metabolic needs that oral ingestion cannot meet. Total nutritional admixture (TNA) system combines IV lipids with the base TPN solution. This admixture is often referred to as three-in-one solution because it contains dextrose, amino acids, and lipids. TPN solutions that contain more than 10% dextrose may be infused only in a central line. Indications for TPN include cancer, chronic nausea, and vomiting of any etiology, prolonged bowel rest, anorexia nervosa, massive burns, and GI disorders such as inflammatory bowel disease, bowel obstruction, or fistula.

 Time Frame
Intratherapy

▣▪▪▪▪▪ DIAGNOSTIC CLUSTER

Collaborative Problems

△ PC: Pneumothorax, Hemothorax, or Hydrothorax
△ PC: Air Embolism
▲ PC: Sepsis
▲ PC: Hyperglycemia
▲ PC: Metabolic Complications

Nursing Diagnoses

▲ High Risk for Infection related to catheter's direct access to bloodstream Disturbed Self-Concept related to inability to ingest food

✳ High Risk for Activity Intolerance related to deconditioning

△ High Risk for Ineffective Therapeutic Regimen Management related to insufficient knowledge of home care, signs and symptoms of complications, catheter care, and follow-up care (laboratory studies)

▲ This diagnosis was reported to be monitored for or managed frequently (75%–100%).
△ This diagnosis was reported to be monitored for or managed often (50%–74%).
✳ This diagnosis was not included in the validation study.

Discharge Criteria

Before discharge, the client or family will

1. Demonstrate proper catheter care and TPN administration at home.
2. Discuss strategies for incorporating TPN management into ADLs.
3. Verbalize precautions for medication use.
4. Relate causes, prevention, and treatment of hypoglycemia and hyperglycemia.
5. State signs and symptoms that must be reported to a health care professional.

Collaborative Problems

Potential Complication: Pneumothorax, Hemothorax, or Hydrothorax

Potential Complication: Air Embolism

Potential Complication: Sepsis

Potential Complication: Hyperglycemia

Potential Complication: Metabolic Complications

Nursing Goal

The nurse will detect early signs and symptoms of (a) pneumothorax, hemothorax, or hydrothorax, (b) air embolism, (c) sepsis, (d) hyperglycemia, and (e) metabolic complications, and will intervene collaboratively to stabilize the client.

Indicators

- Alert, calm, oriented (a, b, c, d, e)
- Respirations 16–20 breaths/min (a, b, e)
- Respirations relaxed, rhythmic (a, b, e)
- Pulse 60–100 beats/min (a, b, e)
- BP >90/60, <140/90 mmHg (a, b, e)
- Temperature 98.5–99°F (c)
- Flat neck veins (b)
- Skin usual color, dry, warm (a, b, e)
- No complaints of chest pain (a, b)
- Urine output >5 mL/kg/h (d, e)
- Specific gravity 1.005–1.030 (d, e)
- Urine negative for glucose (d, e)
- Negative blood cultures (c)
- Intact insertion site (c)
- No drainage at insertion site (c)
- No or minimal weight loss (d)
- Phosphorous 3.0–4.5 mg/dL (e)
- Calcium 8.5–10.5 mg/dL (e)
- Aspartate transaminase (AST) 7–21 u/L (e)
- Alanine transaminase (ALT) 5–35 u/L (e)
- Sodium 135–145 mEq/L (e)
- Magnesium 1.5–2.5 mEq/L (e)
- Potassium 3.5–5.0 mEq/L (e)
- Total cholesterol <200 mg/dL (e)
- Triglycerides (e)
  - Male 40–160 mg/dL
  - Female 35–135 mg/dL
- Blood glucose <140 mg/dL (e)
- Prealbumin 3–7 (e)
- Serum ammonia 20–120 µg/dL (e)
- Blood urea nitrogen 5–25 mg/dL (e)
- Creatinine 0.7–1.4 mg/dL (e)
- Oxygen saturation (SaO_2) >94% (e)
- Carbon dioxide ($PaCO_2$) 35–45 mm/Hg (e)
- Arterial pH 7.35–7.45 (e)
- White blood cell count 4800–10,000/mm^3 (c)

Interventions	Rationales
1. Monitor for signs and symptoms of pneumothorax, hemothorax, and hydrothorax: a. Acute chest pain b. Dyspnea	1. Pneumothorax, which is the most common complication of subclavian catheter placement, can result from puncture or laceration of the pleura or lung. In most cases the air leak is self-limiting and pneumothorax resolves spontaneously; some cases require aggressive intervention. The less common complications—hemothorax and hydrothorax—can occur from perforation of a great vessel during catheter insertion. It commonly is diagnosed when the physician cannot obtain a free flow of blood in the syringe.
2. During cannulation of subclavian catheter procedure, maintain client in Trendelenburg position with head turned to the side.	2. Trendelenburg position before and during subclavian catheter insertion provides maximum vein distention and minimizes risk of complications.
3. Assist with radiography after cannula placement.	3. A chest x-ray film confirms catheter placement and helps rule out complications.

(continued on page 758)

Interventions	Rationales
4. Monitor for signs and symptoms of air embolism during dressing and IV tubing changes and on accidental separation of IV connections: a. Acute, sharp chest pain b. Dyspnea c. Cyanosis d. Tachycardia e. Neck vein distention f. Hypotension	4. Air embolism can occur with IV tubing changes, with accidental tubing separations, and during catheter insertion and disconnection. For example, client can aspirate as much as 200 mL of air from a deep breath during subclavian line disconnection. Entry of air into the circulatory system can block blood flow and cause cardiac arrest.
5. Secure proximal catheter connection with a Luer-locking IV set and tape all connections.	5. These precautions can help prevent accidental disconnection.
6. Instruct client to perform Valsalva maneuver during IV tubing disconnections.	6. Valsalva maneuver with breath-holding minimizes air aspiration and reduces risk of embolism.
7. Explain potential problems with tubing separation and instruct client to crimp tubing near entry site if it occurs.	7. Immediate action can prevent air embolism.
8. Monitor for signs and symptoms of sepsis or catheter-related infection: a. Fever b. Chills c. Altered mental status d. Increased WBC count e. Sudden glucose intolerance f. Local signs of infection at insertion site g. Positive blood cultures	8. The high glucose concentration of the TPN solution and frequent catheter manipulation put the client at high risk for infection.
9. Monitor for signs and symptoms of hyperglycemia: a. Kussmaul respirations b. Polyuria c. Low urine specific gravity d. Glycosuria e. Mental status changes (e.g., lethargy or disorientation) f. Elevated serum glucose g. Weight change	9. Osmotic diuresis can result from inability to compensate for rapid instillation of high-glucose solution. The subsequent rise in serum glucose causes fluid shifts to the vascular compartment in an attempt to dilute the hyperosmolar glucose concentration. Increased fluid volume along with the exogenous source is lost rapidly in urine. If unrecognized and untreated, this condition can progress rapidly to nonketotic hyperglycemic coma.
10. Monitor for metabolic complications related to carbohydrate (CHO) content of TPN: a. Hyperglycemia (increased blood sugar, glycosuria) b. Hypoglycemia c. Hyperglycemic hyperosmolar, nonketotic dehydration (HHNKD): • Increased blood glucose • Increased urine output • Increased serum sodium • Changes in mental status	10. a. The high CHO content of TPN makes hyperglycemia the most common metabolic complication. b. Abrupt discontinuation of TPN can cause hypoglycemia. c. HHNKD is a risk with rapid infusion to those with mild diabetes, renal insufficiency, or congestive heart failure.
11. Monitor blood glucose level every 2 hours during and after discontinuation of TPN. Report changes and early signs and symptoms of HHNKD.	11. Fluctuations in blood glucose level need to be detected early.
12. Monitor for metabolic complications related to protein content of TPN:	12. The protein content in TPN can cause amino acid imbalance and azotemia (increased BUN and creatinine). The

(continued on page 759)

Interventions	Rationales
a. Increased BUN b. Increased creatinine c. Increased serum ammonia d. Increased AST e. Increased ALT f. Change in mental status	amount of protein produces increased urea that a compromised kidney (e.g., older adult, preexisting renal insufficiency) cannot excrete. People with hepatic insufficiency cannot metabolize certain amino acids: this causes increased ammonia levels and hepatic encephalopathy.
13. Monitor for metabolic complications related to lipid content, especially triglyceride level.	13. Clients who cannot metabolize more lipids experience hypertriglyceridemia. Rapid infusion can precipitate this condition.
14. Monitor for gallbladder dysfunction commonly shown by dyspepsia.	14. Likely due to the lack of gallbladder contraction, clients receiving TPN are predisposed to developing gallbladder sludge and/or gallstones from therapy (Onizuka et al., 2001).
15. Monitor for metabolic acidosis: a. Hyperkalemia b. Decreased thiamin levels c. Decreased biotin levels d. Decreased pH e. Decreased or normal $PaCO_2$ f. Headache, confusion g. Decreased BP h. Cold, clammy skin i. Increased respiratory rate and depth	15. Metabolic acidosis is produced by loss of bicarbonate or excess acid in extracellular fluid caused by excessive GI or renal losses, inadequate acetate in solution, impaired renal function, and inadequate thiamin and biotin intake.

 Related Physician-Prescribed Interventions

Intravenous Therapy. Nutritional solution; additives (e.g., insulin)
Laboratory Studies. Serum albumin; prealbumin; thyroxine-binding prealbumin; CBC; electrolytes; liver enzymes; serum transferrin; amino acid profile; glucose, BUN, and PT; 24-hour creatinine excretion; arterial blood gases
Diagnostic Studies. Chest x-ray film
Therapies. Daily weights; anthropometric measurements; catheter site care

Documentation

Flow records
  Vital signs
  Intake and output
  Weight
  Serum glucose
  Urine specific gravity
  Catheter site
Progress notes
  Unusual complaints

Nursing Diagnoses

High Risk for Infection Related to the Catheter's Direct Access to Bloodstream

NOC Infection Status, Wound Healing: Primary Intention, Immune Status

Goal

The client will continue to be free of infection.

Indicators

- Verbalize understanding of precautions for catheter care.
- Report any need for additional dressing changes.

NIC Infection Control, Wound Care, Incision Site Care, Health Education

Interventions	Rationales
1. Use aseptic technique and follow appropriate protocols when changing catheter dressings, IV tubing, and solutions. Change insertion site dressing when wet, soiled, or nonocclusive.	1. Aseptic technique can prevent contamination.
2. Avoid administering other IV solutions piggybacked into the TPN/TNA line unless otherwise ordered.	2. Risk of bacterial contamination increases with additional IV junctions, stopcocks, and ports. To minimize risk, TPN/TNA line should be used exclusively for that purpose unless otherwise ordered.
3. Discontinue lipid emulsions and change infusion tubing immediately after infusion.	3. Lipid emulsions and IV tubes should be discontinued promptly because of microbial contamination.
4. Secure proximal IV connections with a Luer-locking set, if possible.	4. This precaution can help to prevent disconnection and subsequent contamination.
5. Securely tape all IV connections.	5. Securing with tape helps to prevent tissue trauma resulting from catheter manipulation.
6. Teach client the following: a. The importance of proper catheter care b. The need to notify nurse when dressing becomes soiled or nonadherent c. How to crimp tubing to stop flow should it become accidentally disconnected	6. Client's understanding of care and precautions can improve compliance and reduce risk of complications.

Documentation

Flow records
    Dressing and tubing changes
    Condition of IV insertion site

High Risk for Disturbed Self-Concept Related to Inability to Ingest Food

NOC Quality of Life, Depression Level, Self-Esteem, Coping

Goal

The client will participate in self-care and grooming activities.

Indicators

- Share feelings related to lack of oral ingestion.
- Verbalize the necessity of continued TPN therapy.

NIC Hope Instillation, Mood Management, Values Clarification, Counseling, Referral, Support Group, Coping Enhancement

Interventions	Rationales
1. Encourage client to verbalize concerns related to lack of oral ingestion.	1. Sharing helps to identify and clarify client's concerns and problems; this guides nurse in planning effective interventions.
2. Explore possible alternatives to oral ingestion or substitute diversional activities.	2. Substituting activities for meals may help to reduce sense of loss related to lack of oral intake.
3. Provide regular feedback on progress and positive reinforcement on appearance and weight gain.	3. Feedback and reinforcement promote self-esteem and encourage continued compliance.
4. Arrange for visits from others on parenteral nutrition, if feasible.	4. Sharing with others in the same situation allows mutual validation and support.
5. If permitted, allow client to taste—but not swallow—desired foods.	5. Placing food in mouth without swallowing may help to satisfy the client's need to taste and smell food.

Documentation

Progress notes
Dialogues

High Risk for Activity Intolerance Related to Deconditioning

NOC Activity Tolerance

Goal

The client will maintain current activity level and make progress toward improved conditioning.

Indicators

• Verbalize the need for participation in progressive activity.
• Demonstrate correct performance of isometric and ROM exercises.

NIC Activity Therapy, Energy Management, Exercise Promotion, Sleep Enhancement, Mutual Goal Setting

Interventions	Rationales
1. Initiate an appropriate activity and exercise regimen that may include the following: a. Active or passive ROM b. Isometric exercises c. Chair-setting d. Trapeze use e. Progressive ambulation	1. Progressive activity or exercise promotes metabolism of TPN/TNA solution into muscle rather than into fat and promotes muscle strengthening.
2. Advance activity according to improved tolerance.	2. Excessive activity beyond limits of tolerance can cause activity intolerance and hypoxia.
3. Emphasize importance of activity during TPN/TNA therapy, and discuss exercises that client can perform without assistance (e.g., walking).	3. Client's understanding can promote compliance with the activity and exercise program.

Documentation

Progress notes
Activity level
Exercises performed

High Risk for Ineffective Therapeutic Regimen Management Related to Insufficient Knowledge of Home Care, Signs and Symptoms of Complications, Catheter Care, and Follow-up Care (Laboratory Studies)

NOC Compliance Behavior, Knowledge: Treatment Regimen, Participation: Health Care Decisions, Treatment Behavior: Illness or Injury

Goal

The goals for this diagnosis represent those associated with discharge planning. Refer to the discharge criteria.

NIC Anticipatory Guidance, Learning Facilitation, Risk Identification, Health Education, Teaching: Procedure/Treatment

Interventions	Rationales
1. Reinforce teaching about TPN/TNA and the infusion and catheter insertion procedures.	1. Client's understanding can reduce misconceptions and encourage participation in care.
2. Encourage client and family to ask questions and express concerns about TPN/TNA therapy.	2. Sharing concerns and questions identifies learning needs and misconceptions; this allows nurse to address problem areas.
3. Using understandable terms, explain nutritional constituents of TPN/TNA solution and how the solution meets nutritional needs.	3. Understanding TPN/TNA constituents and their purpose can encourage compliance with therapy.
4. Discuss reasons for continued diagnostic tests: daily weights, urinalysis, and laboratory tests.	4. Ongoing monitoring is needed to evaluate therapy and nutritional status.
5. Teach and evaluate learning with return demonstration: a. Aseptic technique b. Preparation and storage of TPN/TNA solution c. Preparation of infusion tubing d. Use of pump e. Discontinuation of infusion f. Heparinization of the catheter g. Catheter care h. Dressing changes	5. Many clients and families can perform home TPN/TNA without outside assistance. Proper technique is mandatory to prevent infection and air in infusion line.
6. Teach about hyperglycemia: a. Signs and symptoms: nausea, weakness, thirst, headaches, elevated blood glucose level b. Prevention: maintain prescribed rate; avoid increasing rate to "catch up" c. Treatment: consult with physician for possible insulin supplement	6. Because TPN/TNA solution contains high glucose concentrations, sudden changes in rate can increase blood glucose levels.
7. Teach about hypoglycemia: a. Signs and symptoms: sweating, pallor, palpitations, nausea, headache, shaking feeling, hunger, blurred vision	7. During TPN/TNA infusion, the body produces insulin in response to high glucose concentrations. Too much insulin in TPN/TNA or too-rapid discontinuation of TPN/TNA can produce hypoglycemia.

(continued on page 763)

Interventions	Rationales
b. Prevention: avoid stopping TPN/TNA too abruptly; slow TPN/TNA rate gradually to allow the body to decrease insulin production c. Treatment: glass of orange juice, teaspoon of honey	
8. Teach client or family to report the following: a. Fever, malaise b. Redness or purulent drainage at catheter insertion site c. Unstable blood glucose level	8. Early detection of complications enables prompt intervention to minimize their seriousness.
9. Teach client to keep records of the following: a. Weight b. Temperature c. Amount and infusion rate of TPN/TNA d. Serum glucose level (if advised to monitor) e. Any problems f. Oral intake	9. Accurate records aid in evaluating the safety and effectiveness of TPN/TNA therapy.
10. Refer to a home health care agency for follow-up care.	10. The initial home care visit evaluates suitability for home TPN/TNA by considering client's ability, environment, financial needs, and support system. Subsequent visits are needed to assess client's nutritional status, blood glucose levels, laboratory results, insertion site, and catheter patency.
11. Provide a list of required equipment, supplies, and available sources.	11. Planning can prevent shortages and improper substitutions.

Documentation

Discharge summary record
    Client and family teaching
    Outcome achievement or status
    Referrals, if indicated

REFERENCES/BIBLIOGRAPHY

Acton, A. (2004). When we leave the hospital: A patient's perspective of burn injuries. *British Medical Journal, 329*, 504–506.

Agency for Health Care Policy and Research (AHCPR). (1992). *Pressure ulcers in adults: Prediction and prevention: Clinical practice guideline 3*. Washington, DC: AHCPR, Public Health Service, U.S. Department of Health and Human Services.

Agency for Health Care Policy and Research (AHCPR). (1994). *Evaluation and management of early HIV infection Clinical practice guideline 7*. Washington, DC: AHCPR, Public Health Service, U.S. Department of Health and Human Services.

Alcoholics Anonymous. (2008). *A brief guide to Alcoholics Anonymous. Welcome to Alcoholics Anonymous*. Retrieved January 1, 2008, from www.aa.org.

Allen, D. (2006). Cataract and surgery for cataract. *British Medical Journal, 333*, 128–132.

ALLHAT officers and coordinators for the ALLHAT collaborative research group. (2002). *Journal of the American Medical Association, 288*, 2981–2997.

Allibone, L. (2003). Nursing management of chest drains. *Nursing Standard, 17*(22), 45–54.

Altizer, L. L. (1998). Degenerative disorder. In A. B. Maher, S. W. Salmond, & T. A. Pellino. *Orthopedic nursing* (2nd ed.). Philadelphia: W. B. Saunders.

Altizer. L. (2004, November). Compartment Syndrome. *Orthopaedic Nursing, 23*(6), 391–396.

American Academy of Otolaryngology-Head and Neck Surgery. (2007). *Throat cancer and neck dissection*. Retrieved November 20, 2007, from www.entnet.org.

American Association of Neuroscience Nurses (AANN). (2006). *Guide to the care of the patient with craniotomy post-brain tumor resection*. Retrieved September, 2007, from www.aann.org.

American Cancer Society. (2007a). *Breast reconstruction after mastectomy*. Retrieved November 5, 2007, from http://www.cancer.org/docroot/CRI/content/CRI_2_6X)Breast_Reconstruction_After_Mastectomy_5.asp.

American Cancer Society. (2007b). *Detailed Guide: Laryngeal and hypo laryngeal cancer: What happens after treatment for laryngeal and hypo laryngeal cancer?* Retrieved November 20, 207, from http://www.cancer.org.

American Head and Neck Society. (2007). *Neck Dissection*. Retrieved Novemeber 20, 2007, from www.ahns.info.

American Heart Association. (2003). *Let's talk about stroke and aphasia*. Retrieved November 18, 2007, from http://www.americanheart.org/downloadable/stroke/1079557856294500073%20ASA%20Strokeaphasia.pdf.

American Heart Association (2004a). *Overview of stroke systems plans*. Retrieved November 18, 2007, from http://www.strokeassociation.org/presenter.jhtml?identifier=3028498.

American Heart Association. (2004b). *What is carotid endarectomy?* Retrieved November 17, 2007, from http://www.americanheart.org/downloadable/heart/110065676921546%20WhatIs CarotidEdarterect.pdf.

American Heart Association. (2005). *Heart Disease and Stroke Statistics: 2005 Update*. Dallas, Tex: American Heart Association.

American Heart Association. (2007a). *Bypass surgery, coronary artery*. Retrieved November 7, 2007, from http://www.americanheart.org/presenter.jhtml?indentifier=4484.

American Heart Association. (2007b). *Let's talk about complications after stroke*. Retrieved November 18, 2007, from http://www.americanheart.org/downloadable/stroke/1181161981749500068%20ASA%20ComplicationsStrk_4-07.pdf.

American Heart Association. (2007c). *Let's talk about emotional changes after stroke*. Retrieved from November 18, 2007, from http://www.strokeassociation.org/downloadable/stroke/1181162441922250-0070%20ASA%20EmtnlChgsAftrStrk_4-07.pdf.

American Heart Association. (2007d). *Let's talk about living at home after stroke*. Retrieved from November 18, 2007, from http://www.americanheart.org/downl;oadable/stroke/1181162926046500072%20ASA%20LivingHome AfterStrk_4-07.pdf.

American Heart Association. (2007e). *What is stroke?* Retrieved November 18, 2007, from http://www.stroke association.org/presenter.jhtml?identifier=3030066.

American Speech-Language-Hearing Association. (2007). *Laryngeal Cancer*. Retrieved November 20, 2007, from http://www.asha.org/public/speech/disorderslaryngealCancer.htm.

American Spinal Injury Association (ASIA). (2007). *Spinal cord injury information*. Retrieved December 12, 2007, from http://www.asia-spinalinjury.org.

American Stroke Association. (2004). *Overview of stroke systems plan*. Retrieved November 18, 2007, from http://www.strkeassociation.org/presenter.jhtml?identifier=3028498.

American Stroke Association. (2007). *What is stroke?* Retrieved November 18, 2007, from http://www.stroke association.org/presenter.jhtml?identifier=3030066.

Annon, J. S. (1976). The PLISS T model: A proposed conceptual scheme for the behavioral treatment of sexual problems. *Journal of Sexual Education and Therapy, 2,* 211–215.

Arcangelo, V., & Peterson, A. (2005). Pharmacotherapeutics for advanced practice (2nd ed). Philadelphia: Lippincott Williams & Wilkins.

Armstrong, J. A., & McCaffrey, R. (2006). The effects of mucositis on quality of life. *Clinical Journal of Oncology Nursing, 10*(1), 53–56. Retrieved January 24, 2008, from http://ensco.waldenu.edu/ehost/pdf?vid=68&hid=104&sid=781c7c0c-696c-44ec-9c5d-f6382763aca4%40sessionmgr106.

Aronow, W. S. (2005). Management of peripheral arterial disease. *Cardiology in Review, 13*(2), 61–68.

Arthritis Foundation. (2008). *Take control we can help.* Retrieved January 02, 2008, from http://www.arthritis.org/index.php.

Astle, S. M. (2005). Restoring electrolyte balance. *RN, 68*(5), 34–39.

Bader, M. K., & Lillejohns, L. R. (2004). *American Association of Neuroscience Nurses: Core curriculum for neuroscience nursing* (4th ed.). St. Louis, MO: Saunders.

Badger, T., Braden, & Michel, M. (2001). Depression burden, self-help. Interventions and side effects experience in women receiving treatment for breast cancer. *Oncology Nursing Forum, 28*(3), 567–574.

Bailey, P. P. (2008). Asthma. In T. M. Buttaro, J. Trybulski, P. P. Bailey, & J. Sandberg-Cook (Eds.), *Primary care: A collaborative practice* (3rd ed., pp. 398–422). St. Louis, MO: Mosby.

Baird, M. S., Keen, J. H., & Swearingen, P. L. (2005). *Manual of critical care nursing: Nursing interventions and collaborative management* (5th ed.). St. Louis, MO: Elsevier/Mosby.

Ballas, S., & Delengowski, A. (1993). Pain measurement in hospitalized adults with sickle cell painful episodes. *Annals of Clinical and Laboratory Science, 23*(5), 358–361.

Band, J. D., Alonso-Echanove, J., & Gaynes, R. (2007). *Prevention of intravascular catheter-related infections.* Retrieved January 15, 2008, from www.uptodate.com.

Bard, M. R., Goettler, C. E., Toschlog, E. A., Sagraves, S. G., Schenarts, P. J., Newell, M. A., et al. (2006). Alcohol withdrawal syndome: Turning minor injuries into a major problem. *The Journal of Trauma Injury, Infection and Critical Care, 61*(6), 1441–1446.

Barnason, S., Zimmerman, L., Nieveen, J., & Hertzog, M. (2006). Impact of a telehealth intervention to augment home health care on functional and recovery outcomes of elderly patients undergoing coronary artery bypass grafting. *Heart & Lung: Journal of Acute & Critical Care, 35*(4), 225–233.

Barsevick, A. M., Much, J., & Sweeney, C. (2000). Psychosocial responses of cancer. In S. L. Groenwald, M. H. Frogge, M. Goodman, & C. Yarbro (Eds.), *Cancer nursing: Principles and practice* (5th ed.). Boston: Jones and Bartlett.

Bartlett, J. G., & Finkbeiner, A. K. (2001). *The guide to living with HIV infection* (6th ed.). Baltimore: The Johns Hopkins University Press

Bauer, C., Hents, G., Ducrocq, X., Nicolas, M., Oswald-Mammosser, M., Steib, A., et al. (2007). Lung function after lobectomy: A randomized, double-blinded trial comparing thoracic epidural ropivacaine/sufentanil and intravenous morphine for patient controlled analgesia [Review]. *Anesthesia & Analgesia, 105*(1), 238–244.

Bauldoff, G., Hoffman, L., Sciurba, F., & Zullo, T. (1996). Home based upper arm exercises training for patients with chronic obstructive pulmonary disease. *Heart and Lung, 25*(4), 288–294.

Bautista, L., Cesar, J., & Sumpaico, M. (2007). Stevens-Johnson from hemodialysis-associated hypersensitivity reaction in a 61-year-old male. *World Allergy Organization Journal.*

Beese-Bjurstrom, S. (2004). Aortic aneurysms & dissections. *Nursing 2004, 34*(2), 36–41.

Begelman, S. M. (2002). *Venous thromboembolism facts.* Cleveland clinics. Retrieved December 2, 2007, from http://www.clevelandclinicmeded.com.

Bernstein, C. N., & Leslie, W. D. (2004). Review article: osteoporosis and inflammatory bowel disease. *Alimentary Pharmacology & Therapeutics, 19*(9), 941-952. Retrieved January 21, 2008, from, http://ebsco.waldenu.edu/ehost/pdf?vid=vid57hid=112%sid=b2fae363-688a4e54-96d6-e87fofde711c%40sessionmgr103.

Bhardwaj, A., Mirski, M. A., & Ulatowski, J. A. (2004). *Handbook of neurocritical care.* Totowa, NJ: Humana Press, Inc.

Bick, C. (2003). Intermittent claudication. *Nursing Standard, 17*(42), 45–52.

Black, J. (2005). *Medical-surgical nursing: Clinical management for positive outcomes* (7th ed.). St. Louis, MO: Saunders.

Black, P. (2000). Practical stoma care. *Nursing Standard, 14*(41), 47–55.

Blom, E. D. (2000). Current status of voice restoration following total laryngectomy. *Oncology, 14*(6), 915–929.

Boardman, M. B. (2008). Chronic obstructive pulmonary disease. In T. M. Buttaro, J. Trybulski, P. P. Bailey, & J. Sandberg-Cook (Eds.), *Primary care: A collaborative practice* (3rd ed., pp. 433–443). St. Louis, MO: Mosby.

Bodenheimer, T., MacGregor, K., & Sharifi, C. (2005). Helping patients manage their chronic conditions. Retrieved January 10, 2007, from www.chef.org/publications.

Bonham, P.A. (2006). Get the LEAD out: Noninvasive assessment for lower extremity arterial disease using ankle brachial index and toe brachial index measurements. *Journal of Wound Ostomy Continence Nursing, 33,* 30–41.

Boron, W. F., & Boulpaep, E. L. (2005). *Medical physiology: A cellular and molecular approach.* Philadelphia: Elsevier/Saunders.

Bosmans, J. C., Suurmeijer, T. P. B. M., Hulsink, M., van der Schans, C. P., Geertzen, J. H. B., & Dijkstra, P. U. (2007). Amputation, phantom pain and subjective well-being: A qualitative study. *International Journal of Rehabilitation Research, 30,* 1–8.

Boulware, L. E., Daumit, G. L., & Frick, K. D. (2001). An evidence-based review of patient-centered behavioral interventions for hypertension. *American Journal of Preventive Medicine, 21,* 221–32.

Branson, J., Goldstein, W. (2001). Sequential bilateral total knee arthroplasty. *AORN Journal, 73*(3), 608, 610, 613.

BreastCancer.org. (2007). *The role of surgery in breast cancer treatment.* Retrieved November 5, 2007, from http://www.breastcancer.org/treatment/surgery/index.jsp.

Brown, M. (2000). Lupus erythematosus and nutrition: A review of the literature. *Journal of Renal Nutrition, 10,* 70–183.

Brown, M. A., & Powell-Cope, G. (1991). AIDS family caregiving transitions through uncertainty. *Nursing Research, 40*(6), 338–345.

Brox, A. C., Fillion, K.B., Zhang, X., Pilote, L., Obrand, D., Haider, S., et al. (2003). Inhouse cost of abdominal aortic aneurysm repair in Canada and the United States. *Archives of Internal Medicine, 163*(20), 2500–2504.

Bullock, B., & Henze, R. (2000). *Focus on pathophysiology.* Philadelphia: Lippincott Williams & Wilkins.

Burger, C. (2004). Hyperkalemia: When serum K+ is not okay. *American Journal of Nursing, 104*(10), 66–70.

Burr, J., Azuara-Blanco, A., & Avenell, A. (2004). *Medical versus surgical interventions for open angle glaucoma.* Retrieved January 2, 2007, from Cochrane Database of Systematic Reviews.

Bushkin, E. (1993). Signposts of survivorship. *Oncology Nursing Forum, 20*(6), 869–875.

Butler, D., Turkal, N., & Seidl, J. (1992). Amputation: Preoperative psychological preparation. *Journal of American Board of Family Practice, 5*(1), 69–73.

Butler, L., Downe-Wambolt, B., Marsh, S., Bell, D., & Jarvi, K. (2000). Behind the scenes: Partners' perceptions of quality of life post radical prostatectomy. *Urologic Nursing, 20*(4), 254–258.

Calhoun, J., Bal, B. S., & Yin, L. (2007). *Pathogenesis of osteomyelitis.* Retrieved November 14, 2007, from UptoDate.com.

Calvert, E., Penner, M., Younger, A., & Wing, K. (2007). Transmetatarsal amputations. *Techniques in foot and ankle surgery, 6*(3), 140–146.

Caplan, L. R. (2007). *Overview of the evaluation of stroke.* Retrieved November 14, 2007, from UpToDate.com.

Carbone, A., Palleschi, G., Conte, A., Bova, G., Iacovelli, E., Bettolo, R. M., et al. (2006). Gabapentin treatment of neurogenic overactive bladder. *Clinical Neuropharmocology, 29*(4), 206–214.

Carek, P. J., Dickerson, L. M., & Sack, J. L. (2001). Diagnosis and management of osteomyelitis. *American Family Physician, 63*(12).

Carosella, C. (1995). *Who's afraid of the dark?* New York: Harper Collins.

Carr, E. (2005). Head and Neck Malignancies. In C. H. Yarbo, M. H. Frogge, & M. Goodman (Eds.), *Cancer nursing: Principles and practice* (6th ed.). Boston: Jones and Bartlett.

Casey, K. (1997). Malnutrition associated with HIV/AIDS. Part two: Assessment and interventions. *Journal of the Association of Nurses in AIDS Care, 8*(5), 39–48.

Casswell, D., & Cryer H. G. (1995) When the nurse and the doctor don't agree. *Journal of Cardiovascular Nursing, 9,* 30–42.

Castner, D., & Douglas, C. (2005). Put the spotlight on identifying and responding to renal problems to help your patient stave off major complications. *Nursing 2005, 35*(12), 58–54.

Centers for Disease Control. (2000). Guidelines for prevention of transmission of HIV and hepatitis B virus to health care and public safety workers. *MMWR, 49,* 7–11.

Centers for Disease Control. (2008). Updated US Public Health Service guidelines for management of occupational exposure to HIV and recommendations for post-exposure prophylaxis. *MMWR, 54*(RR09), 1–17.

Challacombe, B., & Dasgupta, P. (2007). Reconstitution of the lower urinary tract by laparoscopic robotic surgery. *Current Opinion in Urology, 17,* 390–395.

Chapman, D., & Moore, S. (2005). Breast cancer. In C. Yarbo, M. H. Frogge, & M. Goodman (Eds.), *Cancer nursing: Principles and practice* (6th ed.). Boston: Jones & Bartlett.

Cheng, D. M. D., Allen, K. M. D., Cohn W. M. D., Connolly, M. M. D., Edgerton, J. M. D., Falk, V. M. D., et al. (2005). Endoscopic vascular harvest in coronary artery bypass grafting surgery: A meta-analysis of randomized trials and controlled trials. *Innovations: Technology 7 Techniques in Cardiothoracic & Vascular Surgery, 1*(2), 61–74.

Cheskin, L., & Lacy, B. (2003). Selected gastrointestinal problems: Bleeding, diarrhea, abdominal pain. In L. R. Barker, J. Burton, & P. D. Aieve (Eds.), *Principles of ambulatory medicine* (6th ed.). Philadelphia: Lippincott Williams & Wilkins.

Chester, M., Wasko, M., Hubert, H., Lingala, V., Elliot, J., Luggen, M., et al. (2007). Hydroxychloroquine and risk of diabetes in patients with Rheumatoid Arthritis. *Journal of the American Medical Association, 298*(2), 187–193.

Chin, T., Sawamura, S., & Shiba, R. (2006). Effect of physical fitness on prosthetic ambulation in elderly amputees. *American Journal of Physical Medicine & Rehabilitation, 85*(12), 992–996.

Chojnowski, D. (2005). Peripheral arterial disease: Danger! Slow blood flow ahead. *Nursing made Incredibly Easy,* (July/August), 4–17.

Cimprich, B. (1992). Attentional fatigue following breast cancer surgery. *Research in Nursing and Health*, *15*, 199–207.

Clark, J. (2006). Ileostomy guide, United Ostomy Association. Retrieved November 20, 2007, from http://www.cancer.org/docroot/CRI/content/CRI_2_6x_Ileostomy.asp.

Cole, R. P., & Ash, J. (2007). Benzodiazepine administration and need for medical ventilation in delirium tremens. *Critical Care Medicine*, *35*(7), 1810–1811.

Collett, K. (2002). Practical aspects of stoma management. *Nursing Standard*, *17*(8), 45–52.

Colwell, J. C., & Beitz, J. (2007). Survey of wound, ostomy and continence (WOC) nurse clinicians on stomal and peristomal complications. *Journal of Wound, Ostomy and Continence Nursing*, *34*(1), 57–69.

Corley, M., Minick, P., Elswick, R., & Jacobs, M. (2005). Nurse moral distress and ethical work environments. *Nursing Ethics*, *12*(4), 381–389.

Cotter, J., Bixby, M., & Morse, B. (2006). Helping patients who need a permanent pacemaker. *Nursing 2006*, *36*(8), 50–54.

Coughlin, A. M., & Parchinsky, C. (2006). Going with the flow of chest tube therapy. *Nursing 2006*, *36*(3), 36–42.

Coyne, D. W. (2007). Use of Epoetin in Chronic Renal Failure. *Journal of the American Medical Association*, *297*(15), 1713–1716.

Cruz, D. N., Brickel, H. M., Wysolmerski, J. J., Gundberg, C. G., Simpson, C. A., Kliger, A. S., et al. (2002). Treatment of osteoporosis and osteopenia [Electronic Version]. *American Journal of Transplantation*, *2*(1), 62–67. Retrieved January 21, 2008, from http://ebsco.waldenu.edu/ehost/pdf?vid=5&hid=106&sid=b2fae363-688a-4e54-96d6-e87f0fde711c%40sessionmgr103.

Cukierman, T., Gatt, M. E., Hiller, N., Chajek-Shaul, T. (2005, August 4). Fracture diagnosis. *New England Journal of Medicine*, *353*, 509–514.

Cutilli, C. C. (2005). Health literacy: What you need to know. *Orthopedic Nursing*, *24*(3), 227–231.

Dadd, M. (1983). Self care for side effects. *Cancer Nursing*, *6*, 63–66.

Damianos, A., & McGarrity, T. (1997). Treatment strategies for Helicobacter pylori infection. *American Family Physician*, *55*(8), 2765–2774.

Davies, P. (2002, March). Guarding your patient against ARD. *Nursing*, *32*(3), 36-42. Retrieved January 14, 2008, from http://web.ebscohost.com/ehost/detail?vid=8&hid=106&sid=c7e5d2b4-a****27f-fdf75c59b820%40sessionmgr106.

Da Vinci Hysterectomy (2007). *Da Vinci hysterectomy*. Retrieved Novemebr 19, 2007, from http://www.davincihysterectomy.com/davincihysterectomy/index.aspx.

Deglin, J. H., & Vallerand, A. H. (2007). *Davis's drug guide for nurses* (10th ed.). Philadephia: F. A. Davis Company.

de Leon, D. G., & Spiegler, P. (2005). The role of prone positioning in the management of hypoxemic acute respiratory failure. *Clinical Pulmonary Medicine*, *12*, 128–134.

Denis, P. (2004, September). Effect of intraocular pressure and arterial blood pressure variations on glaucoma. *Journal of Ophthalmology*, *27*(2), 2S27–2S32.

Denys, P., Schurch, B., & Fraczek,. S. (2005). Poster 59: Management of nuerologic bladder with focal administration of botulinum toxin A: Minimizing risks associated with increased detrusor pressure. *Journal of Pelvic Medicine & Surgery*, *11*(Supplement 1), S52–S53.

DePew, C. L., & McCarthy, M. S., (2007). Subglottic secretion drainage. *Advanced Critical Care*, *18*(4), 366–379.

Dewey, R., Delley, R., & Shulman, L. (2002). A better life for patients with Parkinson's disease. *Patient Care*, *36*(7).

Dillingham, T. (2007). Musculoskeletal rehabilitation: Current understandings and future directions. *American Journal of Physical Medicine and Rehabilitation*, *86*, S19–S28.

Dillion, P. M. (2007). Assessing the respiratory system. In P. M. Dillion (Ed.), *Nursing health assessment: A critical thinking case studies approach* (2nd ed., pp. 393–436). Philadephia: F. A. Davis.

Dinwiddie, L., Burrows-Hudson, S., & Peacock, E. (2006). Stage 4 chronic kidney disease: Preserving kidney function and preparing patients for stage 5 kidney disease. *American Journal of Nursing*, *106*(9), 40–51.

Drews, R. E. (2007). *Superior vena cava syndrome*. Retrieved January 15, 2008, from www.Uptodate.com.

Dudas, S. (1993). Altered body image and sexuality. In S. L. Groenwald, M. H. Frogge, M. Goodman, & C. Yarbro (Eds.), *Cancer nursing: Principles and practice* (3rd ed.). Boston: Jones and Bartlett.

Dudek, S. (2005). *Nutritional handbook for nursing practice* (5th ed.). Philadelphia: Lippincott Williams & Wilkins.

Eachempati, S., Wang, J., Hydo, L., Shou, J., & Barie, P. (2007). Acute renal failure in critically ill surgical patients: Persistent lethality despite new modes of renal replacement therapy. *The Journal of Trauma: Injury, Infection Critical Care*, *63*(50), 987–993.

Early, L. M., & Poquette, R. (2000). Bladder and kidney cancer. In S. L. Groenwald, M. H. Frogge, M. Goodman, & C. H. Yarbro (Eds.), *Cancer nursing: Principles and practice* (5th ed.). Boston: Jones and Bartlett.

ECG. (2006). *ECG interpretation: An incredibly easy pocket guide*. Ambler, PA: Lippincott Williams & Wilkins.

Edelman, C., & Mandle, C. (2007). *Health promotion throughout the lifespan*. St. Louis, MO: Mosby.

Eisenberg, P. (1990). Monitoring gastric pH to prevent stress ulcer syndrome. *Focus on Critical Care*, *17*(4), 316–322.

Ellerhorst-Ryan, J. M. (2000). Infection. In S. Groenwald, M. Frogge, M. Goodman, & C. Yarbro (Eds.), *Cancer nursing: Principles and practice* (5th ed.). Boston: Jones and Bartlett.

Elpern, E., Covert, B., & Kleinpell, R. (2005). Moral distress of staff nurses in a medical intensive care unit. *American Journal Critical Care*, *14*(6), 523–530.

Epilepsy Foundation. (2007). *What is Epilepsy? Frequently asked questions.* Retrieved December 17, 2007, from http://epilepsyfoundation.org/about/faq/index.cfm.

Esche, C.A. (2005). Resiliency: a factor to consider when facilitating the transition from the hospital to home in older adults. *Geriatric Nursing, 26*(4), 218–222.

Eslinger, P. (2002). Empathy and social-emotional factors in recovery from stroke. *Current Opinion in Neurology, 15*(1), 91–97.

Evans, B. (2005). Best practice protocols: VAP prevention. *Nursing Management,* (December), 10–15.

Ewing, J. A. (1984). Detecting alcoholism: The CAGE questionnaire. *Journal of American Medical Association, 252,* 1905–1907.

Fineman, L. D., LaBrecque, M. A., Shih, M., & Curley, M. A. Q. (2006). Prone positioning can be safely performed in critically ill infants and children. *Pediatric Critical Care Medicine, 7*(5), 413–422.

Flaskerud, J., & Ungrarski, P. (1999). *HIV/AIDS: A guide to nursing care* (3rd ed.). Philadelphia: W. B. Saunders.

Fletcher, L. (2006). Management of patients with intermittent claudication. *Nursing Standard, 20*(31), 59–65.

Foltz, A. (2000). Nutritional disturbances. In S. Groenwald, M. Frogge, M. Goodman, & C. Yarbro (Eds.), *Cancer nursing: Principles and practice* (5th ed.). Boston: Jones and Bartlett.

Foo, N. P., & Lin, H. J. (2005). Delayed perforation of right ventricle with cardiac tamponade: A complication of pacemaker implantation. *European Journal of Emergency Medicine, 12,* 89–91.

Forsythe, B. & Faulkner, K. (2004). Overview of the tolerability of Gefitinin (IRESSA) Monotherapy: Clinical experience in non-small-cell-lung cancer [Electronic version]. *Drug Safety, 27*(14), 1081–1092. Retrieved January 26, 2008, from http://ebsco.waldenu.edu/ehost/pdf?vid=144&hid=102&sid=781c7c0c-696c-44ec-9c5d-f6382763aca4%40sessionmgr106.

Franklyn, J., & Sheppard, M. (1990). Thyroxine replacement treatment and osteoporosis. *British Medical Journal, 300,* 693–694.

Fraser, J., Mullany, D., & Traber, D. (2007). Inhalation lung injury in patients with severe thermal burns. *Contemporary Critical Care, 4*(9), 1–11.

Freidburg, C., Igneri, P., Satorelli, K., & Rogers, F. (2007). Effects of differences in percent total body surfaces area estimation on fluid resuscitation of transferred burn patients. *Journal of Burn Care & Research, 28*(1), 42–48.

French, K., Beynon, C., & Delaforce, J. (2007). Alcohol is the true "Rape Drug." *Nursing Standard, 21*(29), 26–27.

Gill, J., Quisel, A., Rocca, P., & Walters, D. (2003). Diagnosis of systemic lupus erythematosus. *American Family Physician, 68*(11), 2179–86.

Ginzler, E., & Tayar, J. (2004). *Systemic lupus erythematosus.* Retrieved December 29, 2007, from http://rheumatolgy.org/public/factsheets/sle_new.asp.

Gladman, D. D. (1996). Prognosis and treatment of systemic lupus erythematosus. *Current Opinions in Rheumatology, 8,* 430-437.

Gobel, B. H. (2005). Bleeding disorder. In S. Groenwald, M. Frogge, M. Goodman, & C. Yarbro (Eds.), *Cancer nursing: Principles and practice* (6th ed.). Boston: Jones and Bartlett.

Goodman, M., & Hayden, B. K. (2000). Chemotherapy: Principles of administration. In C. H. Yarbo, M. H. Frogge, & M. Goodman, *Comprehensive cancer nursing review* (6th ed.). Boston: Jones and Bartlett.

Gordon, A. J. (2006). Identification and treatment of alcohol-use disorders in the perioperative period. *Post Graduate Medicine, 199*(2), 46–55.

Goshorn, J. (2000). Management of patients with urinary and renal dysfunction. In S. Smeltzer & B. Bare (Eds.), *Brunner & Suddarth's textbook of medical-surgical nursing* (9th ed.). Philadelphia: Lippincott Williams & Wilkins.

Gorski, L. A. (October 2002). Effective teaching of home IV therapy [Electronic version]. *Home Healthcare Nurse, 20*(10), 666–674. Retrieved January 15, 2008, from http://gateway.tx.ovid.com.library.gcu.edu:2048/gw2/ovidweb.cgi.

Graf, J., & Janssens, U. (2007). Recognizing shock: Who cares, and when? *Critical Care Medicine, 35*(11), 2651–2652.

Graul, T. (2002). Total joint replacement: Baseline benchmark data for interdisciplinary outcomes management. *Orthopaedic Nursing, 21*(3), 57–67.

Greelish, J., Mohler, E., & Fairman, R. (2006a). *Carotid edarectomy in asymptomatic patients.* Retrieved November 14, 2007, from UpToDate.com.

Greelish, J., Mohler, E., & Fairman, R. (2006b). *Carotid edarectomy: Preoperative evaluation; surgical technique; and complications.* Retrieved November 14, 2007, from UpToDate.com.

Griffin-Broan, J. (2000). Diagnostic evaluation, classification, and staging. In C. Yarbo, M. H. Frogge, M. Goodman, & S. Groenwald (Eds.), *Cancer nursing: Principles and practice* (5th ed.). Boston: Jones and Bartlett.

Groenwald, S. L., Frogge, M., Goodman, M., & Yarbro, C. (Eds.). (2005). *Cancer nursing: Principles and practice* (6th ed.). Boston: Jones and Bartlett.

Haire, W. D. (2007). *Catheter-induced upper extremity venous thrombosis.* Retrieved January 15, 2008, from www.UpToDate.com.

Hamilton, H. (2006). Complications associated with venous access devices: Part one. *Nursing Standard, 8*(26), 43–50. Retrieved January 7, 2008, from http://ebscohost.com/ehost/pdf?vid=140&hid=106&sid=c7e5d2b4-a693-4480-a27f-fdf75c59b820%40sessionmgr106.

Hanna, D. (2004). Moral Distress: The state of the science. *Research and Theory for Nursing Practice: An International Journal, 18*(1), 73–9.

Hansen, L. B., & Vondracek, S. F. (2004). Prevention and treatment of nonpostmenapausal osteoporosis. *American Journal of Health-System Pharmacy, 61*(24), 2637–2654.

Happ, M. B., Swigert, V. A., Tate, J. A., Arnold, R. M., Serelka, S. M., & Hoffman, L. A. (2007). Family presence and surveillance during wearing from prolonged mechanical ventilation. *Heart & Lung, 36*(1), 47–57.

Harmanli, O. H., Khilnani, R., Dandolu, V., & Chatwani, A. J. (2004). Narrow pubic arch and increased risk of failure for vaginal hysterectomy. *Obstetric Gynecology, 104*(4), 697–700.

Harris, L. (2000). Head and neck malignancies. In C. Yarbro, M. Frogge, M. Goodman, & S. Groenwald (Eds.), *Cancer nursing: Principles and practice* (5th ed.). Boston: Jones and Bartlett.

Harvey, S., & Whelan, C. A. (2008). Pneumonia. In T. M. Buttaro, J. Trybulski, P. P. Bailey, & J. Sandberg-Cook (Eds.), *Primary Care: A Collaborative Practice* (3rd ed., pp.466–475). St. Louis, MO: Mosby.

Haugen, V., Bliss D. Z., & Savik, K. (2006). Perioperative factor that affect long-term adjustments to an incontinent ostomy. *Journal of Wound, Ostomy and Continence Nursing, 33*(5), 525–535.

Haughney, A. (2004). Nausea and vomiting in end-stage cancer: these symptoms can be treated most effectively if the underlying cause is known. *American Journal of Nursing, 104*(11), 40–48.

Hayes, D. L. (2007). *Modes of cardiac pacing: Nomenclature and selection.* Retrieved January 15, 2008, from www. UpToDate.com.

Haynes, V. L. (1996). Caring for the laryngectomy patient. *American Journal of Nursing, 96*(5), 16B–16K.

Hector, D., Miguel, A., & Sebastian, D. (2006). Endoscopic treatment of postoperative bronchopleural fistula and prolonged air leaks. *Journal of Bronchology, 13*(2), 67–71.

Heinrich, L. (1987). Care of the female rape victim. *Nurse Practitioner, 12*(11), 9–27.

Held, & Warmkessel, J. (2005). Prostate cancer. In C. Yarbo, M. Frogge, & M. Goodman (Eds.), *Cancer nursing: Principles and practice* (5th ed.). Boston: Jones and Bartlett.

Hernigou, P., Bachir, D., Galacteros, F. (2003). The national history of symptomatic osteonecrosis in adults with sickle cell disease. *The Journal of Bone and Joint Surgery, 85*(3), 500–504.

Hickey, J. V. (2003). *The clinical practice of neurosurgical nursing* (5th ed.) Phildephia: Lippincott Williams & Wilkins.

Hilderley, L. (2000). Radiotherapy. In S. Groenwald, M. Frogge, M. Goodman, & C. Yarbro (Eds.), *Cancer nursing: Principles and practice* (5th ed.). Boston: Jones and Bartlett.

Hillman, S. S., Hedrick, M. S., Withers, P. C., & Drewes, R. C. (2004). Lymph pools in the basement, sump pumps in the attic: The anuran dilemma for lymph movement [Electronic version]. *Physiological & Biochemical Zoology, 77*(2), 161–173. Retrieved January 21, 2008, from http://ebsco.waldenu.edu/ehost/pdf?vid=11&hid=8&sid=758d5251-92bc-4582-bf2c-72c0983df20a%40sessionmgr7.

Himiak, L. (2007). *The amputee community continues to face undue hardships and discrimination.* Retrieved November 13, 2007, from http://nursing.advanceweb.com/Editorial/Content/Editorial.aspx?CC=100852&CP=2.

Hirsch, A. T., Haskal, Z. J., Hertzer, N. R., Dalal, G. W., Graagor, M. A., Halperin, J. L., et al. (2006). ACC/AHA guidelines for the management of patients with peripheral arterial disease (lower extremity, renal mesenteric, and abdominal aortic). *Journal of Vascular Inerventional Radiology,* (17), 1383–1398.

Ho-Shing, D. (2000). Treating glaucoma with drainage devices and pericardial grafts. *AORN, 71*(6), 1234, 1237, 1239–1240, 1243–1244, 1247–1248, 1251–1252, 1255–1256, 1259–1261.

Hoskins, C. N., & Haber, J. (2000). Adjusting to breast cancer. *American Journal of Nursing, 100*(4), 26–33.

Huffman, G. B. (2002). Evaluating and treating unintentional weight loss in the elderly [Electronic Version]. *American Family Physician, 65*(4). Retrieved January 18, 2008, from http://web.ebscohost.com/ehost/detail?vid=4%hid=106&sid=c7e5d2b4-a****3-4480-a27f-fdf75c59b820%40sessionmgr106.

Hunt, S. A., Baker, D. W., Chin, M. H., et al. (2001). ACC/AHA guidelines for the evaluation and management of chronic heart failure in the adult: Executive summary: A report of the American College of Cardiology/ American Heart Association Task Force on Practice Guidelines (Committee to Revise the 1995 Guidelines for the Evaluation and Management of Heart Failure). *Journal of the American College of Cardiology, 38,* 2101–2113.

Hunter, M., & King, D. (2001). COPD: Management of acute exacerbations and chronic stable disease. *American Family Physician, 64*(4), 603–612.

Hunter, K. F., Moore, K. N., & Glazner, C. M. A. (2007). Conservative management for postprostectomy urinary incontinence [Systematic Review]. *Cochrane Database of Systematic Reviews, 3.*

Hyland, J. (2002). The basics of ostomies. *Gastroenterology Nursing, 25*(6), 241–244.

International League Against Epilepsy, (2007). *Classifications of seizures.* Retrieved December 17, 2007, from http://www.ilae-epilepsy.org.

Institute for Healthcare Improvement, (n.d.). *Implement the ventilator bundle.* Retrieved January 14, 2007, from http://www.ihi.org/IHI/Topics/CriticalCare/IntensiveCare/Changes/ImplementtheVentilatorBundle.htm.

Jablonski, R. (2001). Discovering asthma in the older adult. *The Nurse Practitioner, 25*(1), 14, 24–25, 29–32+.

James, M. L. (2007). Prostate cancer (early). In G. F. G. (Ed.), *Clinical Evidence.* London: BMJ Publishing Group Ltd.

Jenkins, T. (2002). Sickle cell anemia in pediatric intensive care unit. *AACN Clinical Issues, 13*(2), 154–168.

Jennings-Ingle, S. (2007). The sobering facts of alcohol wiothdrawal. *Nursing Made Incredibly Easy, 5*(1), 50–60.

Johns Hopkins Breast Cancer Center. (2007). *Johns Hopkins decision of plastic and reconstructive surgery: Breast reconstruction*. Retrieved November 5, 2007, from http://www.hopkinsbreastcenter.org/services/patientcare/plasticsurgery.shtml.

Johnson, J. E., Rice, V., Fuller, S., & Endress, P. (1978). Sensory information instruction in coping strategy and recovery from surgery. *Research in Nursing and Health, 1*(1), 4–17.

Johnson, N., Barlow, D., Lethaby, A., Travender, E., Curr, L., & Garry, R. (2005). Methods of hysterectomy: Systematic review and meta-analysis of randomized controlled trials. *British Medical Journal, 330*(7506), 1478.

Joint National Committee 7. (2004, August). *Complete report: The seventh report of the Joint Committee on prevention, detection, and treatment of high blood pressure*. US Department of Health and Human services; National Institute of Health; National Heart ,Lung and Blood Institute; National High Blood Pressure Education Program. NIH Publication no.04-5230.

Joint National Committee. (2007). *Clinical practice guidelines for hypertension prevention, screening, counseling and management*. Retrieved November 5, 2007, from http://mahealthcare.com/practice_guidelines/hypertension.pdf.

Joque, L., & Jotai, A. (2005).Total parenteral nutrition in cancer patients: Why and when? [Electronic version]. *Nutrition in Critical Care, 8*(2), 89–92. Retrieved January 6, 2008, from http://web.ebscohost.com/ehost.com/pdf?vid=113&hid=106&sid=c7e5d2b4-a****3-4480-a27f-fdf75c59b820%40sessionmgr106.

Junkin, J., & Beitz, J. M. (2005). Sexuality and the person with a stoma. *Journal of Wound, Ostomy and Continence Nursing, 32*(2), 121–128.

Kannel, W. B. & Belanger, A. J. (1991). Epidemiology of heart failure. *American Heart Journal, 121,* 951–957.

Kantaff, P., Carroll, P., D'Amico, A., Isaacs, J., Ross, R., & Schertt. (2001). *Prostate cancer: Principles and practice.* Philadelphia: Lippincott Williams & Wilkins.

Kaplan, J. E., Masur, H., & Holmes, K. K. (2002). USPHS Infectious Disease Society of America: Guidelines for preventing opportunistic infections in HIV infected groups. *MMWR, 51*(RR8), 1–52.

Kappas-Larson, P., & Lathrop, L. (1993). Early detection and intervention for hazardous ethanol use. *Nurse Practitioner, 18*(7), 50–55.

Karchmer, A. W. (2007). *Infection of cardiac pacemakers and implantable cardioverter-defibrillators.* Retrieved January 15, 2008, from www.UpToDate.com.

Katz, A. (2006). What have my kidneys got to do with my sex life? The impact of late stage chronic kidney disease on sexual function. *American Journal of Nursing, 106*(9), 81–83.

Katz, J. (1996). The role of the sympathetic nervous system in phantom limb pain. *Physical Medicine and Rehabilitation: State of the Art Reviews, 10*(1), 153–175.

Katz, P. (2003). Peptic ulcer disease. In L. R. Baker, J. Burton, & P. Zieve. *Principles of ambulatory medicine* (6th ed.). Philadelphia: Lippincott Williams & Wilkins.

Kawada, E., Moridaira, K., Itoh, K., Hoshino, A., Tamura, J. & Morita, T. (2006). Long-term bedridden elderly patients [Electronic version]. *Annals of Nutrition & Metabolism, 50*(5), 420–424. Retrieved January 21, 2008, from http://ebsco.waldenu.edu/ehost/pdf?vid=11&hid=102&sid=b2fae363-688a-4e54-96d6-e87f0fde711c%40sessionmgr103.

Kee, J. L. (2005). *Handbook of laboratory & diagnostic tests with nursing implications* (5th ed.). New Jersey: Pearson Education, Prentice Hall.

Khraim, F. M. (2007). The wider scope of video-assisted thoracoscopic surgery. *AORN Journal, 85*(6), 1199–1208.

King, D., & Pippin, H. J. (1997). Community-acquired pneumonia in adults. *American Family Physician, 56*(2), 544–50.

Kirkeby-Garstad, I., Wisloff, U., Skogvoll, E., Stolen, T., Tjonna, A. E., Stenseth, R., et al. (2006). The marked reduction in mixed venous oxygen saturation during early mobilization after cardiac surgery: The effect of posture or exercise? *Anesthesia & Analgesia, 102*(6), 1609–1616.

Koelling, T. M., Chen, R. S., Lubwama, R. N., L'Italien, G. J., & Eagle, K. A. (2004). The expanding national burden of heart failure in the United States: the influence of heart failure in women. *American Heart Journal, 147,* 74–78.

Kok, N., Alwayn, I., Tran, K., Hop, W., Weimar, W., & Ijzermans, J. (2006). Psychosocial and physical impairment after mini-incision open and laparoscopic donor nephrectomy: A positive study [Electronic version]. *Transplantation, 82*(10), 1291–1297. Retrieved November 4, 2007, from http://gateway.uk.ovid.com/gw1/ovidweb.cgi.

Krebs, L. U. (2000). Sexual and reproductive dysfunction. In S. L. Groenwald, M. H. Frogge, M. Goodman, & C. Yarbro (Eds.), *Cancer nursing: Principles and practice* (5th ed.). Boston: Jones and Bartlett.

Kress, J. P., Hall, J. B. (2006). Sedation in the mechanically ventilated patient. *Critical Care Medicine, 34*(10), 2541–2546.

Kupecz, D. (2000). Intermittent claudication treatment. *The Nurse Practitioner, 25*(5), 112–115.

Kuriakose, A. (2008). Using the synergy model as best practice in endotracheal tube suctioning of the critically ill patients. *Dimensions of Critical Care Nursing, 27*(1), 10–15.

Ladd, A., Jones, H. H., & Otanez, O. (2003). *Osteomyelitis.* Retrieved November 17, 2007, from http://osteomyelitis.standford.edu.

Lash, A. & Lusk, B. (2004) Systemic Lupus Erythematosus in the Intensive Care Unit. *Critical Care Nurse. 24*(2), 56–65.

Leenerts, M. H., Teel, C. S., & Pendelton, M. K. (2002). Building a model of self-care for health promotion in aging [Electronic version]. *Journal of Nursing Scholarship, 34*(4), 355–361. Retrieved January 14, 2008, from http://web.ebscohost.com/ehost/detail?vid=21&hid=106&sid=c7e5d2b4-a****3-4480-a27f-fdf75c59b820%40session mgr106.

Lehmann, O. J., Bunce, C., Maurino, V., Khaw, P. T., Wormald, R., & Barton, K. (2000). Risk factors for development of post-trabeculectomy endophthalmitis. *British Journal of Ophtalmology, 84*(12), 1349–1353.

Lehne, R.A. (2004). *Pharmacology for nursing care* (5th ed.). St. Louis, Missouri: Saunders.

Lejeune, M., & Howard-Fain, T. (2002). Caring for patients with increased intracranial pressure. *Nursing 2007, 32*(11), 32cc1–32cc5.

Lemke, J. R., Kasprowicz, K., & Worral, P. S. (2005). Intermittent catheterization for patients with neurogenic bladder: Sterile versus clean: Using evidence-based practice at the staff nurse level. *Journal of Nursing Care Quality, 20*(4), 302–306.

Lennie, T., Christman, S., & Jadack, R. (2001). Educational needs and altered eating habits following a total laryngectomy. *Oncology Nursing Forum, 28*(4), 667–674.

Leukemia & Lymphoma Society. (2007a). *Hairy cell leukemia*. Retrieved November 16, 2007, from http://www.leukemia-lymphoma.org/all_page?itemid=8507.

Leukemia & Lymphoma Society. (2007b). *Leukemia*. Retrieved November 16, 2007, from http://www.leukemia-lymphoma.org/all_page?itemid=7026.

Lew, D. P., & Waldvogel, F. A. (2004) Osteomyelitis. *Lancet, 364*(9431), 369–379.

Lewis, S. M., Heitkemper, M., Dirksen, S. R., O'Brien, P. G., Giddens, J. F., & Bucher, L. (2004). *Medical surgical nursing: Assessment and management of clinical problems* (6th ed.). St. Louis, MO: Mosby.

Licker, M., de Perrot, M., Spiliopoulos, A., Robert, J., Diaper, J., Chevalley, C., et al. (2003). Risk factors for acute lung injury after thoracic surgery for lung cancer. *Anesthesia & Analgesia, 97*(6), 1558–1565.

Lindqvist, O., Widmark, A., & Rasmussen, B. H. (2006). Reclaiming wellness—living with bodily problems, as narrated by men with advanced prostate cancer. *Cancer Nursing: An International Journal for Cancer Care, 24*(9), 327–337.

List, M. A. (1996). Longitudinal assessment of quality of life in laryngeal cancer patients. *Head and Neck, 18*, 1–10.

Lopez-Bushnell, K., Gary, G., Mitchell, P., & Reil, E. (2004). Joint replacement and case management in indigent hospitalized patients. *Orthopaedic Nursing, 23*(2), 113–117.

Lord, R., & Dayhew, J. (2001). Visual risks factors for falls in older people. *American Journal of Geriatric Society, 49*, 58–64.

Lussier-Cushing, M., Repper-Del, J., Mitchell, M. T., Lakatos, B. E., Mahoud, F., & Lipkis-Oralando. (2007). Is your medical/surgical patient withdrawing from alcohol? *Nursing 2007, 37*(10), 50–55.

Lynn-McHale Wiegand, D. J., & Carlson, K. K. (2005). *AACN procedure manual for critical care*. St. Louis, MO: Elsevier.

Mackowaik, P. (2007). *Diagnosis of osteomyelitis in adults*. Retrieved November 14, 2007, from UpToDate.com.

Maclean, C., Louie, R., Leake, B., McCaffery, D., Paulus, H., Brook, R., et al. (2000). Quality of care for patients with rheumatoid arthritis. *The Journal of the American Medical Association, 284*(8), 984–992.

Maghsoudi, H., Asyani, Y., & Ahmadian, N. (2007). Electrical and lightning injuries. *Journal of Burn Care & Research, 28*(2), 255–261.

Maher, K. (2005). Radiation therapy: Toxicities and management. In C.H. Yarbro, M. H. Frogge, & M. Goodman (Eds.), *Cancer Nursing: Principle and Practice* (6th ed.). Boston: Jones & Bartlett.

Maklebust, J. (1990). Assisting with adjustment following ostomy surgery. *Hospital Home Health, 7*(7), 91–94.

Maklebust, J., & Sieggreen, M. (2001). *Pressure ulcers: Guidelines for prevention and nursing management* (3rd ed.). West Dundee, IL: SN Publications.

Malabanan, A. O. (2008). Osteoporosis. In T. M. Buttaro, J. Tyrbulski, P. P. Bailey, & J. Sandberg-Cook (Eds.), *Primary care: A collaborative practice* (3rd ed., pp. 996–1005). St. Louis, MO: Mosby.

Maliski, S., Heilemann, M. S., & McCorkle, R. (2001). Mastery of postprostatectomy incontinence and impotence: His work, her work, our work. *Oncology Nursing Forum, 28*(6), 985–992.

Mallinson, R. K. (1999). The lived experince of AIDS-related multiple losses by HIV-negative gay men. *Journal of Association of Nurses in AIDS Care, 10*(5), 22–31.

Margaretten, M., Kohlwes, J., Moore, D., & Bent, S. (2007). Synovial lactic acid and septic arthritis. *The Journal of the American Medical Association, 298*(1), 40.

Martin, C. G., & Turkelson, S. L. (2006). Nursing care of the patient undergoing coronary artery bypass grafting. *Journal of Cardiovascular Nursing, 21*(2), 109–117.

Masoudi, F. A., Havranek, E. P., Krumholz, H. M. (2002). The burden of chronic congestive heart failure in older persons: Magnitude and implications for policy and research. *Heart Failure Review, 7*, 9–16.

Massie, B. M. & Shah, N. B. (1997). Evolving trends in the epidemiologic factors of heart failure: Rationale for preventive strategies and comprehensive disease management. *American Heart Journal, 133*, 703–712.

Mattano, L. A. (2004). *Strategic approaches to osteoporosis in pediatric transplantation*. Retrieved January 21, 2008, from http://ebsco.waldenu.edu/ehostpdf?vid=5&hid=106&sid=b2fae363-688a-4e54-96d6-e87f0fde711c%40session mgr103.

Mattar, K., & Finelli, A. (2007). Expanding the indications of laparoscopic radical nephrectomy [Electronic version]. *Current Opinion in Urology, 17*(2), 88–92. Retrieved November 4, 2007, from http://www.kidney.org.

Mauer, K. A., Abrahams, E. B., Arslanian, C., Schoenly, L., & Taggart, H. M. (2002). National practice patterns for the care of the patient with total joint replacement. *Orthopedic Nursing, 21*(3), 37–47.

McGrory, B., Callaghan, J., Kraay, M., Jacobs, J., Robb, W., & Wasielewski, R. (2005). Editorial: Minimally invasive and small-incision joint replacement surgery—What surgeons should you consider. *Clinical Orthopaedics and Related Research, 440,* 251–254.

McKinley, M. (2005). Alcohol withdrawal syndrome: Overlooked and mismanaged? *Critical Care Nurse, 25*(3), 40–49.

Merbs, S., Grant, M., & Iliff, N. (2004). Simple outpatient postoperative analgesia using an orbital catheter after enucleation. *The Journal of the American Medical Association, 122*(3), 349–352.

Merck Manual Online Library. (2005). *Osteomyelitis*. Retrieved November 17, 2007, from http://www.merck.com/mmpe/sec04/ch039/ch039d.html.

Miller, C. A. (2004). *Nursing care of older adults* (4th ed.). Philadelphia: Lippincott Williams & Wilkins.

Miller-Hoover, S. (2005). Juvenile idiopathic arthritis: Why do I have to hurt so much? *Journal of Infusion Nursing, 28*(6), 385–391.

Mitchell, M., Mohler, E., & Carpenter, J. (2007). *Acute arterial occlusion of the lower extremity*. Retrieved November 14, 2007, from UpToDate.com.

More, K. N., Truong, V., Estey, E., & Voaklander, D. C. (2007). Urinary incontinence after prostatectomy: Can men at risk be indentified preoperatively? *The Journal of Wound, Ostomy and Continence.*

Morgan, E. (2005). When critical limb ischemia strikes: Find out how to intervene when ischemia threatens life and limb. *Nursing 2005, 35*(8), 32cc31–32cc34.

Morris, D. (2005). Independent nurse: Clinical – Prescribing – Prescribing for osteoporosis. *General Practitioner*, July 1, 97–102. Retrieved January 20, 2008, from http://ebsco.waldenu.edu/ehost/detail?vid=4&hid=115&sid=55fdd3ae-a6d5-4629-8fa9-fd6330627fcf%40sessionmgr103.

Mueller, A. C., & Bell, A. E. (2008). Electrolye update: Potassium, chloride, and magnesium. *Nursing Critical Care, 3*(1), 5–7.

Mulhauser, G. (2007). *Welcome to the CAGE questionnaire, a screening test for alcohol dependence*. Retrieved January 1, 2008, from http://counsellingresource.com/quizzes/alcohol-cage/index.html.

Murphy, S.A. (1993). Coping strategies of abstainer from alcohol up to three years post-treatment. *Image: Journal of Nursing Scholarship, 25*(2), 87.

Nagel, C. L., Markie, M. B., Richards, K. C., & Taylor, J. L. (2003). Sleep promotion in hospitalized elders. *Medical and Surgical Nursing, 12*(5), 279–290. Retrieved January 14, 2008, from http://web.ebscohost.com/ehost/results?vid=17&hid=106&sid=c7e5d2b4-a****3-4480-a27f-fdf75c9b820%40sessionmgr106.

Namias, N. (2007). Advances in burn care. *Current Opinions in Critical Care, 13*(4), 405–410.

National Cancer Institute. (2003a). *Stem cell transplantation*. Retrieved November 16, 2007, from http://www.cancer.gov/cancertopics/wyntk/leukemia/page16.

National Cancer Institute. (2003b). *Types of leukemia*. Retrieved November 16, 2007, from http://www.cancer.gov/cancertopics/wyntk/leukemia/page5.

National Cancer Institute. (2007). *Lymphedema management*. Retrieved November 5, 2007, from http://www.cancer.gov/cancertopics/pdq/supportivecare/lymphedema/HealthProfessional/page2.

National Cancer Institute. (2008). *Support and resources*. Retrieved January 2, 2008, from http://www.cancer.gov/cancertopics/support.

National Cholesterol Education Program. (2002). Expert panel on detection, evaluation and treatment of high cholesterol in adults. *Circulation, 106,* 413–421.

National Health Consensus Development Panel on Osteoporosis Prevention, Diagnosis, and Therapy. (2001). Osteoporosis prevention, diagnosis, and therapy [Comment]. *Journal of the American Medical Association, 285*(6), 785–795.

National Institute of Arthritis and Musculoskeletal and Skin Diseases. (2003). *Lupus*. Retrieved December 30, 2007, from http://www.niams.nih.gov/Health_Info/Lupus/default.asp.

National Institute of Arthritis and Musculoskeletal and Skin Diseases. (2008) *Health information page*. Retrieved January 07, 2008, from http://www.naims.nih.gov/Health_Info/Fibromyalgia /fibrmyalgia_ff.asp.

National Institutes of Health (NIH). (2000). Optimal calcium intake. *U.S. Department of Health and Human Services, NIH Consensus Statement, 12*(4), 1–31.

National Institute of Neurological Disorders and Stroke. (2007). Guillain-Barre Syndrome information page. Retrieved December 2, 2007, from http://ninds.nih.gov/disorders/gbs/gbs.htm.

National Kidney Foundation. (2007). *Facts about chronic kidney disease*. Retrieved November 4, 2007, from www.kidney.org.

National Library of Medicine. (2006). *Leukemia*. Retrieved November 16, 2007, from http://www.nlm.nih.gov/medlineplus/tutorials/leukemia/htm/index.htm.

National Spinal Cord Injury Association. (2007). *National Spinal Cord Injury Association*. Retrieved December 12, 2007, from http://www.spinalcord.org.

Nettina, S. M. (2006). *Lippincott manual of nursing practice* (8th ed.). Ambler, PA: Lippincott Williams & Wilkins.

Newman, D. K., Kennelly, M. J., Lemack, G. E., & McIlwain, M. (2007). Transdermal oxybutynin treatment for neurogenic bladder: Patient safety and QOL. *The Journal of Wound, Ostomy and Continence Nursing, 34*(3S), S64.

Newmarch, C. (2006). Caring for the mechanically ventilated patient: Part one. *Nursing Standard, 20*(17), 54–64.

Nguyen, T., Gwynn, R., Kellerman, S. Begier, E., Garg, R., Pfeiffer, et al. (2008). Population prevalence of reported and unreported HIV and related behaviors among the household adult population in New York City, 2004. *AIDS: Official Journal of the International AIDS Society, 22*(2), 281–287.

Nichols, R. I. (1991). Surgical wound infections. *American Journal of Medicine, 91*(Suppl. 3B), 54–64.

Nighorn, S. (1988). Narcissistic deficits in drug abusers: A self-psychological approach. *Journal of Psychosocial Nursing & Mental Health Services, 26*(9), 22–26.

Ninot, G., Fortes, M., Leymarie, S., Burn, A., Poulain, M., Desplan, J., et al. (2002). Effects of an intensive-period inpatient rehabilitation programme on the perceived physical self in moderate chronic obstructive pulmonary disease patients [Electronic version]. *International Journal of Rehabilitation Research, 25*(1), 51–55. Retrieved January 15, 2008, from http://web.ebscohost.com/ehost/detail?vid=23&hid=106&sid=c7e5d2b4-a****3-4480-a27f-fdf75c59b820%40sessionmgr106.

O'Connell, J. B., & Bristow, M. R. (1994). Economic impact of heart failure in the United States: Time for a different approach. *Journal of Heart and Lung Transplant,*13, S107–112.

Ofman, U. S. (1993). Psychosocial and sexual implications of genitourinary cancer. *Seminars in Oncology Nursing, 9*, 286–292.

Olek, M. J. (2007a). *Comorbid problems associated with multiple sclerosis in adults*. Retrieved November 1, 2007, from UpToDate.com.

Olek, M. J. (2007b). *Diagnosis of multiple sclerosis in adults*. Retrieved November 1, 2007, from UpToDate.com.

Olek, M. J. (2007c). *Epidemiology, risk factors, and clinical features of multiple sclerosis in adults*. Retrieved November 1, 2007, from UpToDate.com.

Olek, M. J. (2007d). *Treatment of progressive multiple sclerosis in adults*. Retrieved November 1, 2007, from UpToDate.com.

Oliveira-Filho, J., & Koroshetz, W. J. (2007). *Initial assessment and management of acute stroke*. Retrieved November 14, 2007, from UpToDate.com.

Oliver, M. J. (2007). Chronic hemodialysis vascular access: Types and placement. Retrieved January 15, 2008, from www.UpToDate.com.

Onizuka, Y., Mizuta, Y., Isomoto, H., Takeshima, F., Murase, K., Miyazaki, M., et al. (2001). Sludge and stone formation in the gallbladder in bedridden elderly patients with cerebrovascular disease: influence of feeding method [Electronic version]. *Journal of Gastroenterology, 36*(5), 330–337. Retrieved January 5, 2008, from http://web.ebscohost.com/ehost/pdf?vid=132&hid=106&sid=c7e5d2b4-a****3-4480-a27f-fdf75c59b820%40sessionmgr106.

Ottawa Eye Institute. (2006). *How cataract eye surgery is done*. Retrieved January 5, 2008, from http://www.eyeinstitute.net/cat-howsurgery.html.

Pace, R. C. (2007). Fluid management in patients on hemodialysis. *Nephrology Nursing Journal, 34*(5), 557–559.

Pajeau, A. (2002). Identifying patients at high risk of ischemic stroke. *Patient Care, 36*(5), 36–51.

Paparella, P., Sizzi, O., De Benedittis, F., Rossetti, A., & Paparella, R. (2004). Vaginal hysterectomy in generally considered contraindications to vaginal surgery. *Archives of Gynecological Obstetrics, 270*(2), 104–109.

Parikh, S., Koch, M., & Naraysn, R. (2007). Traumatic brain injury. *International Anesthesiology Clinics, 45*(3), 119–135.

Parker-Frizzell, J. (2005). Acute stroke. *AACN Clinical Issues, 16*(4), 421–440.

Parkinson's Disease Foundation (2007). *Parkinson's disease: An overview. What is Parkinson's Disease?* Retrieved December 10, 2007, from http://www.pdf.org/AboutPD.

Patsy, B. M., Smith, N. L., & Siscovick, D. S. (1997). Health outcomes associated with antihypertensive therapies used as first-line agents, *Journal of the American Medical Association, 277*, 739–45.

Pearce, J. M. (2007). Documenting peritoneal dialysis. *Nursing2007, 37*(10), 28.

Piasecki, P. A. (2000). Bone and soft tissue sarcoma. In S. Groenwald, M. Frogge, M. Goodman, & C. Yarbro (Eds.), *Cancer nursing: Principles and practice* (5th ed.). Boston: Jones and Bartlett.

Pickering, T. (1996). Recommendations for the use of home (self) and ambulatory blood pressure monitoring. American Society of Hypertension ad hoc Panel. *American Journal of Hypertension, 0*, 1–11.

Pieper, B., & Mikols, C. (1996). Predischarge and postdischarge concerns of persons with an ostomy. *The Journal of WOCN, 23*(2), 105–109.

Piette, J. D. (2005). *Using telephone support to manage chronic disease*. Retrieved January 6, 2007, from http://www.chef.org/topics/chronicdisease/index.cfm.

Pontieri-Lewis, V. (2006). Basics of ostomy care. *Medical and Surgical Nursing, 15*(4), 199–202.

Porth, C. M. (2006). Disorders of ventilation and gas exchange. In C. M. Porth (Ed.), *Pathophysiology: Concepts of altered health states* (7th ed., pp. 689–724). Philadelphia: Lippincott Williams & Wilkins.

Porth, C. M. (Ed.). (2006). *Pathophysiology: Concepts of altered health states* (6th ed.). Philadelphia: Lippincott Williams & Wilkins.

Powell-Cope, G., & Brown, M. A. (1992). Going public as an AIDS family caregiver. *Social Science & Medicine, 34*(5), 571–580.

Pruitt, W. C., & Jacobs, M. (2006). The ins and outs of mechanical ventilation. *LPN 2006, 2*(2), 18–27.

Purdue, G. F. (2007). American Burn Association presidential address 2006 on nutrition: Yesterday, today, and tomorrow. *Journal of Burn Care & Research, 28*(1), 1–5.

Ray, R. I. (2000). Complications of lower extremity amputations. *Topics in Emergency Medicine, 22*(3), 35–42.

Reddy, L. S. (2006). Heads up on cerebral bleeds. *ED Inside,* 4–9.

Redemann, S. (2002). Modalities for immobilization. In A. B. Maher, S. W. Salmond, & T. A. Pellino (Eds.), *Orthopedic nursing* (3rd ed., p. 303). Philadelphia: W. B. Saunders.

Redman, B., & Thomas, S. (1996). Patient teaching. In J. Kulbshek & J. McCloskey (Eds.), *Nursing interventions* (2nd ed.). Philadelphia. W. B. Saunders.

Redmond, A., & Doherty, E. (2005). Peritoneal Dialysis. *Nursing Standard, 19*(40), 55–65.

Redmond, A., McDevitt, M., & Barnes, S. (2004). Acute renal failure: recognition and treatment in ward patients. *Nursing Standard,* 18(22), 46–55.

Respiratory Function and Therapy. (2006). In E. J. Mills (Ed.), *Lippincott Manual of Nursing Practice* (8th ed.). Ambler, PA: Lippincott Williams & Wilkins.

Richbourg, L., Thorpe, J. M., & Rapp. C. G. (2007). Difficulties experienced by the ostomate after hospital discharge. *Journal of Wound, Ostomy and Continence Nursing, 34*(1), 70–79.

Rigdon, J. L. (2006). Robotic-assisted laparoscopic radical prostatectomy. *AORN, 84*(5), 759–762, 764, 766–770.

Rogers, B. (2005). Looking at lymphoma and leukemia. *Nursing 2005, 35*(7), 56–64.

Rolim de Moura, C., Paranhos, A., Jr., & Wormald, R. (2007). Laser trabeculoplasty for open angel glaucoma [Systematic Review]. *Cochrane Database of Systematic Reviews* (4).

Rollnick, S., Mason, P., & Butler, C. (2000). *Health behavior change: A guide for practitioners*. Edinburgh, United Kingdom: Churchill Livingstone.

Roman, M., Weinstein, A., & Macaluso, S. (2003). Primary spontaneous pneumothorax. *Medical and Surgical Nursing, 12*(3), 161–169.

Rosamond, W., Flegal, K., Friday, G., Furie, K., Go, A., Grenlund, K., et al. (2007). Heart disease and stroke statistics—2007 update: A report from the American Heart Association Statistics Committee and Stroke Statistics Committee. *Circulation, 115,* e70–e171.

Rudolph, D. (1992). Limb loss in the elderly peripheral vascular disease patient. *Journal of Vascular Nursing, 10*(3), 8–13.

Sacco, R. L., Adams, R., Albers, G., Alberts, M. J., Benavente, O., Furie, K., et al. (2006). Guidelines for prevention of strokes in patients with ischemic stroke or transient ischemic attach: A statement for healthcare professionals from the American Heart Association/American Stroke Association Council on Cardiovascular Radiology and Intervention: The American Academy of Neurology affirms the value of this guideline. *Stroke, 37,* 577–617.

Salmond, S. (Ed.). (1996). *Core curriculum for orthopedic nursing* (3rd ed.). Pitman, NJ: National Association of Orthopedic Nurses.

Salmond, S. (1998). Infections of musculoskeletal system. In A. B. Maher, S. Salmond, & T. Pellino (Eds.), *Orthopedic nursing* (2nd ed.). Philadelphia: W. B. Saunders.

Sampson, H. W. (2002). Alcohol and other factors affecting osteoporosis risk in women [Electronic version]. *Alcohol Research and Health, 26*(4), 292–298. Retrieved January 20, 2008, from http://ebsco.waldenu.edu/ehost/pdf?vid=6&hid=102&sid=55fdd3ae-a6d5-4629-8fa9-fd330627fcf%40sessionmgr103.

Santoni-Reddy, L. (2006). Heads up on cerebral bleeds. *ED Insider,* (Spring), 4–9.

Saxon, L. A., Kumar, U. N., & DeMarco, T. (2007). *Cardiac resynchronization therapy (biventricular pacing) in heart failure*. Retrieved January 15, 2008, from www.UpToDate.com.

Scales, K., & Pilsworth, J. (2007). A practical guide to extubation. *Nursing Standard, 22*(2), 44–48.

Schmiege, S. J., Aiken, L. S., Sander, J. L., & Gerend, M. A. (2007). Osteoporosis prevention among young women: Psychosocial models [Electronic version]. *Health Psychology, 26*(5), 577–587. Retrieved January 21, 2008, from http://ebsco.waldenu.edu/ehost/pdf?vid=38&hid=113&sid=55fdd3ae-a6d5-4629-8fa9-fd6330627fcf%40session mgr103.

Schmidt, L. M. (2004). Herbal remedies: The other drugs your patients take [Electronic version]. *Home Healthcare Nurse, 22*(3), 169–175. Retrieved January 17, 2008, from http://gateway.tx.ovid.com.library.geu.edu:2048/gw2/ovidweb.cgi.

Schoen, D. C. (2004). Osteoporosis. *Orthopaedic Nursing, 23*(4), 261–266.

Schummer, W., Schummer, C., & Schelenz, C. (2003). Case report: the malfunctioning implanted venous access device [Electronic version]. *British Journal of Nursing, 12*(4), 210–214. Retrieved January 5, (2008), from http://web.ebscohost.com/ehost/pdf?vid=139&hid=106&sid=c7e5d2b4-a693-4480-a27f-fdf75c59b820%40session mgr106.

Schur, P. H. (2007). *Patient information: Systemic lupus erythematosus (SLE)*. Retrieved November 1, 2007, from UpToDate.com.

Schur, P. H., & Gladman, D. D. (2007). *Overview of the clinical manifestations of systemic lupus erythematosus*. Retrieved November 1, 2007, from UpToDate.com.

Schur, P. H., & Khoshbin, S. (2007). *Neurologic manifestations of systemic lupus erythematosus*. Retrieved November 1, 2007, from UpToDate.com.

Schur, P. H. & Moschella, S. L. (2007). *Cutaneous manifestations of systemic lupus erthematosus*. Retrieved Novemeber 1, 2007, from UpToDate.com.

Schur, P. H., & Wallace, D. J. (2007). *Overview of the therapy and prognosis of systemic lupus erythematosus*. Retrieved November 1, 2007, from UpToDate.com.

Schwamm, L. H., Pancioli, A., Acker, J. E., Goldstein, L. B., Zorowitz, R. D., Shephard, T. J., et al. (2005). Recommendations for the establishment of stroke systems of care: Recommendations from the American Stroke Association's Task Force on the development of stroke systems. *Stroke, 36,* 690–703.

Seaward-Hersh, A. (2004). Ensuring best practice in the treatment of peritonitis and exit site infection. *Nephrology Nursing Journal, 31*(5), 585–586.

Shah, T., Sharma, R., Mehta, H., Rau, R., & Solanki, P. (2002). Another indication for chest tube after pneumonectomy [comment]. *Texas Heart Institute Journal, 29*(3), 232.

Sheahan, S. L. (2002). How to help older adults quit smoking [Electronic version]. *Nurse Practitioner, 27*(12), 27–34. Retrieved January 15, 2008, from http://web.ebscohost.com/ehost/results?vid=14&hid=106&sid=c7e5d2b4-a****3-4480-a27f-fdf75c59b820%40sessionmgr106.

Shelton, B. K. (2005) Infection. In C. H. Yarbo, M. H. Frogge, & M. Goodman (Eds.), *Cancer nursing: Principles and practice* (6th ed.) Boston: Jones & Bartlett.

Sheth, K. (2007). Increased intracranial pressure. Retrieved November 18, 2007, from http://www.nlm.nih.gov/medlineplus/ency/article/000793.htm.

Shigehiko, U., Kellum, J., Bellomo, R., Doig, G., Morimatsu, H., Morgera, S., et al. (2005). Acute renal failure in critically ill patients. *The Journal of the American Medical Association, 294*(7), 813–818.

Shirato, S. (2005). How CAM helps systemic lupus erythematosus. *Holistic Nursing Practice, 19*(1), 36–39.

Sieggreen, M. (2006). A contemporary approach to peripheral arterial disease. *The Nurse Practitioner, 31*(7), 14–25.

Sieggreen, M. (2007). Recognize acute arterial occulasion. *Nursing 2007 Critical Care, 2*(5), 50–59.

Sims, J. M. (2006). An overview of asthma [Electronic version]. *Dimensions of Critical Care Nursing, 25*(6), 264–268. Retrieved November 30, 2007, from http://gateway.tx.ovid.com.library.gcu.edu:2048/gw2/ovidweb.cgi.

Singh, V., Devgan, L., Bhat, S., & Milner, S. (2007). The pathogenesis of burn wound conversion. *Annals of Plastic Surgery, 59*(1), 109–115.

Sirey, J., Raue, P. J., & Alexopoulos, G. S. (2007). An intervention to improve depression care [Electronic version]. *International Journal of Geriatric Psychiatry, 22,* 154–159. Retrieved January 15, 2008, from http://web.ebscohost.com.ehost/pdt?vid=25&hid=106&sid=c7e5d2b4-a****3-1100 a27f fdf75 c59b820%40sessionmgr106.

Sirocky, M. B. (2002). Pathogenesis of bacteriuria and infection in the spinal cord injured patient. *American Journal of Medicine, 113*(Supplement 1A), 67S–79S.

Sjogren's Syndrome Foundation. (2008). Home page. Sjogren's Syndrome Foundation. Retrieved January 02, 2008, from http://www.sjogrens.org.

Slinger, P. D. (2003). Acute lung injury after pulmonary resection: More pieces of the puzzle. *Anesthesia & Analgesia, 97*(6), 1555–1557.

Smith, M. (2007). Intensive care management of patients with subarachnoid hemorrhage. *Current Opinion in Anesthesiology, 20*(5), 400–407.

Smith-DiJulio, K. (2001). Rape. In E. Varcarolis (Ed.), *Foundations of psychiatric mental health nursing* (4th ed.). Philadelphia: W. B. Saunders.

Society for Vascular Surgery. (2007). *Amputation*. Retrieved November 13, 2007, from http://vascularweb.org/_CONTRIBUTION_PAGES/Patient_Information/NorthPoint/Amputation.html.

Solomon, J., Yee, N., & Soulen, M. (2000). Aortic stent grafts: An overview of devices, indications and results. *Applied Radiology Supplement, 7,* 43–51.

Sommers, M. S., Johnson, S. A., & Beery, T. A. (2007). *Diseases and disorders: A nursing therapeutics manual* (3rd ed.). Philadelphia: F. A. Davis Company.

Spratto, G., & Woods, A. (2007). *2007 Edition PDR nurse's drug handbook*. Thomas Delmar Learning.

Stajduhar, K. I., Martin, W. L., & Barwich, D. (2008). Factors influencing family caregivers ability to cope with providing end-of-life cancer at home. *Cancer Nursing: An International Journal for Cancer Care, 31*(1), 77–85.

Stanbridge, R., Hon, J. K. F., Bateman, E., & Roberts, S. (2007). Minimally invasive anterior thoracotomy for routine lung cancer resection. *Innovations, 2*(2), 76–83.

Stevens, R. H. (1992). Patients who have undergone bone marrow transplantation: Their quest for meaning. *Oncology Nursing Forum, 19*(6), 899–905.

Strobik, Y. (2007). Protocols, practice and patients: The case of alcohol withdrawal. *Critical Care Medicine, 35*(3), 955.

Sublett, C. M. (2007). Critique of 'Effects of advanced practice nursing on patient and spouse depressive symptoms, sexual function, and marital interaction after radical prostatectomy.' *Urology Nursing, 27*(1), 78–80.

Sullivan, M. J., & Hawthorne, M. H. (1996). Nonpharmacologic interventions in the treatment of heart failure. *Journal of Cardiovascular Nursing, 10*(2), 47–57.

Surgeryencyclopedia. (2007). Enucleation, eye: definition, purpose, demographics, description, diagnostics/preparation. Retrieved January 15, 2008, from http://www.Surgeryencyclopedia.com/CeFi/Enucleation-eye.html.

Surgical Procedures. (2004). In J. D. Crapo, J. Glassroth, J. B. Karlinsky, & T. E. King (Eds.), *Baum's Textbook of Pulmonary Disease* (7th ed). Philadelphia: Lippincott Williams & Wilkins.

Susan B. Komen for the Cure. (2007a). *Anatomy of breast cancer-Updated: Mastectomy.* Retrieved November 5, 2007, from http://cms.komen.org/komen/aboutbreastcancer/treatment/s_002819?ssSourceNodeld=298&ssSource Siteld=Komen.

Susan B. Komen for the Cure. (2007b). *Enucleation, eye.* Retrieved November 5, 2007, from http://cms.komen.org/komen/aboutbreastcancer/treatment/s_002819?ssSourceNodeld=298&ssSourceSiteld=komen.

Susan B. Komen for the Cure. (2007c). *Lymphedema.* Retrieved November 5, 2007, from http://cms.komen.org/komen/aboutbreastcancer/aftertreatment/3-6-3?ssSourceNodeld=301&ssSourceSiteld=Komen.

Susan B. Komen for the Cure (2007d). *Sex and sexuality.* Retrieved November 5, 2007, from http://cms.komen.org/komen/aboutbreastcancer/aftertreatment/3-3-4?ssSourceNodeld=301&ssSourceSiteld=Komen.

Swanson, M. C. (2004). Encouraging adherence to treatment regimen in a CCPD patient. *Nephrology Nursing Journal, 31*(1), 80.

Tapasi, S., & Harmeet, S. (2007). Noninfectious complications of peritoneal dialysis. *Southern Medical Journal, 100*(1), 54–58.

Tewari, A., Peabody, J., Sarle, R., Balakrishnan, G., Hemal, A., Shrivastava, A., et al. (2002). Technique of Da Vinci robot-assisted anatomic radical prostatectomy. *Urology, 60*(4), 569–572.

Thomas, K., Burton, D., Withrow, L. & Adkisson, B. (2004). Impact of a preoperative education program via interactive telehealth network for rural patients having total joint replacement. *Orthopaedic Nursing, 23*(1), 39–44.

Thomson, N. (2002). *Renal Nursing.* (2nd ed.). London, UK: Bailliere Tindall.

Thoracoscopy (Pleuroscopy). (2004). In C. Jeffrey (Ed.), *Baum's Textbook of Pulmonary Disease* (7th ed.). Philadelphia: Lippincott Williams & Wilkins.

Tinetti, M. E. (2003). Preventing falls in the elderly persons. *New England Journal of Medicine, 348*(January 3), 42–49.

Titler, M., Dochterman, J., Xie, X., Kanak, M., Fei, Q., Picone, D., et al. (2006). Nursing interventions and other factors associated with discharge disposition in elders patients after hip surgery. *Nursing Research, 55*(4), 231–242.

Torpy, J. (2005). Myasthenia Gravis. *The Journal of the American Medical Association, 293*(15), 1940.

Tschopp, O., Boehler, A., Speich, R., Weder, W., Seifert, b., Russi, E. W., et al. (2002). Osteoporosis before lung tranplantation [Electronic version]. *American Journal of Transplantation, 2*(2), 167–172. Retrieved January 23, 2008, from http://ebsco.waldenu.edu/ehost/pdf?vid=4&hid=112&sid=b2fae363-688a-4e54-96d6-e87f0fde711c%40session103.

United Ostomy Association. (2006). *Urostomy: A guide.* Retrieved October 31, 2007, from http://cancer.org/docroot/CRI/content/CRI_2_6x_Urostomy.asp.

U.S. National Library of Medicine. (2006). *Osteomyelitis.* Retrieved November 17, 2007, from http://www.nlm.nih.gov/medlineplus/ency/article/000437.htm.

United Ostomy Association. (2006) *Urostomy: A guide.* Retrieved October 31, 2007, from http://cancer.org/docroot/CRI/content/CRI_2_6x_Urostomy.asp.

Valente, S. (2004). End-of-life challenges: Honoring autonomy. *Cancer Nursing: An International Journal for Cancer Care, 27*(4), 314–319.

Vass, C., Hirn, C., Sycha, T., Findl, O., Bauer, P., & Schmetterer, L. (2007). *Medical interventions for primary angle glaucoma and ocular hypertension.* Retrieved January 2, 2008, from Cochrane Database of Systematic Reviews 2007.

Vattikuti Urology Institute. (2007). *Vattikuti Urology Institute.* Retrieved November 6, 2007, from http://www.henryfordhealth.org/body.cfm?id=41144.

Vere-Jones, E. (2007). Nursing the survivors of sexual assault. *Nursing Times, 103*(35), 18–19.

Voytas, J. J., Kowalski, D., Wagner, S., Carlson, A., & Maddens, M. (2004). Eye care in the skilled nursing facility: A pilot study of prevalence and treatment patterns of the glaucoma. *Journal of the American Medical Directors Association, 5*(3), 156–160.

Wagner, K. D., Johnson, K., & Kidd, P. S. (2006). *High Acuity Nursing* (4th ed.). Upper Saddle River, NJ: Prentice Hall.

Walker, C., Hogstel, M. O., Curry, L. (2007). Hospital discharge of older adults: how nurses can ease the transition. *American Journal of Nursing, 107*(6), 60–70.

Walker, M. D., Babbar, R., Opotowsky, A., McMahon, D. J., Lui, G. & Bilezikian, J. P. (April 2007). Determinants of bone mineral density in Chinese-American women. *Osteoporosis International, 18*(4), 471–478.

Walker, W. E. (2002). Hazards of chest tubes after pneumonectomy. *Texas Heart Institute Journal, 29*(1), 72; author reply 72–73.

Ward, G. E., Rennie, D. J., & Harper, W. (1998). Multidisciplinary assessment of outcome after hip fracture surgery. *British Journal of Therapy and Rehabilitation, 5*(1).

Warner, C. (2001). The use of orthopaedic perioperative autotransfusion (OrthoPAT™) system in total joint replacement surgery. *Orthopaedic Nursing, 20*(6), 29–32.

Weaver, T., & Narsavage, G. (1992). Physiological and psychological variables related to functional status in chronic obstructive pulmonary disease. *Nursing Research, 41*(5), 286–291.

Webb, R. T., Lawson, A. L., & Neal, D. E. (1990). Clean intermittent self-catheterization in 172 adults. *British Journal of Urology, 65*(1), 20–23.

Whelton, S. P., Chin, A., Xin, X., & He, J. (2002). Effect of aerobic exercise on blood pressure: A meta-analysis of randomized, controlled trials. *Ann Intern Med, 136*, 493–503.

Wickham, R., and Keenan, A. K. (2005). Hypercalcemia. In C. Yarbro, M. Frogge, M. Goodman (Eds.), *Cancer nursing: Principles & practice* (6th ed.). Boston: Jones and Bartlett.

Wiesel, P. (2000). Gut focused behavioral treatment (biofeedback) for constipation and fecal incontinence in multiple sclerosis. *Journal of Neurology, Neurosurgery, and Psychiatry, 69*(2), 24003.

Wilkes, G. (2005). Colon, rectal and anal cancers. In C. H. Yarbo, M. H. Frogge, & M. Goodman (Eds.), *Cancer Nursing: Principles and Practices* (6th ed.). Boston: Jones and Bartlett.

Williamson, D. F., Serdula, M. K., & Anda, R. F. et al. (1992). Weight loss in adults: Goals, duration, and rate of weight loss. *American Journal of Public Health, 82*(9), 1251–1257.

Williamson, V, C. (1992). Amputation of the lower extremity: An overview. *Orthopaedic Nursing, 11*(2), 55–65.

Wilson, L. D. (2007). Clinical practice: Superior vena cava syndrome with malignant causes. *New England Journal of Medicine, 356*(18), 1862–1869.

Wing, L. M. H., Reid, P. (2003). A comparison of outcomes with angiotensinconverting-enzyme inhibitors and diuretics for hypertension in the elderly. *New England Journal of Medicine, 348*, 583–592.

Women's Health. (2005). Women's support center for rape victims www.womenshealth.gov.

Wong, S. & Ciliska. (2003). Intentional weight loss was associated with lower mortality, whereas unintentional weight loss was associated with increased mortality. *Evidence-Based Nursing, 6*(4). Retrieved January 15, 2008, from http://ebn.bmj.com/cgi/reprint/6/4/121.

Wright, I. (2007). Cerebral aneurysm-treatment and perioperative nursing care. *AORN, 85*(6), 1172–1182.

Wujcik, D. (2005). Leukemia. In C. Yarbro, M. Frogge, & M. Goodman (Eds.), *Cancer nursing: Principles and practice* (6th ed.). Boston: Jones and Bartlett.

Yates, P. C. (1993). Toward a reconceptualization of hope for patients with a diagnosis of cancer. *Journal of Advanced Nursing, 18*(4), 701–708.

Yetzer, E. A. (1996). Helping the patient through the experience of an amputation. *Orthaepedic Nursing, 15*(6), 45–49.

Yetzer, E., Kauffman, G., & Sopp, F. (1994). Development of a patient education program for new amputees. *Rehabilitation Nursing, 19*(6) 355–358.

Zaetta, J., Mulilu, E., & Baum, P. (2007) *Indications for percutaneous interventional procedures in the in the patient with claudication.* Retrieved November 14, 2007, from UpToDate.com.

Zalon, M. (2004). Correlates of recovery among older adults after major abdominal surgery. *Nursing Research, 53*(2), 99-106.

Zebrack, B. (2000). Quality of Life of long-term survivors of leukemia and lymphoma. *Journal of Psychosocial Oncology, 18*(4), 39–59.

Zeller, J., Lym, C., & Glass, R. M. (2007). Septic arthritis. *The Journal of the American Medical Association, 297*(13), 1405–1407.

Zepf, B. (2002). Outcomes after total versus subtotal abdominal hysterectomy. *New England Journal of Medicine, 347*, 1318–1325.

Zurakowski, T., Taylor, M., & Bradway, C. (2006). Effective teaching strategies for the older adult with urologic concerns. *Urologic Nursing, 26*(5), 355–360.

LIST OF NIC INTERVENTIONS AND NOC OUTCOMES

Nursing Interventions Classification (NIC) Labels[1]

Abuse Protection Support
Abuse Protection Support: Child
Abuse Protection Support: Domestic Partner
Abuse Protection Support: Elder
Abuse Protection Support: Religious
Acid-Base Management
Acid-Base Management: Metabolic Acidosis
Acid-Base Management: Metabolic Alkalosis
Acid-Base Management: Respiratory Acidosis
Acid-Base Management: Respiratory Alkalosis
Acid-Base Monitoring
Active Listening
Activity Therapy
Acupressure
Admission Care
Airway Insertion and Stabilization
Airway Management
Airway Suctioning
Allergy Management
Amnioinfusion
Amputation Care
Analgesic Administration
Analgesic Administration: Intraspinal
Anaphylaxis Management
Anesthesia Administration
Anger Control Assistance
Animal-Assisted Therapy
Anticipatory Guidance
Anxiety Reduction
Area Restriction
Aromatherapy
Art Therapy
Artificial Airway Management
Aspiration Precautions
Assertiveness Training
Asthma Management
Attachment Promotion
Autogenic Training
Autotransfusion

Bathing
Bed Rest Care
Bedside Laboratory Testing
Behavior Management
Behavior Management: Overactivity/Inattention

Behavior Management: Self-Harm
Behavior Management: Sexual
Behavior Modification
Behavior Modification: Social Skills
Bibliotherapy
Biofeedback
Birthing
Bladder Irrigation
Bleeding Precautions
Bleeding Reduction
Bleeding Reduction: Antepartum Uterus
Bleeding Reduction: Gastrointestinal
Bleeding Reduction: Nasal
Bleeding Reduction: Postpartum Uterus
Bleeding Reduction: Wound
Blood Products Administration
Body Image Enhancement
Body Mechanics Promotion
Bottle Feeding
Bowel Incontinence Care
Bowel Incontinence Care: Encopresis
Bowel Irrigation
Bowel Management
Bowel Training
Breast Examination
Breastfeeding Assistance

Calming Technique
Cardiac Care
Cardiac Care: Acute
Cardiac Care: Rehabilitative
Cardiac Precautions
Caregiver Support
Case Management
Cast Care: Maintenance
Cast Care: Wet
Cerebral Edema Management
Cerebral Perfusion Promotion
Cesarean Section Care
Chemical Restraint
Chemotherapy Management
Chest Physiotherapy
Childbirth Preparation
Circulatory Care: Arterial Insufficiency
Circulatory Care: Mechanical Assist Device

[1]From Bulechek, G., Butcher, H., & Dochterman, J. M. (Eds.). (2008). *Nursing interventions classification (NIC): Iowa intervention project* (5th ed.). St. Louis, MO: Mosby. Reprinted with permission.

Circulatory Care: Venous Insufficiency
Circulatory Precautions
Circumcision Care
Code Management
Cognitive Restructuring
Cognitive Stimulation
Communicable Disease Management
Communication Enhancement: Hearing Deficit
Communication Enhancement: Speech Deficit
Communication Enhancement: Visual Deficit
Community Disaster Preparedness
Community Health Development
Complex Relationship Building
Conflict Mediation
Constipation/Impaction Management
Consultation
Contact Lens Care
Controlled Substance Checking
Coping Enhancement
Cost Containment
Cough Enhancement
Counseling
Crisis Intervention
Critical Path Development
Culture Brokerage
Cutaneous Stimulation

Decision-Making Support
Defibrillator Management: External
Defibrillator Management: Internal
Delegation
Delirium Management
Delusion Management
Dementia Management
Dementia Management: Bathing
Depositional Testimony
Developmental Care
Developmental Enhancement: Adolescent
Developmental Enhancement: Child
Dialysis Access Maintenance
Diarrhea Management
Diet Staging
Discharge Planning
Distraction
Documentation
Dressing
Dying Care
Dysreflexia Management
Dysrhythmia Management

Ear Care
Eating Disorders Management
Electroconvulsive Therapy (ECT) Management
Electrolyte Management
Electrolyte Management: Hypercalcemia
Electrolyte Management: Hyperkalemia
Electrolyte Management: Hypermagnesemia
Electrolyte Management: Hypernatremia
Electrolyte Management: Hyperphosphatemia

Electrolyte Management: Hypocalcemia
Electrolyte Management: Hypokalemia
Electrolyte Management: Hypomagnesemia
Electrolyte Management: Hyponatremia
Electrolyte Management: Hypophosphatemia
Electrolyte Monitoring
Electronic Fetal Monitoring: Antepartum
Electronic Fetal Monitoring: Intrapartum
Elopement Precautions
Embolus Care: Peripheral
Embolus Care: Pulmonary
Embolus Precautions
Emergency Care
Emergency Cart Checking
Emotional Support
Endotracheal Extubation
Energy Management
Enteral Tube Feeding
Environmental Management
Environmental Management: Attachment Process
Environmental Management: Comfort
Environmental Management: Community
Environmental Management: Home Preparation
Environmental Management: Safety
Environmental Management: Violence Prevention
Environmental Management: Worker Safety
Environmental Risk Protection
Examination Assistance
Exercise Promotion
Exercise Promotion: Strength Training
Exercise Promotion: Stretching
Exercise Therapy: Ambulation
Exercise Therapy: Balance
Exercise Therapy: Joint Mobility
Exercise Therapy: Muscle Control
Eye Care

Fall Prevention
Family Integrity Promotion
Family Integrity Promotion: Childbearing Family
Family Involvement Promotion
Family Mobilization
Family Planning: Contraception
Family Planning: Infertility
Family Planning: Unplanned Pregnancy
Family Presence Facilitation
Family Process Maintenance
Family Support
Family Therapy
Feeding
Fertility Preservation
Fever Treatment
Financial Resource Assistance
Fire-Setting Precautions
First Aid
Fiscal Resource Management
Flatulence Reduction
Fluid/Electrolyte Management
Fluid Management

Fluid Monitoring
Fluid Resuscitation
Foot Care
Forensic Data Collection
Forgiveness Facilitation

Gastrointestinal Intubation
Genetic Counseling
Grief Work Facilitation
Grief Work Facilitation: Perinatal Death
Guided Imagery
Guilt Work Facilitation

Hair Care
Hallucination Management
Health Care Information Exchange
Health Education
Health Literacy Enhancement
Health Policy Monitoring
Health Screening
Health System Guidance
Heat/Cold Application
Heat Exposure Treatment
Hemodialysis Therapy
Hemodynamic Regulation
Hemofiltration Therapy
Hemorrhage Control
High-Risk Pregnancy Care
Home Maintenance Assistance
Hope Inspiration
Hormone Replacement Therapy
Humor
Hyperglycemia Management
Hypervolemia Management
Hypnosis
Hypoglycemia Management
Hypothermia Induction
Hypothermia Treatment
Hypovolemia Management

Immunization/Vaccination Management
Impulse Control Training
Incident Reporting
Incision Site Care
Infant Care
Infection Control
Infection Control: Intraoperative
Infection Protection
Insurance Authorization
Intracranial Pressure (ICP) Monitoring
Intrapartal Care
Intrapartal Care: High-Risk Delivery
Intravenous (IV) Insertion
Intravenous (IV) Therapy
Invasive Hemodynamic Monitoring

Journaling

Kangaroo Care

Labor Induction
Labor Suppression
Laboratory Data Interpretation
Lactation Counseling
Lactation Suppression
Laser Precautions
Latex Precautions
Learning Facilitation
Learning Readiness Enhancement
Leech Therapy
Limit Setting
Lower Extremity Monitoring

Malignant Hyperthermia Precautions
Massage
Mechanical Ventilation Management: Invasive
Mechanical Ventilation Management: Noninvasive
Mechanical Ventilatory Weaning
Medication Administration
Medication Administration: Ear
Medication Administration: Enteral
Medication Administration: Eye
Medication Administration: Inhalation
Medication Administration: Interpleural
Medication Administration: Intradermal
Medication Administration: Intramuscular (IM)
Medication Administration: Intraosseous
Medication Administration: Intraspinal
Medication Administration: Intravenous (IV)
Medication Administration: Oral
Medication Administration: Rectal
Medication Administration: Skin
Medication Administration: Subcutaneous
Medication Administration: Vaginal
Medication Administration: Ventricular Reservoir
Medication Management
Medication Prescribing
Medication Reconciliation
Meditation Facilitation
Memory Training
Milieu Therapy
Mood Management
Multidisciplinary Care Conference
Music Therapy
Mutual Goal Setting

Nail Care
Nausea Management
Neurologic Monitoring
Newborn Care
Newborn Monitoring
Nonnutritive Sucking
Normalization Promotion
Nutrition Management
Nutrition Therapy
Nutritional Counseling
Nutritional Monitoring

Oral Health Maintenance

Oral Health Promotion

Oral Health Restoration

Order Transcription

Organ Procurement

Ostomy Care

Oxygen Therapy

Pacemaker Management: Temporary

Pacemaker Management: Permanent

Pain Management

Parent Education: Adolescent

Parent Education: Childrearing Family

Parent Education: Infant

Parenting Promotion

Pass Facilitation

Patient Contracting

Patient-Controlled Analgesia (PCA) Assistance

Patient Rights Protection

Peer Review

Pelvic Muscle Exercise

Perineal Care

Peripheral Sensation Management

Peripherally Inserted Central (PIC) Catheter Care

Peritoneal Dialysis Therapy

Pessary Management

Phlebotomy: Arterial Blood Sample

Phlebotomy: Blood Unit Acquisition

Phlebotomy: Cannulated Vessel

Phlebotomy: Venous Blood Sample

Phototherapy: Mood/Sleep Regulation

Phototherapy: Neonate

Physical Restraint

Physician Support

Pneumatic Tourniquet Precautions

Positioning

Positioning: Intraoperative

Positioning: Neurologic

Positioning: Wheelchair

Postanesthesia Care

Postmortem Care

Postpartal Care

Preceptor: Employee

Preceptor: Student

Preconception Counseling

Pregnancy Termination Care

Premenstrual Syndrome (PMS) Management

Prenatal Care

Preoperative Coordination

Preparatory Sensory Information

Presence

Pressure Management

Pressure Ulcer Care

Pressure Ulcer Prevention

Product Evaluation

Program Development

Progressive Muscle Relaxation

Prompted Voiding

Prosthesis Care

Pruritus Management

Quality Monitoring

Radiation Therapy Management

Rape-Trauma Treatment

Reality Orientation

Recreation Therapy

Rectal Prolapse Management

Referral

Relaxation Therapy

Religious Addiction Prevention

Religious Ritual Enhancement

Relocation Stress Reduction

Reminiscence Therapy

Reproductive Technology Management

Research Data Collection

Resiliency Promotion

Respiratory Monitoring

Respite Care

Resuscitation

Resuscitation: Fetus

Resuscitation: Neonate

Risk Identification

Risk Identification: Childbearing Family

Risk Identification: Genetic

Role Enhancement

Seclusion

Security Enhancement

Seizure Management

Seizure Precautions

Self-Awareness Enhancement

Self-Care Assistance

Self-Care Assistance: Bathing/Hygiene

Self-Care Assistance: Dressing/Grooming

Self-Care Assistance: Feeding

Self-Care Assistance: IADL

Self-Care Assistance: Toileting

Self-Care Assistance: Transfer

Self-Efficacy Enhancement

Self-Esteem Enhancement

Self-Hypnosis Facilitation

Self-Modification Assistance

Self-Responsibility Facilitation

Sexual Counseling

Shift Report

Shock Management

Shock Management: Cardiac

Shock Management: Vasogenic

Shock Management: Volume

Shock Prevention

Sibling Support

Skin Care: Donor Site

Skin Care: Topical Treatments

Skin Surveillance

Sleep Enhancement

Smoking Cessation Assistance

Social Marketing
Socialization Enhancement
Specimen Management
Spiritual Growth Facilitation
Spiritual Support
Splinting
Sports-Injury Prevention: Youth
Staff Development
Staff Supervision
Subarachnoid Hemorrhage Precautions
Substance Use Prevention
Substance Use Treatment
Substance Use Treatment: Alcohol Withdrawal
Substance Use Treatment: Drug Withdrawal
Substance Use Treatment: Overdose
Suicide Prevention
Supply Management
Support Group
Support System Enhancement
Surgical Assistance
Surgical Precautions
Surgical Preparation
Surveillance
Surveillance: Community
Surveillance: Late Pregnancy
Surveillance: Remote Electronic
Surveillance: Safety
Sustenance Support
Suturing
Swallowing Therapy

Teaching: Disease Process
Teaching: Footcare
Teaching: Group
Teaching: Individual
Teaching: Infant Nutrition 0–3 Months
Teaching: Infant Nutrition 4–6 Months
Teaching: Infant Nutrition 7–9 Months
Teaching: Infant Nutrition 10–12 Months
Teaching: Infant Safety: 0–3 Months
Teaching: Infant Safety: 4–6 Months
Teaching: Infant Safety: 7–9 Months
Teaching: Infant Safety: 10–12 Months
Teaching: Infant Stimulation: 0–4 Months
Teaching: Infant Stimulation: 5–8 Months
Teaching: Infant Stimulation: 9–12 Months
Teaching: Preoperative
Teaching: Prescribed Activity/Exercise
Teaching: Prescribed Diet
Teaching: Prescribed Medication
Teaching: Procedure/Treatment
Teaching: Psychomotor Skill
Teaching: Safe Sex
Teaching: Sexuality
Teaching: Toddler Nutrition: 13–18 Months
Teaching: Toddler Nutrition: 19–24 Months
Teaching: Toddler Nutrition: 25–36 Months
Teaching: Toddler Safety: 13–18 Months

Teaching: Toddler Safety: 19–24 Months
Teaching: Toddler Safety: 25–36 Months
Teaching: Toilet Training
Technology Management
Telephone Consultation
Telephone Follow-Up
Temperature Regulation
Temperature Regulation: Intraoperative
Therapeutic Play
Therapeutic Touch
Therapy Group
Thrombolytic Therapy: Management
Total Parenteral Nutrition (TPN) Administration
Touch
Traction/Immobilization Care
Transcutaneous Electrical Nerve Stimulation
    (TENS)
Transfer
Transport: Interfacility
Transport: Intrafacility
Trauma Therapy: Child
Triage: Disaster
Triage: Emergency Center
Triage: Telephone
Truth Telling
Tube Care
Tube Care: Chest
Tube Care: Gastrointestinal
Tube Care: Umbilical Line
Tube Care: Urinary
Tube Care: Ventriculostomy/Lumbar Drain

Ultrasonography: Limited Obstetric
Unilateral Neglect Management
Urinary Bladder Training
Urinary Catheterization
Urinary Catheterization: Intermittent
Urinary Elimination Management
Urinary Habit Training
Urinary Incontinence Care
Urinary Incontinence Care: Enuresis
Urinary Retention Care

Validation Therapy
Values Clarification
Vehicle Safety Promotion
Venous Access Devices (VAD) Maintenance
Ventilation Assistance
Visitation Facilitation
Vital Signs Monitoring
Vomiting Management

Weight Gain Assistance
Weight Management
Weight Reduction Assistance
Wound Care
Wound Care: Burns
Wound Care: Closed Drainage
Wound Irrigation

Nursing Outcomes Classifications (NOC) Approved for Clinical Testing[2]

Abuse Cessation
Abuse Protection
Abuse Recovery: Emotional
Abuse Recovery: Financial
Abuse Recovery: Physical
Abuse Recovery: Sexual
Abuse Recovery: Status
Abusive Behavior Self-Restraint
Acceptance: Health Status
Activity Tolerance
Adaption to Physical Disability
Adherence Behavior
Aggression Control
Allergic Response: Localized
Allergic Response: Systemic
Ambulation
Ambulation: Wheelchair
Anxiety Self-Control
Anxiety Level
Appetite
Aspiration Prevention
Asthma Self-Management

Balance
Blood Glucose Control
Blood Loss Severity
Blood Transfusion Reaction Control
Body Image
Body Mechanics Performance
Body Positioning: Self-Initiated
Bone Healing
Bowel Continence
Bowel Elimination
Breastfeeding Establishment: Infant
Breastfeeding Establishment: Maternal
Breastfeeding: Maintenance
Breastfeeding: Weaning

Cardiac Disease Self-Management
Cardiac Pump Effectiveness
Caregiver Adaptation to Patient
    Institutionalization
Caregiver Emotional Health
Caregiver Home Care Readiness
Caregiver Lifestyle Disruption
Caregiver-Patient Relationship
Caregiver Performance: Direct Care
Caregiver Performance: Indirect Care
Caregiver Physical Health
Caregiver Stressors
Caregiver Well-Being
Caregiving Endurance Potential

Child Adaptation to Hospitalization
Child Development: 1 Month
Child Development: 2 Months
Child Development: 4 Months
Child Development: 6 Months
Child Development: 12 Months
Child Development: 2 Years
Child Development: 3 Years
Child Development: 4 Years
Child Development: Preschool
Child Development: Middle Childhood
Child Development: Adolescence
Circulation Status
Client Satisfaction: Access to Care Resources
Client Satisfaction: Caring
Client Satisfaction: Communication
Client Satisfaction: Continuity of Care
Client Satisfaction: Cultural Need Fulfillment
Client Satisfaction: Functional Assistance
Client Satisfaction: Physical Care
Client Satisfaction: Protection of Rights
Client Satisfaction: Psychological Care
Client Satisfaction: Safety
Client Satisfaction: Symptom Control
Client Satisfaction: Teaching
Client Satisfaction: Technical Aspects of Care
Coagulation Status
Cognitive
Cognitive Orientation
Comfort Level
Comfortable Death
Communication
Communication: Expressive
Communication: Receptive
Community Competence
Community Disaster Readiness
Community Health Status
Community Health Status: Immunity
Community Risk Control: Chronic Disease
Community Risk Control: Communicable Disease
Community Risk Control: Lead Exposure
Community Risk Control: Violence
Community Violence Level
Compliance Behavior
Concentration
Coordinated Movement
Coping

Decision Making
Depression Level
Depression Self-Control
Diabetes Self-Management
Dialysis Access Integrity

---

[2]From Moorhead, S., Johnson, M., Maas, M., & Swenson, E. (Eds.). (2008). *Nursing outcomes classification* (4th ed.). St. Louis, MO: Mosby. Reprinted with permission.

Dignified Life-Closure
Discharge Readiness: Independent Living
Discharge Readiness: Supported Living
Distorted Thought Self-Control

Electrolyte & Acid–Base Balance
Endurance
Energy Conservation

Fall Prevention Behavior
Falls Occurrence
Family Coping
Family Functioning
Family Health Status
Family Integrity
Family Normalization
Family Participation in Professional Care
Family Physical Environment
Family Resiliency
Family Support During Treatment
Fear Level
Fear Level: Child
Fear Self-Control
Fetal Status: Antepartum
Fetal Status: Intrapartum
Fluid Balance
Fluid Overload Severity

Grief Resolution
Growth

Health Beliefs
Health Beliefs: Perceived Ability to Perform
Health Beliefs: Perceived Control
Health Beliefs: Perceived Resources
Health Beliefs: Perceived Threat
Health Orientation
Health Promoting Behavior
Health Seeking Behavior
Hearing Compensation Behavior
Hemodialysis Access
Hope
Hydration
Hyperactivity Level

Identity
Immobility Consequences: Physiological
Immobility Consequences: Psycho-Cognitive
Immune Hypersensitivity Control
Immune Hypersensitivity Response
Immune Status
Immunization Behavior
Impulse Self-Control
Infection Severity
Infection Severity: Newborn
Information Processing

Joint Movement: Active
Joint Movement: Ankle
Joint Movement: Elbow
Joint Movement: Fingers
Joint Movement: Hip
Joint Movement: Knee
Joint Movement: Neck
Joint Movement: Passive
Joint Movement: Shoulder
Joint Movement: Spine
Joint Movement: Wrist

Kidney Function
Knowledge: Body Mechanics
Knowledge: Breastfeeding
Knowledge: Cardiac Disease Management
Knowledge: Child Physical Safety
Knowledge: Conception Prevention
Knowledge: Diabetes Management
Knowledge: Diet
Knowledge: Disease Process
Knowledge: Energy Conservation
Knowledge: Fall Prevention
Knowledge: Fertility Promotion
Knowledge: Health Behavior
Knowledge: Health Promotion
Knowledge: Health Resources
Knowledge: Illness Care
Knowledge: Infant Care
Knowledge: Infection Control
Knowledge: Labor & Delivery
Knowledge: Maternal-Child Health
Knowledge: Medication
Knowledge: Ostomy Care
Knowledge: Parenting
Knowledge: Personal Safety
Knowledge: Postpartum Maternal Health
Knowledge: Preconception Maternal Health
Knowledge: Pregnancy
Knowledge: Prescribed Activity
Knowledge: Sexual Functioning
Knowledge: Substance Use Control
Knowledge: Treatment Procedure(s)
Knowledge: Treatment Regimen

Leisure Participation
Loneliness Severity

Maternal Status: Antepartum
Maternal Status: Intrapartum
Maternal Status: Postpartum
Mechnical Ventilation Response: Adult
Mechnical Ventilation Weaning Response: Adult
Medication Response
Memory
Mobility
Mood Equilibrium

Motivation
Muscle Function

Nausea and Vomiting: Control
Nausea and Vomiting: Disruptive Effects
Nausea and Vomiting Severity
Neglect Cessation
Neglect Recovery
Neurological Status
Neurological Status: Autonomic
Neurological Status: Central Motor Control
Neurological Status: Consciousness
Neurological Status: Cranial Sensory/
   Motor Function
Neurological Status: Spinal Sensory/
   Motor Function
Newborn Adaptation
Nutritional Status
Nutritional Status: Biochemical Measures
Nutritional Status: Body Mass
Nutritional Status: Energy
Nutritional Status: Food & Fluid Intake
Nutritional Status: Nutrient Intake

Oral Hygiene
Ostomy Self-Care

Pain: Adverse Psychological Response
Pain: Disruptive Effects
Pain Control
Pain Level
Parent–Infant Attachment
Parenting: Adolescent Physical Safety
Parenting: Early/Middle Childhood
Parenting: Infant/Toddler Physical Safety
Parenting: Psychological Safety
Parenting: Social Safety
Parenting Performance
Participation in Health Care Decisions
Personal Autonomy
Personal Health Status
Personal Safety Behavior
Personal Well-Being
Physical Aging
Physical Fitness
Physical Maturation: Female
Physical Maturation: Male
Play Participation
Post-Procedure Recovery Status
Prenatal Health Behavior
Preterm Infant Organization
Psychomotor Energy
Psychosocial Adjustment: Life Change

Quality of Life

Respiratory Status: Airway Patency
Respiratory Status: Gas Exchange
Respiratory Status: Ventilation

Rest
Risk Control
Risk Control: Alcohol Use
Risk Control: Cancer
Risk Control: Cardiovascular Health
Risk Control: Drug Use
Risk Control: Hearing Impairment
Risk Control: Sexually Transmitted Diseases
   (STDs)
Risk Control: Tobacco Use
Risk Control: Unintended Pregnancy
Risk Control: Visual Impairment
Risk Detection
Role Performance

Safe Home Environment
Seizure Control
Self-Care Status
Self-Care: Activities of Daily Living (ADL)
Self-Care: Bathing
Self-Care: Dressing
Self-Care: Eating
Self-Care: Grooming
Self-Care: Hygiene
Self-Care: Instrumental Activities of Daily
   Living (IADL)
Self-Care: Non-Parenteral Medication
Self-Care: Oral Hygiene
Self-Care: Parenteral Medication
Self-Care: Toileting
Self-Direction of Care
Self-Esteem
Self-Mutilation Restraint
Sensory Function Status
Sensory Function: Cutaneous
Sensory Function: Hearing
Sensory Function: Proprioception
Sensory Function: Taste & Smell
Sensory Function: Vision
Sexual Functioning
Sexual Identity
Skeletal Function
Sleep
Social Interaction Skills
Social Involvement
Social Support
Spiritual Health
Stress Level
Student Health Status
Substance Addiction Consequences
Suffering Severity
Suicide Self-Restraint
Swallowing Status
Swallowing Status: Esophageal Phase
Swallowing Status: Oral Phase
Swallowing Status: Pharyngeal Phase
Symptom Control
Symptom Severity

Symptom Severity: Perimenopause
Symptom Severity: Premenstrual Syndrome (PMS)
Systemic Toxin Clearance: Dialysis

Thermoregulation
Thermoregulation: Newborn
Tissue Integrity: Skin & Mucous Membranes
Tissue Perfusion: Abdominal Organs
Tissue Perfusion: Cardiac
Tissue Perfusion: Cerebral
Tissue Perfusion: Peripheral
Tissue Perfusion: Pulmonary
Transfer Performance

Treatment Behavior: Illness or Injury

Urinary Continence
Urinary Elimination

Vision Compensation Behavior
Vital Signs

Weight: Body Mass
Weight Control
Will to Live
Wound Healing: Primary Intention
Wound Healing: Secondary Intention

CLINICAL SITUATIONS INDEX

NURSING DIAGNOSES INDEX

A

Activity Intolerance

High Risk for

related to deconditioning, in total parenteral nutrition, 761–762

related to claudication, in peripheral arterial disease, 112–113

related to fatigue and inadequate oxygenation for activities, in chronic obstructive pulmonary disease, 129–130

related to insufficient oxygenation for activities of daily living (ADLs) secondary to cardiac tissue ischemia, prolonged immobility, narcotics or medications, in acute coronary syndrome, 105–106

related to pain and weakness secondary to anesthesia, tissue hypoxia, and insufficient fluid and nutrient intake, in surgical client, 477–478

Acute Pain. *See* Pain, Acute

Airway Clearance, Ineffective

High Risk for, related to relaxation of tongue and gag reflexes secondary to disruption in muscle innervation, in seizure disorders, 294–295

related to excessive and tenacious secretions, in chronic obstructive pulmonary disease, 128–129

related to increased mucus production, tenacious secretions, and bronchospasm, in asthma, 121–122

related to increased secretions and diminished cough secondary to pain and fatigue, in thoracic pulmonary surgery, 642–644

Anxiety

related to anticipated surgery and unfamiliarity with preoperative and postoperative routines and postoperative sensations, in carotid endarterectomy, 512–513

related to breathlessness and fear of suffocation, in chronic obstructive pulmonary disease, 131

related to fear of embarrassment secondary to having a seizure in public, in seizure disorders, 295–296

related to impending pacemaker insertion and prognosis, 127–129

related to impending surgery and insufficient knowledge of preoperative routines, intraoperative activities, and postoperative self-care activities, in thoracic pulmonary surgery, 638–639

related to impending surgery and perceived negative effects on life style, in cranial surgery, 555–556

related to insufficient knowledge of postoperative routines, postoperative sensations, and crutch-walking techniques, in amputation, 487–488

related to lack of knowledge of colostomy care and perceived effects on life style, 527–528

related to lack of knowledge of ileostomy care and perceived negative effects on life style, 591–592

related to lack of knowledge of impending surgical experience and implications of condition on life style, in laryngectomy, 613–614

related to lack of knowledge of urostomy care and perceived negative effects on life style, 657–658

related to loss of control, memory losses, and fear of withdrawal, in alcohol withdrawal syndrome, 447–448

related to perceived effects of injury on life style and unknown future, in spinal cord injury, 304–305

related to prescribed chemotherapy, insufficient knowledge of chemotherapy, and self-care measures, 685–686

related to prescribed radiation therapy and insufficient knowledge of treatment and self-care measures, 752–753

related to sudden injury, treatment, uncertainty of outcome, and pain, in thermal injuries, 343–344

related to unfamiliar environment, routines, diagnostic tests, treatments, and loss of control, in hospitalization, 64–65

related to unfamiliar hospital environment, uncertainty about outcomes, feelings of helplessness and hopelessness, and insufficient knowledge about cancer and treatment, 409–410

related to upcoming insertion of catheter/port and insufficient knowledge of procedure, with long-term venous access devices, 715–716

related to upcoming surgery and insufficient knowledge of routine preoperative and postoperative activities, in prostatectomy, 630

Anxiety/Fear

related to perceived mastectomy and prognosis, 504–506

related to surgical experience, loss of control, unpredictable outcome, and insufficient knowledge of preoperative routines, postoperative exercises and activities, and postoperative changes and sensations, 465–467

Anxiety/Fear (individual, family)

related to unfamiliar situation, unpredictable nature of condition, fear of death, negative effects on life style, or possible sexual dysfunctions, in acute coronary syndrome, 103–104

Aspiration, High Risk for

related to position of tube and client, in enteral nutrition, 704–705

Autonomic Dysreflexia, High Risk for

related to reflex stimulation of sympathetic nervous system below the level of cord injury secondary to loss of autonomic control, in spinal cord injury, 308–309

B

Body Image, Disturbed, High Risk for

related to changes in appearance, in corticosteroid therapy, 696–697

related to perceived negative effects of amputation and response of others to appearance, 489–490

Bowel Incontinence: Areflexia

related to lack of voluntary sphincter control secondary to spinal cord injury involving sacral reflex arc (S2-S4), 314–316

Bowel Incontinence: Reflexic

related to related to lack of voluntary sphincter control secondary to spinal cord injury above the eleventh thoracic vertebra (T11), 312–314

Breathing Pattern, Ineffective, High Risk for

related to immobility, pressure, and pain, in peritoneal dialysis, 742–743

C

Caregiver Role Strain, High Risk for

related to AIDS-associated shame/stigma and uncertainty about course of illness and demands on the caregiver, 394–395

Chronic Pain. *See* Pain, Chronic

Comfort

Altered, related to catheter insertion, instillation of dialysis solution, outflow suction, and chemical irritation of peritoneum, in peritoneal dialysis, 743–744

Impaired

related to cold intolerance secondary to decreased metabolic rate, in hypothyroidism, 172

related to demyelinated areas of the sensory tract, in multiple sclerosis, 263–264

related to pruritus secondary to accumulation of bilirubin pigment and bile salts, in cirrhosis, 150

Impaired: Cramping, Distention, Nausea, Vomiting

related to type of formula, administration rate, route, or formula temperature, in enteral nutrition, 702–703

COLLABORATIVE PROBLEMS INDEX

The prefix Potential Complication (PC) has been omitted for easier use of the index only.

COLLABORATIVE PROBLEMS INDEX

Note: Page numbers followed by f and t indicate figures and tables, respectively. Those followed by b indicate boxed material.

A

Abdominal aortic aneurysm resection, 480–485
Abdominal hysterectomy, 584
Abscess
  bone, in osteomyelitis, 376–377
  in inflammatory bowel disease, 195–198
Acid–base balance. *See also* Diabetic ketoacidosis; Metabolic
      acidosis
  in asthma, 119–121
  in chronic obstructive pulmonary disease, 127
  in cirrhosis, 147
Acidosis. *See also* Ketoacidosis, diabetic
  in acute renal failure, 213–217
  in chronic renal failure, 221–228
  in thermal injuries, 336–343
Acquired immunodeficiency syndrome (AIDS), 385–399
Action
  direct, 33, 33t
  inhibition of, 33t, 33–34
Acute arterial thrombosis, in peripheral arterial disease, 111–112
Acute chest syndrome, in sickle cell disease, 319–322
Acute coronary syndrome, 99–110
  recurrent, 100–103
Acute kidney failure (AKF), 212–219
Acute lung injury, in thoracic surgery, 639–642
Acute lymphocytic leukemia (ALL), 433–434
Acute myelogenous leukemia (AML), 433
Acute organic psychosis, in hypothyroidism, 169–172
Acute pulmonary edema, in thoracic surgery, 639–642
Acute renal failure, 212–219
  intrarenal, 212
  in pancreatitis, 181–185
  postrenal, 212
  prerenal, 212
Acute respiratory distress syndrome, in pancreatitis, 181–185
Acute respiratory failure, in Guillain-Barré syndrome, 252–254
Adaptation, 32
Addendum care plan, 15, 15f–16f, 17
Addendum diagnoses, 18
  in care plan, 59
Adolescent(s). *See also* Children
  growth retardation, in inflammatory bowel disease, 196–198,
      205
Adrenocorticotropic hormone (ACTH), malignancy and, 408
Adult respiratory distress syndrome, in cerebrovascular acci-
      dent (stroke), 238–242
AIDS. *See* Acquired immunodeficiency syndrome
Air embolism
  in hemodialysis, 708–711
  long-term venous access devices and, 714
  in total parenteral nutrition, 756–759
Airway obstruction
  in carotid endarterectomy, 513–515
  upper, with thermal injury, 338
Albumin, serum, in chronic renal failure, 225–226
Alcohol
  abuse, and pancreatitis, 183, 187–188
  and fracture risk, 382
  and Parkinson disease, 288
  and peptic ulcer disease, 209
Alcohol hallucinosis, in alcohol withdrawal syndrome, 442–444
Alcohol withdrawal syndrome, 441–449
  in pancreatitis, 183
Alendronate, 384
Alkalosis, in acute renal failure, 215
Allergies, in hemodialysis, 708–711
Alopecia, in client with cancer, 412
Alpha-fetoprotein, malignancy and, 409
Ambulatory surgery. *See* Same-day surgery
Amenorrhea, in chronic renal failure, 229–230

Amputation, 485–496
  above knee, 485
  below knee, 485
  hip disarticulation, 485
  knee disarticulation, 485
  in osteomyelitis, 376–377
  Syme, 485
  transmetatarsal, 485–486
Amputation site hematoma, 488–489
Analgesics, for pain in end-stage cancer, 424–425
Anal stretch maneuver, 279
Anaphylaxis/anaphylactic reaction
  in chemotherapy, 680–685
  in hemodialysis, 708–711
Anastomosis disruption, in arterial bypass grafting in lower
      extremity, 498–503
Anemia
  in chronic renal failure, 219, 221–228
  in hemodialysis, 708–711
  in hypothyroidism, 171
  in inflammatory bowel disease, 195–198
  in sickle cell disease, 319–322
Aneurysm
  abdominal aortic, ruptured, 481–482
  resection, 481–482
Anger
  as coping strategy, 34–35
  in grief work, 107
Angina, unstable, 99–110
Ankylosing spondylitis, in inflammatory bowel disease, 205
Anorexia, in HIV/AIDS, 399
Anorexia nervosa, and fracture risk, 381
Antacid therapy, 210
Anticoagulant therapy, 668–672
Anticonvulsants, for pain in end-stage cancer, 424
Antidiuretic hormone (ADH), malignancy and, 408
Antidiuretic hormone secretion, inappropriate, in cranial
      surgery, 557–562
Antiplatelet agents, 668
Anxiety
  in chronic illness, 35
  versus fear, 35
  state, 41
  in surgical client, 40
  trait, 41
  types of, 35, 36b
Aorta, abdominal, aneurysm resection, 480–485
Aortoenteric fistula, in abdominal aortic aneurysm resection,
      482–484
Aphasia, stroke and, 242–243
Aplastic crisis, in sickle cell disease, 320–321
Apraxia, stroke and, 242–243
Arm, fractures of, 356
Arrhythmias. *See* Dysrhythmias
Arterial bypass grafting
  coronary artery, 540–553
  in lower extremity, 497–503
Arterial thrombosis, acute, in peripheral arterial disease, 111–112
Arthritis
  in inflammatory bowel disease, 205
  rheumatoid, 360–375
  septic, in inflammatory joint disease, 362–364
  septic (infectious, bacterial), 360–375
Arthroplasty, 647–655
Asians, fracture risk in, 382
Aspiration
  in myasthenia gravis, 270–272
  in Parkinson disease, 286–289
  in pneumonia, 144
  in seizure disorders, 293–294
Aspirin, risks with, 209, 211